Orthopaedic Rotations Survival Guide

Orthopaedic Rotations Survival Guide

In Cooperation With

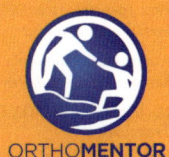

EDITORS

Amiethab A. Aiyer, MD, FAAOS, FAOA
Chief, Foot and Ankle Service
Associate Professor, Department of Orthopaedics
Faculty Affiliate, Center for Innovative Leadership
Johns Hopkins University Carey Business School
Director, Orthopaedic Medical Student Education
Director, UME to GME Transition
The Johns Hopkins University School of Medicine
Baltimore, Maryland

William N. Levine, MD, FAAOS, FAOA
Frank E. Stinchfield Professor and Chairman
Department of Orthopedic Surgery
Chief, Shoulder Service, Co-Director, Center for Shoulder, Elbow and Sports Medicine
Head Team Physician, Columbia University
36th President, American Shoulder and Elbow Surgeons
Editor-in-Chief, Journal of the American Academy of Orthopaedic Surgeons (JAAOS)
NYP/Columbia University Medical Center
New York, New York

ASSOCIATE EDITORS

Jonathan R. Kaplan, MD, FAAOS
Partner, Orthopaedic Specialty Institute
Orthopaedic Surgeon
Hoag Orthopedic Institute
Orange, California

Matthew A. Varacallo, MD
Chief of Sports Medicine Department
Director of Orthopedic Robotic Surgery
Sports Medicine/Joint Reconstruction
Penn Highlands Healthcare System
DuBois, Pennsylvania

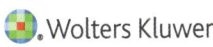 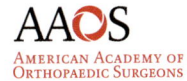

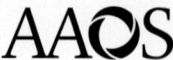

AMERICAN ACADEMY OF ORTHOPAEDIC SURGEONS

Board of Directors, 2023-2024

Kevin J. Bozic, MD, MBA, FAAOS
President

Paul Tornetta III, MD, PhD, FAAOS
First Vice President

Annunziato Amendola, MD, FAAOS
Second Vice President

Michael L. Parks, MD, FAAOS
Treasurer

Felix H. Savoie III, MD, FAAOS
Past President

Alfonso Mejia, MD, MPH, FAAOS
Chair, Board of Councilors

Joel L. Mayerson, MD, FAAOS
Chair-Elect, Board of Councilors

Michael J. Leddy III, MD, FAAOS
Secretary, Board of Councilors

Armando F. Vidal, MD, FAAOS
Chair, Board of Specialty Societies

Adolph J. Yates, Jr, MD, FAAOS
Chair-Elect, Board of Specialty Societies

Michael P. Bolognesi, MD, FAAOS
Secretary, Board of Specialty Societies

Lisa N. Masters
Lay Member

Evalina L. Burger, MD, FAAOS
Member at Large

Chad A. Krueger, MD, FAAOS
Member at Large

Toni M. McLaurin, MD, FAAOS
Member at Large

Monica M. Payares, MD, FAAOS
Member at Large

Thomas E. Arend, Jr, Esq, CAE
Chief Executive Officer (ex-officio)

Staff

American Academy of Orthopaedic Surgeons

Anna Salt Troise, MBA, *Chief Commercial Officer*

Hans Koelsch, PhD, *Director, Publishing*

Lisa Claxton Moore, *Senior Manager, Editorial*

Steven Kellert, *Senior Editor*

Wolters Kluwer Health

Brian Brown, *Director, Medical Practice*

Matt Hauber, *Senior Content Editor, Acquisitions*

Stacey Sebring, *Senior Development Editor*

Anthony Gonzalez, *Editorial Coordinator*

Kirsten Watrud, *Product Marketing Manager*

Catherine Ott, *Production Project Manager*

Stephen Druding, *Manager, Graphic Arts & Design*

Margie Orzech-Zeranko, *Senior Manufacturing Coordinator*

TNQ Technologies, *Prepress Vendor*

Orthopaedic Rotations Survival Guide

The material presented in *Orthopaedic Rotations Survival Guide* has been made available by the American Academy of Orthopaedic Surgeons (AAOS) for educational purposes only. This material is not intended to present the only, or necessarily best, methods or procedures for the medical situations discussed, but rather it is intended to represent an approach, view, statement, or opinion of the author(s) or producer(s), which may be helpful to others who face similar situations. Medical providers should use their own, independent medical judgment, in addition to open discussion with patients, when developing patient care recommendations and treatment plans. Medical care should always be based on a medical provider's expertise that is individually tailored to a patient's circumstances, preferences and rights.

Some drugs or medical devices demonstrated in AAOS courses or described in AAOS print or electronic publications have not been cleared by the US Food and Drug Administration (FDA) or have been cleared for specific uses only. The FDA has stated that it is the responsibility of the physician to determine the FDA clearance status of each drug or device he or she wishes to use in clinical practice and to use the products with appropriate patient consent and in compliance with applicable law.

Furthermore, any statements about commercial products are solely the opinion(s) of the author(s) and do not represent an AAOS endorsement or evaluation of these products. These statements may not be used in advertising or for any commercial purpose.

All rights reserved. No part of this publication may be reproduced, stored in a retrieval system, or transmitted, in any form, or by any means, electronic, mechanical, photocopying, recording, or otherwise, without prior written permission from the publisher.

ISBN: 978-1-9751-7386-9

Library of Congress Control Number: Cataloging in Publication data available on request from publisher.

Printed in Mexico

Published 2024 by the American Academy of Orthopaedic Surgeons

9400 West Higgins Road

Rosemont, Illinois 60018

Copyright 2024 by the American Academy of Orthopaedic Surgeons

Contributors

S. Elizabeth Ames, MD, FAAOS
Professor and Program Director
Department of Orthopaedics and Rehabilitation
University of Vermont College of Medicine
Burlington, Vermont

Tessa Balach, MD, FAAOS
Professor of Orthopaedic Surgery
Vice Chair of Education
Residency Program Director
Department of Orthopaedic Surgery and Rehabilitation Medicine
The University of Chicago Medicine and Biological Sciences
Chicago, Illinois

Matthew Blue, MD
Orthopaedic Surgeon
Olathe Health
Olathe, Kansas

Robert H. Brophy, MD, FAAOS
Professor, Department of Orthopaedic Surgery
Washington University School of Medicine
St. Louis, Missouri

Charles Cassidy, MD, FAAOS
Professor and Chair
Department of Orthopaedics
Tufts Medical Center and Tufts University School of Medicine
Boston, Massachusetts

Cara A. Cipriano, MD, MSc, FAAOS
Associate Professor and Chief, Orthopaedic Oncology
Director, Undergraduate Medical Education
Department of Orthopaedic Surgery
University of Pennsylvania
Philadelphia, Pennsylvania

Sheila Ann Conway, MD, FAAOS, FAOA
Professor and Vice Chair of Education
Department of Orthopaedic Surgery
University of Miami Miller School of Medicine
Miami, Florida

Seth D. Dodds, MD, FAAOS
Professor and Chief, Hand and Upper Extremity Surgery
Associate Program Director, Orthopaedic Surgery
Department of Orthopaedics
University of Miami Miller School of Medicine
Miami, Florida

Yoshimi Endo, MD
Associate Attending Radiologist and Director of Ultrasound Education
Department of Radiology and Imaging
Hospital for Special Surgery
Associate Professor of Clinical Radiology
Weill Medical College of Cornell University
New York, New York

Contributors

Lauren E. Geaney, MD, FAAOS
Associate Professor
Department of Orthopedic Surgery
University of Connecticut
Farmington, Connecticut

Diane Ismat Ghanem, MD
Postdoctoral Research Fellow
Department of Orthopaedic Surgery, Division of Trauma
Johns Hopkins Hospital
Baltimore, Maryland

Aaron Gipsman, MD
Division of Sports Medicine
NYU Langone Orthopedics
New York, New York

Graham Goh, MD
Orthopaedic Surgery Resident
Department of Orthopaedic Surgery
Boston University Medical Center
Boston, Massachusetts

Theodore T. Guild, MD
Harvard Combined Orthopaedic Residency Program
Boston, Massachusetts

Melvyn A. Harrington, Jr, MD, FAAOS, FAOA
Professor, Residency Program Director
Adult Reconstruction Fellowship Director
Vice Chair for Diversity and Inclusion
Department of Orthopedic Surgery
Baylor College of Medicine
Houston, Texas

Giselle M. Hernandez, DMed, FAAOS
Assistant Professor
Department of Orthopaedics-Trauma Division
University of Miami Miller School of Medicine
Miami, Florida

MaCalus V. Hogan, MD, MBA, FAAOS, FAOA
David Silver Professor and Chair
Chief, UPMC Orthopaedic Service Line
Senior Medical Director, Orthopaedic and Musculoskeletal Services
UPMC Health Plan
University of Pittsburgh School of Medicine - UPMC
Department of Orthopaedic Surgery and Bioengineering
Katz Graduate School of Business
Pittsburgh, Pennsylvania

Ginger E. Holt, MD, FAAOS
Professor, Orthopaedic Surgery
Vanderbilt Medical Center
Nashville, Tennessee

Charles M. Jobin, MD, FAAOS
Louis U. Bigliani Associate Professor of Orthopedic Surgery
Department of Orthopedic Surgery
Columbia University Irving Medical Center
New York, New York

Jonathan R. Kaplan, MD, FAAOS
Partner, Orthopaedic Specialty Institute
Orthopaedic Surgeon
Hoag Orthopedic Institute
Orange, California

Mara S. Karamitopoulos, MD, FAAOS
Pediatric Orthopedic Surgeon
Clinical Associate Professor, Orthopedic Surgery
Associate Program Director, Orthopedic Surgery Residency Program
Hassenfeld Children's Hospital at NYU Langone Health
New York, New York

Monica Kogan, MD, FAAOS, FAOA
Associate Professor
Department of Orthopaedic Surgery
Rush University Medical Center
Chicago, Illinois

John Y. Kwon, MD
Chief, Foot and Ankle Service
Department of Orthopaedic Surgery
Massachusetts General Hospital
Associate Professor, Harvard Medical School
Boston, Massachusetts

Joseph D. Lamplot, MD
Assistant Professor
Department of Orthopaedic Surgery
Emory University
Atlanta, Georgia

Dawn M. LaPorte, MD, FAAOS
Professor and Vice Chair, Education
Department of Orthopaedic Surgery
Johns Hopkins University
Baltimore, Maryland

William N. Levine, MD, FAAOS, FAOA
Frank E. Stinchfield Professor and Chairman
Department of Orthopedic Surgery
Chief, Shoulder Service, Co-Director, Center for Shoulder, Elbow and Sports Medicine
Head Team Physician, Columbia University
36th President, American Shoulder and Elbow Surgeons
Editor-in-Chief, Journal of the American Academy of Orthopaedic Surgeons (JAAOS)
NYP/Columbia University Medical Center
New York, New York

Danielle C. Marshall, MD
Orthopaedic Surgery Resident, PGY4
University of Miami/Jackson Memorial Hospital
Miami, Florida

Samir Mehta, MD, FAAOS
Chief, Division of Orthopaedic Trauma and Fracture Care
Associate Professor of Orthopaedic Surgery
Hospital of the University of Pennsylvania
Philadelphia, Pennsylvania

Emmanuel Menga, MD, FAAOS
Associate Professor of Orthopaedics and Neurosurgery
Department of Orthopaedic Surgery and Rehabilitation
University of Rochester School of Medicine and Dentistry
Rochester, New York

Julianne Munoz, MD, FAAOS
Assistant Professor
UHealth Sports Medicine
Department of Orthopaedics
University of Miami Miller School of Medicine
Miami, Florida

Brian I. Nwannunu, MD
Orthopaedic Surgeon
Alpha Orthopedics and Sports Medicine
McKinney, Texas

Javad Parvizi, MD, FRCS, FAAOS
James Edwards Professor of Orthopaedic Surgery
Sidney Kimmel School of Medicine
Rothman Institute at Thomas Jefferson University
Philadelphia, Pennsylvania

Contributors

Hollis G. Potter, DMed
Attending Radiologist and Chairman, Department of Radiology and Imaging and
The Coleman Chair, MRI Research
Hospital for Special Surgery
Professor of Radiology
Weill Medical College of Cornell University
New York, New York

Brian Scannell, MD, FAAOS
Associate Professor of Pediatric Orthopaedic Surgery Atrium Health
Pediatric Orthopaedic Surgery, OrthoCarolina
Charlotte, North Carolina

Nicole S. Schroeder, MD, FAAOS
Professor, Department of Orthopaedic Surgery, UCSF
Chief, Hand and Upper Extremity
Associate Vice Chair of Education, Undergraduate Medical Education
Academy Chair in Orthopaedic Surgery
UCSF Academy of Medical Educators
San Francisco, California

Alexandra K. Schwartz, MD, FAAOS
Professor of Clinical Orthopedic Surgery
Chief, Orthopedic Trauma
Fellowship Director
UCSD Department of Orthopedic Surgery
Clinical Professor
San Diego, California

Babar Shafiq, MD, MSPT, FAAOS, FAOA
Director, Orthopaedic Bone Health Center
Associate Director, Residency Program
Associate Professor, Department of Orthopaedic Surgery, Trauma Division
Johns Hopkins School of Medicine
Baltimore, Maryland

Carolyn M. Sofka, MD, FACR
Attending Radiologist
Hospital for Special Surgery
Professor of Radiology
Weill Medical College of Cornell University
New York, New York

Eric Strauss, MD, FAAOS
Division of Sports Medicine
NYU Langone Orthopedics
New York, New York

Robert Z. Tashjian, MD, FAAOS
Ezekiel R. Dumke, Jr. Presidential Endowed Professor
Vice Chair for Research
Department of Orthopaedics
University of Utah
Salt Lake City, Utah

Matthew A. Varacallo, MD
Chief of Sports Medicine Department
Director of Orthopedic Robotic Surgery
Sports Medicine/Joint Reconstruction
Penn Highlands Healthcare System
DuBois, Pennsylvania

Fernando E. Vilella, MD, FAAOS
Director, Orthopaedic Trauma Service
University of Miami, Miller School of Medicine
Ryder Trauma Center
Jackson Memorial Hospital
Miami, Florida

Preface

Thank you for beginning your exploratory journey into orthopaedics—we are thrilled to share this textbook with you. The concept behind the *Orthopaedic Rotations Survival Guide* has been inspired by you—the students, residents, and colleagues—with whom we have worked alongside and from whom we have learned so much. The editorial team has carefully curated content experts who are leaders in their fields and dedicated educators genuinely committed to advancing your understanding of orthopaedics.

Along with each of the content experts, the editorial team is passionate about encouraging your interest in orthopaedics. The *Orthopaedic Rotations Survival Guide* represents an extension of our commitment to your interest in musculoskeletal patient care. Furthermore, whether you are considering a career in orthopaedic surgery, physical therapy, athletic training, or otherwise, the goal of this text is to provide you with a "one-stop shop" resource for high-yield information as you move between learning experiences in the clinic or in the operating room.

The primary goal of this text is to provide readily accessible information on topics that are high yield for anyone interested in orthopaedics. The text is designed to teach key principles in musculoskeletal education ranging from history and physical examination pearls to important nuances of planning and advanced imaging, to surgical approach considerations across all major orthopaedic subspecialties. Each chapter is accompanied by select recent literature to further broaden your breadth of knowledge.

We would like to thank the AAOS and Wolters Kluwer for their support during the development of this text. We would also like to extend a special debt of gratitude to all the authors who devoted significant time and effort to the writing of each chapter. Finally, we would like to thank all of you for joining us on this novel educational journey.

Amiethab A. Aiyer, MD, FAAOS, FAOA
William N. Levine, MD, FAAOS, FAOA
Editors

Jonathan R. Kaplan, MD, FAAOS
Matthew A. Varacallo, MD
Associate Editors

Contents

Contributors v
Preface x

Chapter 1

The Orthopaedic Physical Examination 1

Matthew A. Varacallo, MD, Jonathan R. Kaplan, MD, FAAOS

Chapter 2

Imaging 5

Yoshimi Endo, MD, Carolyn M. Sofka, MD, FACR, Hollis G. Potter, DMed

Chapter 3

I Fell and Cannot Get Up—Lower Extremity Trauma 45

Alexandra K. Schwartz, MD, FAAOS, Samir Mehta, MD, FAAOS, Giselle M. Hernandez, DMed, FAAOS, Theodore T. Guild, MD, John Y. Kwon, MD, Fernando E. Vilella, MD, FAAOS, Danielle C. Marshall, MD, Diane Ismat Ghanem, MD, Babar Shafiq, MD, MSPT, FAAOS, FAOA

Chapter 4

I Fell and Cannot Use My Upper Extremity 168

Robert Z. Tashjian, MD, FAAOS, Nicole S. Schroeder, MD, FAAOS

Chapter 5

My Shoulder Hurts—Now What? 223

William N. Levine, MD, FAAOS, FAOA, Julianne Munoz, MD, FAAOS

Chapter 6

My Elbow Hurts 270

Charles M. Jobin, MD, FAAOS, Charles Cassidy, MD, FAAOS

Preface xiii

Chapter 7

My Hand Hurts 313

Dawn M. LaPorte, MD, FAAOS, Seth D. Dodds, MD, FAAOS

Chapter 8

My Hip Hurts 345

Aaron Gipsman, MD, Eric Strauss, MD, FAAOS, Matthew A. Varacallo, MD

Chapter 9

My Knee Hurts 387

Joseph D. Lamplot, MD, Robert H. Brophy, MD, FAAOS

Chapter 10

I Need a Joint Replacement 440

*Melvyn A. Harrington, Jr, MD, FAAOS, FAOA,
Javad Parvizi, MD, FRCS, FAAOS, Matthew Blue, MD,
Graham Goh, MD, Brian I. Nwannunu, MD*

Chapter 11

My Foot and Ankle Hurt 496

*Lauren E. Geaney, MD, FAAOS, Jonathan R. Kaplan, MD, FAAOS,
MaCalus V. Hogan, MD, MBA, FAAOS, FAOA*

Chapter 12

Spine—My Back Is Killing Me 556

S. Elizabeth Ames, MD, FAAOS, Emmanuel Menga, MD, FAAOS

Chapter 13

Tumor ABCs 586

*Tessa Balach, MD, FAAOS, Cara A. Cipriano, MD, MSc, FAAOS,
Sheila Ann Conway, MD, FAAOS, FAOA, Ginger E. Holt, MD, FAAOS*

Chapter 14

Pediatrics 609

Monica Kogan, MD, FAAOS, FAOA, Brian Scannell, MD, FAAOS, Mara S. Karamitopoulos, MD, FAAOS

Index 679

1 The Orthopaedic Physical Examination

Matthew A. Varacallo, MD
Jonathan R. Kaplan, MD, FAAOS

Introduction

Although the orthopaedic examination will be covered in depth in each chapter as it pertains specifically to the key components of a particular topic or body part, this chapter will present the general approach to the orthopaedic evaluation.

The orthopaedic evaluation is a systematic process that examination should follow in a clear, concise, and reproducible pattern to ensure both efficiency and accuracy. In addition to a thorough history, the orthopaedic examination is critical to aid in the evaluation, diagnosis, and treatment of the patient.

Inspection and Observation

- Findings can dictate perspective for the remainder of the physical examination
- Assessment of patient in clinical setting
  - Reasonable distance given setting (office, trauma bay, etc)
  - Multiple views/angles for comprehensive assessment
- Gait pattern (if applicable)
- Region/extremity soft-tissue integrity (open wounds, obvious deformity)

Dr. Varacallo or an immediate family member serves as a paid consultant to or is an employee of Arthrex, Inc. Dr. Kaplan or an immediate family member has received royalties from Novastep; serves as a paid consultant to or is an employee of Medline, Novastep, and Vilex; has stock or stock options held in GLW Medical Innovation; and serves as a board member, owner, officer, or committee member of American Orthopaedic Foot and Ankle Society.

- Limb and joint alignment
- Skin assessment
  - Edema, swelling
  - Ecchymosis
  - Discoloration (dusky, pale, etc)
  - Abrasions
  - Open wounds, lacerations
  - Compartment swelling/pressure (firm, compressible, etc)

Palpation

- Important to palpate relevant anatomy, landmarks to elicit focal (versus) diffuse versus pain in a specific region/joint
- Work from proximal to distal direction to organize systematic approach
- Varying degrees of pressure depending on clinical presentation
  - For example, in setting of known fracture, aggressive palpation over the fracture site causes the patient a significant amount of pain and is not necessary.
- Contralateral assessment
  - Palpation of "normal" and compare with "abnormal"

Range of Motion

- Important to assess the joint above and below the region/joint of interest
  - For example, a knee examination should always include an evaluation of mobility and function of the ipsilateral hip and ankle.
- Range of motion (ROM) categories and positions
  - ROM categorical comparison can be useful in diagnosing various orthopaedic conditions.
    - For example, adhesive capsulitis of the shoulder yields both limited active range of motion (AROM), active assisted range of motion (AAROM), and passive range of motion (PROM), whereas an isolated full-thickness rotator cuff tear may lead to full PROM but limited AROM.
  - AROM: the patient actively moves the joint
    - Helpful for the examiner to stand in front of the patient and demonstrate the ROM planes for evaluation

- AAROM: the patient uses the contralateral extremity to move the affected extremity
- PROM: the examiner performs the motion of the joint
  - Care is taken in the traumatic setting to avoid aggressive jerking or pushing the joint into positions causing unnecessary pain for the patient.
- Relevant positions for assessment of ROM may include standing, sitting, supine, prone, and lateral decubitus.
- Comprehensive plane of motion evaluation
  - Depending on the joint in consideration, all planes of motion should be assessed (flexion, extension, rotation, etc).

Neurovascular Evaluation

- **Motor**
  - Includes focused muscle subgroup analysis to identify each individual muscle or groups of muscles
  - Grading examination
    - Grade 0: Complete paralysis
    - Grade I: Flicker/contraction
    - Grade II: Movement with gravity eliminated
    - Grade III: Movement against gravity, no resistance
    - Grade IV: Movement against gravity and resistance
    - Grade V: Movement/power is normal (compare with contralateral)
- **Sensory**
  - Evaluation involves assessment of sensation along the skin dermatomes for any deficits and additional special evaluation can be performed with Semmes-Weinstein monofilament testing for any other neuropathic deficits.
- **Vascular**
  - Assess for strength of pulses, capillary refill, and overall skin turgor and warmth within the extremity/distally

Provocative Maneuvers and Special Tests

- Important to use and apply the various available sensitive and specific testing maneuvers to diagnose specific pathologies
- Special testing used in tandem with the aforementioned findings and in addition to diagnostic imaging if applicable

- Will be discussed throughout the chapters in this book and will be critical in aiding in the diagnosis and treatment of the orthopaedic patient

Other Takeaways
- Serial examinations can be of benefit to help with determining diagnoses.
- Remember to think outside of the box; various medical conditions can present with musculoskeletal complaints.
- A thorough history and physical examination are critical to the treatment of patients.

2

Imaging

Yoshimi Endo, MD • Carolyn M. Sofka, MD, FACR
Hollis G. Potter, DMed

Introduction

Proper evaluation of a patient presenting with orthopaedic complaints almost always includes imaging. Although there are other imaging modalities, the most commonly used and thus probably the most important for the orthopaedic surgeon to be comfortable interpreting are radiography, CT, and MRI. It is important to review the most pertinent pearls or knowledge drops that will be useful for interpreting these three imaging modalities, both for orthopaedic residents and surgeons already in practice.

Radiography

Radiography is the mainstay of orthopaedic imaging, whether the setting is the emergency department or the outpatient clinic. A firm grasp of radiographic interpretative skills is crucial to the orthopaedic surgeon. Therefore, it is important to be mindful of the following principles.

Dr. Sofka or an immediate family member serves as a paid consultant to or is an employee of OSSIO Ltd. Dr. Potter or an immediate family member has stock or stock options held in Imagen and has received research or institutional support from GE Healthcare, GE/NBA, National Institutes of Health (NIAMS & NICHD), and Siemens. Neither Dr. Endo nor any immediate family member has received anything of value from or has stock or stock options held in a commercial company or institution related directly or indirectly to the subject of this chapter.

Always Obtain at Least Two Views

Radiation safety is a primary consideration with any imaging examination. It is desirable to obtain as few radiographs as possible to limit unnecessary radiation exposure as summarized in the ALARA (<u>a</u>s <u>l</u>ow <u>a</u>s <u>r</u>easonably <u>a</u>chievable) concept,[1] especially in young or pregnant patients.

It serves no benefit, however, if only one radiograph is obtained, yet the single view is nondiagnostic. For example, it is not uncommon for intramedullary split fractures in the digits to be occult on one view. Similarly, in the postoperative patient, a percutaneous pin reducing a metatarsal fracture may look perfect on the AP view but may be completely missing purchase of the bone on the lateral view. Ideally, obtaining two views at 90° to one another (frontal and lateral) is recommended (**Figures 1** and **2**).

Make Sure the Images Include Everything They Should

It is important when reviewing radiographs to ensure that the appropriate anatomy is included completely on the radiograph. If

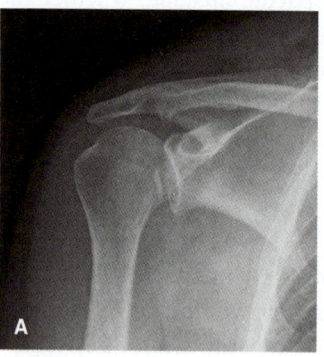 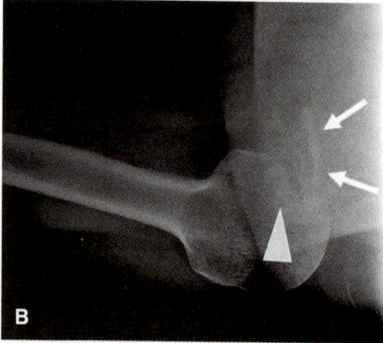

Figure 1 **A**, Neutral frontal radiograph of the right shoulder demonstrates relatively normal glenohumeral alignment, but the joint space is markedly narrowed with overlap of the humeral head and glenoid. **B**, Axillary view from the same patient clearly demonstrates the fixed posterior dislocation of the humeral head (arrows = glenoid) with a reverse Hill-Sachs fracture deformity (arrowhead). Subtle posterior shoulder dislocations can be missed on radiographs if only frontal views are obtained.

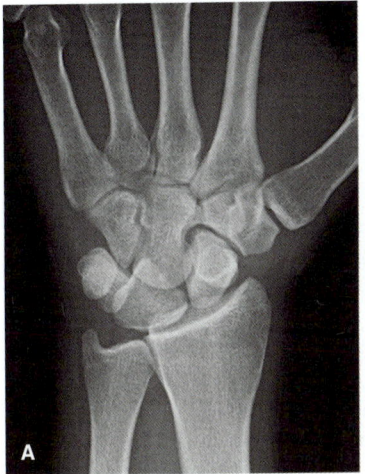 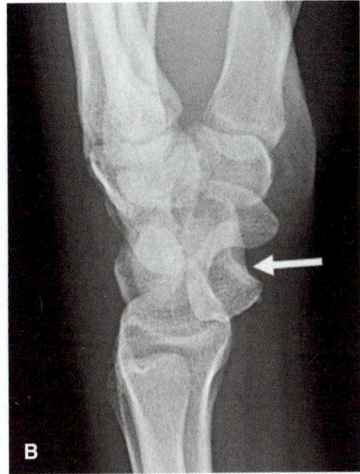

Figure 2 **A**, PA view of the wrist in a patient with trauma demonstrates no obvious fracture. **B**, The lateral view, however, clearly demonstrates the volarly dislocated and rotated lunate (arrow) reflecting a lunate dislocation. Malalignment of the carpal bones can be missed on radiographs if only a frontal view is ordered.

the radiographs are incomplete or poor in quality, the diagnosis may be incomplete as well.

Cervical spine radiographs should include the entire cervical spine from C1 to C7. If the patient's shoulders are large or otherwise obscuring the lower cervical spine, then additional views such as a swimmer's lateral view should be obtained. For the swimmer's lateral view, one arm is lifted up and forward while the other is forced down, as if overhead swimming. This is especially important in the setting of trauma where acute fractures can be hidden. If the entire cervical spine still cannot be visualized despite these maneuvers, there should be a very low threshold for ordering CT.

When reviewing radiographs after an arthroplasty, the entire prosthesis needs to be included on the radiograph to evaluate for subtle periprosthetic lucency or fracture. In complex knee arthroplasty revision cases, additional dedicated radiographs of the femur

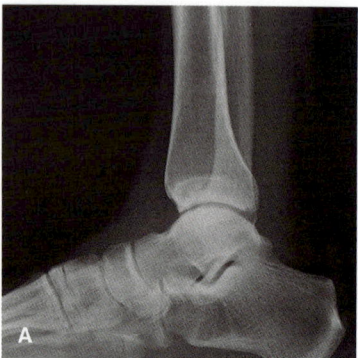 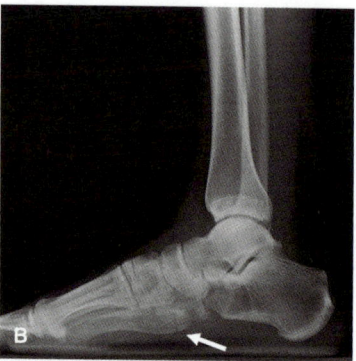

Figure 3 **A**, Lateral view of the ankle after an ankle sprain. On initial review, no obvious osseous abnormality is noted, but the plantar surface of the foot is cut off. **B**, Repeat lateral view, with a more appropriate field-of-view to include most of the foot including the base of the fifth metatarsal, clearly demonstrates the nondisplaced avulsion fracture (arrow).

or tibia may be required. Care should also be taken to ensure that lateral views are true laterals; lateral views can often be suboptimal, because of either pain or poor technologist positioning of the patient. If lateral views, notably of the elbow or ankle, are malpositioned, intra-articular effusions or subtle nondisplaced fractures can be overlooked (**Figure 3**).

Insignificant Findings Could Be Just the Tip of the Iceberg

It is common when reviewing radiographs to look for the big things—that is, fracture, arthritis, and tumor. Beginning early in an orthopaedic surgeon's career, being diligent is imporant when evaluating radiographs, as subtle findings may reflect a larger pathologic process[2] (**Figure 4**).

In the knee, a small bone fragment next to the medial patellar facet may represent an osteochondral fracture in the setting of a patellar dislocation rather than a degenerative intra-articular body. A small fleck of bone in the proximal first web space of the foot may be indicative of disruption of the Lisfranc ligament, which can lead to chronic midfoot articular surface malalignment and the development of early arthritis.

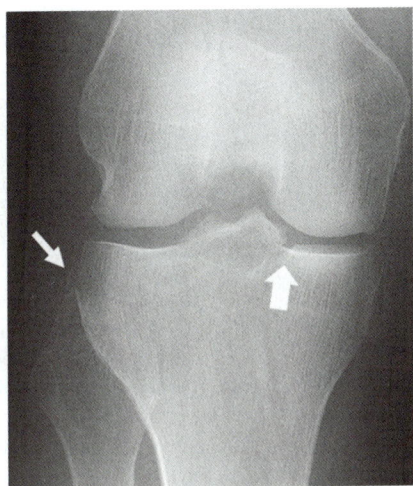

Figure 4 AP view of the knee of a patient after a skiing injury demonstrates a subtle cortical avulsion injury of the lateral tibial plateau (thin arrow), representing a Segond fracture, which has been shown to have a high association with anterior cruciate ligament (ACL) tears. Avulsion fracture of the tibial spine (thick arrow) reflects the ACL injury.

Have a Basic Knowledge of Less Commonly Obtained Radiographic Views

There are numerous radiographic views beyond basic frontal and lateral projections, each providing unique and specific information regarding a certain condition[3,4] (**Figure 5; Table 1**).

Some of the more commonly obtained uncommon views include the external, or reverse, oblique view of the foot to better visualize the medial navicular tuberosity and assess for the presence of an accessory navicular, the false profile view of the hip to better see anterior uncoverage or overcoverage of the femoral head, and the elongated femoral neck lateral view to identify a cam morphology of the femoral head–neck junction in femoroacetabular impingement.

Manipulate the Images to See More: Adjust Window/Level, Magnify

One of the many advantages of picture archiving and communication systems (PACS) as opposed to routine hard-copy radiographs

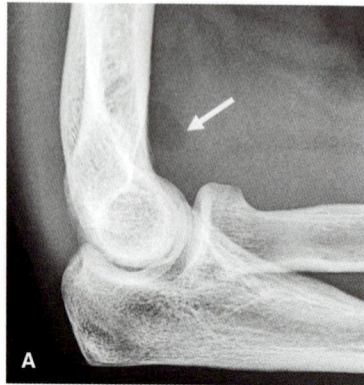 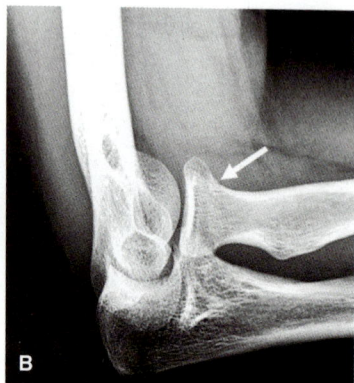

Figure 5 **A**, Lateral view of the elbow demonstrates an intra-articular effusion (arrow) but no fracture. **B**, The radial head or Coyle trauma view obtained with a slightly more lordotic projection with the x-ray beam directed 45° toward the shoulder now demonstrates the periosteal reaction (arrow) associated with a subtle nondisplaced fracture of the radial neck.

TABLE 1 Additional Helpful Radiographic Views

View	Indication
Stryker notch (shoulder)	Chronic dislocation/instability, sensitive for Hill-Sachs lesions
Coyle trauma (elbow)	Suspected radial head fracture
Carpal tunnel (wrist)	Suspected hook of the hamate fracture
Scaphoid (wrist)	Suspected scaphoid fracture
Judet (pelvis)	Suspected acetabular fracture
False profile (hip)	Dysplasia, anterior uncoverage or overcoverage of the femoral head
Elongated femoral neck lateral (hip)	Femoroacetabular impingement
Broden view (foot)	Intra-articular extension of calcaneal fracture into the subtalar joint
Reverse oblique (foot)	Presence of an accessory navicular

is that the images can be magnified and manually manipulated to pick up subtle findings. Although it is impossible to zoom in and meticulously inspect the cortices of every bone on every image, there are some settings where adjusting the viewing parameters might be beneficial.

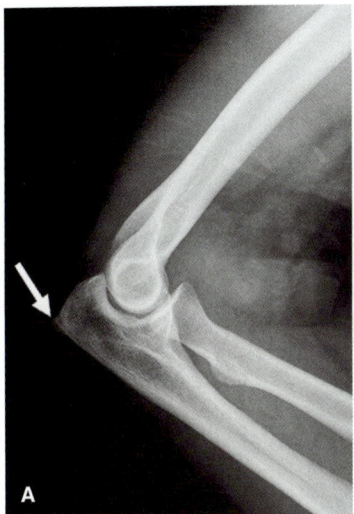 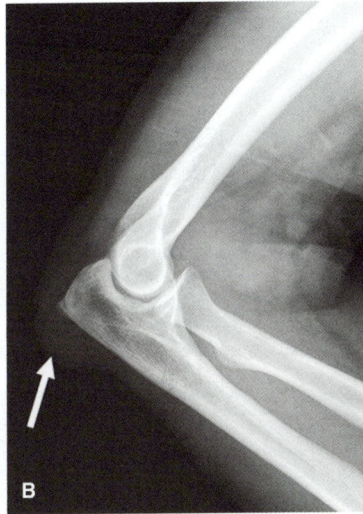

Figure 6 **A**, Routine lateral view of the elbow shown as sent to the picture archiving and communication system. Minimal enthesopathic change is seen at the triceps insertion (arrow). **B**, When windowed properly to look at the soft tissues, the associated olecranon bursitis is clearly seen (arrow).

In the emergency setting, it is imperative to window the images appropriately to be able to view the soft tissues in addition to the osseous structures (**Figure 6**). Soft-tissue swelling can reveal areas of trauma, and in pediatric patients, soft-tissue swelling about an open and otherwise radiographically normal physis is a Salter-Harris I injury until proven otherwise.

Look at Everything on the Radiograph: Unexpected Findings May Be Crucial

Radiographs may be looked at for a specific reason: to find a fracture, evaluate the alignment of a prosthesis, or assess the degree of arthritis; yet other structures on the radiograph may demonstrate findings that have important implications for the patient's health.

Cervical spine and shoulder radiographs will often demonstrate portions of the lungs where incidental pulmonary lesions may be seen (**Figure 7**). Ribs are visible on radiographs of the shoulder,

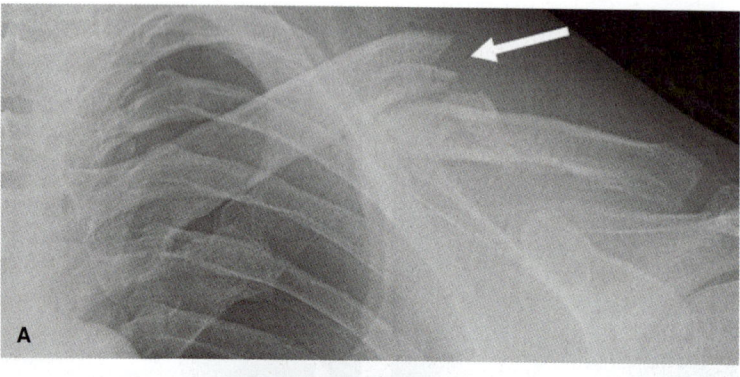

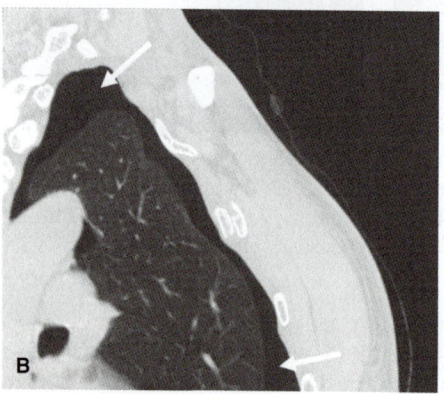

Figure 7 **A,** Frontal view of the left clavicle demonstrates an acute midshaft fracture (arrow). Nothing is seen in the adjacent lung but the absence of *anything* is concerning. **B,** Coronal reformatted image from CT scan of the left shoulder confirms the presence of a pneumothorax (arrows).

clavicle, or even the humerus, and associated rib fractures should not be missed in the setting of trauma. Observing extensive vascular calcifications on radiographs of the lumbar spine or leg in a patient with claudication could indicate more of a vascular problem than spinal stenosis or arthritis.

Compare With Prior Radiographs If Available

If there are any prior studies of the same body part, these should be compared. There are situations where even relatively acute traumatic

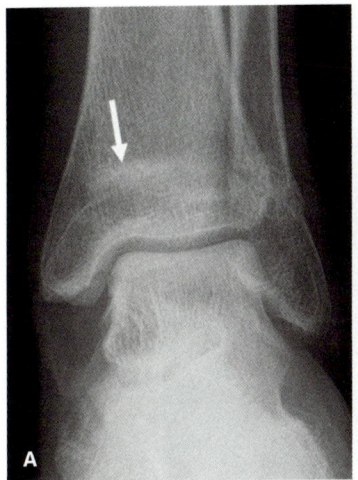 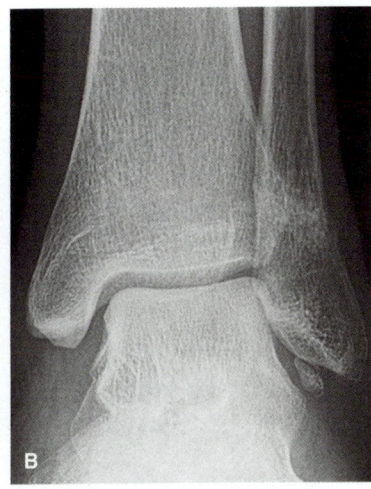

Figure 8 A, AP view of the ankle of a patient presenting for routine follow-up of a distal fibular fracture with persistent pain. **B**, Radiograph 6 weeks prior. Looking at the current AP view in isolation, it is difficult to appreciate the insufficiency fracture of the distal tibia (arrow) as it can easily be dismissed as the physeal scar. Only when comparing with the prior study is it clear the finding is a fracture and is new.

changes can only be appreciated when comparing with a normal prior study. Subtle stress or insufficiency fractures notably can be very difficult to appreciate in isolation (**Figure 8**).

Be Mindful of Laterality

It seems simple, but when reviewing multiple radiographs throughout a busy day, right versus left can get confused—whether the technologist mislabeled the radiographs, they appear on the PACS incorrectly, or the orthopaedic surgeon is distracted or fatigued. Bilateral radiographs should be reviewed the same way every time in terms of right versus left.

Another situation when laterality can become confusing is when reviewing oblique views of the cervical or lumbar spines. Oblique views are either right or left anterior oblique, where the nondependent side is the side being profiled. Radiographs can be

Chapter 2: Imaging

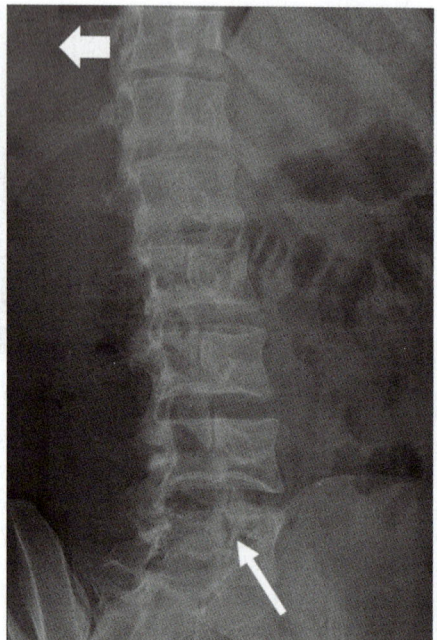

Figure 9 Right anterior oblique (also called left posterior oblique) view of the lumbar spine demonstrates unilateral left spondylolysis of L5 (thin arrow). The right side of the patient is correctly labeled on the film (thick arrow), even though this view is obtained to better assess the left side of the spine.

marked by the technologist by indicating either the dependent or nondependent side and it is important to be mindful of this (**Figure 9**).

Have a Knowledge of Normal Anatomy

It is hard to detect abnormal findings on radiographs if it is not known what normal looks like. This is usually most problematic in the pediatric population. There is some variability in the appearance of normal physes and epiphyses in children, which is compounded by the fact that these same physes and epiphyses can become injured and look even more abnormal.

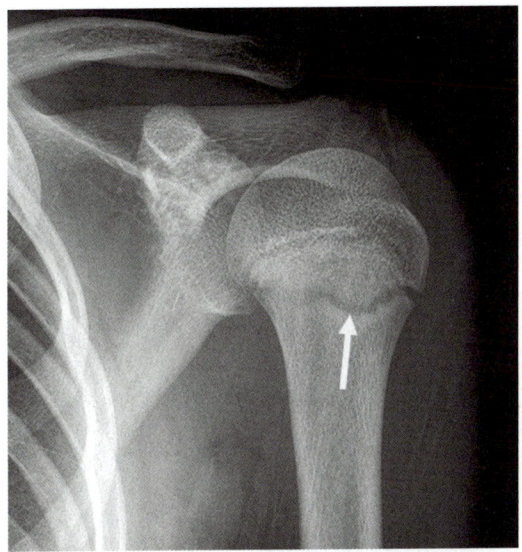

Figure 10 Frontal radiograph of the shoulder in a pediatric patient demonstrates the normal appearance of the proximal humeral physis, with a somewhat undulating contour (arrow).

One classic example is the proximal humeral physis in a child and not mistaking the "football helmet strap" appearance on the frontal view for a fracture (**Figure 10**). Although not ideal, views of the contralateral side can always be obtained for comparison.

The elbow can also be problematic. Many use the popular mnemonic "CRITOE" (capitellum; radial head; internal [medial] epicondyle; trochlea; olecranon; external [lateral] epicondyle) when reviewing pediatric elbow radiographs, but it is important to remember that this mnemonic reflects the order of appearance of the ossification centers about the elbow, not the order in which they completely fuse. Therefore, the lateral epicondyle is the last apophysis to appear, but the medial epicondyle is the last to fuse. This is important to remember when reviewing radiographs for possible medial epicondylar avulsion injuries. When in doubt, reference guides and textbooks should be used.

Beware of the Satisfaction of Search

Everyone wants to make the diagnosis and solve the case. It is important to keep in mind, however, that the first abnormality seen may not be the only one; the radiographs require meticulous inspection, especially in the setting of trauma. It is not uncommon to find one obvious fracture but miss the others that may have been clinically unsuspected because of extensive soft-tissue swelling (**Figure 11**).

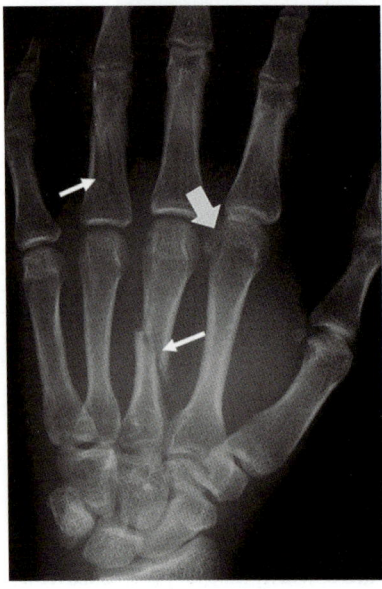

Figure 11 PA view of the hand of a patient with acute trauma demonstrates relatively conspicuous fractures of the shafts of the third metacarpal and proximal phalanx of the ring finger (thin arrows). Less obvious is an osteochondral shear fracture of the ulnar aspect of the head of the second metacarpal (thick arrow). Always keep looking!

Top 10 Knowledge Drops for Your Rotation

1. Always obtain at least two views.
2. Make sure the images include everything they should.
3. Insignificant findings could be just the tip of the iceberg.
4. Have a basic knowledge of less commonly obtained radiographic views.
5. Manipulate the images to see more: adjust window/level, magnify.

6. Look at everything on the radiograph: unexpected findings may be crucial.
7. Compare with prior radiographs if they are available
8. Be mindful of laterality.
9. Have a knowledge of normal anatomy.
10. Beware of the satisfaction of search.

Computed Tomography

CT provides two-dimensional (2D) and three-dimensional (3D) representations of osseous anatomy and therefore can provide important information that radiographs may not. The following pearls or knowledge drops will help the orthopaedic surgeon interpret CT scans accurately and take full advantage of what CT offers in terms of imaging the musculoskeletal system.

Don't Forget the Scout Image and the Accompanying Radiographs

The scout image is a low-resolution radiograph, usually obtained in frontal and lateral projections, acquired at the beginning of the CT study so that the scan can be properly plotted. Most non-radiologists are probably not even aware that these scout images exist, but it is important to inspect them before starting to look at the actual CT scan. The scout images show a larger field of view of the patient, larger than the anatomy that is covered by the CT scan, and can reveal pathologic processes that the CT examination may not. For example, scout images before a CT scan of the lumbar spine will include the entire lower chest, abdomen, and pelvis, and may show such abnormalities as a tumor in the lower lung, calcified mass in the abdomen, or arthritis of the hip. Scout images before a CT scan of one hip will include the pelvis and the contralateral hip and may show abnormalities that would not be included in the CT examination of the hip of interest.

The scout image may provide an easy diagnosis for the patient's complaints or may reveal pathology that was not clinically suspected but is still relevant. It should be noted that medicolegally, the standard of care is that the scout images are reviewed, and malpractice lawsuits have been settled in favor of the patient when an abnormality on a scout image was missed.[5]

Similarly, radiographs of the relevant anatomy obtained either concurrently or before the CT examination should also be reviewed before looking at the CT scan. Because radiographs are a 2D representation of a 3D structure, certain structures, both normal and pathologic, are much more conspicuous on radiographs than CT. Overall alignment of a joint, degree of displacement of a fracture, or integrity of hardware may be easier to assess on radiographs compared with CT.

Use Multiplanar Reformations (Reformats)

Modern multidetector CT allows acquisition of isotropic (3D) volume data and thin, submillimeter slice-thickness images reconstructed in any plane. It is crucial that not just the axial slices but the reformations in these other planes, typically coronal and sagittal, are also reviewed when interpreting a CT image. Fracture lines often do not follow any one plane, and complex fractures will not be adequately evaluated in just one plane (**Figure 12**). Assessment of the degree of height loss of a vertebral compression fracture would not be possible without coronal and sagittal reformations.

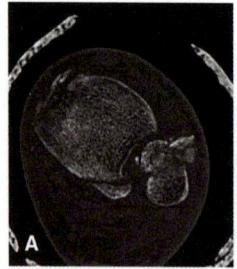 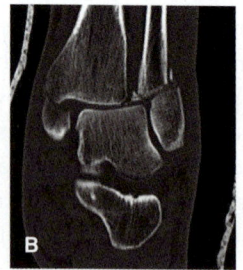 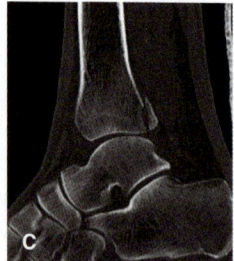

Figure 12 CT images of the ankle in axial (**A**), coronal (**B**), and sagittal (**C**) reformations show a trimalleolar fracture. Multiplanar evaluation allows more accurate interpretation of fracture alignment compared with axial plane only.

It is important to remember that, because these multiplanar reformations are a product of postprocessing after image acquisition, it is possible for the CT technologist to generate additional reformations in other planes if the provided planes do not depict the pathology adequately. Most PACS also have built-in 3D software that allows users to manipulate the images themselves.

Optimize Windowing of the Study

For musculoskeletal CT, the images are sent to the PACS in standard bone windows, in which the Hounsfield unit (HU, numerical unit signifying how dense a structure is on CT) window level and width are optimized to best assess osseous structures. However, evaluation of structures other than bone such as soft tissues or surgical implants such as joint arthroplasties requires manual adjustment of the HU window level and width. For example, adjusting these parameters can reduce the streak artifact around metal and allow better evaluation of the metal as well as the structures around it. For hip arthroplasties, increasing the HU level and widening the window width will allow the differentiation of metal such as titanium from ceramic, and even allow the diagnosis of nondisplaced fractures of ceramic liners[6] (**Figure 13**).

Evaluate the Soft Tissues

Orthopaedic surgeons use CT primarily to evaluate bone because of the exquisite bony detail. However, by changing the windowing to soft-tissue windows, the soft tissues can be evaluated as well. Soft-tissue edema can point to an area of pathology, and soft-tissue emphysema is a sign of penetrating injury, infection with a gas-producing organism, or communication with an injured bowel. Fluid collections, such as a synovial effusion, bursitis, or abscess, can be identified, especially if CT is done with intravenous contrast.

Tendons are more hyperdense (bright) than the rest of the soft tissues and can easily be identified on soft-tissue windows. By developing a habit of looking at all the tendons in every CT scan, tendon ruptures as well as tendon entrapment (**Figure 14**) and tenosynovitis can be diagnosed.

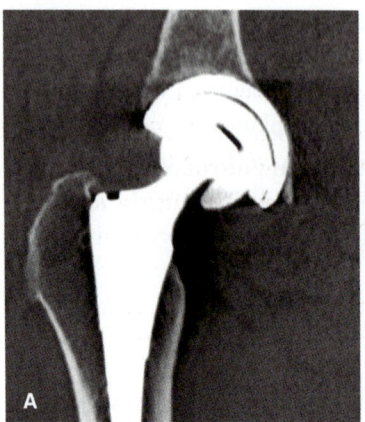 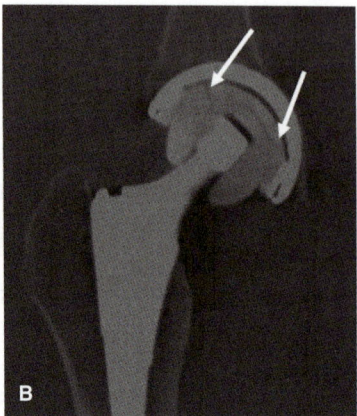

Figure 13 Coronal reformation of CT of the hip with arthroplasty (**A**) in a standard bone window shows both the ceramic femoral head and liner and titanium femoral stem and acetabular cup being much more radiodense (brighter) than bone, and thus indistinguishable from each other. **B**, With the Hounsfield unit window level raised and window width widened, the ceramic components are differentiated from the titanium components, unmasking a nondisplaced fracture of the ceramic liner (arrows).

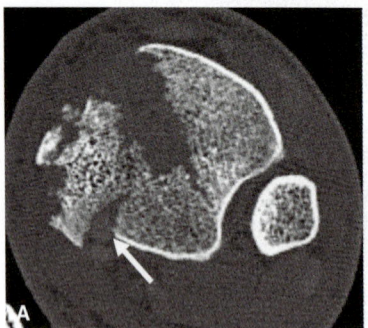 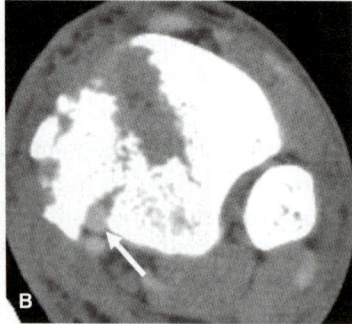

Figure 14 **A**, Axial CT in bone window shows a comminuted fracture of the distal tibia with the posterior tibial tendon (arrow) entrapped between fracture fragments, which is more easily seen in a soft-tissue window (**B**).

Not Just a Fracture: Importance of Fracture Characterization and Complications

CT is very accurate in identifying and characterizing acute fractures. Its multiplanar capability allows assessment of fracture displacement, intra-articular extension, and resultant disruption of the articular surface, which can guide surgical management. In skeletally immature patients, CT will identify physeal involvement in Salter-Harris fractures.

CT is also very useful for distinguishing acute from chronic fractures and fracture nonunion. Sclerotic and smooth margins of a fracture are signs of fracture nonunion. Quantifying the amount of cortical and trabecular bony bridging across a fracture site will help determine whether the fracture is healed and guide removal of hardware. In the pediatric population, traumatic physeal bars as a complication of physeal injury can be identified (**Figure 15**).

Stress fractures, either insufficiency or fatigue fractures, have a characteristic appearance on CT as a linear band of sclerosis

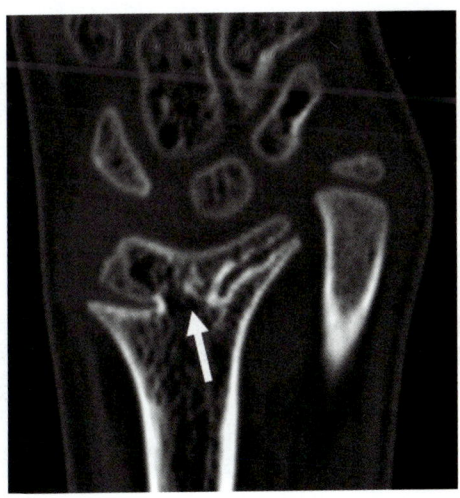

Figure 15 Coronal reformation of a CT scan of the wrist shows a physeal bar (arrow) of the distal radius.

oriented perpendicular to the trabeculae, with or without cortical breach. It is important to recognize stress fractures, as their imaging appearance is different from that of traumatic fractures and because stress fractures are often not clinically suspected.

Know When Contrast is Administered

CT is performed without contrast for routine evaluation of osseous structures. In certain instances, contrast may be administered to answer a specific clinical question, and it is important to become familiar with its appearance on CT.

CT arthrography is performed after iodinated contrast is administered into the joint under ultrasound or fluoroscopic guidance. CT arthrography can be useful in diagnosing intra-articular pathology when the patient has a contraindication to MRI; rotator cuff and labral tears of the shoulder, triangular fibrocartilage complex tears of the wrist, labral tears of the hip, and meniscal tears of the knee, for example, which would not be possible with a standard noncontrast CT scan of the respective joint (**Figure 16**).

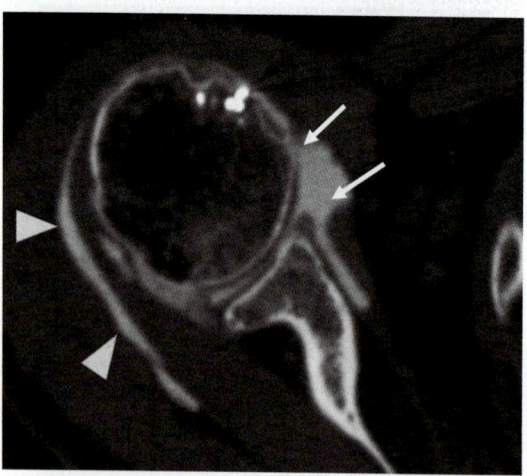

Figure 16 Axial CT arthrography of the shoulder in a patient after subscapularis repair shows absence of the subscapularis tendon (arrows), consistent with retear, and contrast freely extending into the subacromial subdeltoid bursa (arrowheads).

Similarly, CT myelography is CT of the spine performed after intrathecal administration of iodinated contrast under fluoroscopic guidance. Unlike noncontrast CT of the spine, CT myelography allows visualization of the spinal cord and the nerve roots traversing the subarachnoid space, similar to MRI. Compressive lesions of the spinal cord and nerve roots, or traumatic avulsions of the cervical nerve roots (**Figure 17**), can be diagnosed on CT myelography, which would otherwise not be possible on standard noncontrast CT scans.

Contrast can also be administered intravenously as part of CT. Although this is much more commonly done for CT of the chest, abdomen, and pelvis, it is occasionally indicated for joints and extremities as well. CT with intravenous contrast may be performed to assess the vascularity of a soft-tissue mass, to look for arterial injuries, or preoperatively to map out the vasculature in an area of interest.

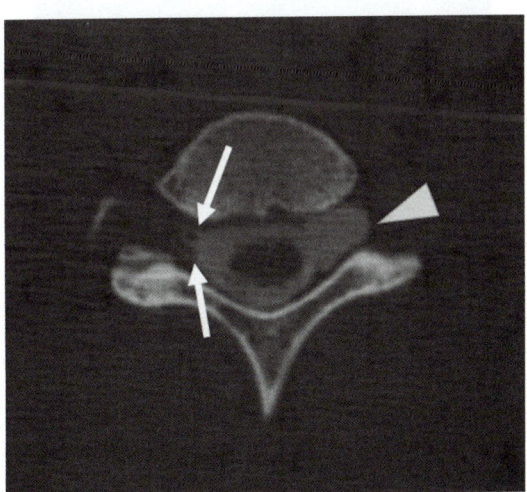

Figure 17 Axial CT myelography of the cervical spine shows a left pseudomeningocele (arrowhead) and absence of the left nerve root, reflecting a traumatic root avulsion from the spinal cord. The uninjured right nerve root is seen (arrows) for comparison.

Beware of Satisfaction of Search

In the radiology community, satisfaction of search refers to the pitfall of being psychologically content with the interpretation of a study when one abnormality is found. It is known that a radiologist is more likely to miss an abnormality on a study if one abnormality has already been found. This is especially true in the setting of trauma when a radiologist notices one fracture but misses the second (**Figure 18**). This pearl also applies to the examining orthopaedic surgeon; patients are more difficult to evaluate when there is accompanying soft-tissue swelling, and pain caused by one fracture can mask the symptoms of a second fracture.

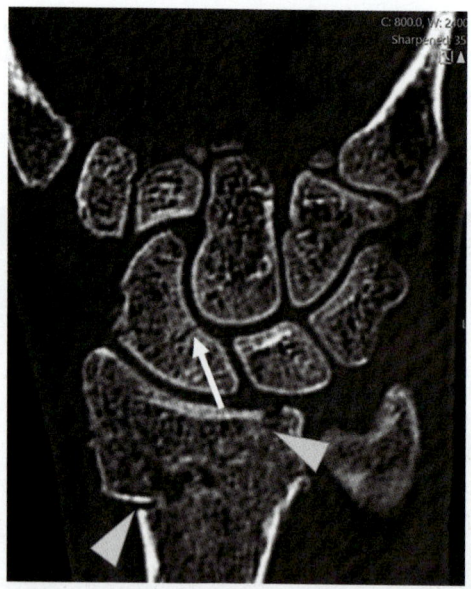

Figure 18 Coronal reformation of a CT scan of the wrist shows a comminuted fracture of the distal radius (arrowheads) and a more subtle, nondisplaced fracture of the waist of the scaphoid (arrow).

Top 10 Knowledge Drops for Your Rotation
1. Don't forget the scout image.
2. Looking at the relevant radiographs before the CT can help avoid missed diagnoses.
3. Use multiplanar reformations (reformats).
4. Optimize windowing of the study.
5. Soft tissue edema and soft tissue emphysema are important clues to injury.
6. Don't forget to look for fluid collections and tendon injuries.
7. Know the differential features of acute vs chronic fractures and fracture nonunion.
8. Stress fractures have a characteristic appearance on CT.
9. Know when contrast is administered.
10. Beware of satisfaction of search.

Magnetic Resonance Imaging

MRI has become an indispensable diagnostic imaging tool for the orthopaedic surgeon because of its exquisite soft-tissue contrast, ability to image cartilage and marrow, and availability of different pulse sequences for problem solving. The following are important pearls and pitfalls to guide the orthopaedic surgeon in accurate interpretation of MRI studies.

Recognize Pulse Sequences

There is no universal set of pulse sequences that all institutions obtain for an MRI of a particular body part. Even for a study as common as an MRI of the knee, each imaging center will acquire its own set of pulse sequences, made up of a combination of fat-suppressed, T1-weighted, T2-weighted, and/or intermediate-weighted fast spin echo sequences, often with inversion recovery and gradient echo (GRE) sequences. All of these pulse sequences differ in terms of signal-to-noise ratio, contrast resolution, and acquisition time (**Table 2**).

Many but not all fat-suppressed sequences are fluid-sensitive, meaning that fluid and edema are bright whereas fat, including marrow fat, is dark gray. An exception is the fat-suppressed T1-weighted sequence, in which fat signal is suppressed and thus is dark gray, but fluid and edema also remain dark, just as in conventional

TABLE 2 Typical MRI Pulse Sequences Used in Orthopaedic Imaging

Pulse Sequence	Advantages	Disadvantages	Signal Intensity of Fat	Signal Intensity of Fluid
Intermediate-weighted FSE	Superb evaluation of articular cartilage Fluid-sensitive	Difficult to identify edema in bone marrow Difficult to characterize pathologic processes of bone marrow in the absence of fat suppression	Bright	Bright
T1-weighted FSE	Can identify pathologic processes of bone marrow	Poor evaluation of articular cartilage and fluid Difficult to identify edema in soft tissues and bone marrow	Bright	Dark
T2-weighted (TE > 50 ms) FSE	Fluid-sensitive	Poor evaluation of articular cartilage, particularly the basilar component Difficult to identify edema in soft tissues or in bone marrow Difficult to identify plastic deformation of ligaments	Bright	Bright
Fat-suppressed T2/proton density-weighted FSE	Fluid-sensitive Can differentiate edema from fat	Inferior signal-to-noise ratio Magnetic field inhomogeneities (eg, from metallic fixation, suture) can lead to artifact/incomplete fat suppression	Dark	Bright
STIR	Fluid-sensitive Can differentiate edema from fat Less susceptible to magnetic field inhomogeneities	Poor anatomic detail Inferior signal-to-noise ratio Longer acquisition time than other forms of fat suppression	Dark	Bright
GRE	Blooming artifact can identify hemosiderin and calcium Increase conspicuity of small bone fragments	Susceptible to metal artifact	Variable	Variable
Gadolinium-enhanced T1-weighted FSE	Assess vascularity of tissue (eg, solid mass versus cyst)	Requires intravenous administration of gadolinium Poor evaluation of articular cartilage	Bright (unless fat-suppressed)	Dark

FSE = fast spin echo, GRE = gradient echo, STIR = short tau inversion recovery, TE = echo time

T1-weighted sequences. Intermediate-weighted sequences (echo time of 30 to 35 ms) are the workhorse for musculoskeletal MRI at most institutions, because of overall high signal-to-noise ratio, conspicuity of fluid and fat, and optimal visualization of grayscale stratification of articular cartilage, which reflects the orientation of the collagen.[7] Intermediate-weighted pulse sequences provide the best differential contrast among fibrocartilage, articular cartilage, and fluid. On T1-weighted sequences, only fat is bright among normal tissues and there is poor contrast between fluid/edema and other tissues. T2-weighted sequences have a similar appearance to intermediate-weighted sequences in musculoskeletal imaging, but evaluation of articular cartilage on T2-weighted imaging is highly suboptimal.

A GRE sequence may be obtained in addition to a routine protocol of fast spin echo sequences. Unlike fast spin echo sequences in which a 90° excitation pulse is applied to flip the magnetization vector of protons into the transverse plane followed by multiple 180° refocusing pulses, in a GRE sequence, the excitation pulse is typically less than 90° and the 180° refocusing pulse is not applied. Without going too much into the physics, hemosiderin products cause blooming, or are accentuated on GRE sequences, and a synovial-based soft-tissue mass that exhibits blooming artifact on GRE sequences is pathognomonic for pigmented villonodular synovitis (**Figure 19**).

For nonradiologists who want to become skilled at interpreting MRI, it is imperative that they become comfortable identifying the various pulse sequences, as structures, both normal and abnormal, will appear different depending on the particular pulse sequence.

Begin With the Fat-Suppressed Sequence, End With the Fat-Suppressed Sequence

Although there are a few exceptions, most pathologies on MRI, especially acute ones, are hyperintense (bright) on the fat-suppressed fluid-sensitive sequence (ie, fat-saturated T2-weighted, fat-saturated intermediate-weighted, or short tau inversion recovery sequence).

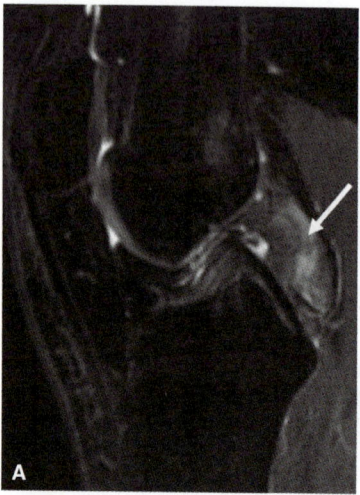 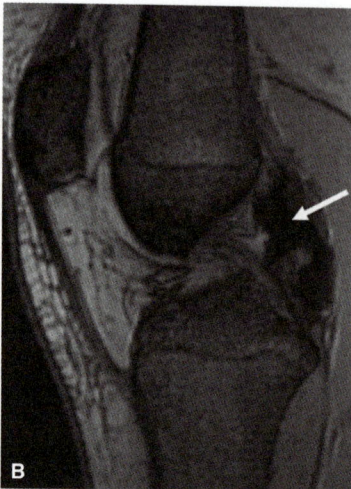

Figure 19 **A**, Sagittal inversion recovery image of the knee shows a heterogeneous synovial-based soft-tissue mass distending the posterior capsule (arrow). **B**, Corresponding gradient echo image shows the mass to become diffusely low signal (blooming) (arrow) because of hemosiderin products, pathognomonic for pigmented villonodular synovitis.

Areas of soft-tissue edema and bone marrow edema initially seen on the fat-suppressed sequence are good areas to first direct attention to on the other pulse sequences, as these areas often show soft-tissue and osseous pathology. The other pulse sequences are used to provide an anatomic explanation for why there is soft-tissue or marrow edema on the fat-suppressed sequence. Finally, before concluding the interpretation, it is prudent to scroll through the fat-suppressed sequence one more time; it is not uncommon to find an additional, more subtle area of soft-tissue edema or marrow edema during this final run through the fat-suppressed sequence, which again needs to be explained by the other pulse sequences and which often ends up being an important finding.

Determine the Cause of Any Bone Marrow Edema

When bone marrow edema (ie, high signal intensity in the marrow on the fat-suppressed fluid-sensitive sequence) is encountered, there

Chapter 2: Imaging

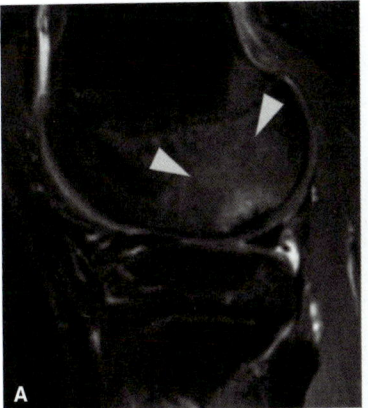 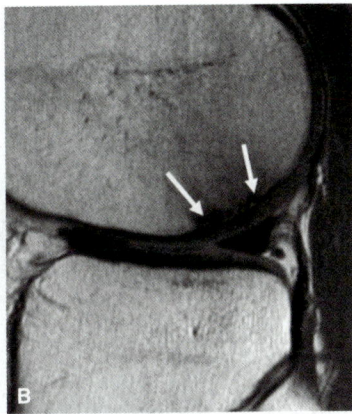

Figure 20 **A**, Sagittal inversion recovery image of the lateral compartment of the knee shows intense marrow edema of the posterolateral femoral condyle (arrowheads), which itself is nonspecific. **B**, Corresponding sagittal intermediate-weighted image shows a thin low signal intensity subchondral line (arrows), reflecting a subchondral fracture.

must be an explanation for it, as there are myriad entities that may result in bone marrow edema.

In the setting of trauma, bone marrow edema may represent a contusion, sequela of avulsion, or an actual fracture. A low signal intensity fracture line will be visible if the marrow edema is due to a fracture (**Figure 20**). A stress reaction from repetitive injury will also present as marrow edema. Geodes (well-defined lytic lesions at the periarticular surfaces, also known as subchondral cysts) and intraosseous ganglion cysts are isointense (same degree of brightness) to fluid and hyperintense (brighter) to marrow edema on fluid-sensitive sequences, but other lesions of bone can have associated marrow edema, including benign and malignant neoplastic processes. Osteoid osteoma characteristically presents with marked marrow edema, but its nidus may be subtle and may result in a delay in diagnosis (**Figure 21**).

Osteoarthritis can result in bone marrow edema in the opposing subchondral regions of the bone, especially if the cartilage loss is full thickness, and this does not necessarily represent a more aggressive process (**Figure 22**).

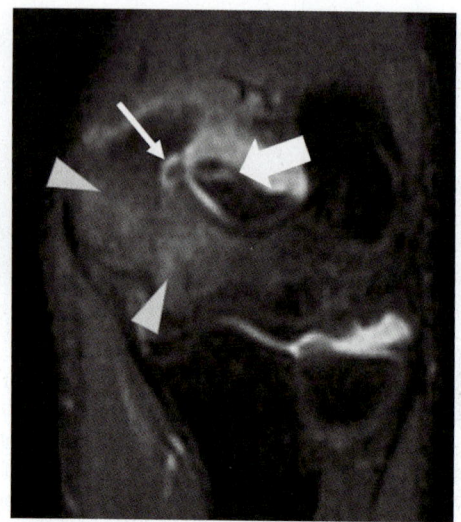

Figure 21 A 23-year-old patient who is a baseball pitcher is suspected of having posteromedial impingement of the elbow. Coronal inversion recovery image of the elbow shows fibrous union through a fractured olecranon osteophyte (thick arrow). There is, however, also intense marrow edema in the medial aspect of the distal humerus (arrowheads) secondary to a subtle osteoid osteoma (thin arrow).

Marrow edema may also represent a reactive process from adjacent extraosseous pathologies. For example, active infectious or inflammatory arthritis will result in a synovitis but can also result in reactive marrow edema of the adjacent bone. Osteomyelitis will result in marrow edema, usually with destructive changes to the bone and surrounding soft-tissue edema.

Know the Distribution of Bone Marrow Edema Associated With Classic Injuries

Bone marrow edema is a sign of osseous injury, and many classic injuries are associated with a particular distribution of marrow edema on the fat-suppressed fluid-sensitive sequence because of the mechanism of injury (**Table 3**).

In the shoulder, bone marrow edema in the posterolateral aspect of the superior humeral head should suggest a Hill-Sachs lesion from anterior dislocation, whereas marrow edema in the

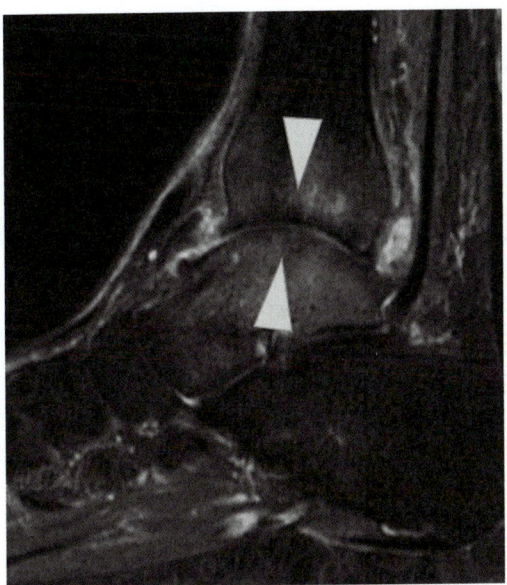

Figure 22 Sagittal inversion recovery image of the ankle shows marrow edema along the subchondral regions of the opposing surfaces of the tibiotalar joint (arrowheads) related to advanced osteoarthritis, although the marrow edema of the talus is more extensive, extending into the body.

anteromedial aspect of the humeral head should suggest a reverse Hill-Sachs lesion from posterior dislocation.

In the knee, marrow edema both in the anterolateral femoral condyle and posterolateral tibial plateau has a high association with anterior cruciate ligament (ACL) tears (**Figure 23**), marrow edema in the anterior aspects of the distal femur and proximal tibia is usually indicative of a hyperextension injury highly associated with ACL tears (**Figure 24**), and marrow edema in the anterolateral femoral condyle and inferomedial patella is associated with a recent patellar dislocation.

In the ankle, marrow edema in the medial aspect of the talar dome is usually indicative of a deltoid injury (**Figure 25**), whereas marrow edema along the tibiotalar joint can be seen with different impingement syndromes.

The association of these patterns of marrow edema with the particular type of injury is because the mechanism of injury for each

TABLE 3 Distribution of Bone Marrow Edema in Key Injuries

Shoulder	
Anterior dislocation	Posterolateral humeral head (Hill-Sachs lesion) and anterior-inferior glenoid
Posterior dislocation	Anteromedial humeral head (reverse Hill-Sachs) and posterior glenoid
Elbow	
Valgus injury	Lateral capitellum and radial head
Triceps avulsion	Olecranon process
Knee	
Anterior cruciate ligament tear	Anterolateral femoral condyle and posterolateral tibial plateau (pivot shift)
Hyperextension (posterior cruciate ligament injury)	Anterior distal femur and proximal tibia
Valgus injury	Lateral femoral condyle and lateral tibial plateau
Varus injury	Medial femoral condyle and medial tibial plateau
Patellar dislocation	Anterolateral femoral condyle and inferomedial patella
Ankle	
Deltoid ligament avulsion	Medial talus
Anterior impingement syndrome	Dorsal talar neck and anterior distal tibia
Lateral subtalar impingement	Lateral talar process and calcaneus at angle of Gissane
Subfibular impingement	Lateral calcaneus and distal fibula

results in bone impaction at those sites (except for marrow edema in the medial talus associated with deltoid avulsion). For example, varus and valgus forces would result in impaction along apposing surfaces over the medial and lateral sides of the joint, respectively (**Figure 24**). Therefore, a firm grasp of the injury mechanism will help in accurately interpreting magnetic resonance images demonstrating these distributions of marrow edema.

Recognize Infection and Its Mimickers

Musculoskeletal infection requires a rapid diagnosis so that antibiotic treatment can be initiated and/or surgical management performed urgently. Musculoskeletal infection may present as cellulitis,

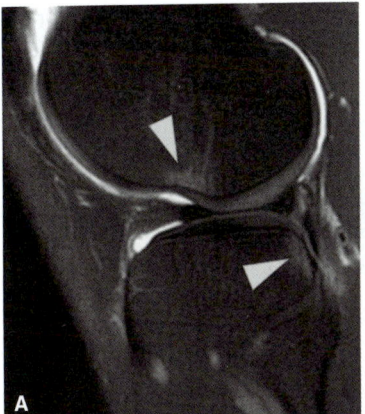
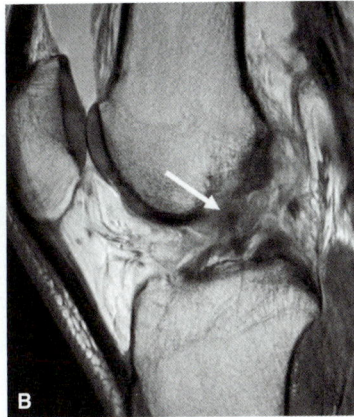

Figure 23 **A**, Sagittal inversion recovery image of the lateral compartment of the knee shows marrow edema in the anterolateral femoral condyle and posterolateral tibial plateau (arrowheads) from tibial translation, which has a high association with anterior cruciate ligament (ACL) injuries. **B**, Corresponding sagittal intermediate-weighted image through the midline of the knee shows an acutely disrupted ACL (arrow).

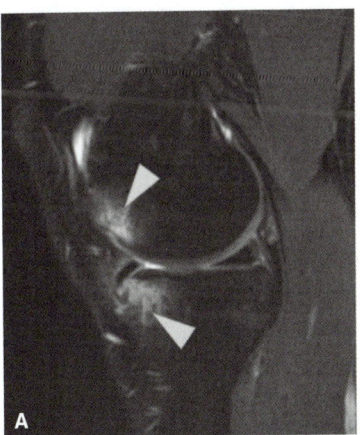
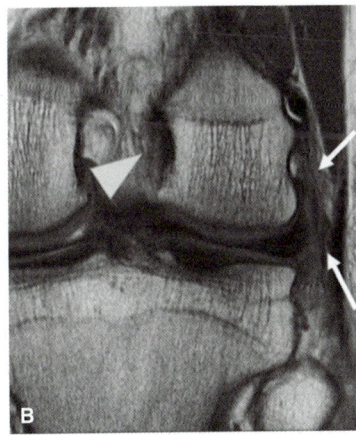

Figure 24 **A**, Sagittal inversion recovery image of the medial compartment of the knee shows marrow edema anteriorly (arrowheads) within the medial femoral condyle and medial tibial plateau, reflecting a combination of hyperextension and varus distraction. **B**, Coronal intermediate-weighted image shows diffuse signal hyperintensity within the fibular collateral ligament (arrow), which was torn because of the varus force, as well as a high-grade anterior cruciate ligament tear (arrowhead).

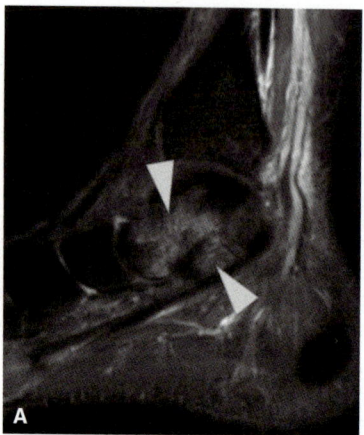 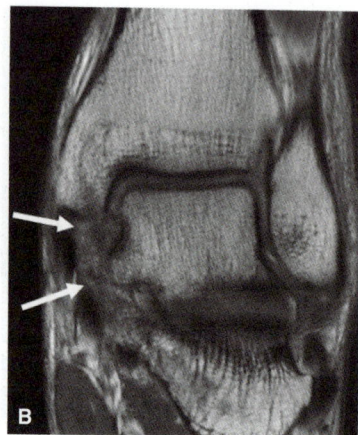

Figure 25 **A**, Sagittal inversion recovery image of the medial side of the ankle shows marrow edema of the body of the talus and sustentaculum tali of the calcaneus (arrowheads) due to deltoid injury. **B**, Straight coronal intermediate-weighted image shows tear of both the superficial and deep fibers of the deltoid ligament (arrows).

fasciitis, pyomyositis, septic tenosynovitis, septic arthritis, or osteomyelitis with/without soft-tissue or intraosseous abscesses. The appearance on MRI varies based on the specific tissue involved. However, diffuse soft-tissue edema or bone marrow edema with fluid in the infected space is a common MRI feature of infection (**Figure 26**). One must have a high index of suspicion as the MRI features can sometimes be subtle.

There are noninfectious entities whose imaging features classically overlap those of septic arthritis and osteomyelitis but which the orthopaedic surgeon may not remember to include in the differential diagnosis. Inflammatory arthritides, gout, and neuropathic arthropathy are three such entities; all three can present with a synovitis, marked periarticular soft-tissue edema, and associated marrow edema (**Figure 27**). Neuropathic arthropathy more commonly consolidates marrow and soft-tissue edema at the joint surface, whereas infection may occur remote from the joint. Image-guided arthrocentesis or even a bone biopsy may be required to confidently exclude infection even if one of these nonseptic diagnoses is favored.

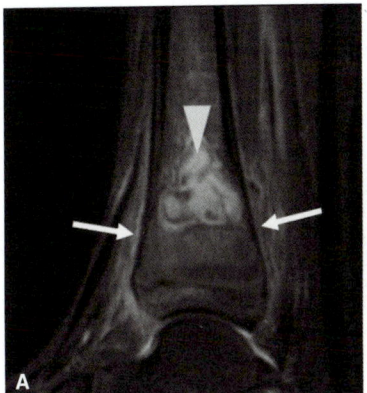
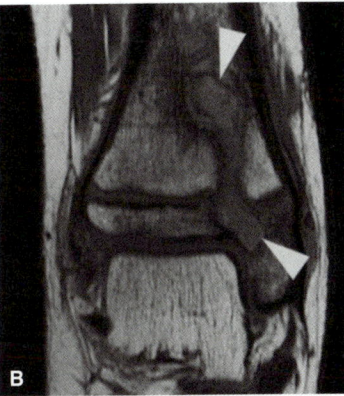

Figure 26 **A**, Sagittal inversion recovery image of the ankle shows an irregular fluid collection in the distal tibia (arrowhead) with surrounding marrow edema pattern and periosteal soft tissue edema (arrows). **B**, On the straight coronal T1-weighted image, this fluid collection violates the physis and extends into the epiphysis (arrowheads). These are consistent with osteomyelitis and intraosseous abscess.

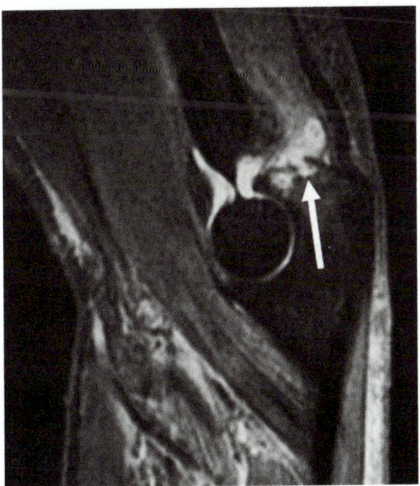

Figure 27 Sagittal inversion recovery image of the elbow shows osseous destruction of the olecranon (arrow) with associated marrow edema, synovitis, and surrounding soft-tissue edema, highly suspicious for osteomyelitis. Aspiration yielded uric acid crystals, consistent with gout rather than infection.

Calcium deposition diseases such as calcium hydroxyapatite deposition disease or calcium pyrophosphate deposition/pseudogout may present with prominent soft-tissue edema and mimic infection. Osteoid osteoma may mimic osteomyelitis on imaging if its central nidus is not identified. After orthopaedic surgery, the host's foreign body reaction to surgical implants can result in a septic arthritis–like appearance on MRI.

Because the delay in diagnosis can result in long-term morbidity, there should be a low threshold for suggesting infection based on the MRI appearances, while also keeping in mind the various mimickers of infection.

Look at the Entire Study for Unexpected Findings

Pathology that is unexpected yet relevant may be visible only at the edge of one image. For example, a portion of the pectoralis major tendon may be visible at the edges of a routine MRI of the shoulder, and if it is torn, it can present clinically similar to a rotator cuff tear. Another example is the visualization of deep vein thrombosis of the calf veins in MRI performed to rule out muscle strains. A pathologic finding may only be visible on the localizer sequence, which is obtained only for the purposes of plotting the subsequent diagnostic sequences. Being systematic and paying attention to all images of all pulse sequences helps one avoid missing such findings.

Chronic Fractures and Nonunion May Not Have Accompanying Bone Marrow Edema

Although the fat-suppressed fluid-sensitive sequence identifies most acute pathologies as an area of soft-tissue edema or bone marrow edema, chronic fractures and fracture nonunion may not contain any marrow edema or soft-tissue edema and thus could be overlooked. Chronic spondylolysis of the pars interarticularis of the lumbar spine is a good example (**Figure 28**). Bone marrow edema, when present, helps direct attention; however, the non-fat-suppressed sequences must be carefully inspected. Persistent bone marrow edema at the site of fracture could be a sign of ongoing healing of the fracture, whereas persistent fracture line and cortical discontinuity without bone marrow edema is a sign of nonunion.

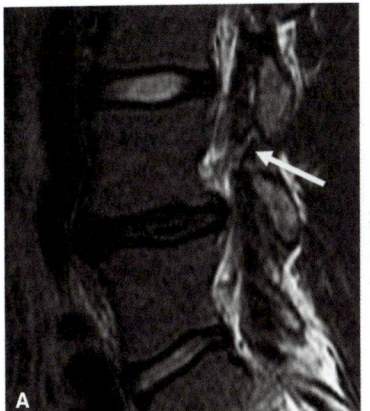 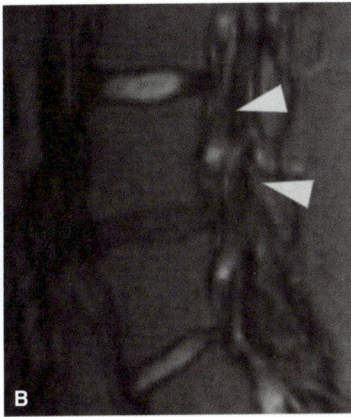

Figure 28 A, Sagittal T2-weighted image of the right side of the lumbar spine shows a discontinuity of the L4 pars interarticularis (arrow) reflecting spondylolysis. **B**, Corresponding inversion recovery sequence shows absence of bone marrow edema (arrowheads), making the spondylolysis much less conspicuous. Although spondylolysis most commonly occurs at L5, more cephalad lumbar involvement can also be seen, particularly in rowers.

Black Bone on All Pulse Sequences is Dead Bone: Do Not Try to Fix It

Cortical bone is black (low signal) on all pulse sequences, and normal cancellous bone will be dark gray on fat-suppressed sequences because marrow fat in the medullary canal is suppressed out or darkened. However, when the medullary canal is diffusely black on all pulse sequences, including the non-fat-suppressed sequences, it indicates the absence of mobile water protons and is thus a sign of bone necrosis with completely devitalized bone that is not suitable for primary repair. This corresponds to diffusely sclerotic bone on radiography and CT.

No matter what the indication is for the MRI, the presence of dead bone is critical to note as it can alter surgical management. If the lunate is diffusely devitalized in the setting of Kienböck disease, or if the proximal pole of the scaphoid is diffusely devitalized in the setting of a fracture of the waist of the scaphoid, surgery may include resection or revascularization attempts. If an osteochondritis

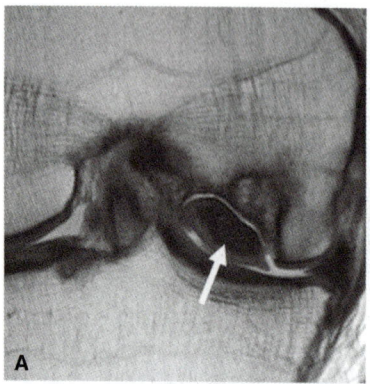 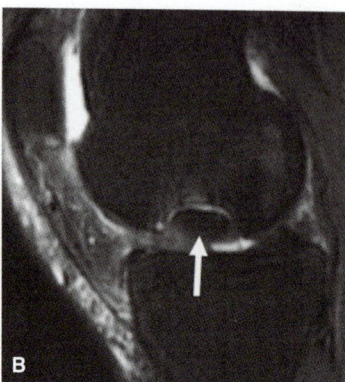

Figure 29 **A**, Coronal intermediate-weighted and (**B**) sagittal inversion recovery images of the knee show an osteochondritis dissecans of the medial femoral condyle with the marrow signal of the lesion being diffusely black (arrows), reflecting devitalized bone. On the corresponding radiograph, the lesion was diffusely sclerotic (not shown).

dissecans lesion is diffusely black (**Figure 29**), fixation may not be a viable option for this avascular structure.

Pay Attention to Articular Cartilage

Noting the integrity of the articular cartilage of the regional joints is critical in all clinical scenarios that led to MRI. Obtaining cartilage-sensitive intermediate-weighted fast spin echo sequences in three planes usually allows adequate evaluation of the articular cartilage, although an additional imaging plane is often helpful if the particular joint of interest courses obliquely relative to the body part being imaged (eg, an oblique axial plane to evaluate the patellofemoral joint of the knee, oblique sagittal plane to evaluate the first carpometacarpal joint as part of MRI of the wrist, and a straight coronal plane through the tibiotalar joint as part of MRI of the ankle) (**Figure 30**).

On intermediate-weighted sequences, signal alterations, including loss of normal gray scale stratification, will be appreciated as the earliest form of cartilage degradation. Macroscopic structural changes will then become apparent, including fibrillation and fissuring of the surface of the cartilage, partial-thickness wear, and

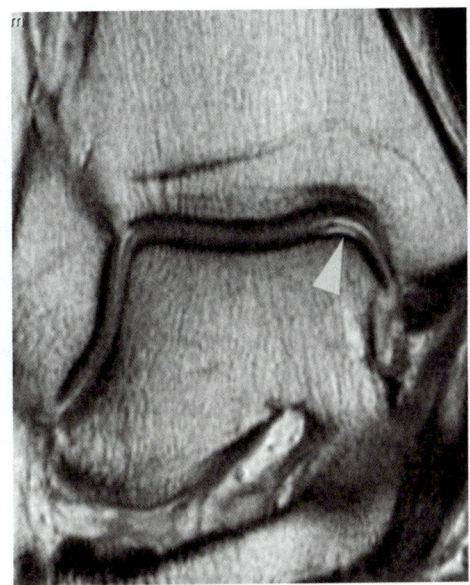

Figure 30 Straight coronal intermediate-weighted image of the ankle shows basilar delamination (arrowhead) of cartilage of the medial talar dome but without disruption of its surface.

finally full-thickness wear of the articular cartilage with disruption of the tidemark. MRI has been validated to be an accurate predictor of arthroscopic findings. More importantly, MRI will also identify areas of basilar delamination in which the surface is not disrupted and thus not easily recognizable arthroscopically (**Figure 30**).

Evaluation of the articular cartilage, just like many other facets of an MRI, is indispensable for preoperative planning. It will determine whether the patient is a candidate for a joint replacement, help the orthopaedic surgeon decide the appropriate cartilage restoration procedure in osteochondral lesions, or may dictate which form of surgical intervention is appropriate (**Figure 31**).

Recognize MRI Artifacts

Artifacts are commonly encountered in musculoskeletal MRI. A patient's inability to lie still will result in generalized blurring,

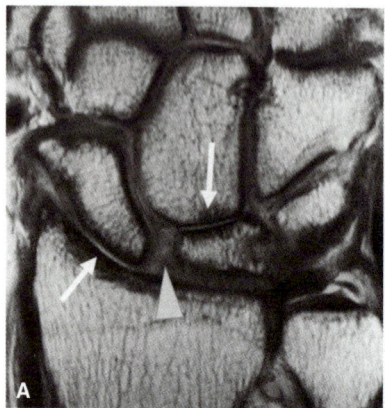
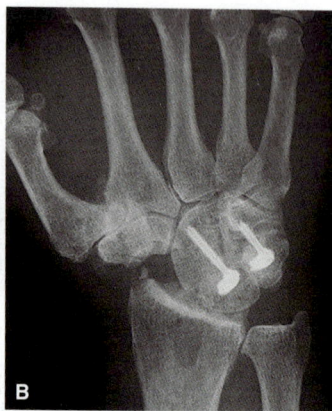

Figure 31 **A**, Coronal intermediate-weighted image of the wrist shows tear of the interosseous scapholunate ligament (arrowhead) and advanced osteoarthritis of both the radioscaphoid and capitolunate articulations (arrows), necessitating scaphoid excision and four-corner fusion rather than scapholunate ligament repair or proximal row carpectomy. **B**, Postoperative radiograph showing scaphoid excision and four-corner fusion.

which is easily recognizable by the person interpreting the magnetic resonance image results and should not be mistaken for pathology albeit it can result in a nondiagnostic examination. Susceptibility artifact from metal implants can result in a large area of signal void, which is also obvious as artifact.

An artifact can become more problematic when it is not obvious as artifact and mistaken for pathology. On fat-suppressed sequences, inhomogeneous fat-suppression can result in artifactual areas of high signal intensity that can mimic marrow edema or soft-tissue edema (**Figure 32**). These are usually in the periphery of the body and have a characteristic appearance but can sometimes lead to confusion. Susceptibility artifact can also create factitious high signal next to metal or suture when metal artifact reduction sequences are not used, for example in bone marrow adjacent to an arthroplasty, and mimic marrow edema. Pulsation artifact from arteries usually extends outside the body and thus is recognizable as artifact, but it can occasionally overlap with an area of interest and be mistaken for injury.

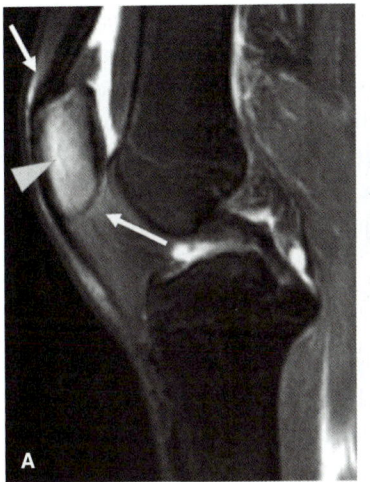 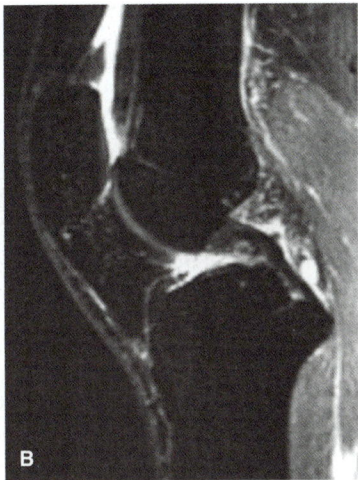

Figure 32 **A**, Sagittal fat-saturated T2-weighted sequence of the knee shows artifactual high signal intensity in the patella (arrowhead), which can occur with frequency-selective fat suppression. Similar high signal in the adjacent soft tissues (arrows) is a clue that the signal in the patella is artifact. **B**, In the sagittal inversion recovery sequence obtained at the same time, there is no longer any increased signal intensity in the patella because of homogenous fat suppression.

If a signal abnormality that may or may not be artifact is noticed by the MRI technologist while the patient is still in the scanner, then additional sequences can be acquired to resolve the issue. If it is noted only after the patient has left the department, then the radiologist must rely on their expertise to determine whether it can confidently be dismissed as artifact or if further imaging is warranted.

Be Familiar With Advanced Imaging

Through research, new MRI pulse sequences are constantly becoming commercially available and familiarity with these new techniques will allow the orthopaedic surgeon to request the most optimal pulse sequences for answering the clinical question. 3D multispectral imaging techniques, such as MAVRIC (multiacquisition with variable resonance imaging combination) or SEMAC (slice encoding for metal artifact correction), are essential for adequate imaging around metal implants, particularly cobalt-chromium. In ultrashort echo time pulse sequences, signal is seen in structures that are signal void in conventional fast spin echo sequences because of low T2 relaxation times (such as knee menisci). Zero echo time imaging is a new technique in which contrast between bone and soft tissues is increased, resulting in CT-like image contrast with superb osseous detail[8] (**Figure 33**).

Quantitative magnetic resonance techniques such as T2 map and T1 rho can detect early changes to tissue structure, for example articular cartilage, even before signal alterations are detected on intermediate-weighted fast spin echo sequences.

In magnetic resonance neurography, attention is directed to the regional nerves of interest; combination of fat-suppressed fluid-sensitive sequences and fast spin echo sequences with anatomic detail allows unprecedented imaging of nerves[9] (**Figure 34**). Diffusion tensor imaging can provide physiologic information about nerves and may aid in assessing for peripheral neuropathy.

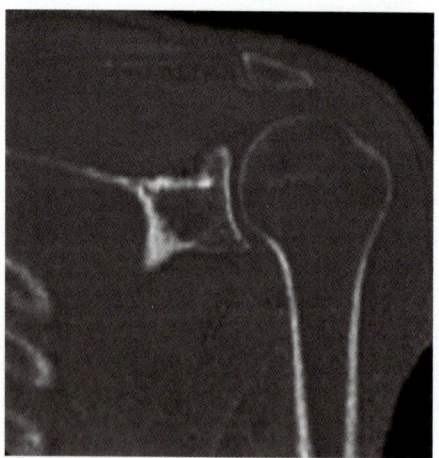

Figure 33 Zero echo time sequence of the shoulder reconstructed in the coronal plane shows conspicuity of bone relative to the soft tissues, similar to a CT scan.

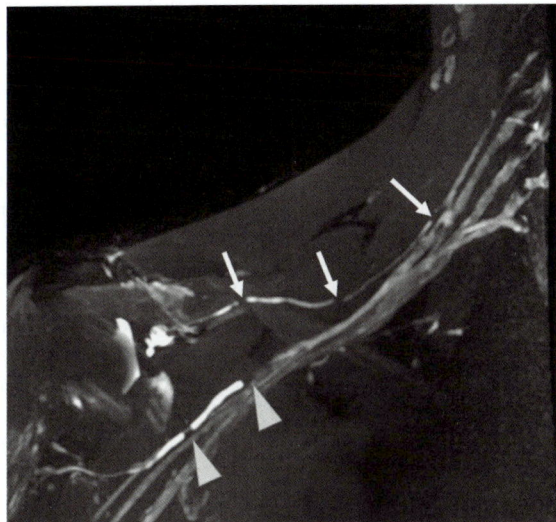

Figure 34 Coronal maximum intensity projection image from magnetic resonance neurography of the brachial plexus shows constrictions along the suprascapular (arrows) and axillary (arrowheads) nerves, representing characteristic inflammatory lesions of Parsonage-Turner syndrome.

Top 10 Knowledge Drops for Your Rotation

1. Recognize pulse sequences.
2. Begin with the fat-suppressed sequence, end with the fat-suppressed sequence.
3. Determine the cause of any bone marrow edema and use it as a clue to the mechanism of injury.
4. Recognize infection and its mimickers.
5. Look at the entire study for unexpected findings.
6. Chronic fractures and nonunion may not have accompanying bone marrow edema.
7. Black bone on all pulse sequences is dead bone; do not try to fix it.
8. Pay attention to articular cartilage.
9. Recognize MRI artifacts.
10. Be familiar with advanced imaging.

References

1. National Council on Radiation Protection and Measurements: *Report No. 107. Implementation of the Principle of as Low as Reasonably Achievable (ALARA) for Medical and Dental Personnel.* NCRP Publications, 1990.
2. Goldman AB, Pavlov H, Rubenstein D: The Segond fracture of the proximal tibia: A small avulsion that reflects major ligamentous damage. *Am J Roentgenol* 1988;151(6):1163-1167.
3. Pavlov H, Burke M, Giesa M, Seager KR, White ET: *Orthopaedist's Guide to Plain Film Imaging.* Thieme Medical, 1999.
4. Broden B: Roentgen examination of the subtaloid joint in fractures of the calcaneus. *Acta Radiol* 1949;31(1):85-91.
5. Daffner RH: Reviewing CT scout images: Observations of an expert witness. *Am J Roentgenol* 2015;205(3):589-591.
6. Endo Y, Renner L, Schmidt-Braekling T, Mintz DN, Boettner F: Imaging of ceramic liner fractures in total hip arthroplasty: The value of CT. *Skeletal Radiol* 2015;44(8):1189-1192.
7. Potter HG, Foo LF: Magnetic resonance imaging of articular cartilage: Trauma, degeneration, and repair. *Am J Sports Med* 2006;34(4):661-677.
8. Breighner RE, Endo Y, Konin GP, Gulotta LV, Koff MF, Potter HG: Technical developments: Zero echo time imaging of the shoulder. Enhanced osseous detail using MR imaging. *Radiology* 2018;286(3):960-966.
9. Sneag DB, Arányi Z, Zusstone EM, et al: Fascicular constrictions above elbow typify anterior interosseous nerve syndrome. *Muscle Nerve* 2020;61(3):301-310.

3. I Fell and Cannot Get Up—Lower Extremity Trauma

Alexandra K. Schwartz, MD, FAAOS • Samir Mehta, MD, FAAOS
Giselle M. Hernandez, DMed, FAAOS
Theodore T. Guild, MD • John Y. Kwon, MD
Fernando E. Vilella, MD, FAAOS • Danielle C. Marshall, MD
Diane Ismat Ghanem, MD • Babar Shafiq, MD, MSPT, FAAOS, FAOA

PELVIC FRACTURES

Introduction

Lower extremity musculoskeletal trauma is increasing in incidence with a bimodal distribution—higher energy fractures in younger patients and lower energy fractures in older patients. These fractures are particularly important to manage and understand because they often require inpatient hospitalization until the fractures are stabilized, because mobilization (ie, discharge) is not possible.

Dr. Schwartz or an immediate family member is a member of a speakers' bureau or has made paid presentations on behalf of Synthes; serves as a paid consultant to or is an employee of OsteoCentric; and has stock or stock options held in OsteoCentric and Zimmer. Dr. Mehta or an immediate family member is a member of a speakers' bureau or has made paid presentations on behalf of Bioventus, DePuy, a Johnson & Johnson Company, and Smith & Nephew; serves as a paid consultant to or is an employee of Smith & Nephew and Synthes; has received research or institutional support from Becton-Dickinson and Synthes; and serves as a board member, owner, officer, or committee member of AO Foundation and Orthopaedic Trauma Association. Dr. Hernandez or an immediate family member serves as a board member, owner, officer, or committee member of Orthopaedic Trauma Association. Dr. Kwon or an immediate family member has received royalties from DJ Orthopaedics, Medline, Paragon 28, and Trimed and serves as a paid consultant to or is an employee of DJ Orthopaedics, Paragon 28, and Restor3D. Dr. Shafiq or an immediate family member is a member of a speakers' bureau or has made paid presentations on behalf of Smith & Nephew; serves as a paid consultant to or is an employee of Bone Foam and Synthes; has received research or institutional support from DePuy, a Johnson & Johnson Company and Synthes; and serves as a board member, owner, officer, or committee member of Orthopaedic Trauma Association. None of the following authors or any immediate family member has received anything of value from or has stock or stock options held in a commercial company or institution related directly or indirectly to the subject of this chapter: Dr. Guild, Dr. Marshall, Dr. Vilella, and Dr. Ghanem.

Pelvic fractures range in severity from low to high energy and affects young to elderly patients. Young patients usually have high-energy injuries, such as those sustained from motor vehicle or motorcycle accidents, and elderly patients, or those with osteoporosis, may sustain a pelvic fracture from a fall from standing position. In young patients these injuries can be life-threatening and require a multidisciplinary approach to treatment. Even in elderly patients, there can be excessive bleeding from a pelvic fracture due to calcified vessels and/or the patient's use of anticoagulants for other medical problems.

Epidemiology

- Incidence: Pelvic fractures represent approximately 3% of skeletal injuries.[1]
- Demographics affected: Pelvic fractures have a bimodal distribution.
  - Young patients typically sustain high-energy injuries, often with associated injuries, with unstable pelvic ring injuries.
  - Elderly patients usually sustain stable injuries from a low-energy mechanism.
- Other pertinent information: Patients who sustain high-energy injuries, such as motor vehicle or motorcycle accidents, pedestrians versus auto, or falls from a height, require a multidisciplinary team approach.
  - This often includes general surgery, orthopaedic surgery, interventional radiology, urology, and critical care.

Pertinent Anatomy/Pathoanatomy

- Soft tissue
  - Arteries are depicted in **Figure 1**.
  - Nerves are depicted in **Figure 2**.
  - Ligaments of the pelvis are depicted in **Figure 3**.
- Bones
  - The bony pelvis is composed of the sacrum, and two innominate bones, each containing the ischium, pubis, and ilium.

Chapter 3: I Fell and Cannot Get Up—Lower Extremity Trauma

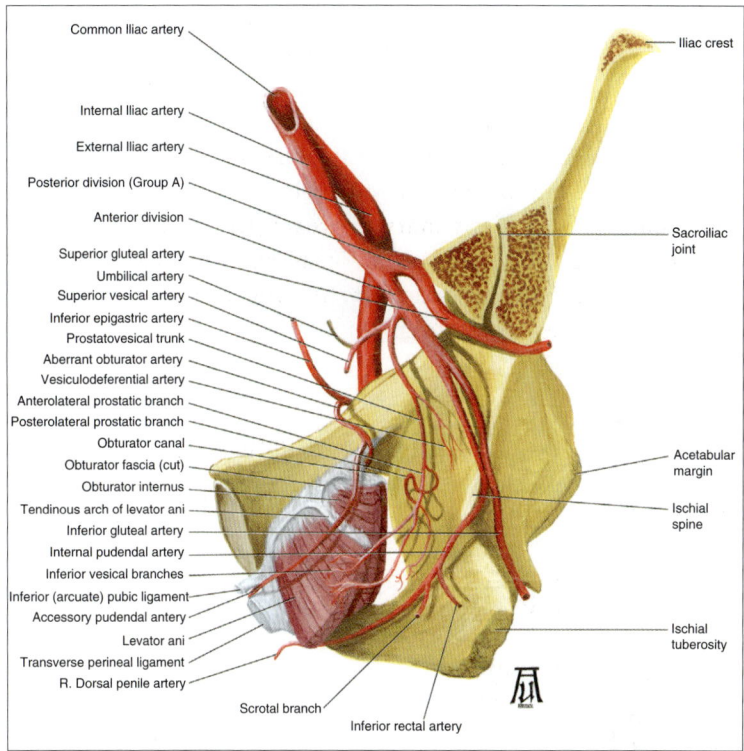

Figure 1 Schematic diagram showing four types of accessory pudendal arteries from a posterolateral view of the pelvis with angiographic views. (Reproduced with permission from Guimares M, ed: *Uflacker's Atlas of Vascular Anatomy*, ed 3. Wolters Kluwer, 2020, Figure 19.22C.)

Pertinent History/Physical Examination Findings

Inspection

- The patient requires a thorough inspection of skin and soft tissues.
  - Attention should be paid to any skin lacerations because they may represent an open fracture.
  - Any extensive ecchymoses or contusions should raise suspicion for a Morel-Lavallée lesion.
    - This is an internal degloving injury, which may be colonized with bacteria, even if it is a closed injury. **Figure 4** depicts the classic appearance of a Morel-Lavallée lesion.

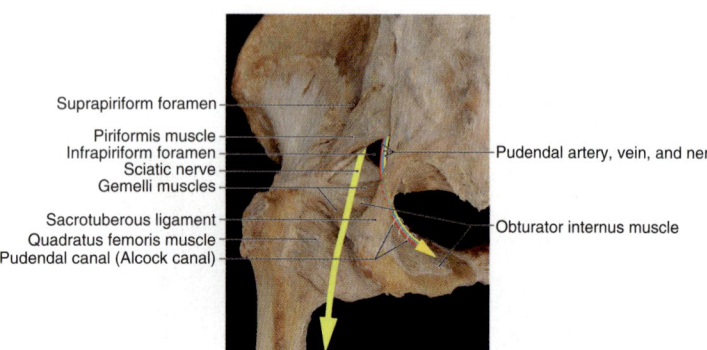

Figure 2 Photograph showing the course of the pudendal nerve, and internal pudendal artery and vein (small arrows) in the female lesser pelvis (posterior aspect). Large yellow arrow = indicated course of the sciatic nerve. (Reproduced with permission from Rohen JW, Yokochi C, Lutjen-Drecoll E, eds: *Photographic Atlas of Anatomy*, ed 9. Wolters Kluwer, 2021, Figure 7.107.)

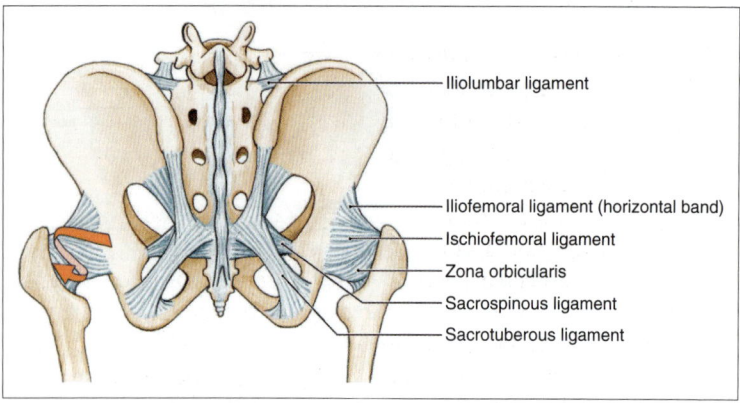

Figure 3 Schematic drawing shows the ligaments of the pelvis and hip joint (posterior aspect). (Reproduced with permission from Rohen JW, Yokochi C, Lutjen-Drecoll E, eds: *Photographic Atlas of Anatomy*, ed 9. Wolters Kluwer, 2021, Figure 4.42.)

- The perineum requires particular attention as any lacerations may also represent an open injury, with trauma to the urethra (blood at the meatus), vagina, or rectum.
- A difference in leg length (vertically unstable pelvic fracture) or difference in rotation (anterior-posterior compression or lateral compression) may be noted.

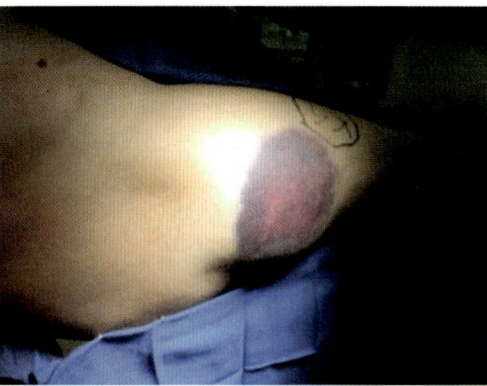

Figure 4 Photograph shows a Morel-Lavallée lesion (skin degloving injury). (Reproduced with permission from Egol KA, Koval KJ, Zuckerman J, eds: *Handbook of Fractures*, ed 6. Wolters Kluwer, 2019, Figure 26.7.)

Palpation

- The pelvis should be palpated to elicit tenderness.
- The pelvis can also be manually stressed to elicit instability.
  - This should be done by one examiner because repeated examinations may dislodge organizing hematoma, which may adversely affect control of bleeding.
  - The pelvis can be stressed using manual compression both with external rotation and internal rotation.
  - According to retrospective data, instability with compression of the pelvis has limited sensitivity for detecting a pelvic fracture (8%) including unstable pelvic fractures (26%).[2] However, when present, such instability is highly specific for both stable and unstable fractures (approximately 99% for each).

Rectal and Vaginal Examination

- Must be performed to rule out an open fracture, as well as palpate for prominent bony fragments, gross blood, and a high-riding prostate

Neurologic Examination

- This is critical for a patient with a pelvic fracture. A detailed sensory and motor examination must be performed. **Figure 5** represents the nerve distributions to the lower extremity.

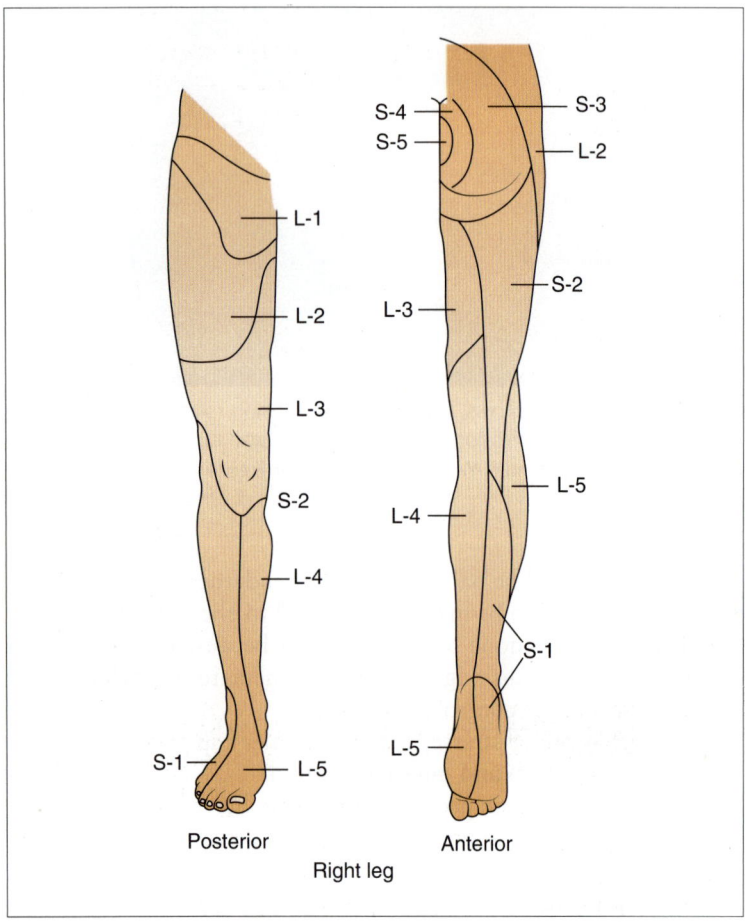

Figure 5 Schematic drawing showing the dermatomes of the leg. (Reproduced with permission from Hickey JV, Strayer AL, eds: *The Clinical Practice of Neurological and Neurological Nursing*, ed 8. Wolters Kluwer, 2019, Figure 16.7.)

Relevant Imaging

- Pertinent radiographic findings
  - Radiographs: Images for a pelvic ring fracture include AP pelvis and inlet/outlet views.

Chapter 3: I Fell and Cannot Get Up—Lower Extremity Trauma

- The AP view is obtained with the patient supine. This image is usually obtained as part of Advanced Trauma Life Support (ATLS) protocol.
  - It should be repeated off the backboard, centered at the midpoint of the pubic symphysis. **Figure 6** represents an AP radiograph of the pelvis.
- Inlet and outlet views: **Figure 7** demonstrates how these images are obtained.
- The inlet view is obtained with the patient supine and the beam is angled 25° to 40° caudad.
  - This view shows anterior/posterior translation of the hemipelvis, as well as narrowing or widening of the pelvic ring.
- The outlet view is obtained with the patient supine and the beam is angled 20° to 40° cephalad.
  - This view demonstrates vertical displacement of the hemipelvis.
- CT is the gold standard modality to assess pelvic ring injuries. CT better delineates fractures seen on plain radiographs. CT can also identify fractures not seen on plain

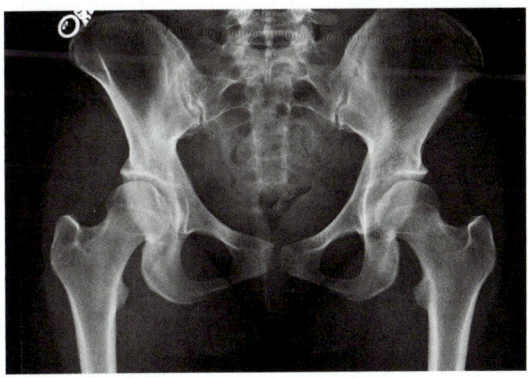

Figure 6 Routine appropriate AP pelvis radiograph. An appropriate AP pelvis radiograph is confirmed by the tip of the coccyx being centered 1 to 3 cm above the pubic symphysis. (Reproduced with permission from Johnson DH, ed: *Operative Arthroscopy*, ed 4. Wolters Kluwer, 2012, Figure 45.13.)

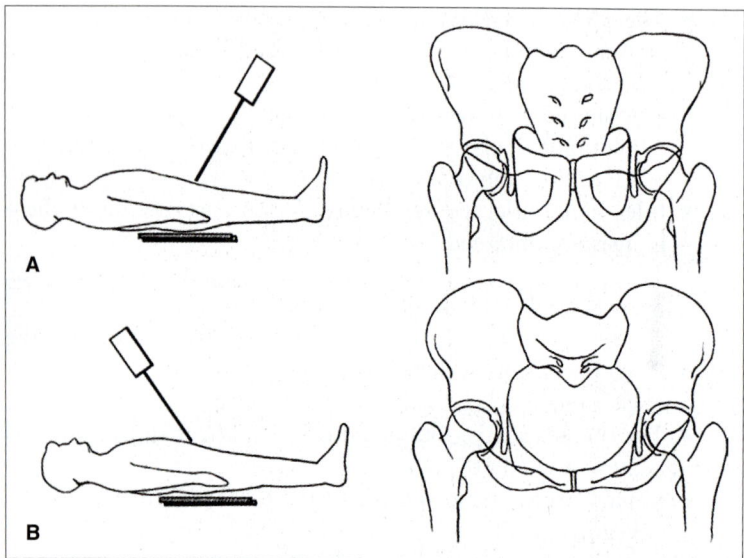

Figure 7 Schematic illustration showing the outlet and inlet views of the pelvis. The outlet view (**A**) is directed in a plane parallel to the rim of the pelvis and perpendicular to the sacrum. The obturator foramina are well visualized. Vertical malalignment is best assessed with this view. The inlet view (**B**) is directed parallel to the anterior sacral cortex and demonstrates the pelvic rim. This view is best for assessing rotational malalignment. (Reproduced with permission from Callaghan JJ, Rosenberg AG, Rubash HE, Clohisy JC, Beaule PE, Della Valle CJ, eds: *The Adult Hip*, ed 3. Wolters Kluwer, 2015, Figure 23.6.)

radiographs, such as sacral fractures. **Figure 8** shows CT images of the pelvis.

- MRI is usually not indicated except for suspected insufficiency fractures. An insufficiency fracture occurs from normal load on abnormal bone, usually osteoporotic bone. This diagnosis should be suspected in elderly patients without any trauma who complain of sacral pain or pelvic pain. Plain radiographs are often negative. If there is high suspicion for an insufficiency fracture, then MRI is indicated. **Figure 9** depicts an insufficiency fracture seen on MRI.

Chapter 3: I Fell and Cannot Get Up—Lower Extremity Trauma

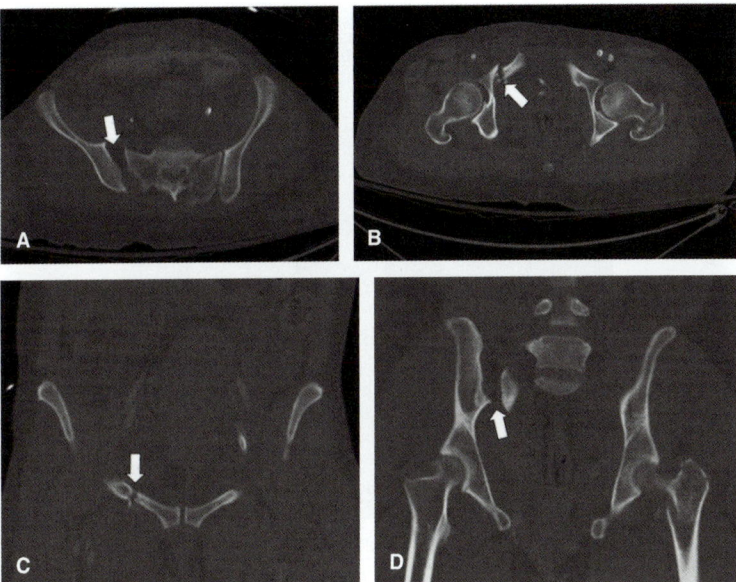

Figure 8 Vertical shear pelvic injury in a 45-year-old man. **A**, Axial CT image shows widening (arrow) of the right sacroiliac joint and a fracture through the left sacrum. **B**, Axial CT image shows a vertically oriented fracture (arrow) of the superior pubic ramus. **C**, Coronal CT image shows a vertically oriented fracture (arrow) of the superior pubic ramus. **D**, Coronal CT image shows widening and superior displacement of the right sacroiliac joint (arrow). (Reproduced with permission from Lee EY, Hunsaker A, Siewert B, eds: *Computed Body Tomography with MRI Correlation*, ed 5. Wolters Kluwer, 2019, Figure 10.68.)

Nonsurgical Measures

- Treatment depends on if the pelvic ring injury is stable or unstable.
- Stable fractures are characterized by disruption in the pelvis in one location.
- Modalities
  - The goal is to have elderly patients with stable pelvic fractures mobilize as early as possible. It is difficult for elderly patients to be non–weight bearing or partial weight bearing; therefore, if the fracture is stable, they are allowed to bear weight as tolerated.

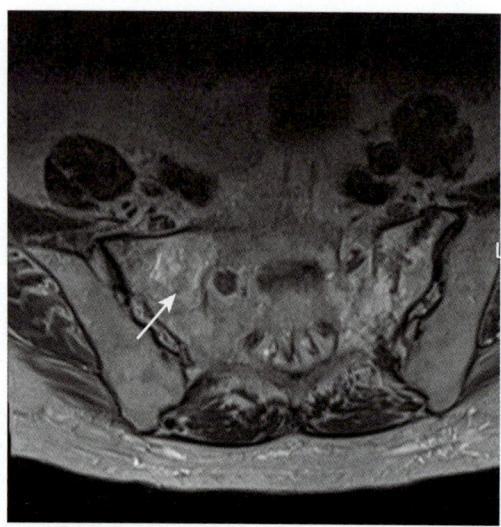

Figure 9 Axial magnetic resonance image showing unilateral sacral insufficiency fracture of the left sacral ala (arrow). Most of the patients affected with pelvic insufficiency fractures are 60 years of age or older, with female predominance.

- Young patients may also be treated nonsurgically, based on their fracture pattern. A study by Bruce et al[3] predicts the risk of displacement based on fracture pattern (**Table 1**). It was concluded that patients with incomplete sacral and ipsilateral rami fractures can be treated nonsurgically and are unlikely to experience fracture displacement. However, consideration for

TABLE 1 Rate of Displacement Based on the Pelvic Ring Fracture Components

Fracture Pattern	Rate of Displacement	Number Displaced	Number of Fractures
Complete sacral fracture + bilateral rami	68%	13	19
Complete sacral fracture + single rami or no rami	30%	6	20
Incomplete sacral fracture + bilateral rami	8%	2	23
Incomplete sacral fracture + unilateral or no rami fracture	zero	0	55

Chapter 3: I Fell and Cannot Get Up—Lower Extremity Trauma

surgical stabilization should be given for complete sacral fractures, especially those with a significant anterior injury.
- Outcomes
  - One of the most recent studies assessing nonsurgical treatment of pelvic ring fractures with less than 1 cm of displacement concluded that acceptable functional outcomes can be expected after nonsurgical management of LC1 pelvic injuries with complete sacral fracture and less than 1 cm initial displacement.[4]

Surgical Intervention

- Indications
  - Key findings on history
    - High-energy trauma in young patients raises the suspicion of an unstable pelvic ring fracture.
  - Key findings on examination
    - Any open fracture of the pelvis warrants immediate and thorough irrigation and débridement and fracture stabilization.
    - Grossly unstable pelvic ring fractures with manual stress are also unstable and are indicated for surgical treatment.
    - A gross leg length discrepancy or gross internal or external rotation of the lower extremity if not associated with a long bone fracture may represent an unstable pelvic ring fracture.
  - Key imaging findings
    - Diastasis of the pubic symphysis greater than 2.5 cm is classically associated with an unstable open-book pelvic fracture. However, the radiograph obtained at the hospital may not represent the true diastasis at the time of injury. Therefore, stress views may be indicated.
    - Other radiographic signs on plain imaging and/or CT include:
      - Sacroiliac displacement greater than 5 mm in any plane
      - A posterior fracture gap
      - Avulsion fracture of L4 or L5 transverse process
      - Avulsion fracture of the lateral border of the sacrum representing an avulsion of the sacrotuberous ligament
      - Avulsion fracture of the ischial spine representing an avulsion of the sacrospinous ligament

- Gross malalignment of the pelvis such as a windswept pelvis or vertically unstable pelvis is also an indication for surgery.
- Top three techniques
  - Indications for particular technique/fixation strategies
    - Posterior pelvic ring injuries: Most sacral fractures and sacroiliac joint injuries are managed with screw fixation.
      - There are different ways to achieve a reduction of the posterior pelvic ring injuries, including closed reduction versus open reduction.
      - Most of these injuries that require open reduction are managed in the prone position with a posterior approach.
      - If the injury can be reduced closed (or does not need a reduction maneuver), the screws can be placed with the patient in the supine or prone position.
    - Anterior pelvic ring injuries

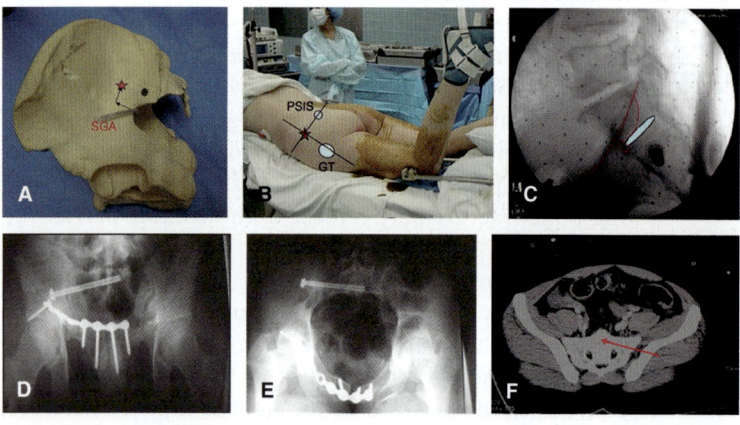

Figure 10 **A**, Photograph showing entry point for sacroiliac (SI) screw on outer table of the ilium. Note proximity to the superior gluteal neurovascular bundle. SGA, superior gluteal artery. **B**, Photograph showing superficial landmarks for percutaneous SI screw placement. PSIS, posterior superior iliac spine; GT, greater trochanter. **C**, Lateral projection of pelvis showing the very narrow safe corridor in S1 as bordered by the iliac cortical density (L5 nerve root), the upper sacral nerve root tunnel, and the vestigial disk space at S1-S2. The iliosacral screw is in S2. **D**, Outlet projection showing path of iliosacral screw for SI joint dislocation. **E**, Inlet projection showing path of iliosacral screw for SI joint dislocation. **F**, Axial CT scan showing correct trajectory through safe corridor in S1 to perform lag technique in reducing the SI joint dislocation.

Chapter 3: I Fell and Cannot Get Up—Lower Extremity Trauma

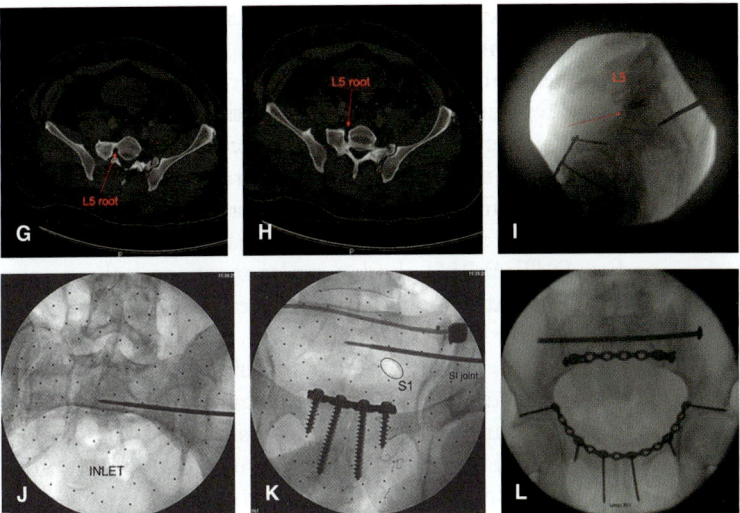

Figure 10 Cont'd **G** and **H**, Axial CT scan showing dysmorphic sacrum with compromised safe corridor. **I**, Lateral intraoperative fluoroscopic image demonstrating an S1 iliosacral screw below the two iliac cortical densities (red arrow). **J**, Intraoperative inlet projection demonstrating the correct trajectory for an iliosacral screw for a sacral fracture now perpendicular to the fracture plane, not the SI joint. **K**, Intraoperative outlet projection demonstrating the correct trajectory for an iliosacral screw for a sacral fracture now perpendicular to the fracture plane, not the sacroiliacl joint. **L**, Intraoperative fluoroscopic AP projection demonstrating the use of a transiliac plate and transsacral screw for fixation of a sacral fracture. (Reproduced with permission from Tornetta P III, ed: *Operative Techniques in Orthopaedic Trauma Surgery*, ed 3. Wolters Kluwer, 2021, Tech Figure 31.4.)

- Symphyseal diastasis is managed with a Pfannenstiel approach and anterior plate fixation.
- Superior ramus fractures that are displaced and require fixation can be managed with either plate or screw fixation. **Figure 10** represents various clinical and radiographic images of pelvic ring fixation.
- Postoperative orders
  - Weight-bearing status: Most unstable pelvic ring fractures that require surgical fixation are non–weight bearing for 6 to 12 weeks postoperatively, depending on the severity of the injury and type of fixation, as well as bone quality.

- Antibiotics: Usually standard 23-hour postoperative prophylactic antibiotics suffice.
- Venous thromboembolism (VTE) prophylaxis: A recent study by Dwyer et al[5] assessed risk of deep vein thrombosis (DVT) after pelvic fracture. Overall, 13,589 patients had a pelvic ring or acetabular fracture and surgical treatment. One hundred thirteen patients (0.83%) had a VTE within 90 days after hospital discharge: 0.51% had a DVT, 0.21% had a pulmonary embolism, and 0.12% had both. Twenty-eight percent of DVTs and 23% of pulmonary embolism occurred more than 35 days after discharge, being evenly distributed out to 90 days. Therefore, overall, DVT developed in fewer than 0.2% of patients and pulmonary embolism was diagnosed in fewer than 0.1% (<0.01% fatal) more than 35 days after the index hospitalization. The study authors concluded that a substantial proportion of VTE events occur more than 35 days after discharge; however, the overall risk is low, with fatal pulmonary embolism being extremely low (<0.01%). Given the diminished VTE risk after 35 days, the decision to further extend antithrombotic drug therapy may be guided by patient-specific factors, such as prolonged immobility.
- Suggested pain regimen: A multimodal pain approach is best to minimize narcotics. This can include acetaminophen, gabapentin, and topical patches. Anti-inflammatory medications are often contraindicated because of chemoprophylaxis for DVT prevention.
- Pearls and pitfalls
  - Potential complications
    - What to look for clinically. A careful and thorough neurologic examination is critical after pelvic fracture fixation. It is also important to monitor wound healing, in particular the open posterior approach.
    - What to look for radiographically. Some advocate for routine postoperative CT scans after pelvic fracture fixation to assess reduction as well as safe hardware placement. Routine follow-up plain radiographs are ordered for

outpatient follow-up to assess healing and guide weight-bearing status.
- Outcomes
  - Kokubo et al[6] studied type B and C pelvic ring fractures (82 patients; mean age 54 years). Age, sex, associated injuries, fracture type, Injury Severity Score rating, and treatment methods were assessed, and Majeed score for functional outcome and radiographic studies at 1 year after injury (short-term) and at final follow-up (long-term), with mean follow-up of 98 months, were analyzed. It was concluded that fracture of lower extremity, nonsurgical therapy, and nerve damage showed significant relationship with unsatisfactory short-term functional outcome. Nerve damage and the pelvic ring displacement over 20 mm were significantly associated with unsatisfactory long-term functional outcome.

Top 10 Knowledge Drops for Your Rotation

1. Young patients with pelvic ring injury are at high risk of hemodynamic instability.
2. Elderly patients may sustain pelvic fracture from low-energy injury.
3. Despite low-energy falls, elderly patients also are at risk of bleeding because of calcified vessels and preinjury use of anticoagulants.
4. A Morel-Lavallée lesion is an internal degloving injury and warrants special attention.
5. Rectal and vaginal examinations are required for pelvic ring fractures to rule out open injury.
6. Appropriate plain radiographs include an AP pelvis as well as inlet and outlet views.
7. CT is the gold standard modality for a pelvic ring injury.
8. Nonsurgical treatment is indicated for stable fractures.
9. Surgical treatment is indicated for unstable fractures.
10. DVT prophylaxis is critical because of risk of DVT and pulmonary embolism.

HIP FRACTURES

Epidemiology

- Incidence and demographics
  - According to Veronese and Maggi,[7] hip fractures are an important and debilitating condition in older people, particularly in women. The epidemiologic data vary between countries, but it is globally estimated that hip fractures will affect approximately 18% of women and 6% of men. Although the age-standardized incidence is gradually decreasing in many countries, this is far outweighed by the aging of the population. Thus, the global number of hip fractures is expected to increase from 1.26 million in 1990 to 4.5 million by the year 2050. The direct costs associated with this condition are enormous because it requires a long period of hospitalization and subsequent rehabilitation. Furthermore, hip fractures are associated with the development of other negative consequences, such as disability, depression, and cardiovascular diseases, with additional costs for society.
- Public health considerations
  - In *The Lancet Public Health*, Papadimitriou et al[8] describe the public health effect of hip fractures on disability-adjusted life years (DALYs) using data from six large cohort studies from Europe and the United States. The results showed that DALYs for hip fracture were 27 per 1,000 individuals, representing an average loss of 2% to 7% of healthy life expectancy. Notably, the effect of hip fractures on DALYs was 2 to 29 times greater than years of life lost due to premature mortality, especially at younger ages (60 to 69 years) and in women. Fear of disability and loss of independence are highly prevalent in older adults. Efforts to address the crisis in the treatment of osteoporosis should emphasize the disability associated with hip fractures and the need to prevent the first hip fracture. Identification of individuals at high risk of hip fracture, such as those with a vertebral fracture, is needed. Fear of the disability associated with hip fracture might persuade women who are more likely to experience hip fracture to seek treatment. The population attributable fraction for major risk factors contributing to the

loss of life years free of disability was calculated. Smoking accounted for 7.5% (95% CI 5.2-9.7) of the total DALYs, followed by no vigorous activity (5.5%, 95% CI 2.1-8.5) and diabetes (2.8%, 95% CI 2.1-4.0).
- Other pertinent information
  - The priority for elderly patients with hip fracture is efficient surgical treatment as soon as the patient is optimized for surgery with an implant and construct that allows for immediate weight bearing.
  - The priority for young patients with both femoral neck and intertrochanteric fractures is an anatomic reduction with appropriate fixation to avoid hardware failure and nonunion.
  - Femoral neck fractures in young patients are considered a surgical urgency.
    - These especially require critical attention to achieve an anatomic reduction and stable fixation; otherwise the fractures are at higher risk of malunion, nonunion, and osteonecrosis.

Pertinent Anatomy/Pathoanatomy

- Soft tissue
  - Nerves/arteries (**Figure 11**)
    - The main blood supply to the femoral head is the posterior femoral circumflex artery. The sciatic nerve is posterior to the hip and the femoral nerve is anterior to the hip.
  - Bony/articular
    - The proximal femur is composed of the femoral head, femoral neck, greater and lesser trochanters, and the intertrochanteric region. The femoral neck is intracapsular, whereas the base of the neck (basicervical region) and intertrochanteric region are extra-articular. The femoral head is covered by cartilage and articulates with the acetabulum.

Pertinent History/Physical Examination Findings

- For elderly patients, a thorough history must include key information.
  - It is very important to rule out syncopal fall leading to the fracture rather than a mechanical fall.

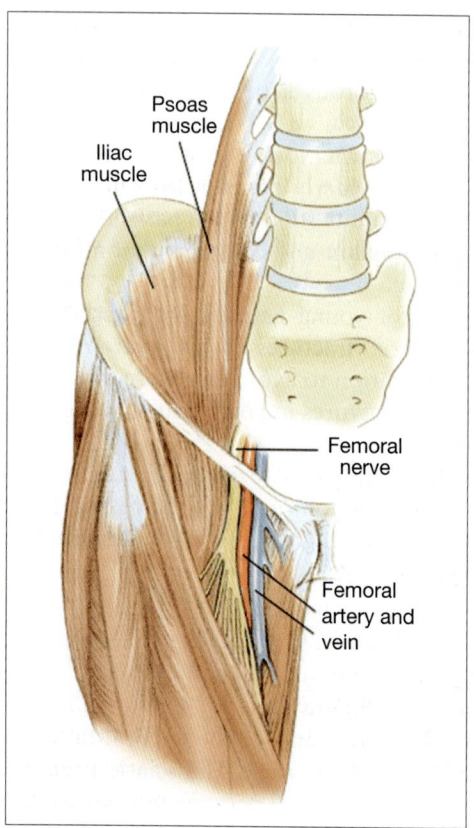

Figure 11 Illustration showing the hip flexor anatomy. The psoas arises from the lumbar spine transverse processes. At the level of the pubic ramus, as it exits the pelvis, it has an intramuscular tendon. Note the proximity of the femoral nerve and artery anteriorly. (Reproduced with permission from Wiesel SW, ed: *Operative Techniques in Orthopaedic Surgery*. Wolters Kluwer, 2010, vol 2, Section 4, Figure 40.1A.)

- Any syncopal symptoms before the fall require an appropriate medical workup before surgery because the fall may be the result of and secondary to a significant comorbidity.
- Determining the patient's function before the fall is also important because it may require a change in the type of implant or arthroplasty used.

- It is important to complete a thorough physical examination, including assessing for contractures of the hip and/or knees.
- If a patient is found with a hip fracture after a prolonged or unknown period of time, a preoperative duplex may be obtained to rule out DVT. One study showed that the incidence of DVT in patients who did not present to the hospital until more than 48 hours after hip fracture was 55%, compared with 6% in those presenting sooner than 48 hours.[9] In another study[10] of 61 consecutive patients admitted for hip fracture, 62% of those who waited to undergo surgery at least 48 hours after hospital admission had preoperative venographic evidence of DVT.

Relevant Imaging

- Pertinent radiographic findings
  - Radiographs: True AP and cross-table lateral radiographs are required for every hip fracture, as well as an AP pelvis and full-length femur radiographs.
    - If the fracture is displaced, a traction and internal rotation view can be helpful to further delineate the fracture pattern.
    - If the patient cannot tolerate traction and internal rotation, an obturator oblique view can be ordered instead.
    - **Figure 12** shows a displaced femoral neck fracture.
  - CT may help elucidate the fracture pattern if plain radiographs are insufficient. They are not routinely required for hip fractures.
  - MRI should be obtained in any patient after fall or trauma with groin pain and concern for hip fracture.
    - A missed hip fracture can lead to disastrous outcomes.
    - Another unique indication for MRI is when an isolated greater trochanter fracture is identified on plain radiographs. A total of 110 patients were identified from 7 published studies. MRI documented isolated greater trochanter fractures diagnosed on initial radiographs in only 11 of 110 patients (10%). In 99 patients (90%), MRI revealed extension of the fracture into the intertrochanteric region. Surgical fixation was necessary for 61 patients, with a pooled percentage of 55%. No complications were observed after surgery.[11]

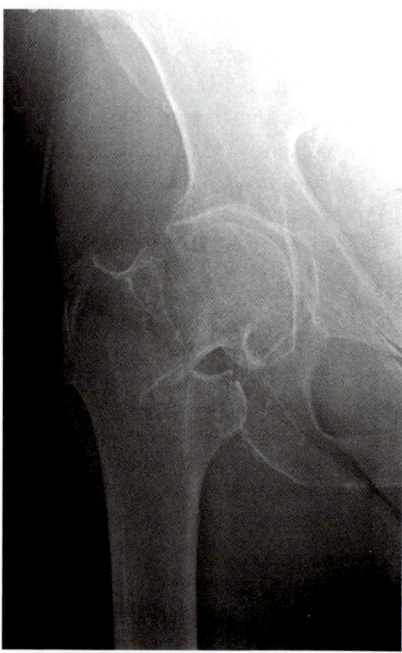

Figure 12 AP radiograph of right hip shows a femoral neck fracture. (Reproduced with permission from Farrell TA, ed: *Radiology 101: The Basics and Fundamentals of Imaging,* ed 5. Wolters Kluwer, 2019, Figure 6.71.)

Nonsurgical Measures

- Modalities
  - Nonsurgical treatment is rarely indicated for hip fractures because of high complication and mortality rates. This is only indicated when the risk of surgery outweighs the risk of nonsurgical treatment.
- Outcomes
  - Patients with hip fracture who were treated nonsurgically had a higher risk of mortality at both 1 (29.8%) and 2 years (45.6%) after fracture ($P < 0.05$). Their risk of mortality was four times higher at 1 year and three times higher at 2 years after fracture than the surgical group.[12]
  - There is also a risk of secondary displacement of nonsurgical femoral neck fractures. If a nondisplaced fracture displaces, the surgery to manage a displaced femoral neck fracture is more complex.

Chapter 3: I Fell and Cannot Get Up—Lower Extremity Trauma

- One study reviewed the records of 593 patients with femoral neck fractures from January 2000 to December 2009. Sixty-one patients (mean age 83.0 years [SD 9.9]) with nondisplaced femoral neck fractures initially received nonsurgical treatment. The occurrence and the time of secondary fracture displacement were documented, as well as demographics and radiologic parameters. Thirty-four fractures (55.7%) showed secondary displacement occurring within the first 12 weeks after initiation of nonsurgical treatment.[13]

Surgical Intervention

- Indications
  - Key findings on history: Number of falls, history of fracture, gait devices, history of hip pain, use of bisphosphonates.
  - Key findings on examination: Shortened, externally rotated limb; check for soft tissue degloving and other orthopaedic injuries.
    - In general, unless there is a medical contraindication, surgery is indicated to reduce risk of postoperative morbidity/mortality.
    - Important clinical findings on physical examination that may influence surgery are significantly contaminated open wounds near surgical sites (uncommon) or vascular injury (uncommon).
    - It is important to note any preexisting contractures before surgery because this may influence surgical approach and/or implants.
- Top three techniques
  - Applied anatomy/approaches
    - Anterior approach: Smith-Petersen approach as shown in **Figure 13**
    - Posterior approach: Kocher-Langenbeck approach as shown in **Figure 14**
    - Anterolateral approach: Watson-Jones approach
    - Lateral approach: Hardinge approach
  - Indications for femoral neck fractures
    - Femoral neck fractures: nondisplaced or valgus impacted
      - These fractures are fixed in situ with either cannulated screws, a sliding hip screw, or newer fixed-angle devices.
    - Femoral neck fractures: displaced or varus alignment

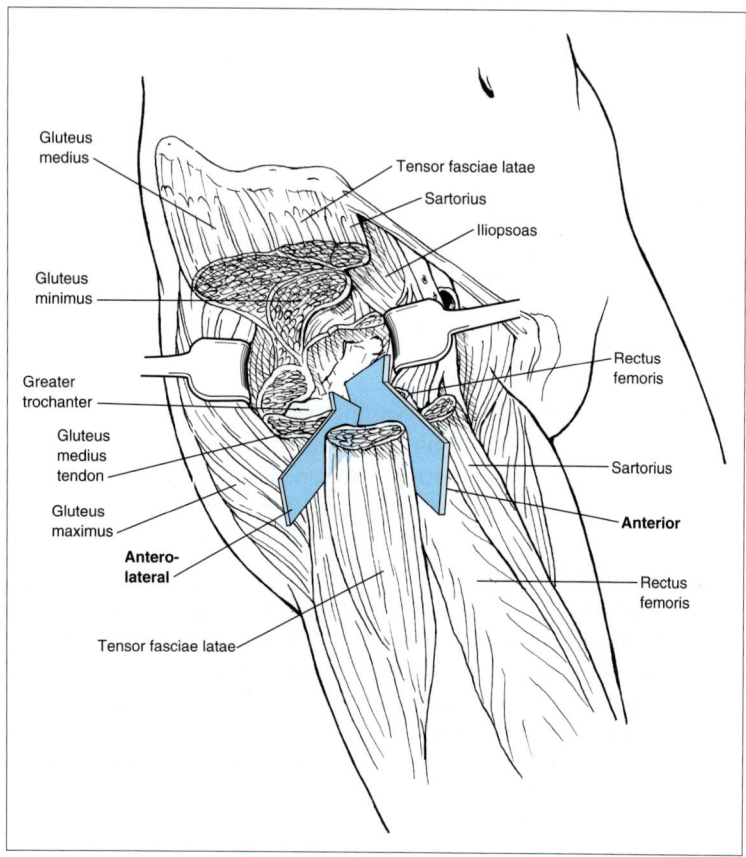

Figure 13 In this illustration, the Smith-Petersen (direct anterior) and the Watson-Jones (anterolateral) approaches to the hip take the same deep interval but pass on different sides of the tensor in their superficial dissections. The anterior approach is well suited for femoral head fractures, while the anterolateral approach is best for irreducible anterior dislocations. (Reproduced with permission from Bucholz RW, Heckman JD, eds: *Rockwood and Green's Fractures in Adults*, ed 5. Lippincott Williams & Wilkins, 2001, Figure 37.29.)

- Young patients (of note, there is no chronologic age criteria; this primarily depends on physiologic age and functional activity): These fractures require an anatomic reduction, which frequently requires an open approach,

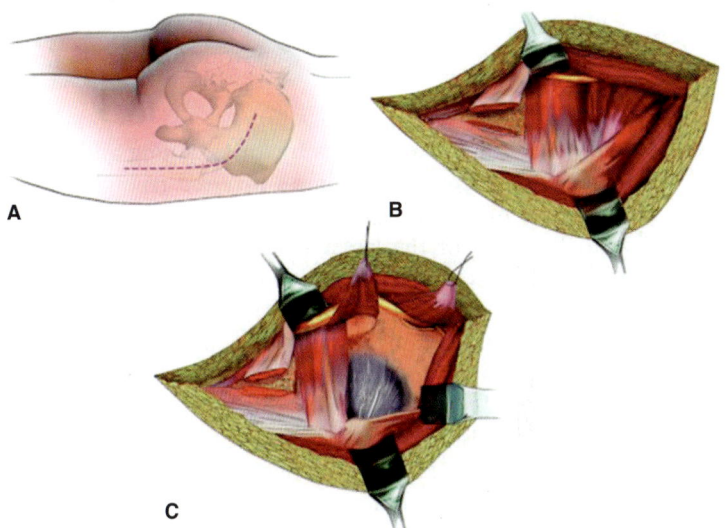

Figure 14 Illustration showing the Kocher-Langenbeck approach. **A**, The skin incision. **B**, The fascia lata and gluteus maximus have been split. The short external rotators are seen with the sciatic nerve lying on the dorsal surface of the quadratus femoris. The gluteus maximus tendon has been transected. **C**, The retroacetabular surface is exposed by transecting the tendons of the piriformis and obturator internus and reflecting them back toward the sciatic notches. (Reproduced with permission from Moed BR, Boudreau JA: Acetabulum fractures, in Tornetta P III, Ricci WM, Ostrum RF, McQueen MM, McKee MD, Court-Brown CM, eds: *Rockwood and Green's Fractures in Adults*, ed 9. Wolters Kluwer, 2019, pp 2081-2179, Figure 50.46A-C.)

usually via the Smith-Petersen approach. At times, an anatomic reduction can be achieved closed. However, the accuracy of the reduction is the most important factor in successful treatment of these fractures.
- Elderly patients
  - Hemiarthroplasty: This surgery removes the fractured femoral head and replaces the native femoral head. This is indicated for low-demand patients, those with dementia, and systemically ill patients.
  - Total hip arthroplasty: This surgery removes and replaces the femoral head as does the hemiarthroplasty, but also resurfaces the acetabulum. This is

indicated for elderly patients who are active, have preexisting arthritis, and can follow postoperative instructions.
- Fixation strategies
  - Nondisplaced, impacted valgus fractures, young and elderly patients: Cannulated screws in an inverted triangle configuration. The most inferior screw should begin at or proximal to the level of the lesser trochanter to minimize risk of iatrogenic fracture. The two superior screws are placed anterior and posterior to one another. The screws should be spread as far apart as possible, ideally within 3 mm of cortical bone when views on cross section of the femoral neck.[14] Cannulated screw fixation of a femoral neck fracture is illustrated in **Figure 15**.
  - Displaced fractures, young patients: Cannulated screws placed in the same technique as above. More vertical fractures may benefit from a sliding hip screw with or without a derotation screw. There are newer fixed angle devices; however, long-term outcomes are still unknown.
  - Displaced femoral neck fractures, elderly patients: Hemiarthroplasty or total hip arthroplasty. **Figure 16** illustrates a hemiarthroplasty of the hip.
  - **Figure 17** demonstrates a total hip arthroplasty.
- Indications for femoral neck fractures
  - Stable, standard obliquity fractures: If nondisplaced, may be treated on a flat top radiolucent table. If displaced, usually treated on a fracture table. These can be treated with either a sliding hip screw or short cephalomedullary nail.
  - Unstable fractures (lateral wall incompetent, significant posteromedial comminution, reverse obliquity, transtrochanteric, subtrochanteric extension) are best treated with a cephalomedullary nail. A short nail can be used for standard obliquity fractures with less than 3 cm distal extension from the lesser trochanter[15] and those with an incompetent lateral wall. A long nail should be used for reverse obliquity, transtrochanteric, and fractures with greater than 3 cm subtrochanteric extension.
  - The classification of intertrochanteric fractures is shown in **Figure 18**.

Chapter 3: I Fell and Cannot Get Up—Lower Extremity Trauma

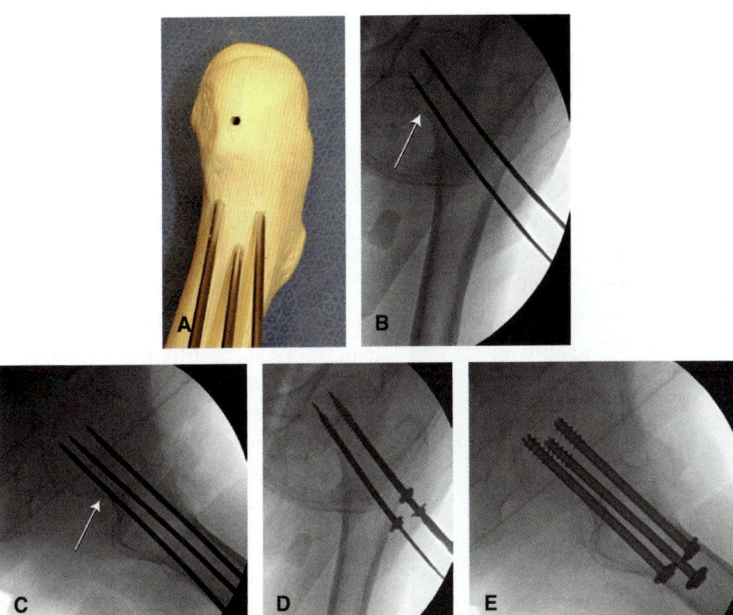

Figure 15 **A**, Sawbones lateral view of the proximal femur showing configuration for three parallel guidewires before placement of cannulated screws. The wire starting points form an inverted triangle. **B**, Intraoperative AP fluoroscopic view showing position and depth of the guidewires. The inferior wire runs right along the inferior cortex of the femoral neck—the calcar (arrow). **C**, Intraoperative lateral fluoroscopic view showing guidewire position. The posterior wire is directly adjacent to and supported by the posterior cortex of the neck (arrow). Care is necessary to ensure that the guidewire does not go outside of the neck and then reenter the femoral head. **D** and **E**, Intraoperative fluoroscopic views demonstrating cannulated screw insertion over guidewires. **D**, AP view showing use of washers in this metaphyseal location. **E**, Lateral view showing parallel insertion and appropriate depth. (Reproduced with permission from Wiesel SW, Albert T, eds: *Operative Techniques in Orthopaedic Surgery*, ed 3. Wolters Kluwer, 2021, Part 2, Tech Figure 6.1.)

- Postoperative orders
  - Weight-bearing status: All postoperative hip fractures except displaced femoral neck fractures in young patients should be allowed to bear weight as tolerated. Displaced femoral neck fractures in young patients require 6 to 12 weeks of

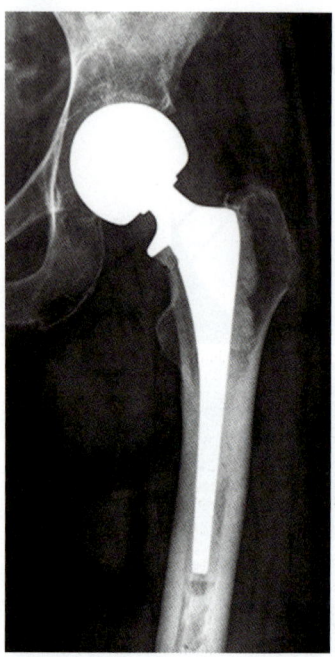

Figure 16 Hemiarthroplasty of the hip joint. AP radiograph of the left hip of a 61-year-old woman, in whom advanced osteonecrosis of the femoral head was diagnosed, following hemiarthroplasty using a bipolar-type prosthesis. The cemented stem of the prosthesis is in neutral position within the femoral shaft. (Reproduced with permission from Greenspan A, Gershwin ME, eds: *Imaging in Rheumatology: A Clinical Approach*. Wolters Kluwer, 2017, Figure 4.2.)

non–weight bearing depending on fracture pattern and type. Patients who undergo arthroplasty via a posterior approach may require 6 weeks of posterior hip precautions, whereas those who undergo an anterior approach may require 6 weeks of anterior hip precautions.

- Antibiotics: Typically, 23 hours of postoperative first-generation cephalosporin, except for those patients with an allergy.
- VTE prophylaxis: This is controversial and ranges from compressive devices to aspirin to low-molecular-weight heparin, or other anticoagulants if the patient has other high-risk comorbidities.
- Suggested pain regimen: A multimodal pain approach is best to minimize narcotics use. This is especially true in elderly patients to minimize the risk of delirium. This can include acetaminophen, gabapentin, and topical patches. Anti-inflammatory medications are often contraindicated because of chemoprophylaxis for DVT prevention.

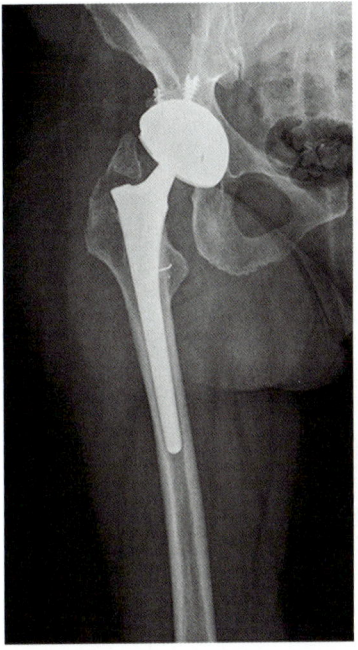

Figure 17 Radiograph of hip after revision total hip arthroplasty. The cup has been revised because careful intraoperative testing revealed loosening, despite radiographs that suggested the cup was well fixed. (Reproduced with permission from Berry DJ, Trousdale RT, Dennis DA, Paprosky WG, eds: *Revision Total Hip and Knee Arthroplasty*. Wolters Kluwer, 2012, Figure 7.9B.)

- Pearls and pitfalls
  - Potential complications
    - What to look for clinically: Postoperatively, the patient should be monitored for appropriate wound healing and to ensure there is no excessive oozing from the wound or into the thigh. The patient should be assessed for blood clots, as well as pressure sores.
    - What to look for radiographically: Follow-up radiographs approximately 6 weeks after surgery should ensure there is no hardware failure and fracture healing, or malposition of the arthroplasty.
- Outcomes
  - A critical review of cohort studies of hip fracture patients reporting outcomes of mobility, participation in domestic and community activities, health or quality of life at 3 months postfracture or longer was conducted by Dyer et al.[16] Thirty-eight studies from 42 publications were

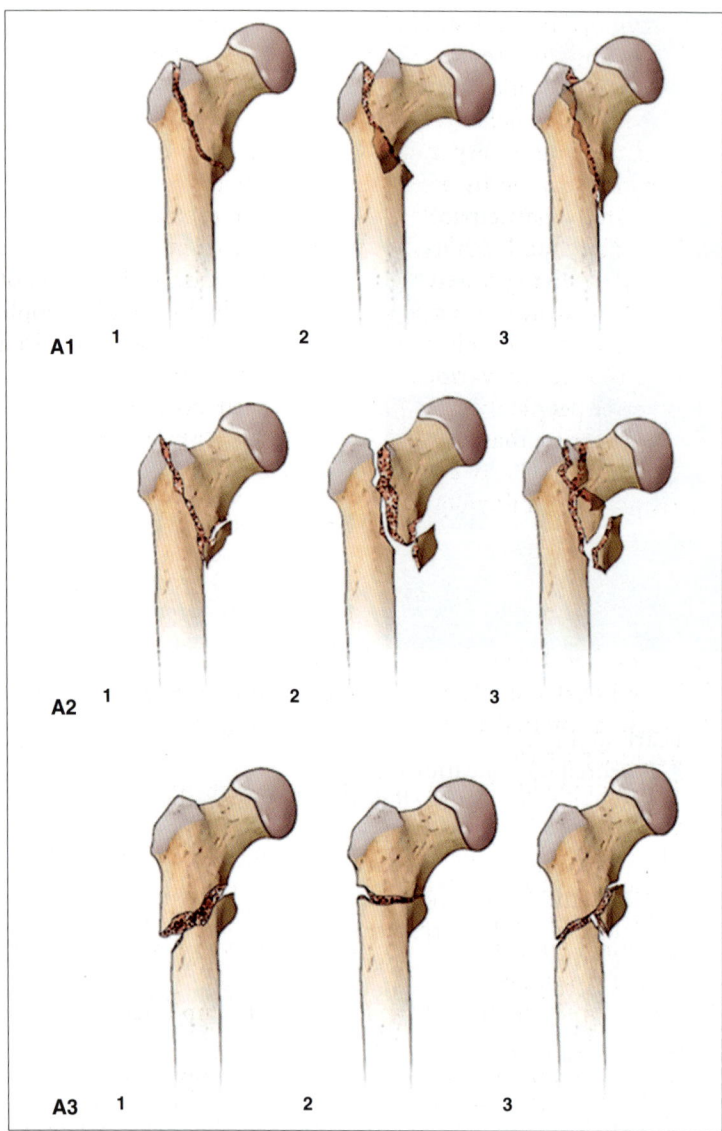

Figure 18 Illustration shows the AO/OTA classification of intertrochanteric hip fractures. (Reproduced with permission from Gardner MJ, ed: *Master Techniques in Orthopaedic Surgery: Fractures*, ed 4. Wolters Kluwer, 2021, Figure 18.1.)

included for review. Hip fracture survivors experienced significantly worse mobility, independence in function, health, quality of life, and higher rates of institutionalization than age-matched control patients. The bulk of recovery of walking ability and activities for daily living occurred within 6 months after fracture. Between 40% and 60% of study participants recovered their prefracture level of mobility and ability to perform instrumental activities of daily living, whereas 40% to 70% regained their level of independence for basic activities of daily living. For people independent in self-care prefracture, 20% to 60% required assistance for various tasks 1 and 2 years after fracture. Fewer people living in residential care recovered their level of function than those living in the community. In Western nations, 10% to 20% of hip fracture patients are institutionalized following fracture.

Top 10 Knowledge Drops for Your Rotation

1. Femoral neck fractures are intracapsular.
2. Basicervical and intertrochanteric fractures are extracapsular.
3. Traction internal rotation view may help better characterize fracture pattern.
4. The goal in elderly patients is to operate as soon as medically stable and use fixation to allow immediate weight bearing.
5. The goal in young patients is anatomic reduction of the femoral neck with stable fixation.
6. MRI should be performed if there is high suspicion for hip fracture despite negative radiographs as well as for all isolated greater trochanter fractures.
7. Delayed presentation to the hospital after hip fracture is associated with a high rate of DVT.
8. Almost all hip fractures are managed surgically because of high morbidity and mortality associated with nonsurgical treatment.
9. Stable intertrochanteric fractures may be managed with a sliding hip screw device.
10. Unstable intertrochanteric fractures require management with a cephalomedullary nail.

TIBIAL PLATEAU FRACTURES

Tibial plateau fractures range in severity from low to high energy and affect both young and elderly patients. Young patients usually have high-energy injuries, such as those sustained from motor vehicle or motorcycle accidents. Elderly patients or those with osteoporosis sustain lower energy injuries, though complex patterns may be present. Goals of care include stabilization with restoration of alignment and early range of motion.

Epidemiology

- Incidence: represent approximately 1% of skeletal injuries[17]
- Demographics affected: have a bimodal distribution
  - Young patients typically sustain high-energy injuries, often with associated soft-tissue injuries.
  - Elderly patients usually sustain a crush injury with low-energy mechanism.
- Other pertinent information: Patients who sustain high-energy injuries during motor vehicle or motorcycle accidents, pedestrians versus auto accidents, or falls from a height are at risk for compartment syndrome. The risk of soft-tissue injury to the structures around the knee can range from 10% to 45%.[18]

Pertinent Anatomy/Pathoanatomy

- Soft-tissue anatomy, including arteries, ligaments, and nerves, is shown in **Figure 19**.
- Bones
  - The tibial plateau is the upper third of the tibia and articulates with the femur and the patella. Its primary function is flexion and extension and, in conjunction with the soft-tissue structures of the knee, it also contributes to rotation and varus/valgus motion.

Pertinent History/Physical Examination Findings

Inspection

- The patient requires a thorough inspection of skin and soft tissues.
  - Attention should be paid to any skin lacerations because they may represent an open fracture.

Chapter 3: I Fell and Cannot Get Up—Lower Extremity Trauma

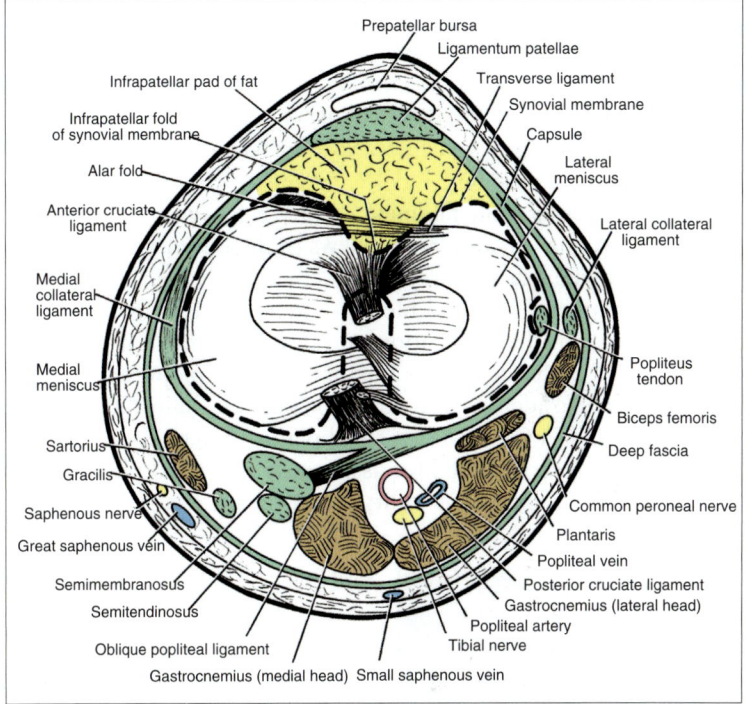

Figure 19 Schematic drawing shows the relations of the right knee joint. (Reproduced with permission from Snell RS, ed: *Clinical Anatomy*, ed 7. Lippincott Williams & Wilkins, 2003, Figure 10.57.)

- There can be a large effusion in the knee consistent with a hemarthrosis from bleeding from the intra-articular fractures.
- Alignment of the limb should be assessed.

Palpation

- A thorough examination of the structures around the knee is critical.
- Stability of the knee will be difficult to assess because of motion through the fracture.
- The compartments of the limb should be assessed with manual palpation, and if necessary, compartment pressure monitoring should be performed.

Neurologic Examination

- This is critical for a patient with a tibial plateau fracture. A detailed sensory and motor examination must be performed with specific emphasis on the peroneal nerve.

Relevant Imaging

- Pertinent radiographic findings
  - Radiographs: AP and lateral views of the knee and the tibia of the involved side (**Figure 20**).
  - CT is the gold standard modality to assess tibial plateau fractures to aid in classification and development of a treatment plan. CT better delineates fractures seen on plain radiographs. CT can also identify fractures not seen on plain radiographs. **Figure 21** is a CT scan of a tibial plateau fracture.
  - MRI can be considered for assessment of a tibial plateau fracture where a soft-tissue injury about the knee is suspected.

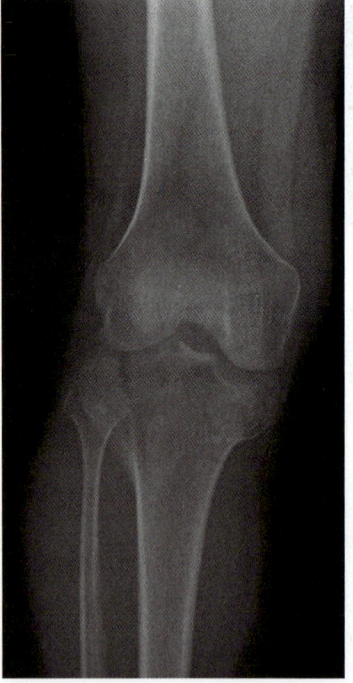

Figure 20 Schatzker type V fracture of the medial and lateral tibial plateau evident on an AP radiograph. (Reproduced with permission from Maniar H, Kubiak EN, Horwitz DS: Tibial plateau fractures, in Tornetta P III, Ricci WM, Ostrum RF, McQueen MM, McKee MD, Court-Brown CM, eds: *Rockwood and Green's Fractures in Adults*, ed 9. Wolters Kluwer, 2019, pp 2623-2685, Figure 61.16.)

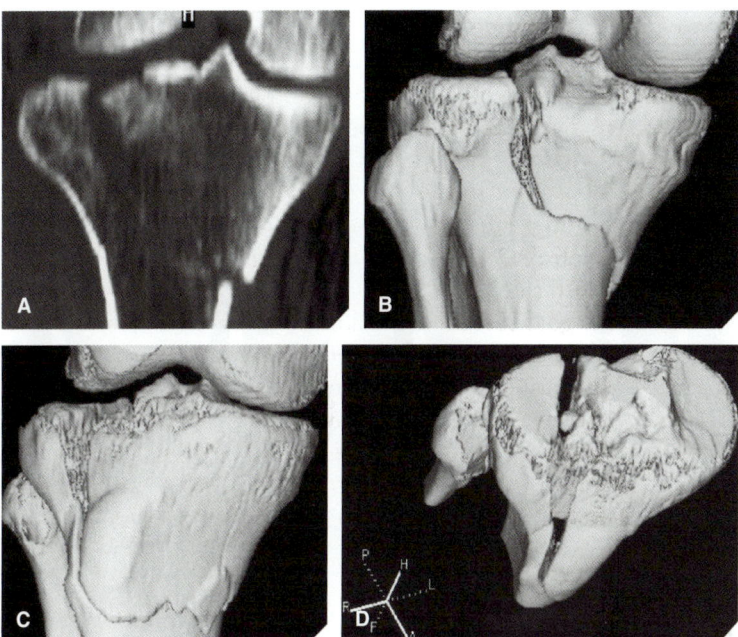

Figure 21 CT and three-dimensional (3D) CT of fracture of the tibial plateau. A 22-year-old man fell down from a tall ladder and injured his right knee. The conventional radiographs demonstrated fracture of the tibial plateau. **A**, Coronal reformatted CT scan shows extension of the lateral tibial plateau fracture into the tibial shaft. **B**, Posterior view of the 3D CT reconstruction shows the fracture line, but the interfragmental split is not well demonstrated. **C**, Anterior view of the 3D reconstruction shows the split better. **D**, Bird's eye view of the 3D CT scan effectively demonstrates the details of the split and comminution of the tibial plateau. (Reproduced with permission from Greenspan A, Beltrain J, eds: *Orthopaedic Imaging: A Practical Approach*, ed 7. Wolters Kluwer, 2020, Figure 9.27.)

- The classification of tibial plateau fractures based on CT and radiographic findings is critical to decision making regarding treatment.[19] The Schatzker classification is commonly used to describe these fractures (**Figure 22**).
  - Type I: lateral plateau split fracture
  - Type II: lateral plateau split-depression fracture

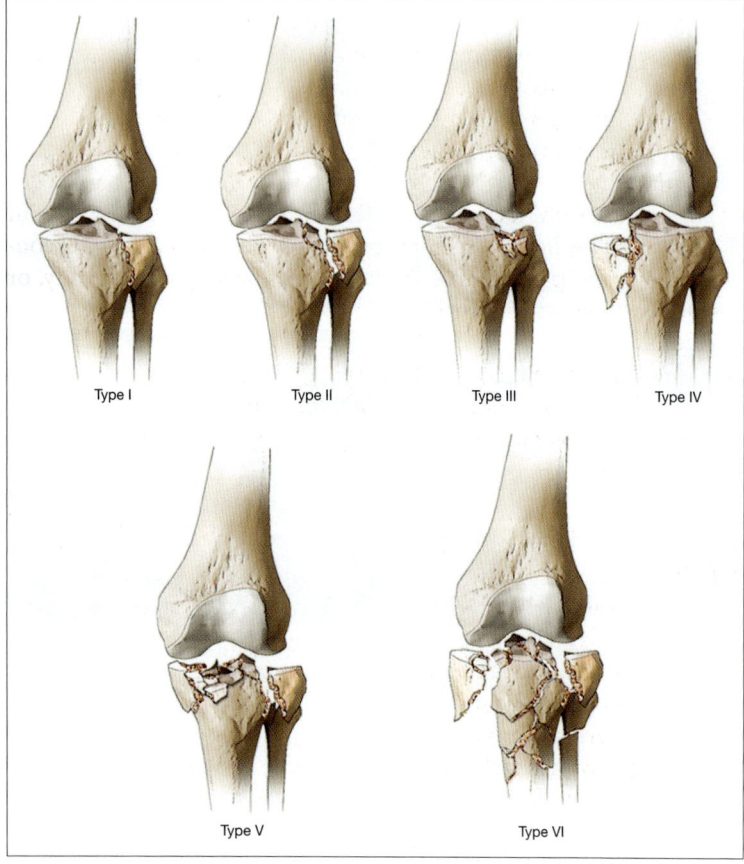

Figure 22 Illustration shows the Schatzker classification of tibial plateau fractures. Type I: lateral plateau split fracture. Type II: lateral plateau split-depression fracture. Type III: lateral plateau depression fracture. Type IV: medial plateau fracture (split or depressed). Type V: bicondylar tibial plateau fracture. Type VI: metaphyseal-diaphyseal disassociation. (Reproduced with permission from Gardner MJ, ed: *Master Techniques in Orthopaedic Surgery: Fractures*, ed 4. Wolters Kluwer, 2020, Figure 26.1.)

- Type III: lateral plateau depression fracture
- Type IV: medial plateau fracture
- Type V: bicondylar tibial plateau fracture
- Type VI: metaphyseal-diaphyseal disassociation

Nonsurgical Measures

- Nonsurgical management includes a period of non–weight bearing for 4 to 6 weeks followed by a graduated increase in weight bearing, a hinged knee brace to allow for protected range of motion, and interval radiographs to monitor healing and alignment.
- There are several factors that affect the decision to treat a patient nonsurgically, including an articular step-off less than 3 mm, condylar widening less than 5 mm, no varus or valgus instability, or severe degenerative arthritis.
- Outcomes
  - Nonsurgical management of tibial plateau fractures with no malalignment, stable ligaments, and no significant articular depression is acceptable as long as early range of motion can be performed.

Surgical Intervention

- Indications
  - Key parameters
    - Articular step-off greater than 3 mm
    - Condylar widening greater than 5 mm
    - Varus or valgus instability
    - Medial tibial plateau fractures
    - Bicondylar tibial plateau fractures
- Top three techniques
  - Acute management
    - Initial treatment in patients with high-energy fractures, fractures with instability, or fractures with soft-tissue compromise is a knee-spanning external fixator (**Figure 23**).
    - The external fixator allows for restoration of length, alignment, and rotation through ligamentotaxis.
  - Definitive management
    - Open reduction and internal fixation (ORIF) with the use of periarticular plates and screws.
      - For lateral tibial plateau fractures, a lateral-based buttress plate is applied through an anterolateral incision.
      - For medial tibial plateau fractures, a medial or posteromedial plate is applied through a medial exposure.

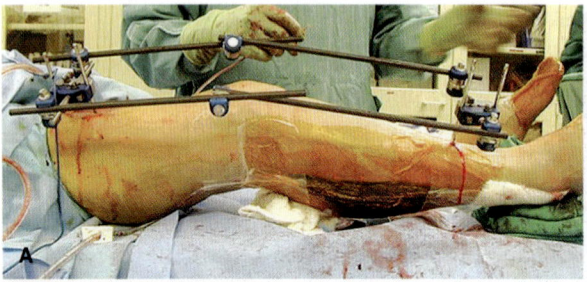 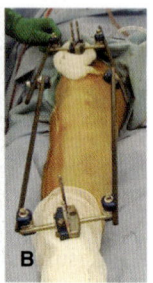

Figure 23 Intraoperative photographs of the lower extremity demonstrate a knee-spanning external fixation frame used to stabilize a bicondylar tibial plateau fracture with associated lower leg compartment syndrome in profile (**A**) and en face (**B**). (Reproduced from Tejwani N, Polonet D, Wolinsky PR: External fixation of tibial fractures. *J Am Acad Orthop Surg* 2015;23[2]:126-130.)

- For bicondylar fractures, the medial and lateral sides are plated through dual incisions (**Figure 24**).
- External fixation/ring fixation with minimally invasive restoration of the articular surface
  - Hybrid fixation uses principles of thin wire fixation in combination with traditional external fixation half-pins.
  - This technique is soft-tissue friendly and may be useful in patients with severe open fractures, poor soft-tissue envelope, or concern for infection.
- Postoperative orders
  - Weight-bearing status: Most patients who require surgical fixation are non–weight bearing for 8 to 12 weeks postoperatively, depending on the severity of the injury and type of fixation as well as bone quality.
  - Antibiotics: Usually standard 23-hour postoperative prophylactic antibiotics suffice.
  - VTE prophylaxis: The risk of a DVT in a low-energy tibial plateau fracture with early range of motion is low and chemoprophylaxis with aspirin is often sufficient. For patients with high-energy injuries or multiple trauma or prolonged immobilization, consideration for higher order therapy such as low-molecular-weight heparin may be indicated.
  - Suggested pain management regimen: A multimodal approach is best to minimize narcotics use. This can include

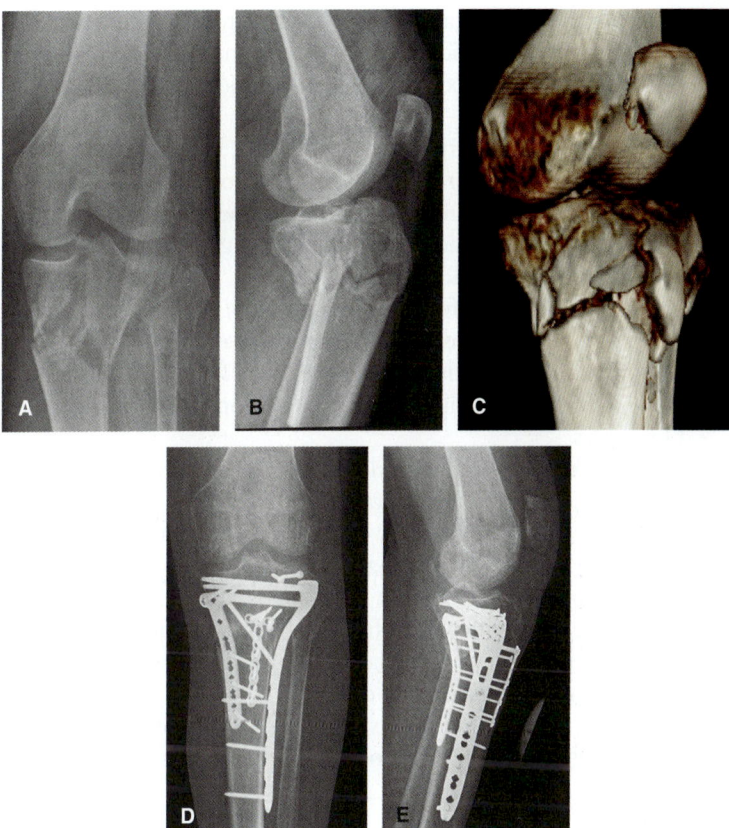

Figure 24 Images show a bicondylar tibial plateau fracture in a 66-year-old man who was injured after being struck by a car. AP (**A**) and lateral (**B**) radiographs showing a complex bicondylar fracture with tubercle involvement. **C**, Three-dimensional CT reconstruction showing comminution about the tibial tubercle, which can preclude the use of screw fixation alone. One-year follow-up AP (**D**) and lateral (**E**) radiographs showing tension band minifragment fixation of the comminuted tubercle after open reduction and internal fixation of the fracture. (Reproduced from Achor TS, Taylor RM: Tibial plateau and shaft fractures, in Grauer JN, ed: *Orthopaedic Knowledge Update® 12*. American Academy of Orthopaedic Surgeons, 2017, p 499, Figure 3.)

acetaminophen, gabapentin, and topical patches. Anti-inflammatory medications are often contraindicated because of chemoprophylaxis for DVT prevention.
- Pearls and pitfalls
  - Potential complications
    - What to look for clinically: It is important to monitor for compartment syndrome in the preoperative and perioperative period in the management of high-energy bicondylar tibial plateau fractures.[20]
    - What to look for radiographically: Intraoperative and postoperative radiographs should be monitored for loss of alignment, especially in osteoporotic fractures or bicondylar fractures in the absence of fixation of the medial side.
- Outcomes
  - The strongest predictor of long-term outcomes after tibial plateau fractures is restoration of alignment with joint stability. Although articular reduction and congruity matter, stability and alignment have been shown to have a greater effect on the development of posttraumatic arthritis.[21]
  - Postoperative infection after ORIF is associated with high-energy injuries (bicondylar fractures), long surgical times, smoking, and pulmonary disease.
  - Patients with ligamentous instability, loss of meniscus, or change in mechanical axis of greater than 5° have worse results.

Top 10 Knowledge Drops for Your Rotation

1. CT is required for classification and surgical planning.
2. Temporizing external fixation is necessary for high-energy tibial plateau fractures.
3. Definitive fixation is most commonly performed through ORIF.
4. High-energy tibial plateau fractures must be monitored for compartment syndrome.
5. The Schatzker classification is one of the most common systems used to describe tibial plateau fractures.
6. Restoration of joint stability and alignment is the most critical factor affecting outcome.
7. Nonsurgical treatment is indicated for fractures with limited joint involvement, stability, and good alignment.

8. Immediate range of motion can be performed after stable fixation of tibial plateau fractures.
9. Patients with articular injuries should remain non–weight bearing for 8 to 12 weeks after fixation.
10. Soft-tissue injuries (meniscus tears, ligament tears) are common in conjunction with tibial plateau fractures.

TIBIAL SHAFT FRACTURES

Tibial shaft injuries are common long bone injuries that are frequently open. They can occur from both higher and lower injury mechanisms although trauma from vehicles is most common.

Epidemiology

- Incidence and demographics
  - Most common long bone fractures; make up approximately 20% of all lower extremity fractures
  - Bimodal distribution, with younger patients often sustaining tibial fractures through high-energy mechanisms and older patients via falls
- Other pertinent information
  - Compartment syndrome is a common complication, occurring in approximately 10% of fractures
    - Compartment syndrome can be diagnosed clinically by using the 5 P's
      - Pain out of proportion to examination (during passive stretching)
      - Pallor (lack of color)
      - Paresthesias
      - Paresis
      - Pulselessness
  - Alternatively, compartment pressures can be quantified and calculated using a compartment pressure monitoring device. If the difference between the diastolic pressure and the intracompartmental pressure is less than 30 (delta P), a fasciotomy is indicated.
  - Open fractures of the tibia are the most common open long bone fractures, with an annual incidence of 3.4 per 100,000.

Pertinent Anatomy/Pathoanatomy

- There are four compartments that make up the tibia. The compartments of the tibia contain arteries, nerves, and muscle. The anatomy of the compartments puts them at risk for compartment syndrome in the setting of trauma to the tibia. Understanding the anatomy of the compartments is critical in assessment of injuries to the tibia or an evolving compartment syndrome (**Figure 25**).

Pertinent History/Physical Examination Findings

- Patients with tibial fractures will typically present immediately after an acute trauma. Determining the mechanism of injury can provide insight in terms of the energy of the injury and also the type of fracture that may be present.
  - Torsional or rotational injuries are typically low energy and result in spiral fractures of the distal tibia (**Figure 26**) and usually an associated fibular fracture.
  - High-energy injuries are associated with comminuted or segmental tibial shaft fractures. This mechanism can result in soft-tissue compromise or open fractures (**Figure 26**).
- Patients will note severe leg pain and an inability to bear weight.
- Physical examination
  - There may be an obvious deformity of the limb with respect to angulation or rotation.
  - The limb should be examined for open wounds, soft-tissue defects, and impending open wounds with threatened skin.
    - The classification system for closed injuries is presented in **Table 2**.
    - The classification for open fractures is presented in **Table 3**. Segmental fractures, barnyard injuries, or grossly contaminated open wounds with bone loss are classified as type III despite the size of the wound.
  - Manual compression can be performed to assess for compartment syndrome, but this method is not reliable. If compartment syndrome is suspected, formal measurement of compartment pressures should be performed.[22]
  - A thorough neurovascular examination should be performed including the deep peroneal nerve, superficial peroneal nerve, sural nerve, tibial nerve, and the saphenous nerve, in addition to dorsalis pedis and posterior tibial pulses.

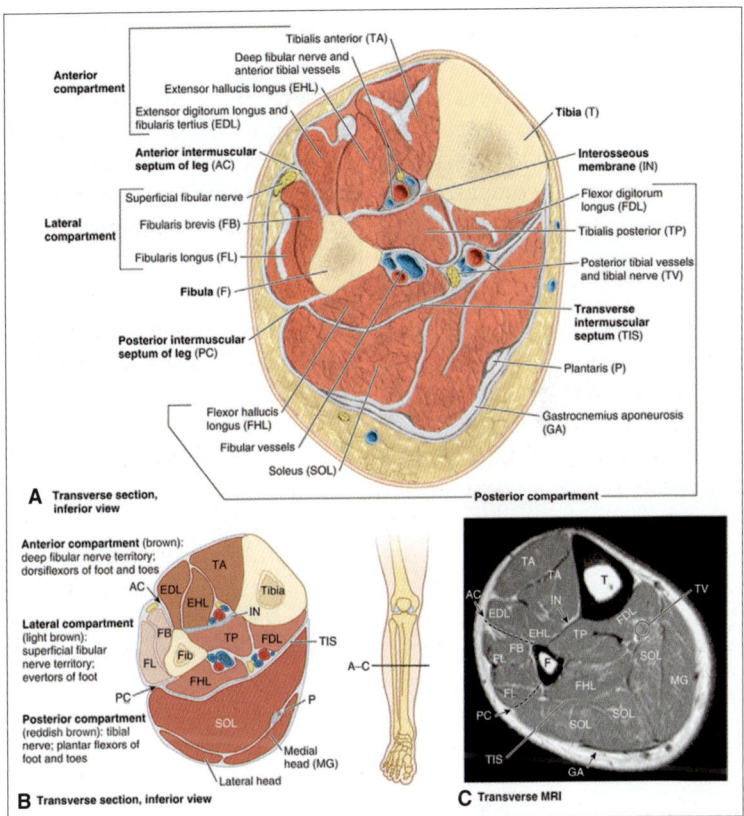

Figure 25 Compartments of leg at midcalf level in transverse anatomic section. **A**, Illustration shows that the anterior (dorsiflexor or extensor) compartment contains four muscles (the fibularis tertius lies inferior to the level of this section). The lateral (fibular) compartment contains two evertor muscles. The posterior (plantarflexor or flexor) compartment, containing seven muscles, is subdivided by an intracompartmental transverse intermuscular septum into a superficial group of three (two of which are commonly tendinous/aponeurotic at this level) and a deep group of four. The popliteus (part of the deep group) lies superior to the level of this section. **B**, Illustration shows the overview of compartments of leg. **C**, Magnetic resonance image of the leg. Abbreviations are defined in the labels for panels A and B. (Panels A and B reproduced with permission from Dalley AF, Agur AMR, eds: *Moore's Clinically Oriented Anatomy*, ed 9. Wolters Kluwer, 2022, Figure 5.56. Panel C reproduced with permission from *The Visible Human Project*. National Library of Medicine; Visible Man 2551.)

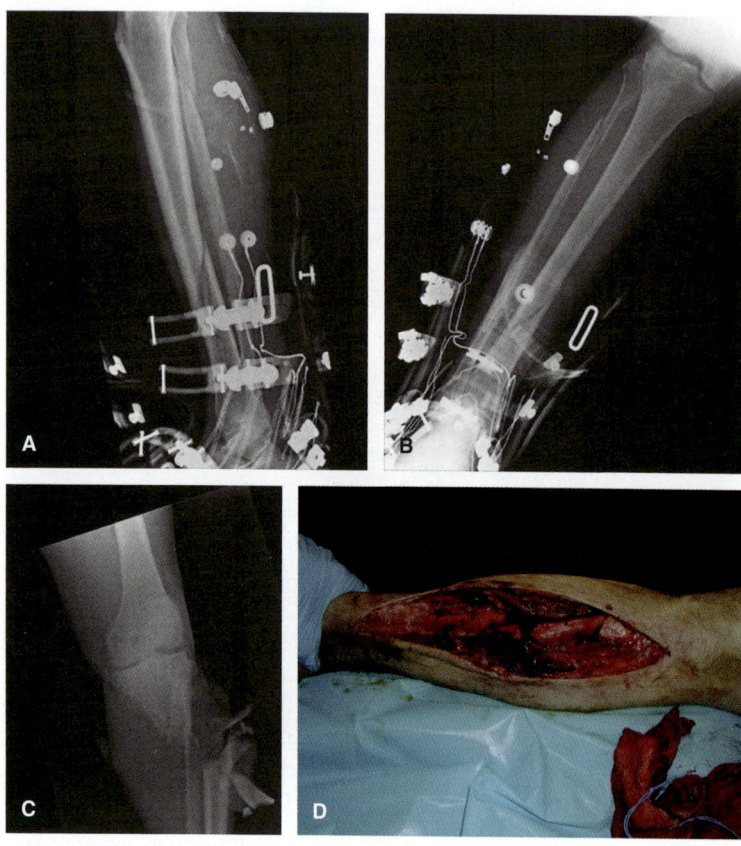

Figure 26 **A**, AP and **B**, lateral radiographs of the tibia revealing a distal third tibia fracture spiraling into the articular surface of tibia from a torsional injury during skiing. **C**, AP radiograph of an open IIIB tibial shaft fracture resulting from a high-energy crush injury. **D**, Photograph showing type IIIB open wound in a tibial shaft fracture. The wound will require flap coverage. (Courtesy of Samir Mehta, MD, FAAOS, Penn Medicine, Philadelphia, Pennsylvania.)

Relevant Imaging

- Full-length AP and lateral radiographs of the tibia should be obtained along with views of the ipsilateral ankle and knee.
- CT of the tibia is indicated if there is concern about proximal or distal extension. Approximately 40% of distal third spiral fractures exit into the articular surface of the distal tibia[23] (**Figure 27**).

TABLE 2 Tscherne Classification of Closed Fracture Soft-Tissue Injury

Grade 0	Injuries from indirect forces with negligible soft-tissue damage
Grade I	Superficial contusion/abrasion, simple fractures
Grade II	Deep abrasions, muscle/skin contusion, direct trauma, impending compartment syndrome
Grade III	Excessive skin contusion, crushed skin or destruction of muscle, subcutaneous degloving, acute compartment syndrome, and rupture of major blood vessel or nerve

TABLE 3 Gustilo-Anderson Classification of Open Tibial Fractures

Type I	Limited periosteal stripping, clean wound <1 cm
Type II	Minimal periosteal stripping, wound >1 cm but <10 cm in length without extensive soft-tissue injury damage
Type IIIA	Significant soft-tissue injury (often evidenced by a segmental fracture or comminution), significant periosteal stripping, wound usually >10 cm in length, no flap required.
Type IIIB	Significant periosteal stripping and soft-tissue injury, flap required due to inadequate soft-tissue coverage (skin graft does not count).
Type IIIC	Significant soft-tissue injury (often evidenced by a segmental fracture or comminution), vascular injury requiring repair to maintain limb viability
	For prognostic reasons, severely comminuted, contaminated barnyard injuries, close-range shotgun/high-velocity gunshot injuries, and open fractures presenting over 24 hours from injury have all been included in the grade III group.

Nonsurgical Measures

- Acute management of tibia fracture includes a thorough assessment of the involved limb and also examination for associated injuries.
  - A reduction of the tibia should be performed to restore length, alignment, and rotation.
  - A posterior splint that can be supplemented with a "U" splint along with a knee immobilizer should be applied.
  - Compartments should be assessed frequently.
  - Neurovascular assessment should be performed postreduction.
  - Open fractures
    - Require immediate antibiotics[24]
      - Cephalosporin given for all open fractures

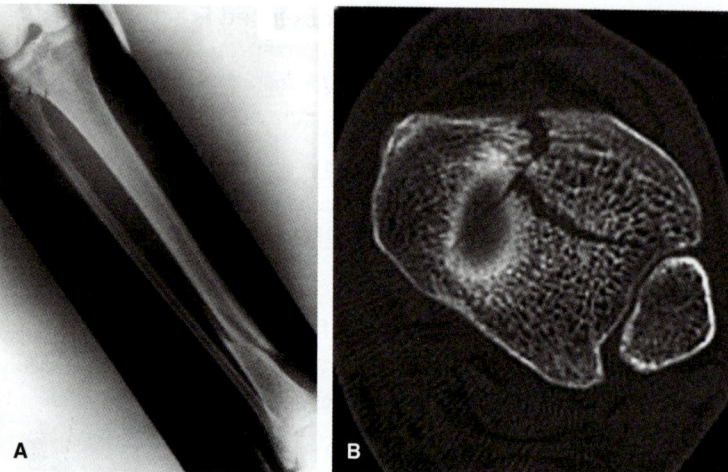

Figure 27 **A**, AP radiograph of a typical tibia and fibula fracture sustained in a characteristic indirect torsional injury to the leg. The patient's fracture resulted from the foot and ankle being fixed while the upper body twisted about the tibia, resulting in the classic spiral oblique fracture from the distal medial cortex up to the superior lateral cortex of the tibia. **B**, CT scan from a 48-year-old man who was involved in a skiing accident. He has a spiral metadiaphyseal tibial fracture with contiguous displaced anterolateral plafond fracture. The surgical tactic included an anterolateral exposure of the distal tibial articular surface with adjunctive percutaneous medial plating to stabilize the metadiaphyseal injury. (Panel A reproduced with permission from Bucholz RW, Heckman JD, eds: *Rockwood & Green's Fractures in Adults*, ed 5. Lippincott Williams & Wilkins, 2001, Figure 5.56B. Panel B reproduced with permission from Wiss D: *Master Techniques in Orthopaedic Surgery: Fractures*, ed 3. Wolters Kluwer, 2012, Figure 31-9C.)

- Aminoglycoside added in type III injuries
- Penicillin added in farm injuries
- Tetanus vaccination status should be confirmed and prophylaxis administered when necessary.
- Large debris should be removed from the open wound.
- The open wound should be irrigated with saline in the emergency department or trauma bay.
- The open wound should be covered with a moist dressing or betadine dressing before splint application.

Chapter 3: I Fell and Cannot Get Up—Lower Extremity Trauma

- Closed reduction and cast immobilization can be considered for closed low-energy injuries with alignment that meets and can be maintained using the following criteria:
  - Less than 10° of rotational malalignment
  - Less than 1 cm of shortening
  - Greater than 50% cortical apposition
  - Less than 10° of AP angulation
  - Less than 5° of varus/valgus angulation
- The patient is placed in a long leg cast initially, which is converted to a functional (patellar tendon bearing) brace at approximately 4 to 6 weeks. However, close follow-up with repeat radiographs to ensure no displacement is necessary, with monitoring of soft tissue, especially in at-risk groups such as patients with diabetes.
- Outcomes
  - Although angulation and rotation can be maintained in a cast, shortening can be difficult to control. There is an increased risk of varus if the fibula is intact (not broken). The nonunion rate is between 1% and 3% for closed treatment of tibia fractures.

Surgical Intervention

- Indications
  - Surgery is indicated for tibial fractures where nonsurgical management cannot maintain necessary alignment and stability.
  - Immediate weight bearing is possible with surgical stabilization, particularly intramedullary nailing.
  - Open fractures require surgical management.
- Top three techniques
  - Débridement and stabilization of open fractures[25]
    - Open tibia fractures require emergent incision, débridement, and irrigation in the operating room.
    - The traumatic wound is extended to allow for débridement of the bone edges sharply followed by copious irrigation with saline (typically, 3 to 9 L).[26]
    - Soft-tissue coverage in type IIB open tibial fractures
      - Proximal third—gastrocnemius rotation flap
      - Middle third—soleus rotation flap
      - Distal third—free flap

- External fixation is indicated for type IIB and IIIC injuries where the soft-tissue envelope is compromised or there is significant bone loss.
  - Polytrauma patients may benefit from damage control orthopaedics with application of an external fixator for tibial shaft fractures.
- Intramedullary nailing
  - Intramedullary nailing of tibial shaft fractures is the standard treatment regimen used for most patients.
  - Insertion of an intramedullary nail for tibial fractures can be performed in a minimally invasive manner using either a suprapatellar or infrapatellar technique (**Figure 28**).
  - The intramedullary nail is usually placed with reaming to allow for placement of a larger device and also to initiate a healing cascade (**Figure 29**).
- ORIF
  - The use of plates and screws for fixation of tibial shaft fractures is usually limited to those fractures that are proximal or distal in the tibial shaft.
  - Modern intramedullary nails allow for treatment of extra-articular proximal and distal third tibial fractures.

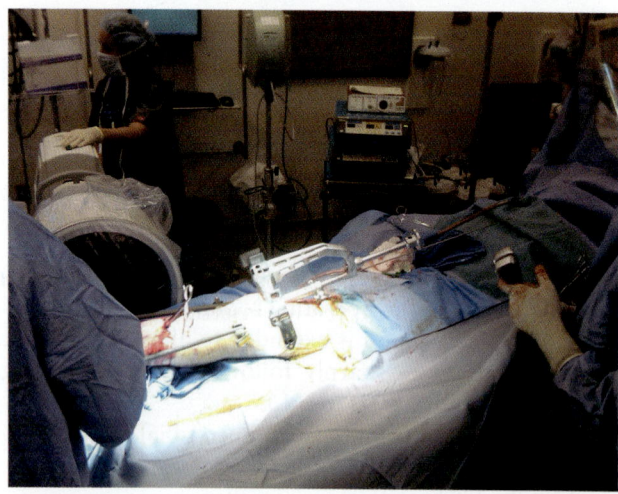

Figure 28 Intraoperative photograph showing the suprapatellar approach to the intramedullary nail of the tibia.

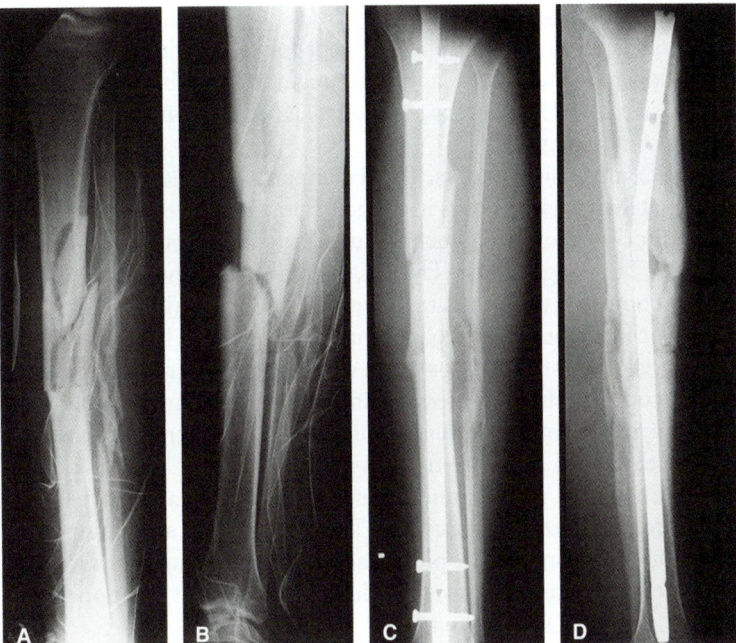

Figure 29 Displaced closed fractures of the tibia shaft, when shortened more than 1 cm or considered to be unstable, are best managed with interlocking nails. **A** and **B**, Preoperative radiographs of a shortened, unstable segmental fracture of the tibia shaft. **C** and **D**, The interlocking nail in place. The screws placed through the holes in the nail proximal and distal to the fracture provide length and rotational stability for the fracture. Nearly all fractures of the femoral shaft in skeletally mature individuals are treated with similar interlocking nails, allowing mobilization of the patient and early range of motion of adjacent joints. (Reproduced with permission from Swiontkowski MF, ed: *Manual of Orthopaedics*, ed 7. Wolters Kluwer, 2012, Figure 26-3.)

- ORIF may be necessary in patients who have preexisting hardware present precluding insertion of a nail (eg, those with total knee arthroplasty)
- Postoperative orders
  - Weight-bearing status: With intramedullary fixation and no involvement of the proximal or distal articular surface of the tibia, immediate weight bearing can be initiated. In situations where there may be proximal or distal extension of the fracture, weight bearing may be limited for 2 to 6 weeks.

- Antibiotics: Typically, 23 hours of postoperative first-generation cephalosporin, except for those with an allergy. In open fractures, the antibiotic regimen may be more aggressive and extended to 48 hours depending on the soft-tissue contamination.
- Compartment checks: Tibial compartments should be assessed at least every 2 hours in the acute postoperative period to monitor for the development of an acute compartment syndrome.
- VTE prophylaxis: This is controversial and ranges from compressive devices to aspirin to low-molecular-weight heparin, or other anticoagulants if the patient has other high-risk comorbidities or has experienced polytrauma. There is concern about aggressive anticoagulation immediately after a tibial fracture because of the risk of increased bleeding leading to a compartment syndrome.
- Suggested pain regimen: A multimodal pain approach is best to minimize narcotics use. This can include acetaminophen, gabapentin, and topical patches. Anti-inflammatory medications are often contraindicated because of chemoprophylaxis for DVT prevention.
- Pearls and pitfalls
  - Potential complications
    - What to look for clinically: The primary complication that is devastating is compartment syndrome and must be a consideration for all tibial fractures, including open fractures, whether they are managed surgically or nonsurgically. Close monitoring and appropriate vigilance is necessary to prevent a catastrophic complication. If compartment syndrome is identified, a two-incision fasciotomy to release all four compartments is indicated (**Figure 30**).
    - What to look for radiographically: Tibial fractures should reveal radiographic union by approximately 6 months. If the patient has persistent pain or other clinical symptoms and radiographs at 6 months show incomplete healing, additional treatment should be considered.
- Outcomes
  - Intramedullary nailing allows for shorter immobilization time, earlier weight bearing, and accelerated healing compared with casting. However, union rates are approximately

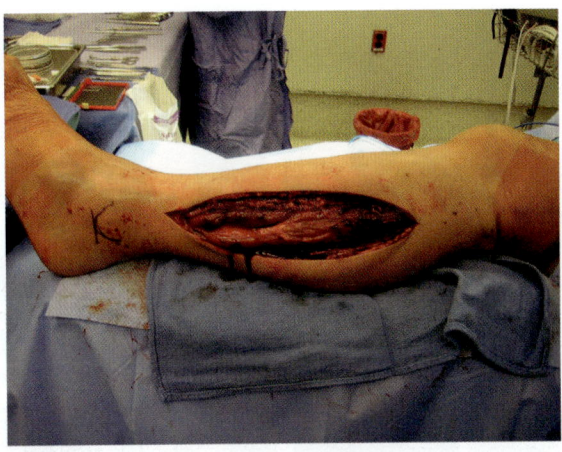

Figure 30 Photograph shows the lateral fasciotomy incision releasing the anterior and lateral compartments in a patient with a tibial shaft fracture and compartment syndrome.

80%.[27] Alignment is improved with suprapatellar nailing compared with infrapatellar nailing.[28] Reaming also has been shown to be beneficial.[29]

- Outcomes of ORIF compared with intramedullary nailing have shown increased radiation exposure, similar rates of union, and increased risk of wound complications and hardware issues as a result of the poor soft-tissue envelope around the tibia.
- Complications associated with tibia fractures include:
  - Nonunion in approximately 10% of patients
    - Risk factors are open fractures, lack of cortical contact of greater than 50%, and fracture gap in a transverse fracture pattern.
  - Malunion is common in proximal third tibia fractures with approximately 50% showing some loss of reduction, typically valgus and procurvatum (**Figure 31**).
  - Open tibial fractures with associated soft-tissue injury can result in infection or amputation (**Table 4**).
  - Anterior knee pain occurs in approximately 30% of patients after intramedullary nailing, more commonly with the infrapatellar approach.

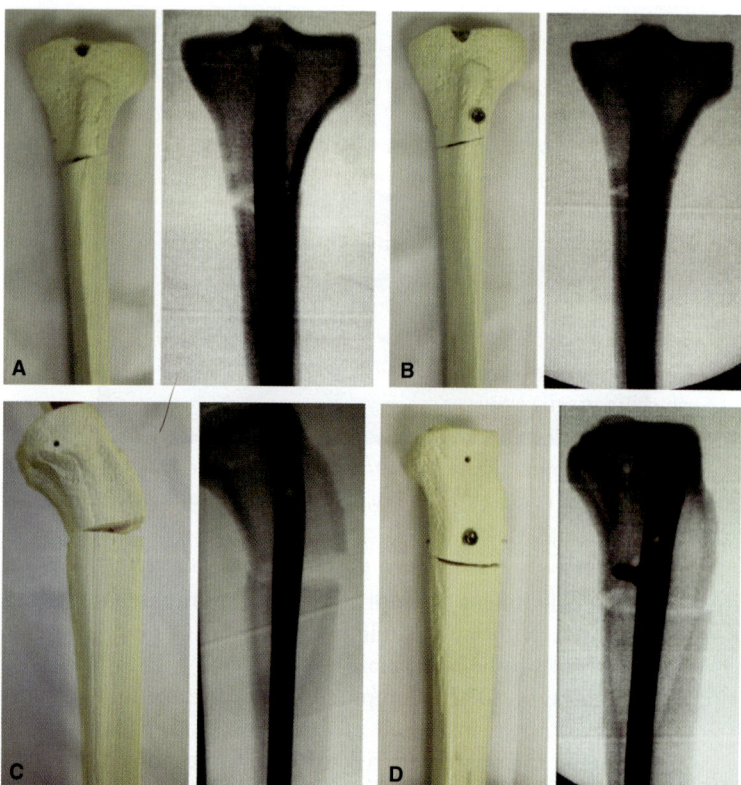

Figure 31 **A** and **B**, AP views, before and after placement of an ideally placed blocking screw in the concavity of the deformity, shifting the nail medially, avoiding valgus deformity. **C** and **D**, Lateral views, before and after placement of an ideally placed blocking screw in the concavity of the deformity, shifting the nail anteriorly, avoiding procurvatum deformity. (Reproduced from Avilucea FR, Yoon RS, Stinner DJ, Langford JR, Mir HR: Lower extremity fractures: Tips and tricks for nails and plates. *Instr Course Lect* 2020;69:433-448.)

TABLE 4 Complication Rates Associated With Gustilo-Anderson Type of Open Fracture

Type	I	II	IIIA	IIIB	IIIC
Infection	zero-2%	2%-7%	10%-25%	10%-50%	25%-50%
Amputation	—	—	—	—	50%

Chapter 3: I Fell and Cannot Get Up—Lower Extremity Trauma

Top 10 Knowledge Drops for Your Rotation

1. Tibial fractures are at risk for compartment syndrome.
2. If a patient has an open tibial fracture with violation of the fascia, compartment syndrome can still occur.
3. There are four compartments of the tibia, each with its own nerve.
4. The most common treatment option for a tibial shaft fracture is intramedullary nailing.
5. If there is no joint involvement, weight bearing can be initiated immediately after stabilization.
6. Open fractures can be classified using the Gustilo-Anderson classification system.
7. Open fractures should be managed with antibiotics immediately as the primary means of infection prevention.
8. Urgent surgical débridement is indicated for open contaminated tibial fractures.
9. CT of the distal tibia should be performed in spiral distal third tibial fractures to determine whether there is articular involvement.
10. Close monitoring and sequential examination are critical in high-energy tibial fractures to identify compartment syndrome.

PILON FRACTURES

The terms pilon and plafond are often used interchangeably, both referring to the weight-bearing portion of the distal tibial articular surface. A pilon fracture is a fracture of the weight-bearing articular portion of the distal tibia. Ankle fractures usually involve the non–weight-bearing portions of the ankle joint, including the medial, lateral, and posterior malleoli. Ankle fractures are typically associated with low-energy twisting mechanisms, whereas pilon fractures are associated with high-energy axial forces.

Epidemiology

- 1% of all lower extremity fractures, 20% are open injuries
- Males age 30 to 45 years
- Associated injuries

- 90% have associated distal fibular fracture
- 30% have an ipsilateral lower extremity injury
- 15% have injuries to the spine, pelvis, or upper extremities

Pertinent Anatomy/Pathoanatomy

- The distal tibia is quadrilateral shaped, with notable bony features including the anterolateral tubercle, posterior tubercle, medial malleolus, and fibular notch.
- The talus lies below the distal tibia and is made up of dense bone.
- The distal tibiofibular syndesmosis is made up of five ligaments, two of which are relevant to pilon fractures: the anterior-inferior and posterior-inferior tibiofibular ligaments (AITFL and PITFL). The AITFL originates from the anterolateral tubercle of the tibia and inserts on the anterior tubercle of the fibula. The PITFL originates from the posterior tubercle of the tibia and inserts on the posterior lateral malleolus[30] (**Figure 32**).

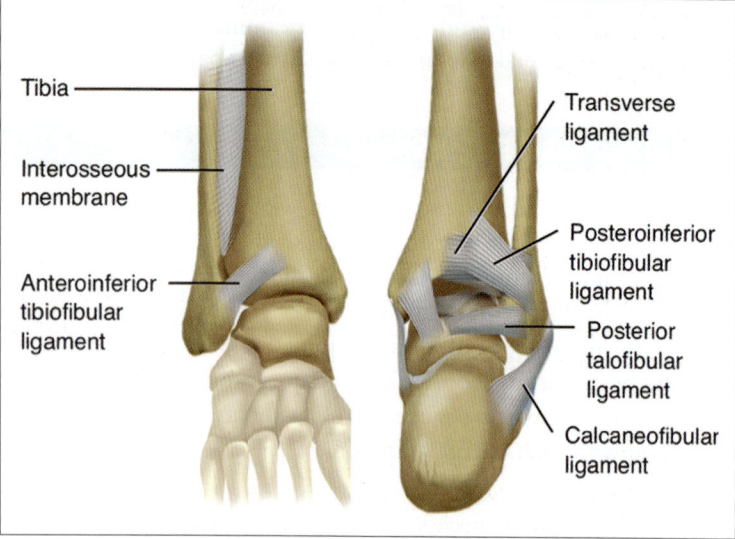

Figure 32 Illustration showing ligamentous anatomy of the ankle joint. (Reproduced with permission from Easley ME, ed: *Operative Techniques in Foot and Ankle Surgery*, ed 3. Wolters Kluwer, 2021. Figure 132.1C.)

- The mechanism of injury is bipartite:[31]
  - High-energy axial force that drives the talus into the distal tibia, resulting in highly comminuted articular fracture. This mechanism is seen in patients who fall from a height or are involved in a motor vehicle accident. This mechanism comprises most of the pilon fractures and is more commonly associated with open injury and other fractures.
  - Low-energy rotational force that results in a distal tibia spiral fracture with minimal articular comminution. This mechanism is seen in patients who were injured during a sporting accident (such as while skiing).

Pertinent History/Physical Examination Findings

- As stated previously, most patients presenting with a pilon fracture have sustained significant high-energy trauma, and thus should be worked up for additional injuries according to ATLS protocols.
- Comorbidities that may affect wound healing (eg, diabetes mellitus, vascular disease, tobacco use, autoimmune disease) as well as surgical planning (eg, blood thinners, osteoporosis, ambulatory status and activity level) should be assessed.
- Pilon fractures are associated with a high rate of wound complications because of the tenuous thin, soft-tissue envelope and high-energy injury mechanism; it is crucial to perform a thorough soft-tissue and neurovascular examination.[30]
  - Soft tissue: Wounds, blisters, ischemic skin, chronic vascular changes, open fractures.
  - Lower extremity neurovascular examination: Palpate other surrounding joints to ensure no other fractures; assess for vascular compromise with pulses, Doppler examination, and/or ankle-brachial index.

Relevant Imaging

- Radiographs—primarily used for diagnosis
  - AP, lateral, and mortise views of the ankle
- CT—almost always necessary to better characterize the fracture and for preoperative planning
  - Classically, in high-energy pilon fractures, there are three or four major fragments that can be appreciated on axial cut[32] (**Figure 33**):

- Medial malleolar fragment
- Anterolateral fragment—due to avulsion of the AITFL; also known as the Chaput fragment
- Posterior fragment—also known as the Volkmann fragment
- Lateral malleolar fragment—also known as the Wagstaffe fragment
  - This fracture pattern is sometimes called the Mercedes-Benz sign
- NOTE: For displaced, comminuted pilon fractures, the best time to perform CT scan is after temporizing external fixation.

Nonsurgical Measures

- Nonsurgical management with long leg casting for 6 weeks and then progression to a fracture brace is rare. It is reserved for nondisplaced low-energy fractures with minimal comminution or for those who are nonambulatory or too infirm to undergo surgical treatment.
- Outcomes are poor, with a high risk of progressive deformity, skin breakdown, and other soft-tissue complications.

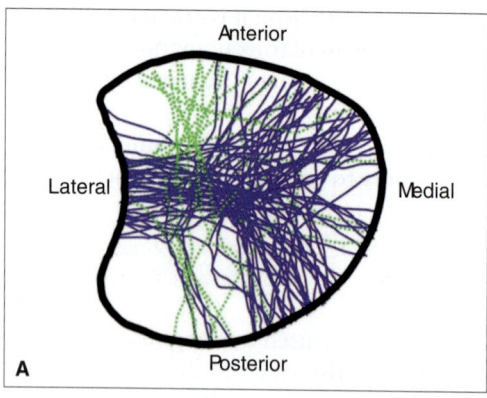

Figure 33 Images of common pilon fracture patterns. **A**, Schematic drawing showing an axial view digital compilation of fracture lines (blue lines) and zones of comminution (green lines) in 38 complete articular pilon fractures. This pilon map reveals the typical pattern of three primary joint fragments.

Chapter 3: I Fell and Cannot Get Up—Lower Extremity Trauma

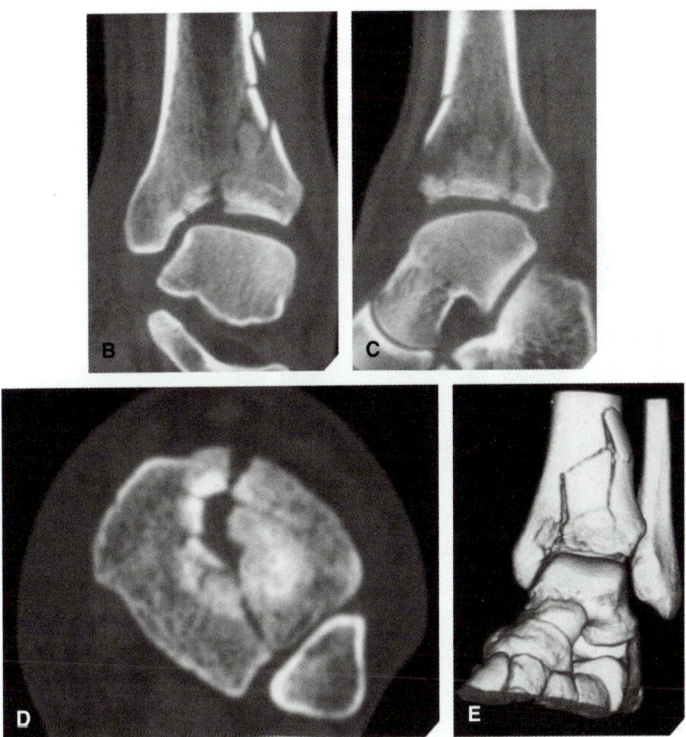

Figure 33 Cont'd **B**, Coronal, **C**, sagittal, **D**, axial, and **E**, 3D reconstructed CT images show characteristic features of pilon fracture in a 30-year-old man who was injured in a motorcycle accident. (Panel A reproduced from Black DA, Spitler CA, Graves ML: Ankle and hindfoot fractures, in Grauer JN, ed: *Orthopaedic Knowledge Update® 12*. American Academy of Orthopaedic Surgeons, 2017, p 544, Figure 3; originally adapted with permission from Cole P, Mehrle R, Bhandari M, et al: The pilon map: Fracture line and comminution zones in OTA/AO type 43C3 pilon fractures. *J Orthop Trauma* 2013;27:e152-e156. Panels B through E reproduced with permission from Greenspan A, Beltran J, eds: *Orthopaedic Imaging: A Practical Approach*, ed 7. Wolters Kluwer, 2020, Figure 10.39.)

Surgical Intervention

- All displaced pilon fractures in patients who can tolerate surgery are indicated for surgical management (**Figure 34**).
  - The key decision is whether the soft tissues surrounding the ankle are too swollen to perform ORIF and close thereafter.

Should this be the case, staged surgery is recommended, whereby temporary reduction and fixation of the fracture with an external fixator is performed.[33]
- Once the soft tissues are amenable to surgery (return of skin wrinkles, blister epithelialization, and ecchymosis resolution),

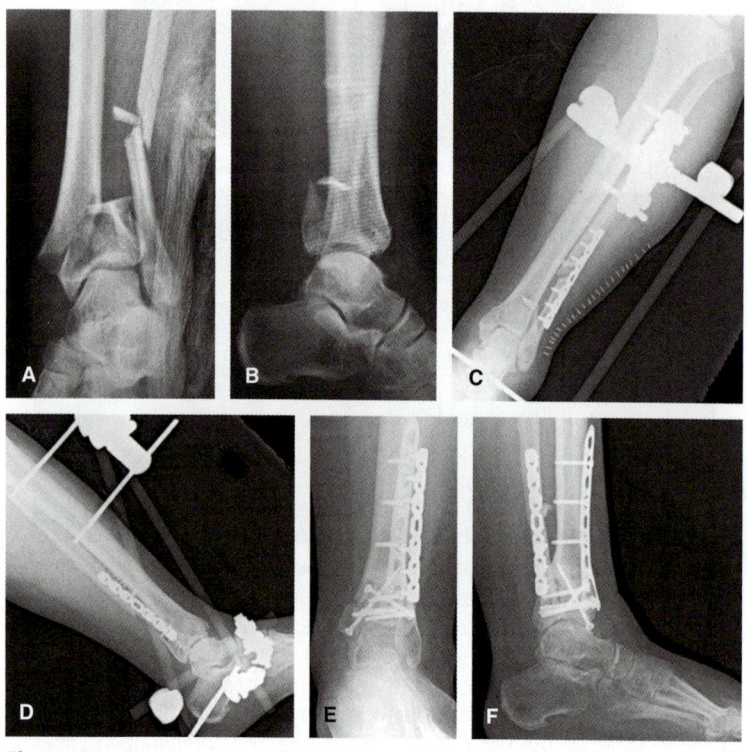

Figure 34 Preoperative AP (**A**) and lateral (**B**) right ankle radiographic views from a patient with well-controlled diabetes who sustained a severely displaced distal tibia and fibula pilon fracture. Early postoperative AP (**C**) and lateral (**D**) right lower extremity radiographic views showing the open reduction and internal fixation (ORIF) of the fibula and closed reduction and stabilization of the tibia pilon fracture with a spanning external fixation device. Postoperative AP (**E**) and lateral (**F**) right lower extremity radiographic views demonstrate an osseous nonunion at the medial malleolus at approximately 6 months after definitive ORIF of the tibia and removal of the spanning external fixator. Patient underwent a revisional reconstructive surgery that consisted of autogenous bone grafting and plating of the medial malleolar fracture fragment.

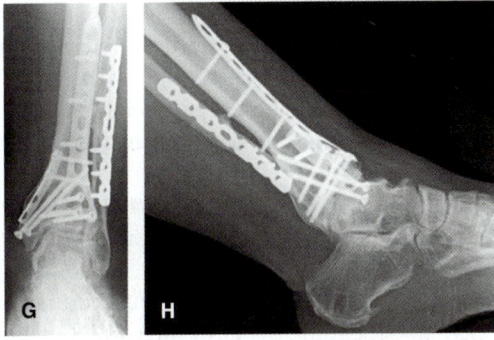

Figure 34 Cont'd Final postoperative AP (**G**) and lateral (**H**) lower extremity radiographic views showing osseous union and anatomic reduction at 4 months follow-up after the revisional surgery. (Reproduced with permission from Zgonis T, ed: *Surgical Reconstruction of the Diabetic Foot and Ankle*, ed 2. Wolters Kluwer, 2017, Figure 25.13.)

usually between 5 and 21 days after injury, patients then may undergo staged ORIF.
- Ankle-spanning external fixation
  - Often simply referred to as a delta frame, an ankle-spanning external fixator bridges the ankle joint to bring the limb out to length and allow the soft tissues to recover. Generally, it consists of four pins and four rods, but techniques vary.[34]
    - Place two pins in the proximal tibia at an adequate distance from the fracture in the sagittal plane, slightly medial to the anterior tibial crest.
    - Attach clamps and connect these two pins with a short rod to form a stable base.
    - Insert a threaded pin from medial to lateral in the calcaneal tuberosity, making sure to avoid injury to the posterior tibial neurovascular bundle.
    - Attach clamps and connect each end of the calcaneal pin to stable base with rods, forming a triangle or delta. Do not tighten clamps yet.
    - Reduce the fracture by manipulating the calcaneal pin, confirm on fluoroscopy, and then tighten the clamps.
    - Finally, place a pin in the first metatarsal shaft from medial to lateral and attach with a clamp and a bar to the stable base. This construct serves to maintain the foot in plantar flexion.

- ORIF
  - A variety of anatomic approaches are used when performing ORIF of a pilon fracture, depending on the fracture pattern and soft-tissue injuries. These approaches include anteromedial, anterolateral, posteromedial, posterolateral, and medial,[35] as demonstrated in **Figure 35**.
    - The anteromedial approach is considered the traditional approach and is used to address medial comminution and large Chaput fragments.
      - Perform a 10-cm longitudinal curved incision on the medial ankle, ending distal to the medial malleolus.
      - Dissect just medial to the tibialis anterior tendon down to bone.
      - Take care to protect the saphenous nerve and long saphenous vein, which run together just anterior to the medial malleolus.
    - The anterolateral approach is used for fractures with lateral comminution, small Chaput fragments, and large Volkmann fragments.[33]
      - The incision is made in line with the fourth metatarsal and extended proximally between the tibia and fibula.
      - Dissect just lateral to the extensor digitorum longus and peroneus tertius.
      - Take care to protect the superficial peroneal nerve during superficial dissection.
  - Once the fracture is exposed, generally the priority is accurate, anatomic reduction of the joint surface. Once stabilized, the articular segment is then attached to the tibial diaphysis, sometimes with the addition of bone graft to fill bony defects.[35]
- Circular frame fixation and primary arthrodesis are other surgical options, but less frequently used. Circular frame fixation is indicated in cases when soft-tissue injury precludes internal fixation. Primary arthrodesis may be performed in rare cases where the fracture is not reconstructable.
- Postoperatively, the patient remains non–weight bearing for 12 to 16 weeks or until radiographic signs of healing are seen. After ORIF, patients are typically immobilized in a short leg

Chapter 3: I Fell and Cannot Get Up—Lower Extremity Trauma

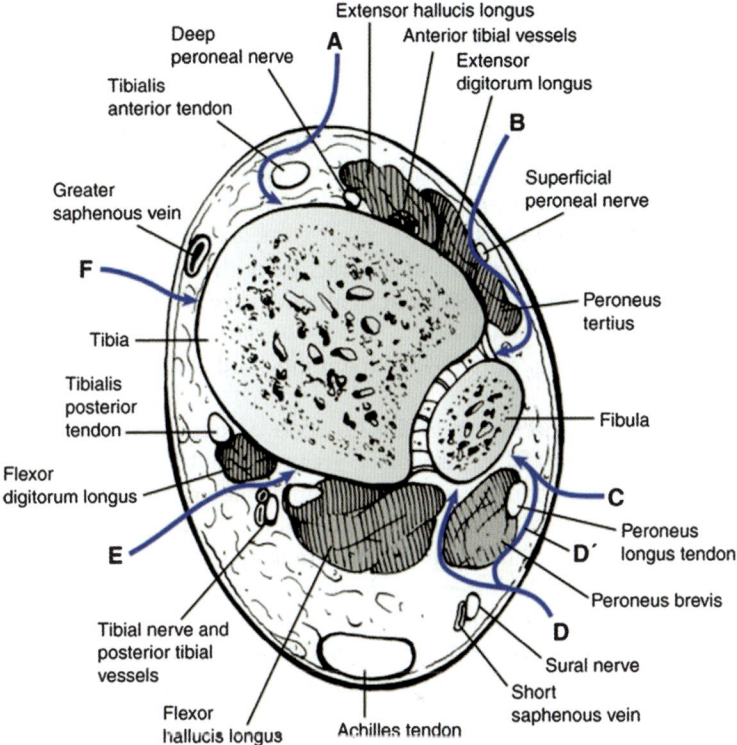

Figure 35 Surgical approaches to a pilon fracture. Axial view of the distal tibia just proximal to the distal tibiofibular syndesmosis demonstrating the relevant local surgical anatomy and surgical approaches for management of distal tibial plafond fractures. A: Anteromedial. B: Anterolateral. C: Posterolateral (fibula). D: Posterolateral (tibia). D′: Posterolateral (fibula). E: Posteromedial. F: Medial. (Reproduced with permission from Court-Brown CM, Heckman JD, McQueen MM, Ricci WM, Tornetta P III, eds: *Rockwood and Green's Fractures in Adults*, ed 8. Wolters Kluwer, 2014, Figure 58-7.)

splint for 2 weeks and then transitioned to a fracture brace to initiate gentle range of motion. Given the severity of the injury and their prolonged non–weight bearing status, it is recommended that patients are placed on VTE prophylaxis until they can move their ankle, although the decision whether to place

the patient on low-dose aspirin versus enoxaparin sodium is a topic of much debate.
- Complications[36]
  - Wound dehiscence (10% to 30% of patients) and infection (5% to 15% of patients) are the most common complications as a result of the high-energy nature of the injury, which leads to significant soft-tissue trauma.
    - Minimize the risk by:
      - Early stabilization of the fracture with external fixation
      - Thorough débridement of all devitalized osseous and soft-tissue elements
      - Avoiding soft-tissue stripping and closing skin on tension
  - Malunion (occurring in 5% to 15% of patients), defined as greater than 10° varus/valgus, greater than 10° procurvatum/recurvatum, and greater than 2 mm articular step-off, is often due to inadequate fracture reduction.
  - Nonunion (occurring in 5% of patients), particularly in highly comminuted fractures and those with significant bone loss or arterial compromise.
  - Posttraumatic arthritis generally develops 1 to 2 years after injury because of cartilage trauma and inadequate articular reduction.
- Outcomes
  - Outcomes correlate with fracture severity and quality of fracture reduction.
  - Studies show long-term outcomes after ORIF for pilon fractures are poor, with diminished scores in all functional domains of the Short Form-36, particularly in physical function, physical role function, and bodily pain.
  - At 5 years postoperatively, a recent study found fewer than 66% of patients returned to baseline physical function and fewer than 50% of patients reached a pain score within one minimal clinically important difference of baseline.[31]
  - Long-term outcomes show poorer quality of life than in patients with pelvic fractures, coronary artery disease, and chronic asthma.[37]

Top 10 Knowledge Drops for Your Rotation

1. Pilon or tibial plafond fractures are intra-articular fractures of the distal tibia that are frequently associated with comminution and significant soft-tissue injury.
2. The most common mechanism of injury is a high-energy axial force resulting from a fall from a height or motor vehicle collision.
3. CT is critical to surgical planning and should be performed after external fixation if a staged reconstruction is planned.
4. On axial CT, high-energy pilon fractures classically have four major fragments: medial malleolar, Chaput, Volkmann, and Wagstaffe.
5. Early external fixation and staged ORIF of pilon fractures is the optimal choice for pilon fractures with significant soft-tissue injury.
6. The anteromedial approach to the ankle involves an incision just medial to the Achilles tendon, and the at-risk structures include the saphenous nerve and long saphenous vein.
7. The anterolateral approach to the ankle lies between the tibia and fibula anteriorly, just lateral to the extensor digitorum longus tendon, and the at-risk structure is the superficial peroneal nerve.
8. Respecting the soft tissues with percutaneous techniques when appropriate, minimal soft-tissue dissection and minimal periosteal stripping reduces postoperative complications.
9. Soft-tissue complications including dehiscence and infection are most common postoperatively.
10. Stiffness, pain, and functional disability are common long-term outcomes of pilon fractures.

LISFRANC INJURY

Lisfranc injuries are rare traumatic bony or ligamentous injuries of the tarsometatarsal (TMT) and intercuneiform joint complex. Specifically, the articulation between the medial cuneiform and base of the second metatarsal is disrupted. The second metatarsal is a critical stabilizer of the midfoot, and thus presents as severe midfoot pain, medial plantar ecchymosis, and instability of the TMT joint. It may be a result of a high-energy axial load or a low-energy twisting force. Treatment is generally indicated with either ORIF or arthrodesis.

Epidemiology

- Fractures are rare, most common in males age 20 to 40 years.
- Approximately 20% of Lisfranc injuries are missed, resulting in delayed treatment, and thus increasing the risk of persistent pain, posttraumatic arthritis, and progressive foot planovalgus deformity.[38]

Pertinent Anatomy/Pathoanatomy

- The midfoot is composed of three columns, the medial (first TMT), middle (second-third TMT), and lateral (fourth-fifth TMT).
- The second metatarsal is recessed between the medial and lateral cuneiforms.
- The TMTs form a Roman arch configuration on cross-section, with the second metatarsal at its apex (**Figure 36**). They are stabilized by dorsal and plantar TMT ligaments.
- The Lisfranc ligament links the medial cuneiform to the base of the second metatarsal on the plantar surface of the foot.[39]
- The unique bony anatomy of the medial midfoot, combined with stout plantar ligaments, creates a stable medial and middle column that both maintains the midfoot arch and enables stable weight bearing.[40]
- Lisfranc injuries are generally the result of a high-energy injury such as a motor vehicle accident, whereby an indirect rotational force and axial load is sustained through a hyper plantarflexed forefoot. However, they can be the result of lower energy twisting injuries in which forceful abduction of the forefoot on the tarsus in equinus results in fracture of the second metatarsal base.[41]
- The resulting pathoanatomy is highly variable, including pure ligamentous injury, bony fracture, or a combination. However, the unifying factor is disruption of the TMT joint complex.
- The Myerson classification is most commonly used to characterize the different Lisfranc injury patterns[42] (**Figure 37**).

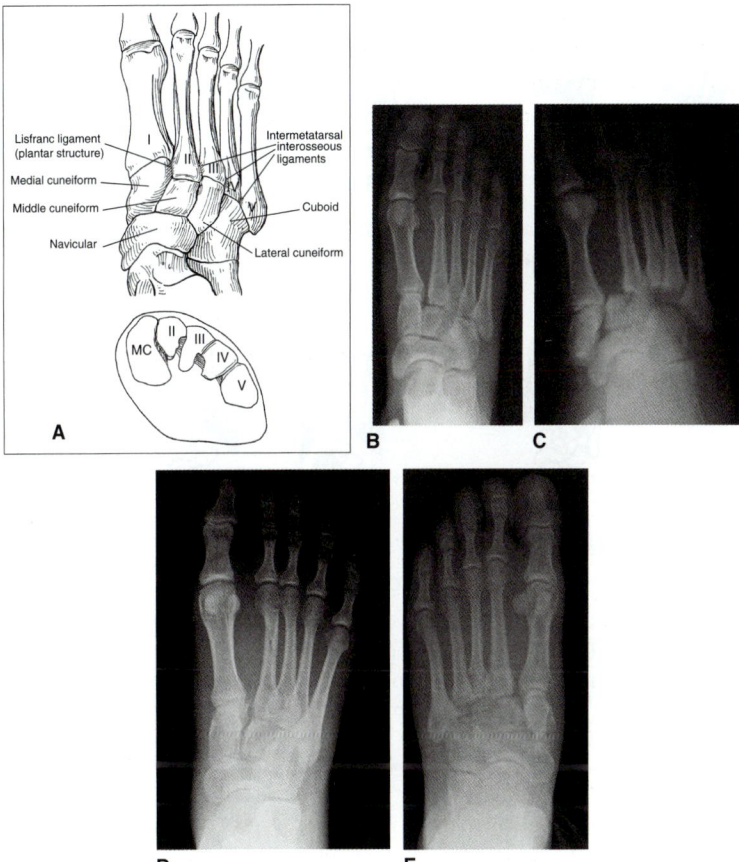

Figure 36 Lisfranc injuries. **A**, Drawing shows dorsal and coronal views of bone, joint, ligament anatomy of Lisfranc complex. **B**, AP radiograph of the foot showing isolated disruption of second TMT joint. **C**, Radiograph showing severe disruption of Lisfranc complex including medial cuneiform. **D**, Radiograph showing a more subtle Lisfranc injury with intercuneiform instability. **E**, Radiograph showing subtle Lisfranc injury with medial cuneiform subluxation and fracture. Note first and second TMT joints are at about the same level. (Reproduced with permission from Kitaoka H, ed: *Master Techniques in Orthopaedic Surgery: The Foot and Ankle*, ed 3. Wolters Kluwer, 2013, Figure 17.1A-E.)

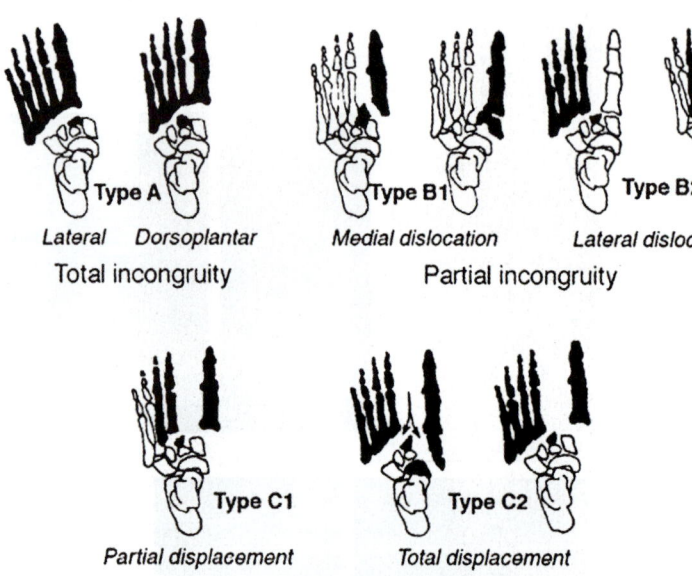

Figure 37 Illustration showing Myerson classification of Lisfranc fracture-dislocations. (Reproduced with permission from Myerson MS, Fisher RT, Burgess AR, et al: Fracture dislocations of the tarsometatarsal joints: End results correlated with pathology and treatment. *Foot Ankle* 1986;6[5]:225-242.)

Pertinent History/Physical Examination Findings

- Diffuse midfoot swelling, pain on palpation of the first TMT joint, and inability to walk are common physical examination findings, but plantar ecchymosis is pathognomonic for this injury[43] (**Figure 38**).
  - If the patient is amenable, instability should be tested. Stabilize the hindfoot with one hand, and with the other attempt to translate the midfoot dorsal and plantar. Subluxation indicates instability.

Relevant Imaging

- AP, oblique, and lateral radiographs of the foot are obtained first. There are five critical radiographic findings that indicate midfoot instability[44] (**Figure 39**):

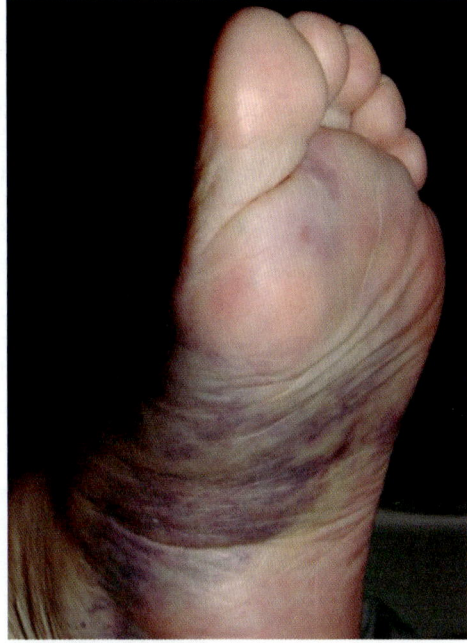

Figure 38 Photograph showing plantar ecchymosis, a common clinical finding associated with a Lisfranc fracture-dislocation. (Reproduced with permission from Tornetta P III, Ricci WM, Ostrum RF, McQueen MM, McKee MD, Court-Brown CM, eds. *Rockwood and Green's Fracture in Adults*, ed 9. Wolters Kluwer, 2019, Figure 67.20.)

- On AP radiograph:
    1. Discontinuity of the medial base of the second metatarsal with the medial side of the middle cuneiform
    2. Widening (>2 mm) between the first metatarsal and medial cuneiform, often accompanied by bony fragment in the first intermetatarsal space, known as the fleck sign
- On lateral radiograph:
    1. Dorsal displacement of the proximal base of the first or second metatarsal greater than 2 mm
- On oblique radiograph:
    1. Discontinuity of the medial base of the fourth metatarsal and medial side of the cuboid
    2. Disruption of the medial column line (line tangential to the medial cuneiform and medial aspect of the navicular)

- Weight-bearing radiographs of the feet can serve as a stress view with a normal comparison to detect subtle unstable Lisfranc injuries.
- CT can be used for preoperative planning in the setting of comminuted bony injuries.
- MRI can be used to confirm injuries that are purely ligamentous.

Nonsurgical Measures

- Nonsurgical management with a controlled ankle motion (CAM) boot or short leg cast for 6 weeks, remaining non–weight bearing during that time, is appropriate for patients with partial Lisfranc injuries, minimally displaced fractures that are stable on weight bearing, or in nonambulatory or very ill patients unable to tolerate surgery.

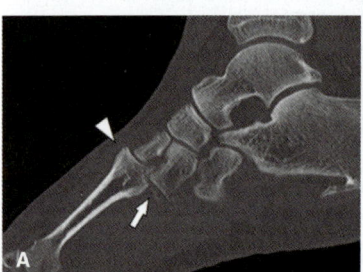
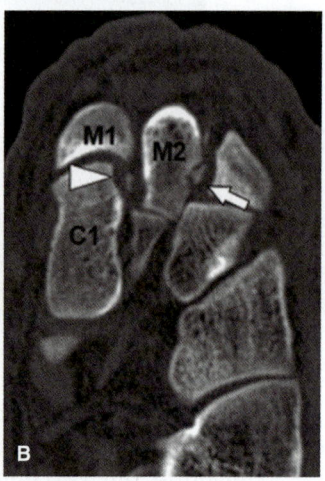

Figure 39 **A**, Sagittal bone window setting CT image shows abnormal dorsal subluxation (arrowhead) of the base of the second metatarsal with respect to the cuneiforms with fracture and impaction of the volar base of the second metatarsal with multifocal small ossific bodies at the tarsometatarsal joint (arrow). **B**, Axial bone window setting CT image better demonstrates the fracture fragments (arrowhead) within the region of the Lisfranc ligament between the first cuneiform (C1) and the base of the second metatarsal (M2) and first metatarsal (M1). Small fractures (arrow) noted at the lateral aspect of the second metatarsal base with mild lateral displacement in keeping with homolateral injury.

Chapter 3: I Fell and Cannot Get Up—Lower Extremity Trauma

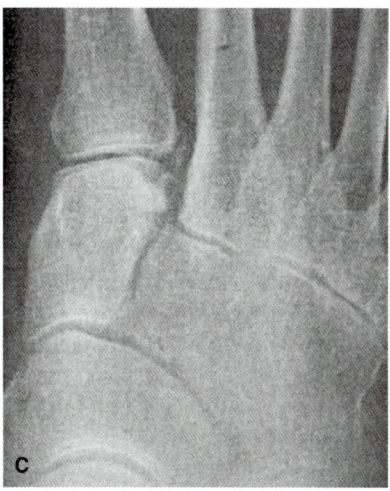

Figure 39 Cont'd **C**, AP weight-bearing radiograph of the foot showing the fleck sign, which indicates avulsion of the origin of the Lisfranc ligament. (Panels A and B reproduced with permission from Lee EY, Hunsaker A, Siewert B, eds: *Computed Body Tomography with MRI Correlation*, ed 5. Wolters Kluwer, 2019, Figure 10-146AB. Panel C reproduced from O'Neil JT, Raikin, SM, Pedowitz DI, eds: Midfoot injuries, in Chou LB, ed: *Orthopaedic Knowledge Update®: Foot and Ankle 6.* American Academy of Orthopaedic Surgeons, 2019, p 354, Figure 8.)

Surgical Intervention

- Surgical management is indicated for unstable or displaced (>2 mm) injuries.
- Surgical options include ORIF versus primary arthrodesis, which is still debated.
  - ORIF[43]
    - The goal of ORIF is to obtain anatomic reduction of the fracture-dislocation of the second metatarsal base. Rigid fixation is used to re-create the stability of the medial and middle columns, whereas flexible temporary fixation is used for the mobile lateral column.
    - A two-incision dorsal approach is most commonly used. The first longitudinal incision is between the first and second metatarsal, in the interval between the extensor hallucis longus and extensor hallucis brevis tendons, allowing for identification of the dorsalis pedis artery and deep peroneal nerve. The second incision is made over the fourth metatarsal.

- Reduction and fixation of the injury generally proceeds proximal to distal and medial to lateral, using a mixture of cortical screws, Kirschner wires, and plates (**Figure 40**).
- Primary arthrodesis of the first, second, and third TMT joints
  - Although controversial, many surgeons perform primary arthrodesis in the setting of pure ligamentous injuries, delayed treatment, or type A or C2 injury patterns.
  - The surgical technique involves exposing all of the TMT joints, removing all cartilage, and fusing the joints with the use of cortical screws and plates.
    - It is important to avoid fusing the fourth and fifth TMT joints if possible because the lateral column is normally mobile and responsible for flexible adaptations when walking on uneven ground.
- Postoperatively, regardless of surgical technique, patients will be immobilized in a cast or CAM boot for 8 to 10 weeks and must remain non–weight bearing. This may be extended for patients who underwent primary arthrodesis until there are radiographic signs of healing.

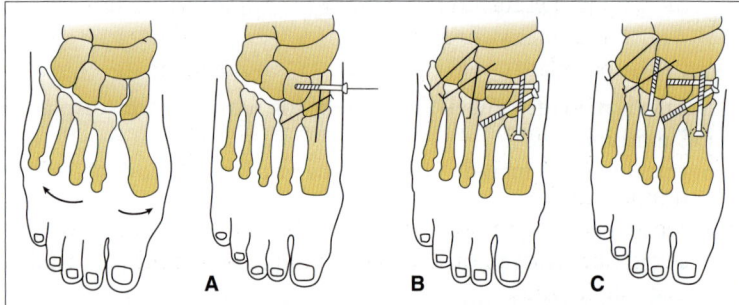

Figure 40 Illustration showing sequence of repair for reduction and stabilization of TMT fracture-dislocations. **A**, Stabilization of the first ray by alignment of the metatarsal, medial cuneiform, and navicular. **B**, Stabilization of the Lisfranc ligament by accurate alignment of the second metatarsal to the medial cuneiform, as well as the medial and middle cuneiforms. **C**, Alignment and stabilization of the third through fifth metatarsal rays. Cannulated screws can be used instead of pins as needed for stability and compression. (Reproduced with permission from Waters PM, Skaggs DL, Flynn JM, eds: *Rockwood and Wilkins' Fractures in Children*, ed 8. Wolters Kluwer, 2014, Figure 33.32.)

Chapter 3: I Fell and Cannot Get Up—Lower Extremity Trauma

- Outcomes
  - Timely accurate diagnosis and anatomic reduction generally result in good outcomes overall, with few activity limitations.
  - Two prospective randomized controlled trials comparing ORIF versus primary arthrodesis reported no difference in functional outcomes between the two techniques; however, there was a substantially higher rate of secondary surgery in the ORIF group (most commonly for elective implant removal).[45]
  - The most common complication is posttraumatic arthritis, most often due to delayed treatment or nonanatomic reduction after ORIF. The same risk factors may lead to malunion. Approximately 75% and 20% of patients undergo hardware removal after ORIF and arthrodesis, respectively.[43]

Top 10 Knowledge Drops for Your Rotation

1. Lisfranc injuries are rare traumatic bony or ligamentous injuries caused by disruption of the articulation between the medial cuneiform and base of the second metatarsal.
2. The Lisfranc ligament links the medial cuneiform to the base of the second metatarsal on the plantar surface of the foot.
3. The unique bony anatomy of the medial midfoot, combined with stout plantar ligaments, is responsible for midfoot stability and arch maintenance.
4. Plantar ecchymosis is pathognomonic for Lisfranc injury.
5. There are five critical radiographic findings that indicate midfoot instability.
6. Weight-bearing radiographs of the bilateral feet can serve as a stress view with a normal comparison to detect subtle unstable Lisfranc injuries.
7. Surgical management is indicated for unstable or displaced (>2 mm) injuries.
8. Surgical options include ORIF versus primary arthrodesis.
9. The goal of ORIF is to obtain anatomic reduction and rigid fixation of the fracture-dislocation of the second metatarsal base.
10. The most common complication is posttraumatic arthritis, most often due to delayed treatment or nonanatomic reduction after ORIF.

ANKLE FRACTURES

Ankle fractures are a common orthopaedic injury that can range from a simple fracture to a very complex and unstable injury. These injuries can happen at any age and can occur as a result of a low-energy or high-energy mechanism.

Epidemiology

- Incidence: approximately 168 fractures per 100,000 people each year[46]
  - Can involve one, two, or three of the malleoli: isolated malleolus fractures—approximately 65%, bimalleolar ankle fractures—approximately 25%, trimalleolar ankle fractures—remaining 5% to 10%[47]
- Most common fracture: lateral malleolus (accounts for approximately 55%)[46]
- Open fractures account for approximately 2% of all ankle fractures; usually from high-energy mechanisms
- Have a bimodal distribution, with occurrences in young, active patients and then in low-demand patients and older people
- Increased incidence in older people as the population continues to age
- Older women more prone to ankle fractures[47]

Pertinent Anatomy/Pathoanatomy

Bones

- Ankle fractures are fractures of the distal portion of specific areas of the tibia and the distal portion of the fibula.
- The three malleoli refer to the lateral malleolus (distal fibula), the medial malleolus, and the posterior malleolus.
- The medial malleolus has an anterior and posterior malleolus.
- The three malleoli surround the talus, which together make up the ankle joint.
- The talus glides between the distal fibula, the medial malleolus, and the distal tibia articular surfaces, also known as the tibial plafond.
- The tibial plafond is concave to accommodate the medial and lateral aspects of the talus and convex slightly in the center portion.

Chapter 3: I Fell and Cannot Get Up—Lower Extremity Trauma

- The distal fibula, or lateral malleolus, also articulates with the lateral portion of the talus and the distal tibia. This creates the distal tibiofibular and tibiotalar joints.
- The talar dome, the portion that articulates with the tibial plafond, is a trapezoid. The anterior portion is 2.5 mm wider than the posterior portion.
- This anatomic difference can create different images on the radiograph depending on if the foot is dorsiflexed or plantarflexed.[47]

Ligaments

- After the bones, the ligaments help stabilize the motion in the ankle.
- There are lateral-based ligaments and medial-based ligaments.
- The four main ligaments commonly discussed on the lateral side are known as the syndesmosis. The syndesmosis provides stability to the lateral aspect of the ankle and allows for rotation of the fibula on the tibia and talus during ankle range of motion. It includes the following ligaments:
  - AITFL
    - Most common cause of ankle sprains are injuries to this ligament
    - Connects the distal fibula to the anterior distal tibia
  - PITFL
    - Strongest stabilizer of the syndesmosis
    - Thicker than the AITFL
    - Connects the posterior malleolus and the distal fibula
  - Transverse tibiofibular ligament (inferior to PITFL)
    - Connects posterior fibula and posterior tibia
  - Interosseous ligament
    - Interosseous membrane stabilized the fibula and the tibia
    - Distal portion of the interosseous membrane
- Other lateral ligaments involved in ankle stability: anterior and posterior talofibular ligament and the calcaneofibular ligament
- Medial ligaments
  - Superficial deltoid ligament
    - Three ligaments that begin at the anterior colliculus of medial malleolus
    - Tibionavicular, tibiocalcaneal, and talotibial ligament

- Deep deltoid ligament
  - Primary stabilizer
  - Spans from the talus and the intercollicular groove[47,48]

Nerves Around the Ankle

- Superficial peroneal nerve
  - Found in the lateral compartment and pierces the fascia approximately 12 cm from distal fibula
  - Motor to the peroneal longus and brevis muscles
  - Sensation to anterolateral distal leg and dorsum of foot[49]
- Sural nerve
  - Sensation to posterolateral ankle and lateral border of foot
  - Sensation to the posterior ankle

Pertinent History/Physical Examination Findings

- History
  - Mechanism of injury—high versus low energy
  - Age and ambulatory status
  - Comorbidities—smoking, diabetes, peripheral vascular disease, neuropathies
- Physical examination
  - Inspection
    - Open wounds or laceration, bruising, swelling, fracture blisters
    - Obvious deformity
  - Palpation
    - Pain around the ankle
    - Stability of the ankle
  - Motor
    - Dorsiflexion, plantar flexion, eversion, and inversion if able
    - Extension and flexion of toes
  - Sensation
  - Vascular—dorsalis pedis, posterior tibialis, and anterior tibial artery

Relevant Imaging

- Radiographs
  - Knee AP and lateral views to look for proximal fibula fractures
  - Ankle: AP, lateral, and mortise
    - AP—Tibiofibular clear space is approximately 6 mm.

- Medial clear space should be less than 5 mm on AP and mortise view.
- Lateral—Fibula is posterior to the tibia, talar dome should be under the tibial plafond, and the talus should not have a shadow.[50]
- Mortise view is obtained with the foot internally rotated approximately 10°.
- Stress views are done to establish the stability of the ankle fracture. This can be done by gravity or with external rotation stress. Both are taken with the mortise view and compared with the stress to see if the medial clear space widens or the tibiofibular space widens. Either test is equally effective.[48,50]
- CT scan
  - Provides more detail about the fractures including fractures of the posterior malleolus or anterior tibia if they are present
  - Can assess the syndesmosis—distal fibula within the groove of the tibia

Classification of Ankle Fractures

- Danis-Weber classification—Based on the location of the fibula fracture (**Figure 41**)
  - Weber A: Fracture of the fibula below the tibial plafond; can include an oblique or vertical fracture of the medial malleolus
  - Weber B: Fracture of the fibula at the syndesmosis; can include fracture of the medial malleolus or posterior malleolus.
  - Weber C: Fracture of the fibula above the syndesmosis; if the medial malleolus is fractured, this more than likely suggests a syndesmotic injury
- Lauge-Hansen classification—Based on the position of the foot and the direction of the force on the ankle at the time of injury
  - Supinated foot—The injury begins at the fibula, extends posteriorly and then ends medially.
    - Supination-adduction (SAD)—Medial displacement of the talus.
      - SAD I: Transverse distal fibula fracture with sprain or avulsion of the talofibular ligament.
      - SAD II: Transverse distal fibula fracture with a vertical medial malleolus fracture. This fracture calls for fixation of the medial malleolus with buttress plate or horizontally placed screws.

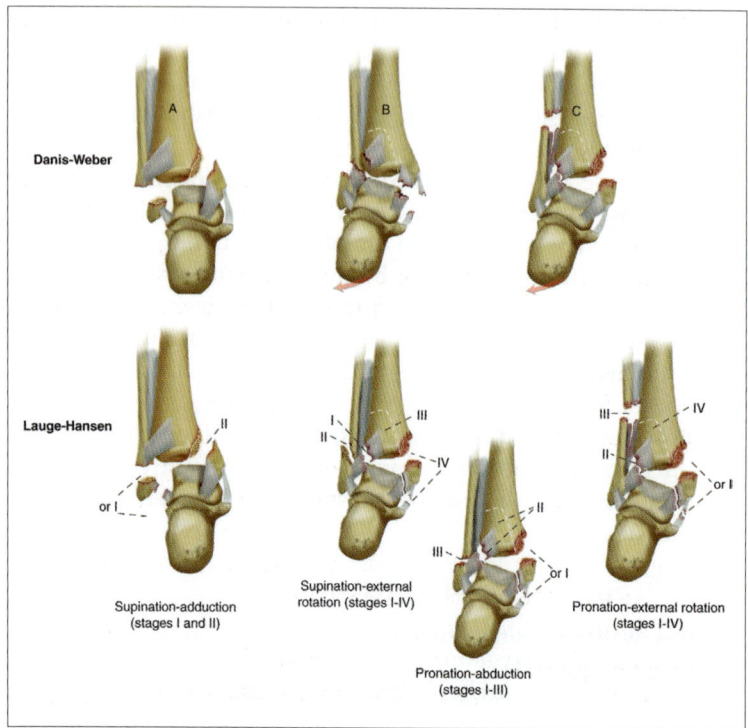

Figure 41 Illustration showing Danis-Weber and Lauge-Hansen ankle fracture classifications. (Reproduced with permission from Brinker MR, ed: *Review of Orthopaedic Trauma*, ed 2. Wolters Kluwer, 2013, Figure 13.4.)

- Supination-external rotation (SER)—most common type of ankle fracture.
  - SER I: Injury to the AITFL with or without fracture to the distal fibula.
  - SER II: Spiral or oblique fracture of the distal fibula that starts inferiorly on the anterior surface and travels superiorly on the posterior aspect of the fibula.
  - SER III: Spiral fracture of the distal fibula with injury to the PITFL or fracture of the posterior malleolus.
  - SER IV: Same as SER III with the addition of injury to the medial malleolus, which is either a transverse fracture or a deltoid ligament tear.

- Pronated foot—Injury begins on the medial side, extends anteriorly, and ends laterally or posteriorly.
  - Pronation-abduction (PAB)
    - PAB I: Isolated transverse fracture of medial malleolus or deltoid ligament disruption.
    - PAB II: Transverse medial malleolus fracture with rupture of syndesmosis. Can have an anterior tibia fracture at AITFL.
    - PAB III: Transverse or oblique medial malleolus fracture with comminuted high fibula fracture. Occurs from bending force.
  - Pronation-external rotation (PER)
    - PER I: Fracture of medial malleolus or disruption of deltoid ligament
    - PER II: Medial malleolus injury with AITFL injury
    - PER III: Medial malleolus fracture, high transverse fibula fracture
    - PER IV: Medial malleolus, high fibula fracture and injury to the PITFL or posterior malleolus
- Maisonneuve ankle fracture
  - Proximal fibula fracture with syndesmotic injury
  - Stress views show widening of the tibiofibular or medial clear space

Initial Management

- Nondisplaced fractures
  - Place in splint: Posterior and a "U" splint to allow for swelling
  - CAM boot—can allow for weight bearing as tolerated if stable ankle fracture
- Displaced
  - Reduction to allow talus to be well positioned in the mortise
  - Well-molded splint with mold inferior to the lateral malleolus and superior to the medial malleolus to prevent talus from translating
- Open fractures
  - Bedside irrigation and débridement of the wound
  - Reduction of the ankle
  - Stabilization with short leg splint
- All necessary imaging should be performed (postreduction radiographs and CT if necessary).

- Inability to achieve appropriate reduction is usually because there is a bony fragment or soft tissue interposed that prevents the reduction.

Nonsurgical Measures

- Stable ankle fractures can be managed nonsurgically (**Figure 42**)
  - Weber A and Weber B that are stable with stress view
  - SER I, SER II, SAD I, nondisplaced medial malleolus
- Patients unable to undergo surgery
- Modalities
  - Splint with posterior slab and a stirrup or "U"
  - Short leg cast
  - CAM boot with weight bearing or non–weight bearing
  - Serial radiographs to monitor reduction

Surgical Intervention

- Indications
  - Unstable ankle fractures
    - Syndesmotic injuries—Maisonneuve fractures
    - Wide mortise on stress view
    - Bimalleolar or trimalleolar ankle fractures (**Figures 43 and 44**)
  - Open ankle fractures

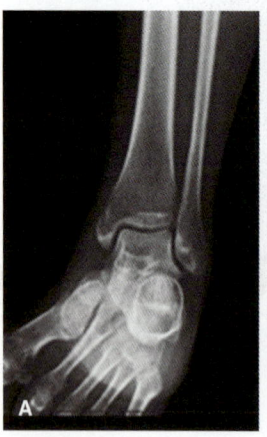
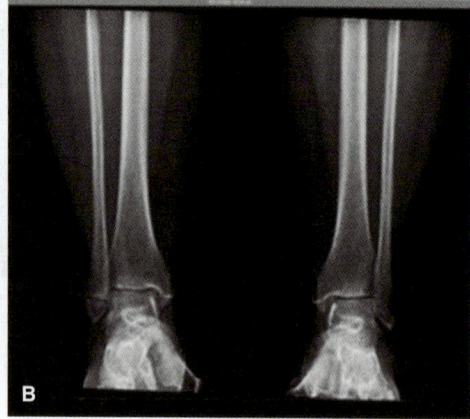

Figure 42 Radiographs showing simple fractures. **A**, Mortise view showing medial malleolus nondisplaced. **B**, AP radiograph showing right nondisplaced lateral malleolus fracture with stable mortise.

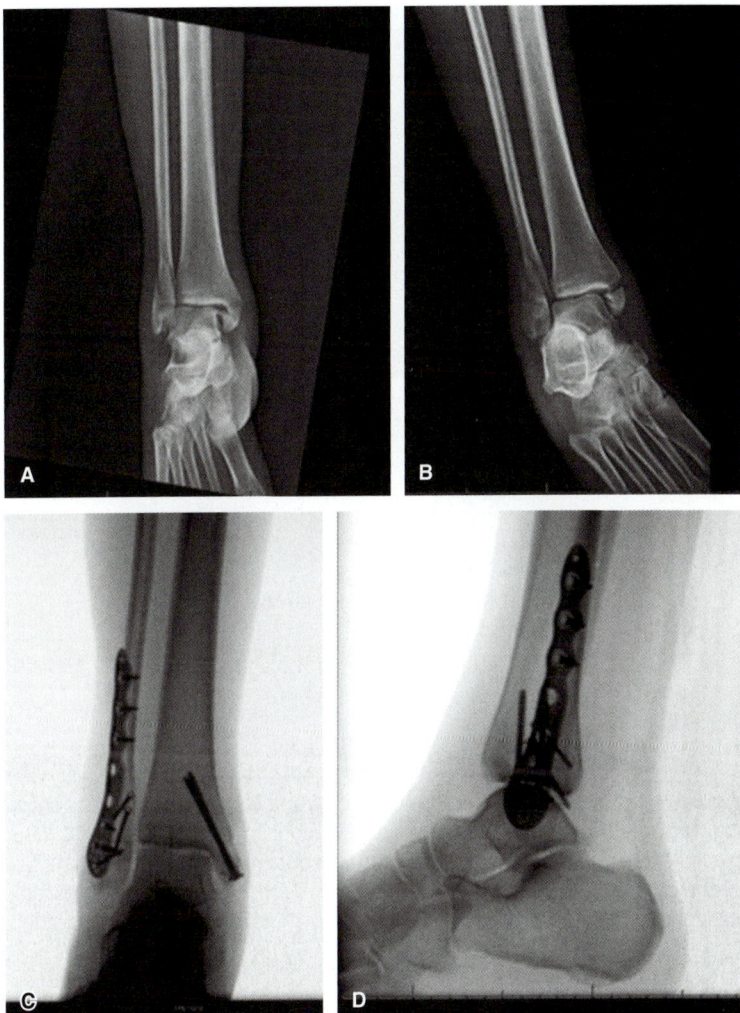

Figure 43 Bimalleolar fracture. Injury radiographs showing spiral distal fibula fracture (**A**) and transverse medial malleolus fracture (**B**). **C** and **D**, Mortise and lateral views, respectively, after open reduction and internal fixation of bimalleolar ankle fracture.

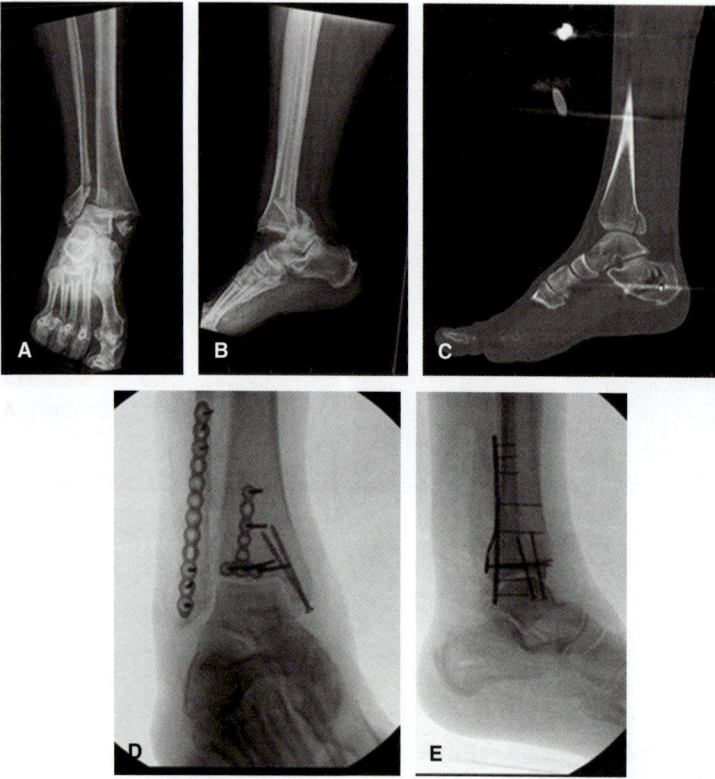

Figure 44 Trimalleolar fracture-dislocation. **A** and **B**, Injury radiographs showing fractures of the lateral, medial, and posterior malleolus fracture. **C**, After placement in an external fixator, CT scan was obtained, which showed the size of the posterior malleolus fracture. **D** and **E**, Mortise and lateral fluoroscopic images after open reduction internal fixation of trimalleolar fracture dislocation.

- Surgical technique
  - Lateral approach—Fixation of the fibula and/or syndesmosis
    - Supine position
    - Incision at or slightly posterior to the fibula
    - Watch out for the superficial peroneal nerve
    - Able to assess the syndesmosis and stabilize the fibula fracture

Chapter 3: I Fell and Cannot Get Up—Lower Extremity Trauma

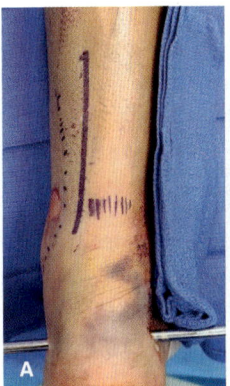 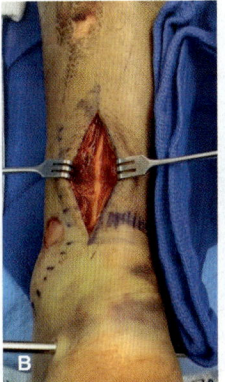 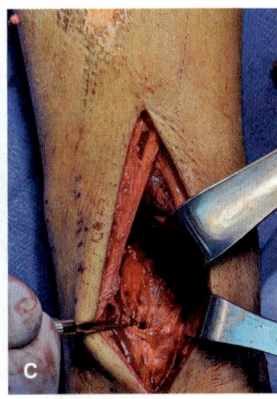

Figure 45 Intraoperative photographs showing posterolateral approach. **A**, Skin incision. **B**, Sural nerve. **C**, Posterior malleolus fragment.

- Posterolateral approach (**Figure 45**)
  - Patient is placed prone.
  - Incision is between the posterior fibula and the Achilles tendon.
  - Deep dissection is between the flexor hallucis longus (FHL) and the peroneal tendons.
  - Have access to the posterior malleolus and fibula through this approach.
  - Sural nerve is at risk.
- Medial approach
  - Curvilinear incision slightly anterior to the medial malleolus
  - Allows for visualization into the medial gutter and the fracture on the medial malleolus if present
  - Saphenous vein is at risk.
- External fixation
  - Stabilization of the fracture if unable to reduce in a splint
  - Allows for swelling to resolve and soft tissue rest if any open wounds, blisters, or abrasions are present before definitive fixation
  - Ankle fracture can be managed with a frame if soft tissues are not amenable to fixation or patient is unable to have definitive fixation.
  - Delta frame is most common with two tibial pins and one transcalcaneal pin.

- Fixation strategies
  - Fibula
    - Fixation with lag screw and neutralization plate
    - Bridge plate when fracture is comminuted
    - Percutaneous screw or fibular intramedullary nail—for transverse fractures
  - Syndesmosis
    - After any fixation of the ankle, the syndesmosis needs to be checked. This can be done with manual stress test, gravity stress, or the Cotton test intraoperatively. In the Cotton test, the fibula is pulled laterally to see if the tibiofibular clear space widens, which would indicate a positive test.[48,50]
    - Screw fixation with plate. Screws can traverse three or four cortices, which includes fibula and one or two cortices of the tibia. Screws are placed in a posterior to anterior angle to reduce the fibula in the groove.
    - Tightrope or suture fixation. Allows for movement of the syndesmosis.
    - Syndesmosis can be reduced with clamp and/or by dorsiflexion of the ankle.
  - Posterior malleolus
    - Percutaneous fixation with screws
    - ORIF with plate to resist shear forces
  - Medial malleolus
    - Percutaneous screws
    - ORIF with screws
    - Can place screws bicortically for increased strength
    - Antiglide plate—most common for vertical fractures
  - Goals of fixation
    - Restore length of the fibula and rotation.
    - Restore relationship of distal fibula with the talus and distal tibia.
    - Stabilize talus under the plafond with no clear space widening with stress. Medial clear space is reassessed when lateral and medial malleoli are well reduced. If medial clear space is still wide, then deltoid ligament or syndesmosis will need to be addressed. Cotton test can be used.
    - On lateral view the talus is well seated under the plafond with no subluxation.

- Fibula is seen on the posterior one-third of the distal tibia.
    - If patient has poor bone quality or other comorbidities that impedes healing, can augment fixation with syndesmotic screws or maintain external fixation.
- Postoperative care
  - Weight bearing
    - Non–weight bearing for 2 to 6 weeks depending on fracture pattern, bone quality, and patient comorbidities. Weight bearing before 2 weeks can lead to wound complications.[51]
    - Remove splint if applied by 2 weeks to start range of motion of the ankle.
    - Start weight bearing in CAM boot when appropriate.
    - Wean from CAM boot as patient progresses with physical therapy.
  - Antibiotics—24 hours if inpatient. Usually not required postoperatively
  - VTE prophylaxis—No gold standard recommendations
  - Pain regimen—Multimodal techniques, including lowest dose of opioid for shortest amount of time, cognitive therapies, regional nerve blocks, and physical therapies such as elevation and ice.[52]

Pearls and Pitfalls

- Initial malreduction of ankle fractures can lead to fracture blisters, soft-tissue complications, and cartilage damage. It is important to reduce any fracture-dislocations to restore anatomic alignment.
- Intraoperative considerations
  - Malreduction of the syndesmosis usually results from fibula being placed too posteriorly in the groove or from external rotation. Can visually inspect the groove to ensure reduction.[50]
  - Have to be careful with fixation of the posterior malleolus to maintain the PITFL attached to the posterior fragment.
  - Medial malleolus fractures commonly have soft tissue interposed in the fracture fragments that needs to be removed for adequate compression.
  - Peroneal tendons need to be protected during fixation of the fibula.
- Postoperative complications
  - Nonunion

- Infection: Increased risk in patients with soft-tissue injury, vascular disease, diabetes, and those who smoke.
- Neuropathy: Damage to superficial peroneal nerve or sural nerve can lead to numbness and tingling around the foot and ankle.
- Posttraumatic arthritis: Patients do well even though approximately 63% of patients have radiographic evidence of arthritis on radiographs.[53]

Top 10 Knowledge Drops for Your Rotation

1. Approximately 55% of all ankle fractures are isolated lateral malleolus fractures.
2. The talar dome is a trapezoid and is wider anteriorly. Therefore, foot must be dorsiflexed to properly assess the medial clear space.
3. A mortise view, which is obtained with the foot internally rotated approximately 10°, allows for assessment of the medial clear space, which should be approximately 4 mm.
4. Supination-external rotation injuries are the most common ankle fractures. A stress view must be obtained to determine stability of lateral malleolus fractures.
5. Posterior inferior tibiofibular ligament is the strongest ligament in the syndesmosis.
6. The purpose of fixation is restoration the fibular length, reduction of the syndesmosis, and restoration the medial gutter to have ankle stability.
7. Superficial peroneal nerve and sural nerve are at risk during surgical approaches.
8. Soft-tissue management is important for good outcomes. Swelling, open wounds, and blisters must be addressed or resolved before undertaking definitive fixation.
9. A period of non–weight bearing after fixation is necessary; however, early range of motion of the ankle improves outcomes and should be encouraged.
10. Patient comorbidities such as smoking, diabetes, and peripheral vascular disease can affect outcomes.

TALAR FRACTURES

With its unique anatomic features and tenuous vascular supply, the talus is considered the second largest tarsal bone (second to the calcaneus).[54] Because of significant bone density, substantial force is required to cause fracture. Most talar fractures (talar neck, body, lateral process, talar head, and posterior process fractures) result from high-energy trauma, such as motor vehicle accidents or falls from a significant height.[55,56] Although they are relatively rare and account for less than 1% of all fractures, understanding fracture pathology and optimal treatment is key to avoiding complications. Most of the talar surface is cartilage, forming multiple joints. This results in little surface area for fracture manipulation and fixation as well as an unforgiving architecture with respect to intolerance for malreduction.[55,57]

Epidemiology

- Incidence
  - Talar fractures are uncommon and are estimated to comprise up to 1% of all fractures and 3% to 6% of foot and ankle fractures.[54-59] The incidence of talar fractures is estimated to be 3.2/100,000 per year.[54] This may be an underestimation because of the limited sensitivity of plain radiographs and subsequently missed diagnoses. They are the second most common hindfoot fractures after calcaneal fractures.
- Demographics
  - Talar fractures appear to occur in patients ranging in age from early 20s to late 30s, with men being up to 7 times more likely to sustain this injury.[54,57-60] The frequency of talar injuries decreases with increasing age.
- The prevalence of talar fractures varies with anatomic location:[57,59]
  - Talar neck fractures are the most common and account for approximately 50% of these injuries.
  - Talar body fractures account for 13% to 61% of talar fractures.
  - Lateral process fractures account for up to 10.4% of talar fractures.
  - Talar head fractures are the least common type, comprising 5% to 10% of all talar fractures.

- Talar neck and body fractures are associated with calcaneal and spine fractures.[54,59]
- Snowboarding is associated with an increased incidence of lateral process fractures.[54,55,57]

Pertinent Anatomy/Pathoanatomy

- Anatomy of the talus (**Figure 46**)
- The talus is a dense weight-bearing bone that constitutes one of the three bones that make up the ankle joint, along with the tibia and fibula, and transmits force between the tibia and the foot.[54-57,60]
- The talus is anatomically divided into three parts: head, neck, and body.[56,57]
  - The body of the talus is trapezoidal. It is covered by the trochlear articular surface, which bears the most significant load per unit area. The body is wider anteriorly, which promotes ankle intrinsic stability. Inferiorly, the subtalar concave surface of the body articulates with the anterior, middle, and posterior facets of the calcaneus.
  - Anterior to the body, the neck does not possess any articular cartilage. It is roughened by ligamentous attachments and the vascular foramina. It has a varus angle of 10° to 44° and a plantarflexed neck-body angle of 5° to 50°. It deviates medially from 15° to 20°.
  - The convex talar head is dome-shaped and articulates with the navicular at the anterior aspect. It is supported by the spring ligament inferiorly, which maintains the plantar arch, the sustentaculum tali posteroinferiorly, and the deltoid ligament medially.
- The medial malleolus (distal part of the tibia) and the lateral malleolus (distal part of the fibula) are located medial and lateral to the talus, respectively.
- There are two bony processes at the talus:
  - The lateral process is wedge-shaped and articulates with the posterior facet of the calcaneus and the lateral malleolus of the fibula, which forms the lateral margin of the talofibular joint.
  - A lateral process fracture, often known as a snowboarder's fracture, is often missed and can be identified with meticulous inspection of an AP or mortise ankle radiograph.[54-57]

Chapter 3: I Fell and Cannot Get Up—Lower Extremity Trauma

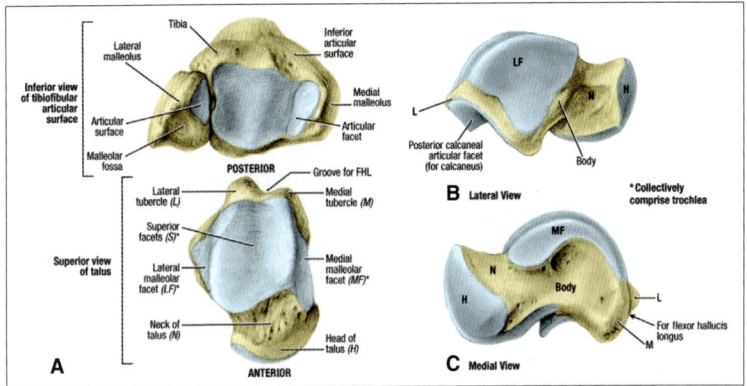

Figure 46 Illustration showing articular surfaces of ankle joint. **A**, Superior view of talus separated from distal ends of tibia and fibula. The superior articular surface of the talus is broader anteriorly than posteriorly. The fully dorsiflexed position is stable compared with the fully plantarflexed position. In plantar flexion, when the tibia and fibula articulate with the narrower posterior part of the superior articular surface of the talus, some side-to-side movement of the joint is allowed, accounting for the instability of the joint in this position. **B**, Lateral view of talus. The triangular lateral facet is for articulation with the lateral malleolus. **C**, Medial view of talus. The comma-shaped medial facet is for articulation with the medial malleolus. (Reproduced with permission from Agur AM, Dalley AF, eds: *Grant's Atlas of Anatomy*, ed 15. Wolters Kluwer, 2016, Figure 6.83.)

- The posterior process consists of a medial and lateral tubercle separated by a groove for the tendon of the FHL.
- A variation of the posterior process is the os trigonum, a bony structure that originates from a secondary ossification center at the posterior lateral tubercle. It is present in up to 50% of normal feet and is frequently mistaken for a fracture.[54-57]
- Soft tissue
  - Myotendinous units: Although many ligaments attach to the talus, it has no muscular or tendinous attachments. Ligaments and surrounding tendons provide the talus with its structural support and stability.
  - The talus is covered in 60% to 70% cartilage and articulates with adjacent bones via capsuloligamentous restraints.[54-57,60]
  - Abundant cartilage limits arterial access to some areas of the bone. Therefore, the vascular supply to the talus is

mainly extraosseous, and capsular disruptions may lead to osteonecrosis.[59,60]
- Nerves/arteries: The blood supply (**Figure 47**) to the talus is a robust antegrade supply.[55,56,60] It includes:
  - Peroneal and dorsalis pedis arteries via artery to the sinus tarsi, which supplies the head and neck
  - Posterior tibial artery via artery of the tarsal canal and via deltoid artery, both of which supply most of the talar body
  - Capsular and ligamentous vessels and intraosseous anastomoses

Pertinent History/Physical Examination Findings

- Patients typically present with a history of high-energy trauma, notably a motor vehicle accident, snowboard landing, or fall from a height.[54-58] They have often experienced polytrauma.

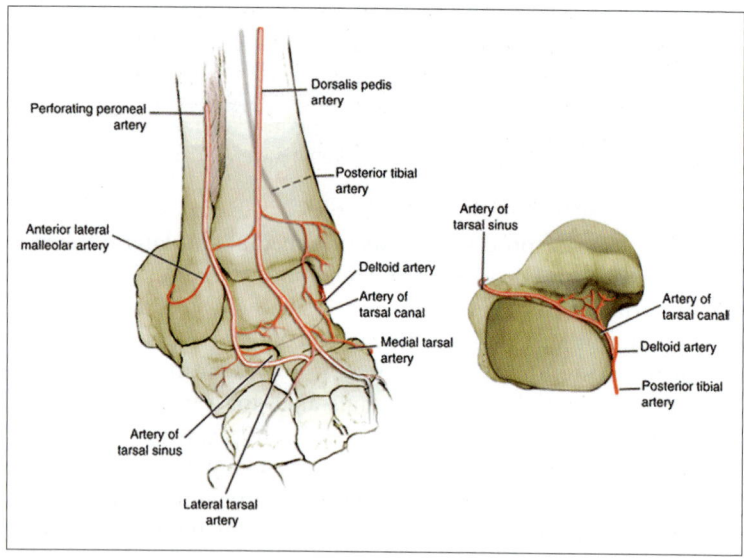

Figure 47 Illustration shows that the talus receives its blood supply from all three main arteries perfusing the foot. The posterior tibial artery is the main contributor to the talar body blood supply. (Reproduced with permission from Gardner MJ, ed: *Master Techniques in Orthopaedic Surgery: Fractures*, ed 4. Wolters Kluwer, 2021, Figure 32.1.)

Chapter 3: I Fell and Cannot Get Up—Lower Extremity Trauma

- Initial assessment should follow the ATLS protocol, prioritizing life-threatening and limb-threatening injuries.[59]
- Patients report pain with weight bearing on the affected extremity.
- On physical examination, diffuse swelling over the dorsal midfoot/midtarsal joint or talar head may be present, with associated tenderness to palpation.[56-58]
- There is painful and limited range of motion at the tibiotalar, subtalar, and midtarsal joints. Dynamic examination may also elicit crepitus.
- Diffuse swelling over the dorsal midfoot/midtarsal joint or talar head may be present, with associated tenderness to palpation.
- The nutcracker sign, known as pain and crepitus with forced plantar flexion, may suggest a fracture of the posterior process. This fracture may also be accompanied by tenderness over the posterior talus and insertion of the Achilles tendon.[54]
- Persistent lateral ankle pain following forced dorsiflexion and eversion injuries to the foot may suggest a fracture of the lateral process, although often misdiagnosed as an ankle sprain.[54,56,57]
- Pain that is worsened with flexion or extension of the FHL tendon may suggest a fracture of the posterolateral tubercle.[54,56]
- A neurovascular examination and skin assessment should always be performed as part of the musculoskeletal examination.
- If the pulses are not palpable due to swelling, evaluation with Doppler ultrasonography may be done to determine if they are present.[57,59]
- Immediate surgical consultation is required for any vascular deficit.

Relevant Imaging

- Radiographs:
  - Plain radiographs are considered the gold standard for initial screening.[54-57]
  - AP, mortise, and lateral radiographs of the ankle should be obtained (**Figure 48**).
  - AP, lateral, and oblique views of the foot should also be obtained.
  - Overpenetration of the foot may be necessary to visualize the tarsal bones adequately, although osseous detail in the forefoot may be obscured.

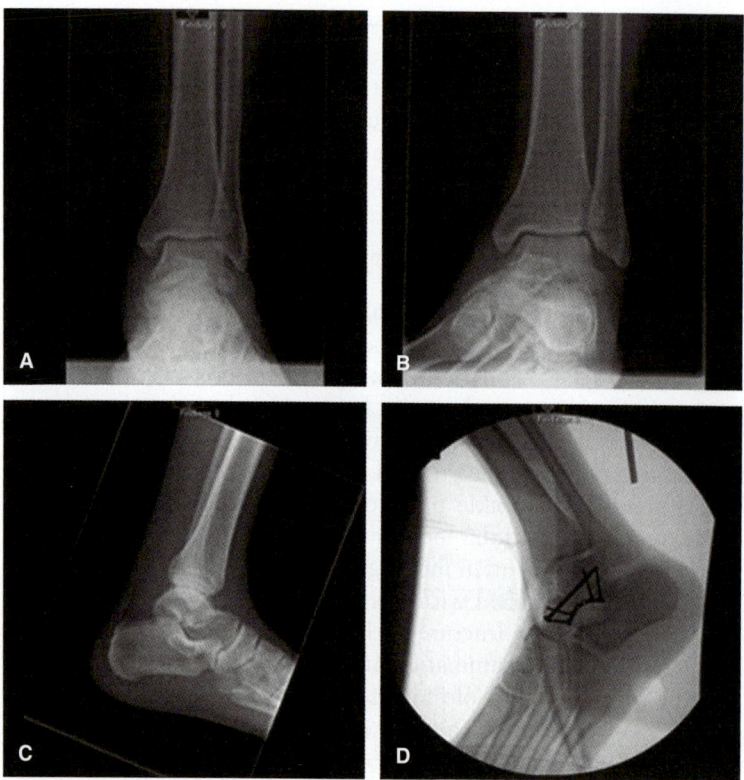

Figure 48 Plain radiographs of a left ankle with talar fracture. **A**, AP view. **B**, Mortise (oblique) view. **C**, Lateral view. **D**, Fluoroscopy, Canale view. (Courtesy of Babar Shafiq, MD, Johns Hopkins Medicine, Baltimore, Maryland.)

- The Canale view (**Figure 49**) is optimal for fractures of the talar neck, which are often oblique to the foot's sagittal plane.[54-57] This specialized view consists in maintaining the ankle in maximum equinus while placing the foot in 15° of pronation and obtaining the radiograph with an angle of 75° cephalad from horizontal.[55-57] Its use has decreased over the years because of the wide availability of CT. Currently, it is mainly used intraoperatively for assessment of reduction and implant position.[57]
- It is important not to mistake the os trigonum.

Chapter 3: I Fell and Cannot Get Up—Lower Extremity Trauma

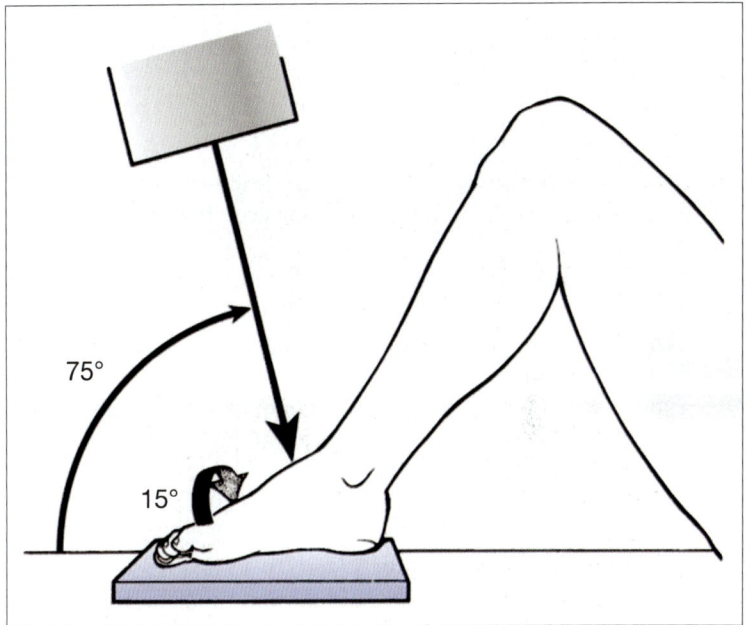

Figure 49 Illustration showing Canale view of the foot. The correct position of the foot for radiographic evaluation is shown. (Reproduced with permission from Court-Brown CM, Heckman JD, McQueen MM, Ricci WM, Tornetta P III, eds: *Rockwood and Green's Fractures in Adults*, ed 8. Wolters Kluwer, 2014, Figure 60.3.)

- It is important to always assess for a lateral process fracture, snowboarder's fracture, on AP and/or mortise views because it may sometimes be occluded.[55-57]
- The sensitivity of detecting talar fractures on plain radiographs is only approximately 74% to 78%.[55,57,60]
- CT[55-57]
  - CT may be performed if clinical suspicion remains high despite negative radiographs.
  - CT helps in making a definitive diagnosis.
  - CT is the best modality to further characterize the talar fracture, determine the degree of displacement and comminution, and gauge any articular involvement.
  - CT may also be used as an aid for surgical planning.

- MRI[57]
  - MRI is not routinely used but might be useful for diagnosis of occult talar fractures.

Talar Fractures Classification

- Anatomic classification: lateral process fractures, posterior process fractures, talar head fractures, talar neck fractures, and talar body fractures.
- Orthopaedic Trauma Association classification of talar fractures:[55]
  - Type A: extra-articular, A1: neck, A2: avulsions
  - Type B: partial articular, B1: lateral half body, B2: medial half body, B3: coronal
  - Type C: articular, C1: simple, C2: complex (multifragmentary)
- Modified Hawkins-Canale classification of talar neck fractures[55,57,58] (**Figure 50**):
  - Type I: nondisplaced with no evidence of subtalar incongruity
    - Best prognosis
    - Lowest risk of osteonecrosis (zero to 13%)
  - Type II: associated subtalar subluxation or dislocation, more often medial than lateral
    - Disruption of at least two sources of blood supply
    - Moderate risk of osteonecrosis (20% to 50%)
  - Type III: associated subtalar and ankle dislocation
    - May further injure the posterior tibial neurovascular bundle
    - All three major arterial sources to the talus are disrupted
    - Moderate to high risk of osteonecrosis (20% to 100%)
  - Type IV: Canale and Kelley—type III with associated talonavicular subluxation or dislocation
    - Disruption of all major arterial sources and head and neck blood supply
    - The highest risk of osteonecrosis (70% to 100%)

Nonsurgical Measures

- Indications
  - True nondisplaced fractures of the lateral or posterior processes, talar head, neck (Hawkins type I), or body, with no evidence of subtalar incongruity (comminution or articular step-off) as determined by CT, may be managed nonsurgically.[54-57]
  - Nondisplaced is defined as a displacement less than 2 mm.[55,56]

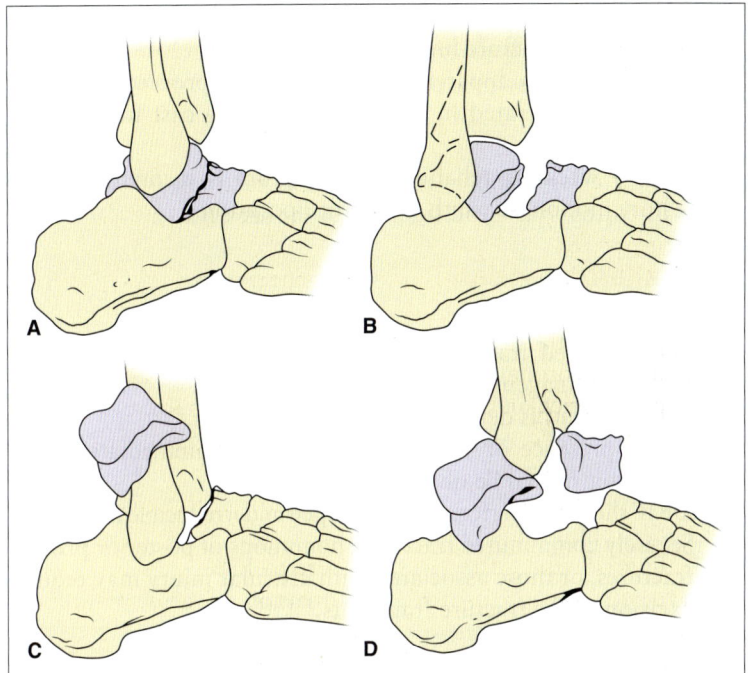

Figure 50 Illustration showing Hawkins classification of talar neck fractures. **A**, Type I, nondisplaced fracture of the talar neck. **B**, Type II, displaced talar neck fracture with subluxation or dislocation of the subtalar joint. **C**, Type III, displaced talar neck fracture with associated dislocation of the talar body from both the subtalar and tibiotalar joints. **D**, Type IV, as suggested by Canale and Kelly, displaced talar neck fracture with associated dislocation of the talar body from subtalar and tibiotalar joints and dislocation of the head and neck fragment from the talonavicular joint. (Reproduced with permission from Waters PM, Skaggs DL, Flynn JM, eds: *Rockwood and Wilkins' Fractures in Children*, ed 9. Wolters Kluwer, 2019, Figure 30.3.)

- Modalities
  - Nonsurgical management consists of a short leg cast or a removable cast boot, molded for longitudinal arch support, to be worn for 6 to 8 weeks.[54-57,61]
  - The patient should remain non–weight bearing until clinical and radiographic evidence of fracture healing is observed. This

includes the absence of tenderness over the fracture site and filling of the fracture line on radiographs.
- Once healing is apparent, the patient may proceed to weight bearing as tolerated in a short leg walking cast for 4 weeks until pain free.
- After 4 weeks, a rehabilitation program is recommended to restore motion, strength, and proprioception.[57]

Surgical Intervention

- Indications
  - For displaced fractures (including Hawkins types II to IV), optimal management is surgical.[60-62]
  - Displacement is defined as greater than 2 mm.[55,56]
  - In the presence of frank joint dislocation, immediate closed reduction should be obtained.
  - ORIF should be performed for all open and irreducible fractures.[61]
  - Severely comminuted fractures, nonunions of posterior process fractures, or those associated with articular injury may require excision of the fracture fragments.[57,61,62]
- Techniques
  - Anatomic reduction
    - Anterolateral approach: This permits visual access to the sinus tarsi, lateral neck, and comminution in the subtalar joint. Beware of inadvertent tarsal sinus artery damage.
    - Posterolateral approach: This is used for optimal access to the lateral tubercle of posterior process or body fractures. The interval is between the peroneus brevis and the FHL tendon. The FHL tendon may be displaced from its groove to ease exposure. It is essential to protect the neurovascular bundle, including the sural nerve.
    - Anteromedial approach: This is usually extended from limited capsulotomy in the anterior-posterior tibial tendon interval. Protection of the saphenous nerve and vein and deltoid artery should be ensured.
    - Posteromedial approach: This allows for the medial tubercle of the posterior process fracture to be accessed, especially when medially displaced. The interval is between the flexor digitorum longus (FDL) and the neurovascular bundle.

- Combined anterolateral and anteromedial approach (**Figure 51**): This is often used for talar neck and/or body fractures and facilitates anatomic reduction.
- ORIF
  - Interfragmentary compression screws alone or in combination with mini-fragment plates are often used.[60]
- Percutaneous wire fixation may be used for temporary stabilization until such time as swelling has resolved sufficiently to allow for ORIF.[56,57,60-62]
- Fragment excisions:[59-62]
  - Occasionally surgical excision of nonviable fracture fragments may be needed.
  - This may include small process fractures that remain symptomatic after healing has occurred and acutely for those fragments that may affect joint stability.
- Outcomes:
  - The prognosis of talar neck fractures and their risk of osteonecrosis heavily depend on displacement at the initial injury and correlate with the modified Hawkins-Canale classification.[54-57,59,60]
  - Talar body fractures have a variable prognosis, with worse outcomes associated with crush/comminuted talar body fractures.[54,55,57]
  - Talar head fractures generally have good outcomes with both surgical and nonsurgical (when indicated) treatment.[54]
- Potential complications:[54-57,59,60]
  - Posttraumatic arthritis
    - It is the most common complication and occurs in 30% to 90% of cases.[59]
    - Like osteonecrosis, it is related to the fracture type, extent of bone injury, degree of comminution, and attempts of fracture reduction.
    - Posttraumatic arthritis is most commonly subtalar or talonavicular, diagnosed via clinical examination and confirmed with radiographs.
  - Osteonecrosis (predominantly of the talar body/dome)
    - It has reduced significantly over the past few decades.
    - It is related to the fracture type and displacement, degree of comminution, extent of soft-tissue injury, and success of surgical reduction.

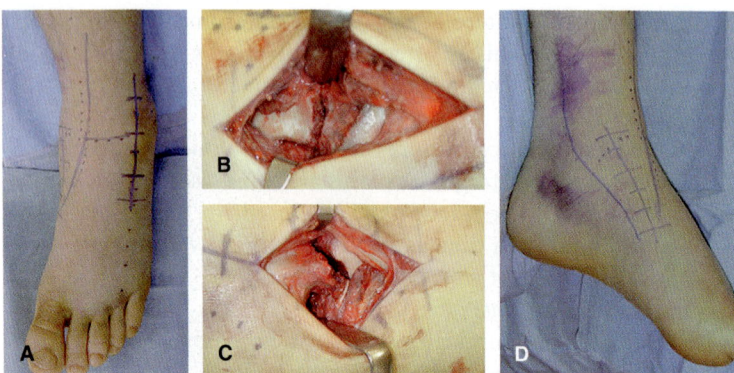

Figure 51 **A**, Photograph showing anteromedial approach to the talus. **B**, Intraoperative photograph showing anteromedial dissection to the talar neck. **C**, Intraoperative photograph showing anterolateral dissection to the talar neck. **D**, Photograph showing anterolateral approach to the talus. (Panels A, C, and D reproduced with permission from Vallier HA, Nork SE, Benirschke SK, et al: Surgical treatment of talar body fractures. *J Bone Joint Surg Am* 2004;86-A[suppl 1, pt 2]:180-192. Panel B adapted from Buckley R, Sands A: Anteromedial approach to the talus. AO Surgery Reference. Available at: https://surgeryreference.aofoundation.org/orthopedic-trauma/adult-trauma/talus/approach/anteromedial-approach-to-the-talus, with permission from Richard Buckley, MD.)

- Look for the Hawkins sign on AP radiographs (**Figure 52**): It is a thin linear subchondral radiolucency that tends to indicate preserved vasculature and talar viability. Hawkins sign is a positive predictive sign but may often be absent, even in well-healing fractures.
- Delayed union or malunion
  - A delayed union of more than 6 months occurs in less than 15% of cases, and malunion rates vary between 25% and 30%.[56,60]
  - It may be managed with rigid open reduction and bone grafting.
  - Clinically, chronic pain may develop from symptomatic nonunion for up to 2 years posttreatment.
  - Nonunions are rare, with reported incidence below 5%.[55]
- Infection
  - The incidence of infection is between 3% and 8%.[55]
  - Clinically, look for signs of infection (eg, edema, erythema, warmth, and systemic symptoms such as fever).

Chapter 3: I Fell and Cannot Get Up—Lower Extremity Trauma

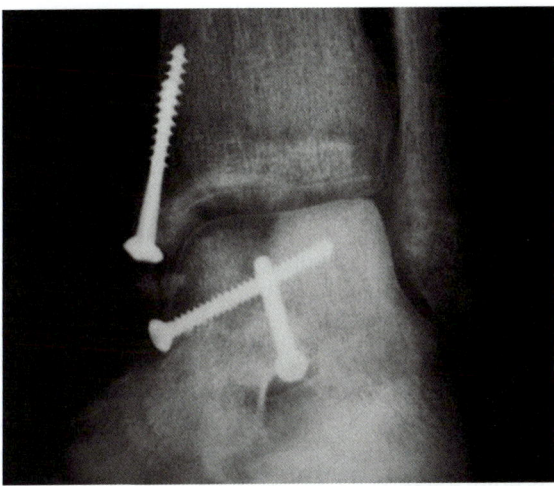

Figure 52 AP radiograph demonstrating osteonecrosis of the lateral half of the body of the talus. Notice the subchondral radiolucency (eg, Hawkins sign) in the medial half of the body of the talus. The sclerotic lateral portion of the body of the talus has evidence of osteonecrosis. (Reproduced with permission from Kitaoka H, ed: *Master Techniques in Orthopaedic Surgery: The Foot and Ankle*, ed 3. Wolters Kluwer, 2013, Figure 28.21.)

Top 10 Knowledge Drops for Your Rotation

1. The talus is the second largest tarsal bone and is also second (to calcaneal fractures) in frequency among all tarsal fractures. It is anatomically divided into three parts, head, neck, and body—neck being the most likely to fracture—and two processes, lateral and posterior.
2. There are seven articulating surfaces: the subtalar surface articulates with the anterior, middle, and posterior facets of the calcaneus; the talar head articulates with the navicular bone and sustentacular tali; and the lateral process articulates with the posterior facet of the calcaneus and the lateral malleolus of the fibula.
3. The blood supply to the talus is a robust antegrade supply: from the posterior tibial artery, dorsalis pedis artery, and perforating peroneal artery.

4. Most talar fractures result from high-energy trauma, such as motor vehicle accidents, snowboard landings, or falls from significant heights.
5. A snowboarder's fracture is a fracture of the lateral process and needs to be meticulously appraised on AP and mortise ankle radiograph to avoid a missed diagnosis.
6. Although often misdiagnosed as an ankle sprain, persistent lateral ankle pain following forced dorsiflexion and inversion injuries to the foot may suggest a fracture of the lateral process.
7. A neurovascular examination and skin condition assessment should always be performed as part of the musculoskeletal examination.
8. Although plain radiographs are considered the gold standard for initial screening, CT has higher sensitivity and may detect occult talar fractures.
9. True nondisplaced fractures (<2 mm with no evidence of subtalar incongruity) may be managed nonsurgically, whereas displaced fractures are to be treated surgically with ORIF/percutaneous fixation and/or fragment excisions.
10. The most common complications are osteonecrosis, posttraumatic arthritis, and delayed union or malunion.

CALCANEUS FRACTURES

Fractures of the calcaneus are serious injuries that often occur as a result of high-energy trauma, such as motor vehicle accidents and falls from a height. Overall, calcaneus fractures are relatively uncommon—representing just 2% of all reported fractures—although they account for 60% of all tarsal fractures.[63] Most of these injuries occur in males between 20 and 40 years of age, thus representing a significant socioeconomic burden to both the patient and society because approximately 20% are unable to return to their prior employment at 1 year postinjury.[64] Although all types of calcaneus fractures may infer morbidity on the patient, intra-articular fractures are particularly severe and therefore it is important to focus on this topic. Disability after calcaneus fracture is compounded by the high rate of concomitant injuries in this patient population, including lower extremity and spine fractures, head injuries, and thoracic organ injury.[65]

Pertinent Anatomy/Pathoanatomy

- The calcaneus supports the foot and also translates vertical load from the lower extremity horizontally into the foot.
- It articulates with two other bones: the talus (superiorly) and the cuboid (anteriorly and distally).
  - It has three important articulations (joint surfaces) on its superior surface: the anterior, middle, and posterior articular facets (**Figure 53**).
  - The smaller anterior and middle facets are usually confluent and primarily support the talar neck and head; the larger saddle-shaped posterior facet supports the talar body.
  - A small groove divides the region between the middle and posterior facets, serving as the insertion point for the inferior extensor retinaculum, the joint capsule of the posterior facet, and the interosseous ligament of the leg. These are important structures for foot and ankle stability because ligaments attach at this nonarticular space on the calcaneus.
- The sustentaculum tali is a medial projection of the calcaneus that supports the talus above and serves as a fulcrum for the FHL passing beneath it to improve its mechanical advantage in great toe dorsiflexion.
  - When placing lateral to medial screws during fixation of a sustentacular fracture, it is important to avoid placing excessively long screws into the sustentaculum because they may endanger the FDL, FHL, or posterior tibial artery, vein, and nerve. Subtalar joint penetration should also be avoided.
- The sinus tarsi is an anatomic space between the anterior facet of the calcaneus and the anterior talus that contains adipose tissue, ligaments, arterial anastomoses, and proprioceptive nerve endings.
- The peroneal tubercle also sits on the lateral wall of the calcaneus and is a bony outcropping surrounded dorsally by the peroneus brevis and plantarly by the peroneus longus.
  - Fractures in this area may entrap or cause tendinitis of the peroneal tendons as a result of fracture callus or inflammation during and after healing.

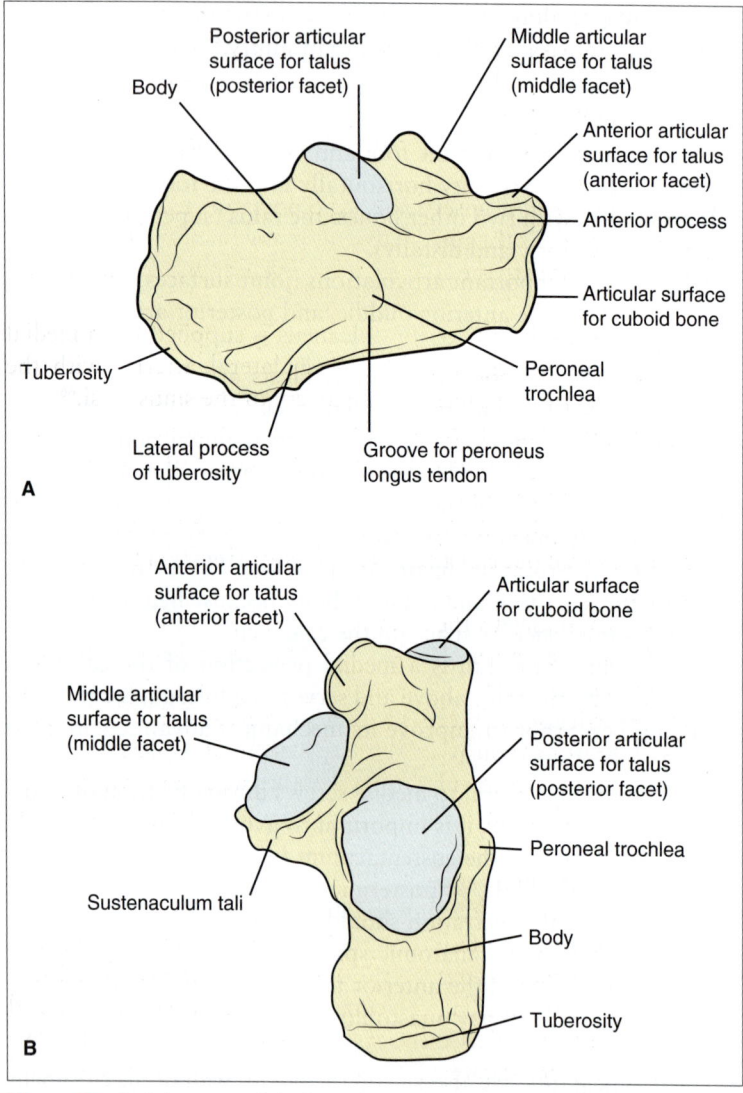

Figure 53 **A**, Schematic of the lateral anatomy of the calcaneus. **B**, Schematic of the coronal anatomy of the calcaneus at the distal level of the sustentaculum tali. (Reproduced with permission from Bucholz RW, Heckman JD, eds: *Rockwood & Green's Fractures in Adults*, ed 5. Lippincott Williams & Wilkins, 2001, Figures 49-1 and 49-4A.)

Chapter 3: I Fell and Cannot Get Up—Lower Extremity Trauma

- Peroneal tendon dislocation is a common concomitant issue, in particular with highly displaced calcaneus fractures.
- The calcaneocuboid joint is the distal articulation of the calcaneus with the cuboid.
  - This articulation provides mobility to the lateral column of the foot.
- The Achilles tendon inserts onto the posterior tuberosity of the calcaneus, as does the plantar fascia on the plantar aspect.
- The blood supply to the calcaneus is from both medial and lateral arteries.
  - Approximately 45% of the calcaneus is supplied from medial arteries of the leg, and 45% from lateral arteries with the remaining 10% supplied by the artery of the sinus tarsi.[66]
  - The medial contribution is predominantly from branches of the posterior tibial artery that supply the medial part of the posterior articulation.
  - The lateral calcaneal artery branches from the posterior tibial artery as well but can also anomalously arise from the peroneal artery.
  - Clinically, injury to the lateral calcaneal artery during the lateral extensile approach to the hindfoot may lead to ischemic soft-tissue necrosis.
  - Severe calcaneus fractures may also result in bleeding from the medial calcaneal arteries into the soft tissues, specifically the quadratus plantae, resulting in compartment syndrome of the foot. This is considered a true orthopaedic emergency.
- Calcaneus fractures occur when a supraphysiologic load is directed through the lower extremity.
- The talus is driven inferiorly into the space between the middle and posterior facets—termed the angle of Gissane (**Figure 54**)—creating an anteromedial fragment consisting of the anterior and middle facets as well as the sustentaculum tali, and a posterolateral fragment consisting of the posterior facet, lateral wall, and calcaneal tuberosity.
  - This primary fracture line develops because of the relatively lateral position of the calcaneus in relation to the axis of the tibia and talar body.

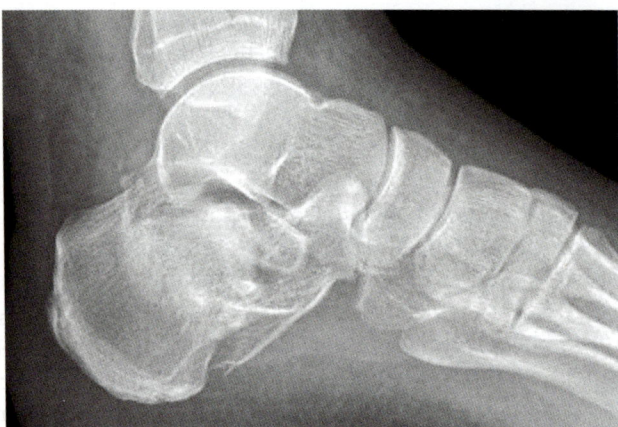

Figure 54 Radiograph showing intra-articular calcaneus fracture with increased critical angle of Gissane. (Reproduced with permission from Kim TS: Fractures of the calcaneus, in Chou LB, ed: *Orthopaedic Knowledge Update®: Foot and Ankle 6*. American Academy of Orthopaedic Surgeons, 2019, p 332, Figure 1.)

- As loading continues, additional secondary fracture lines may divide the calcaneus into as many as five main fragments with variable involvement of the articular facets.
- The sustentaculum tali makes up a large portion of the anteromedial fragment, and historically has been referred to as the constant fragment because of its relatively maintained position to the talus and ankle when fractured.
  - More recent studies have shown that there is a high rate of fractures through the sustentacular fragment and displacement, challenging the theory of constancy.[67,68]
- The posterolateral fragment often displaces laterally as the hindfoot assumes a varus position secondary to the pull of the intact Achilles tendon.
- Comminution of the lateral wall is common and may involve entrapment of the peroneal tendons.

Classification

Broadly, fractures of the calcaneus are categorized as being either intra-articular or extra-articular depending on whether they involve the subtalar joint. Although by strict definition calcaneus fractures

Chapter 3: I Fell and Cannot Get Up—Lower Extremity Trauma

involving the calcaneocuboid joint and/or middle and anterior facets could be considered intra-articular, most of them mainly involve the posterior facet. Approximately 75% of calcaneus fractures are intra-articular.

- Essex-Lopresti[69] first described the pattern of calcaneus fractures on radiographic examination in their seminal 1952 paper on the topic in which a common fracture line originating at the angle of Gissane and exiting out the medial calcaneal cortex was described.
  - The secondary fracture line further classifies the pattern into either a joint-depression or tongue-type fracture based on whether the secondary fracture line exits superiorly through the posterior tuberosity, or posteriorly through the tuberosity (**Figure 55**).
  - The posterior facet in a joint-depression type fracture is completely independent of the calcaneal tuberosity, whereas the two remain in continuity in tongue-type fractures.
  - This classification is helpful in determining whether the fracture may be treated percutaneously (tongue-type) versus with formal ORIF (joint-depression).
- The Sanders classification uses coronal CT to determine the number and position of fracture lines through the posterior articular facet[70] (**Figure 56**).

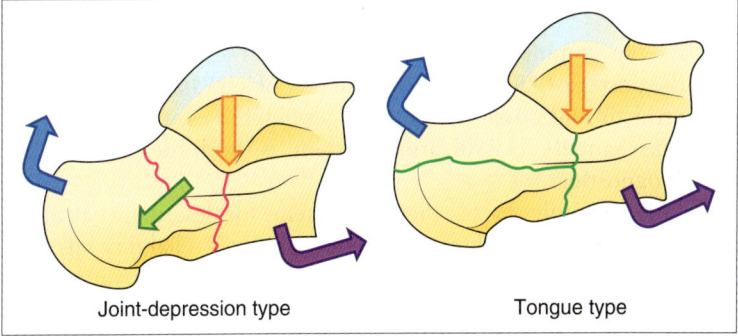

Figure 55 Illustration showing Essex-Lopresti fracture classification. (Redrawn with permission from Kwok HM, Pan NY, Ng FH: Computed tomography for calcaneal fractures: Adding value to the radiology report. *J Clin Imaging Sci* 2021;11:59.)

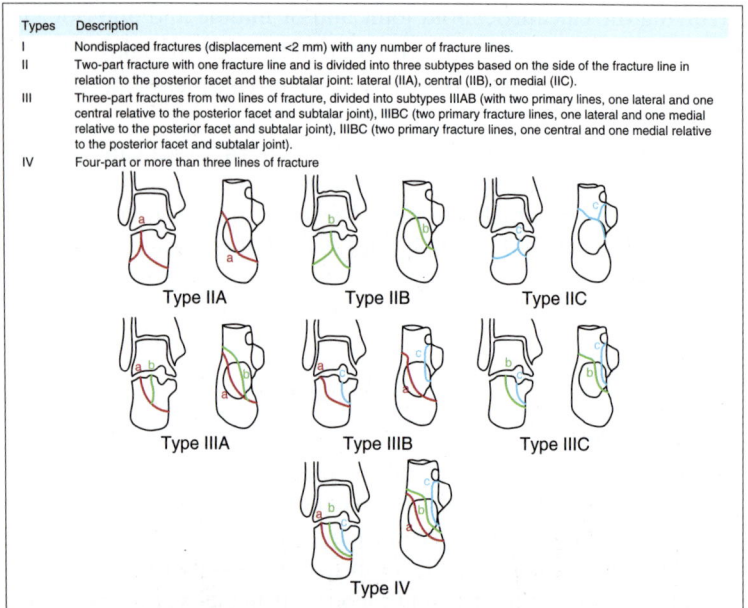

Types	Description
I	Nondisplaced fractures (displacement <2 mm) with any number of fracture lines.
II	Two-part fracture with one fracture line and is divided into three subtypes based on the side of the fracture line in relation to the posterior facet and the subtalar joint: lateral (IIA), central (IIB), or medial (IIC).
III	Three-part fractures from two lines of fracture, divided into subtypes IIIAB (with two primary lines, one lateral and one central relative to the posterior facet and subtalar joint), IIIBC (two primary fracture lines, one lateral and one medial relative to the posterior facet and subtalar joint), IIIBC (two primary fracture lines, one central and one medial relative to the posterior facet and subtalar joint).
IV	Four-part or more than three lines of fracture

Figure 56 Illustration showing Sanders fracture classification. (Redrawn with permission from Kwok HM, Pan NY, Ng FH: Computed tomography for calcaneal fractures: Adding value to the radiology report. *J Clin Imaging Sci* 2021;11:59; originally adapted from Sanders R, Fortin P, DiPasquale T, Walling A: Operative treatment in 120 displaced intraarticular calcaneal fractures. Results using a prognostic computed tomography scan classification. *Clin Orthop Relat Res* 1993;290:87-95.)

- As the comminution—or number of fracture fragments—of the posterior facet increases, the risk of subtalar posttraumatic arthritis and possible future surgery increases.
- The Sanders classification system is both descriptive and prognostic.
- Despite the multiple classification systems for describing calcaneus fractures, both interobserver and intraobserver reliability has been demonstrated to be low, making the ultimate outcomes after these injuries difficult to determine based on fracture type.[71-74]

Pertinent History and Physical Examination Findings

- Evaluation of a patient with a calcaneal fracture begins with a comprehensive history and physical examination.

- The patient's chief complaint should be elicited, as well as information regarding the mechanism of injury (high-energy versus low-energy), location of pain, presence of neurologic symptoms, complaints regarding the ipsilateral knee and hip, back pain, or pain elsewhere in the body, and any history of injury or surgery to the lower extremity.
- Other history points to cover with patients include a comprehensive past medical and surgical history, list of active medications, drug allergies, social history including profession and recreational history, ambulatory status, and smoking status.
- Examination of the patient begins with a concise and efficient orthopaedic survey.
- The upper extremities, spine, and uninjured lower extremity are palpated, gentle range of motion performed, and assessed for neurovascular status.
- Of particular importance is the assessment of the contralateral foot, ankle, and lumbosacral spine for signs of concomitant injury, which is present in 10% to 15% of patients who sustain a calcaneus fracture.
  - Careful palpation of the lumbosacral spine, both midline and paraspinal, should be undertaken and documented.
- The injured extremity is then examined in a focused manner starting at the hip and progressing distally down the extremity.
  - Skin quality should be noted, in particular evidence of any open wounds, abrasions, blisters, ecchymosis, or signs of skin threatening such as blanched, pale skin abutting gross fracture deformity (**Figure 57**).
  - The skin on the back of the heel should be independently assessed for blanching in the setting of tongue-type or calcaneal avulsion fractures, which may ultimately lead to skin necrosis if not managed emergently.
  - Any tenderness to palpation, crepitus, or gross deformity should be noted. The patient's medial and lateral malleoli, fifth metatarsal base, Lisfranc joints, and metatarsals should be gently palpated to identify additional sites of injury.
  - A thorough neurologic examination of the lower extremity including assessment of the saphenous, sural, superficial peroneal, deep peroneal, and plantar nerve distributions should be completed.

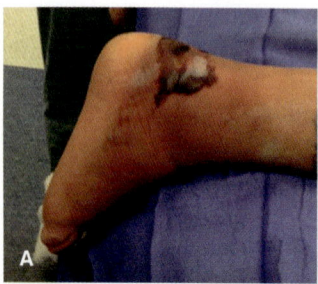 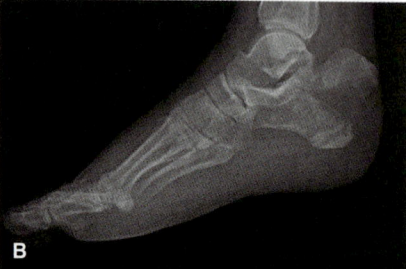

Figure 57 **A**, Photograph and **B**, radiograph show skin threatening related to calcaneus fracture. (Reproduced with permission from Chhabra N, Sherman SC, Szatkowski JP: Tongue-type calcaneus fractures: A threat to skin. *Am J Emerg Med* 2013;31[7]:1151.e3-1151.e4. Copyright © 2013 Elsevier Inc.)

- Palpation of the dorsalis pedis pulse over the dorsal, medial midfoot in the first web space as well as the posterior tibialis pulse just posterior to the medial malleolus should be performed. Capillary refill of all toes should be less than 2 seconds.
- Foot compartment syndrome should be assessed in every patient.
  - Compartment syndrome is a process whereby excessive swelling causes decreased blood flow affecting distal perfusion and can result in tissue hypoxia and necrosis.
  - Palpation of the soft-tissue compartments of the foot with pain out of proportion to the amount of palpation should raise suspicion for compartment syndrome, although this can be unreliable at times.
  - In the foot, compartment syndrome may ultimately lead to long-term problems including claw toe deformities because of necrosis of the intrinsic muscles.
  - Prompt identification of this process is necessary to initiate surgical decompression and avoid long-term sequelae.
- In situations where these fractures occur as a result of a high-energy mechanism, activation of appropriate trauma resources, including the ATLS algorithm, is necessary.
  - At a minimum, patients with high-energy mechanisms of injury should undergo a secondary and tertiary trauma survey to rule out additional injury after other orthopaedic or nonorthopaedic injuries have been temporized or managed.

Chapter 3: I Fell and Cannot Get Up—Lower Extremity Trauma

Relevant Imaging

- For patients with suspected calcaneus fractures, AP, oblique radiographs of the foot as well as AP, mortise, and lateral views of the ankle should be obtained.
- A Harris heel view radiograph is necessary to understand the varus/valgus alignment of the heel, which is performed with the foot in maximal dorsiflexion and the x-ray beam angled 30° to 40° toward the head (cephalad).
- Contralateral heel, foot, and ankle radiographs may also be useful for assessing fracture reduction and the restoration of normal anatomic relationships in the hindfoot during surgical intervention, as previous studies have shown a relative equivalence of osseous anatomy side to side.[75-77]
- For intra-articular fractures that involve the anterior, middle, or posterior facets, CT of the foot is mandatory to allow for appropriate surgical planning including understanding fracture fragment morphology, hardware positioning, and heel alignment.
- Several important radiographic relationships may help to inform both treatment decision making as well as appropriate surgical restoration of anatomy in patients with calcaneus fractures.
  - The Böhler angle, as measured on a lateral radiograph, is defined as the angle between a line drawn from the highest point of the anterior process of the calcaneus to the highest point of the posterior facet, and a line drawn tangentially to the superiormost edge of the tuberosity (**Figure 58**).

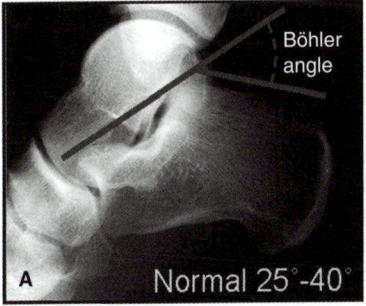 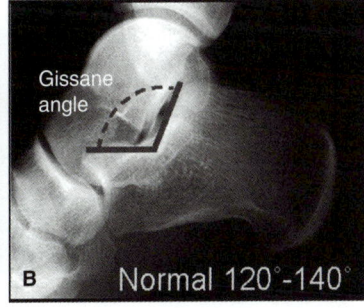

Figure 58 Radiographs showing the Böhler angle (**A**) and critical angle of Gissane (**B**). (Reproduced with permission from Swiontkowski M, ed: *Manual of Orthopaedics*, ed 8. Wolters Kluwer, 2021, Figure 28.2.)

- Normally the Böhler angle is 20° to 40°. This measurement provides an understanding of the loss of calcaneal height and joint depression.
- The critical angle of Gissane is defined as the angle between a line drawn on the dorsal surface of the posterior facet in relation to a line drawn on the dorsal surface of the anterior facet (**Figure 58**).
- This is normally assessed on a lateral foot radiograph and has a normal value between 120° and 145°, any value of which higher than that range indicates collapse of the posterior facet of the calcaneus.
  - In more subtle fractures, both the angle of Gissane and the Böhler angle may appear to be normal, making diagnosis difficult.[78]
- The double density sign refers to the appearance of a fractured posterior facet as it detaches from the sustentaculum tali, creating subtalar incongruity and indicating intra-articular involvement (**Figure 59**).
- CT is necessary to obtain preoperatively.

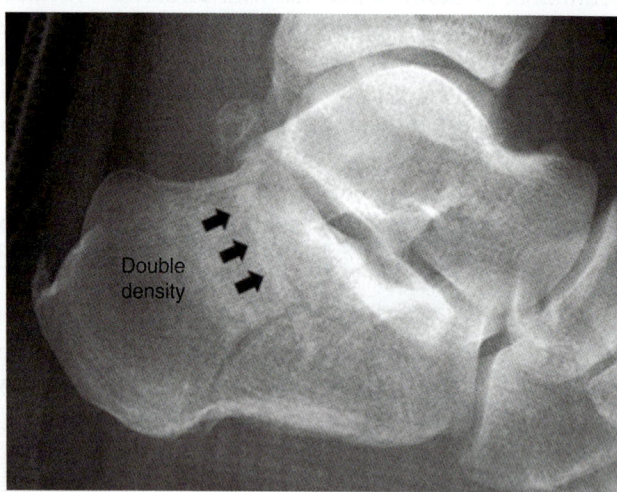

Figure 59 Lateral plain radiograph of a calcaneus fracture demonstrating a double density sign in the tuberosity. (Reproduced with permission from Easley M, ed: *Operative Techniques in Foot and Ankle Surgery*, ed 2. Wolters Kluwer, 2016, Figure 134-2.)

- CT allows for identification of occult injuries and fully elucidates the fracture morphology allowing for appropriate planning of implant needs and construct design.
- Calcaneal articular depression and shortening can both be assessed on the sagittal reformats.
- The coronal plane reformats allow for assessment of heel width, sustentacular fracture morphology, comminution, and fracture pattern evaluation—on which the Sanders classification system described earlier is based.
- Axial slices of the calcaneus provide information on medial and lateral wall comminution, as well as pathologic varus alignment of the calcaneus.
- Finally, CT provides valuable information on calcaneocuboid joint involvement as well as any peroneal tendon subluxation or dislocation that is not apparent on radiographs.
- The utility of three-dimensional reformats for surgical planning continues to be debated.[79-81]

Initial Management

The treatment of calcaneus fractures is predicated on appropriate management of the soft-tissue envelope of the foot and ensuring osseous healing in appropriate alignment.

- Skin threatening is indicated by blanching (restriction of blood flow making the skin pale) of the skin over palpable fracture fragments.
  - In cases where the skin is threatened by displaced fracture fragments or dislocation of the subtalar joint, a closed reduction maneuver should be performed to relieve pressure on the skin and prevent necrosis.
- Compartment syndrome results when severe posttraumatic swelling of the foot becomes so great that it causes collapse of the venous outflow system, increasing internal pressure within compartments of the foot bound rigidly by fascia, and eventually muscle and soft-tissue necrosis.
  - Compartment syndrome is a surgical emergency.
  - Diagnosis is made clinically with severe pain on examination of the soft tissues of the foot, as well as intracompartmental pressure measurements that show less than 30 mm Hg of difference from the diastolic blood pressure.[82]

- When closed reduction does not relieve pressure on the skin, or there is a diagnosis of compartment syndrome, the patient should be taken urgently to the operating room to prevent soft-tissue death and functional morbidity.
- In open fractures, the time from injury to antibiotic administration is the single most important factor in long-term outcomes.[83]
  - Administration of prophylactic antibiotics as well as tetanus vaccination where indicated should be completed as soon as possible.
  - Patients with open fractures should have their wounds gently irrigated with normal saline solution and dressed with a dry sterile dressing.
  - There is no evidence to support the use of high-pressure irrigation or the addition of cleansing agents to the irrigant.[26,84]
  - Patients should be taken to the operating room urgently for irrigation and débridement.
- In the absence of skin threatening or foot compartment syndrome, initial management of all calcaneus fractures should involve the placement of a well-padded bulky Jones dressing and splint.
  - A thick, soft dressing (Jones or first-aid dressing) should be applied primarily to the leg to provide excellent soft-tissue protection of the foot and ankle, over which a plaster splint is then applied (**Figure 60**).
  - Excessive compression with a compression bandage over the splint should be avoided so as to preclude damage to the skin and soft tissues.
- The patient should be encouraged to elevate the extremity with the foot above the level of the heart for the first several days after injury to decrease pain and swelling, as well as minimize risk to the soft tissues.
- The use of intermittent pneumatic pedal compression devices, known as foot pumps, has been shown to significantly reduce edema in the first 48 hours postinjury, as well as to decrease time to return to work.[85,86]
- Rarely, patients with nondisplaced or minimally displaced fractures and mild swelling may be placed into a tall walking boot to protect the extremity and allow for daily skin checks. The patient should remain non–weight bearing on the affected extremity.

Chapter 3: I Fell and Cannot Get Up—Lower Extremity Trauma

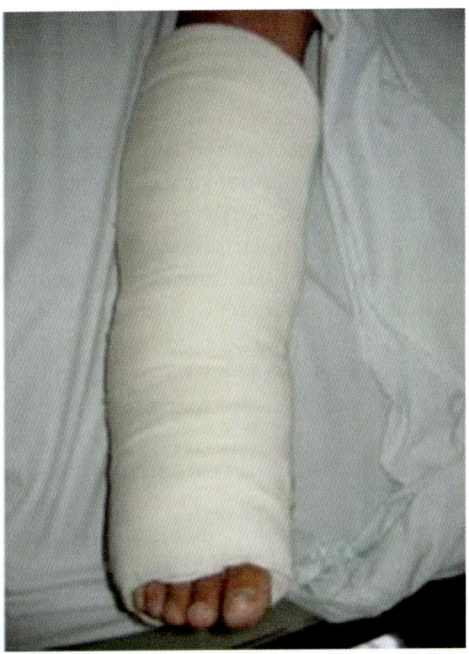

Figure 60 Photograph shows a bulky Jones splint. (Reproduced with permission from Romero ZEE, Cadenas TM, Vargas EJM, et al: Estudio comparativo de la utilidad del vendaje tipo Robert Jones y la férula en "U" en las fracturas de tobillo [Comparison between Robert Jones dressing and "U" splint in ankle fractures] [Article in Spanish]. *Acta Ortop Mex* 2008;22[1]:40-44.)

Treatment

The decision whether to treat a patient with a calcaneus fracture nonsurgically or with surgery is nuanced and depends on multiple patient factors, including fracture characteristics, age, sex, mental and medical comorbidities, profession, smoking history, and workers' compensation status.

- Most of the calcaneal fractures occur in patients between the ages of 20 and 40 years.
- Patient factors that influence treatment decision making include smoking status (smokers have been shown to have up to a 70% complication rate with surgical fixation of fractures) and mental

capacity (those who are unable to abide by non–weight-bearing restrictions postoperatively may fare better with nonsurgical treatment).[87]
- Patients with diabetes and peripheral vascular disease may also have a difficult time healing their surgical incisions and end up with an infection, making nonsurgical treatment more appropriate in some instances.
- Urgent treatment of calcaneus fractures is indicated in those cases where skin and soft-tissue threatening occurs, there is adjacent joint dislocation, or there is a diagnosis of compartment syndrome.
  - Tongue-type fractures of the posterior calcaneal tuberosity are an example of those fractures that often require urgent surgical care.
  - Up to 21% of these fractures can present with skin tenting of the posterior ankle.[88]
  - Treatment of these fractures includes urgent reduction with percutaneously placed wires, over the top of which screws are placed for definitive fixation.
  - Fracture-dislocations warrant urgent open or closed reduction and fixation with plates, screws, or wires to reduce the tension on the soft tissue as well as relieve any pressure on cartilage surfaces to prevent long-term damage and minimize the development of arthritis.
- In cases of compartment syndrome, incisions are made over the top of the major compartments of the foot to release the fascia and allow for swelling without muscle or soft-tissue compromise.
  - These incisions may be left open and then closed at a later date once the swelling has resolved, or the skin may be closed over the top of them after fascial release.
- Open calcaneus fractures should be addressed in a systematic way.
  - Appropriate initial management with antibiotics, tetanus prophylaxis, gentle irrigation, dressing, and splinting is critical in these fractures.
  - Formal irrigation and débridement with provisional fracture reduction in the operating room should occur within 24 hours of receipt of injury to prevent local complications of infection.[89]

Chapter 3: I Fell and Cannot Get Up—Lower Extremity Trauma

- All grossly necrotic tissue should be removed from the wound edges, and the skin incision extended to include the zone of injury.
- Thorough débridement with multiple liters of irrigation should then occur, as well as gentle curettage of the contaminated bone with careful attention being paid not to further strip soft tissues and devitalize bony fragments.
- After that, fixation of the bone should occur by whatever means is appropriate given the fracture type.
- Most cases should undergo temporary pinning or external fixation with definitive ORIF staged at a later date.
- If primary closure of the wound without tension on the soft tissues is possible, antibiotic prophylaxis should be implemented for 24 hours postoperatively.
- When a soft-tissue defect is present, plastic surgery should be involved for appropriate soft-tissue coverage with a flap or soft-tissue advancement within 72 hours, although there is no consensus on this.[90]
  - A vacuum dressing may be applied to the wound in the interim. Regardless, the patient should wear a short leg splint postoperatively to rest the soft-tissue and protect bony fixation.
- Stable intra-articular calcaneus fractures that are nondisplaced or extra-articular fractures that are minimally displaced may be treated nonsurgically.
  - Most commonly this entails splint or cast immobilization with non–weight-bearing activity for 6 weeks or longer based on evidence of healing on interval radiographs.
  - Physical therapy and range of motion exercises are initiated early to mitigate stiffness.
  - There have been several closed reduction methods described in the literature, although these are not routinely used.[91,92]
- Indications for surgical treatment of calcaneal fractures include open fracture, soft-tissue compromise or skin threatening, articular displacement more than 2 mm, or an unacceptable deformity as measured by hindfoot varus, the Böhler angle, or the angle of Gissane.
  - The goals of ORIF are to anatomically reduce the posterior facet and restore as normal calcaneal morphology as possible

while providing a stable fixation construct and allowing the patient to participate in early range of motion—often after several weeks of immobilization.[93]
- Surgical fixation is often delayed 10 to 14 days after injury to allow for resolution of soft-tissue swelling and the return of skin creases about the fracture site, known as the wrinkle sign, so as to avoid undue soft-tissue trauma, wound breakdown, and infection.
- However, minimally invasive surgical techniques (including use of the sinus tarsi approach) have decreased the time to surgery for management of calcaneal fractures demonstrating the benefits of early intervention.[94,95]

- Several different surgical incisions are available for the treatment of calcaneal fractures.
  - The commonly used extensile lateral approach has been described by several authors and involves an approach following the angle of the calcaneus, raising a large lateral soft-tissue flap, and using a combination of independent screws and a laterally based plate to achieve fracture fixation (**Figure 61**).
    - Although excellent visualization of the fracture is possible, a relatively high incidence (up to approximately 30%) of wound healing complications has been reported in the literature.
  - The sinus tarsi approach is a less invasive approach using a smaller incision over the lateral foot starting at the base of the fibula aimed toward the fourth metatarsal base.
    - Although this approach allows for direct access to the posterior facet, other aspects of fracture reduction have to be performed indirectly.
      - Wound healing complications have been demonstrated to be significantly lower (approximately 8% to 12%) compared with the extensile lateral approach.
  - Percutaneous fixation strategies—such as those used for the treatment of tongue-type fractures—are useful for minimizing soft-tissue insult in fractures with large pieces.
    - The use of very small incisions is beneficial for levering fractures into a reduced position and fixation with screws placed over reduction wires or independently.

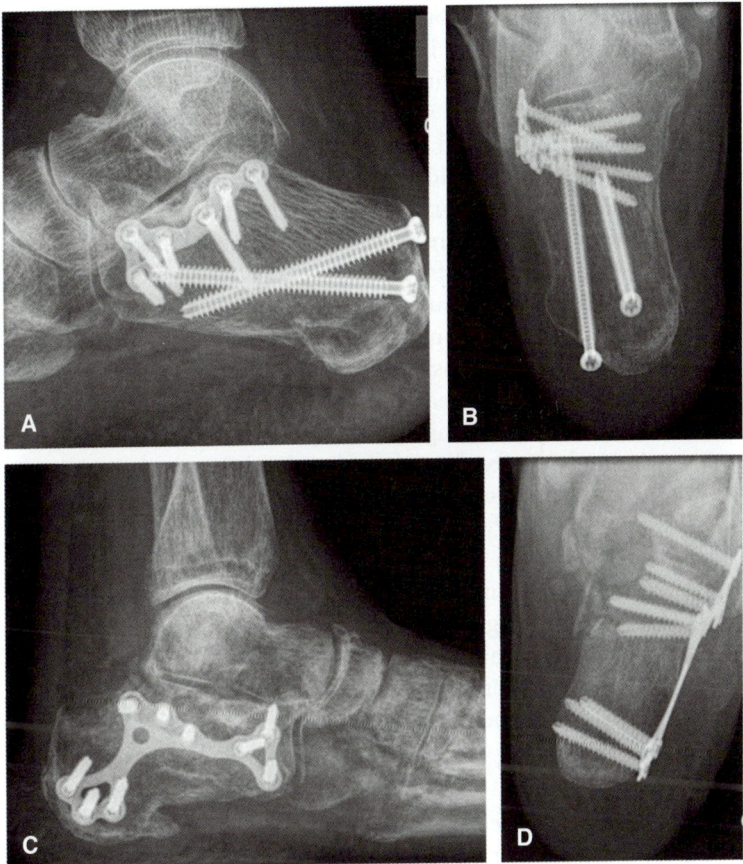

Figure 61 Radiographic examples of calcaneus fracture open reduction and internal fixation (ORIF). **A** and **B**, A tongue-type fracture ORIF. **C** and **D**, An intra-articular fracture ORIF. (Courtesy of John Y. Kwon, MD.)

- The sustentaculum piece may be fixed through a medial approach to the foot if widely displaced.
  - Patients who have concurrent peroneal tendon dislocation or injury should be treated with a repair or reconstruction of the superior peroneal retinaculum at the time of fracture fixation.

- Certain patient populations require specific attention.
  - Patients younger than 14 years have traditionally been treated nonsurgically in a splint or short leg cast for 4 to 6 weeks depending on age.
    - More recently, good outcomes have been shown in several studies in which children were treated with surgical fixation for displaced intra-articular calcaneus fractures.[96-99]
    - Based on this more recent literature, it is recommended that displaced calcaneus fractures be managed with ORIF even in the skeletally immature population.
  - Elderly patients often experience low-energy calcaneus fractures as a result of osteoporosis or a wide variety of medical comorbidities that lead to poor bone health.
  - There are data to suggest that patients older than 50 years who undergo fixation of displaced, intra-articular calcaneus fractures have outcomes similar to those of their younger counterparts.[100]
  - Despite this, in older patients with severe medical comorbidities, low functional demands, or a concurrent smoking history, nonsurgical treatment is recommended to decrease risk of complications.
  - Overall, a patient's age should not be the sole determining factor in treatment decision making.

Outcomes

- Overall, nondisplaced fractures treated nonsurgically with casting demonstrate improved patient-reported functional outcomes compared with intra-articular fractures treated surgically.[101]
- Intra-articular displaced calcaneus fractures are severe injuries, and patients tend to have fair to poor function in the short term.
- Wound healing issues, such as those related to the lateral extensile approach, are a common complication of open treatment of severe calcaneus fractures.
  - Patients treated with minimally invasive approaches such as the single-incision or dual-incision sinus tarsi approach have acceptable fracture alignment and minimal rate of complications.[102]
  - There are data to suggest a higher rate of wound complications in patients treated surgically for calcaneus fractures who

smoke, consistent with known effects of smoking on soft-tissue and bony healing in general.[103]
- Long-term outcome data of intra-articular calcaneus fractures are limited by small sample sizes.
  - Schindler et al[104] reported a complication rate of 29% at 91 months mean follow-up and advocated for the use of primary subtalar joint fusion because of a high (77%) rate of posttraumatic subtalar arthritis. They also found that the risk of nonunion for these fractures although low, was higher in smokers.
  - Potter and Nunley[105] reported that patients who sustained a calcaneus fracture as a result of a motor vehicle accident had worse patient-reported outcomes compared with those who were injured as the result of a fall with a median 12 years of follow-up.
  - Restoration of the normal bony anatomy and minimization of soft-tissue trauma are of paramount importance in improving long-term outcomes.
- Although many relative contraindications for surgery exist, patients who undergo successfully ORIF restoring the articular surface and correcting deformity while avoiding wound-healing complications fare better than those undergoing nonsurgical treatment.

Top 10 Knowledge Drops for Your Rotation

1. Fractures of the calcaneus are severe injuries with significant personal and societal cost and consequences.
2. Patients can have concurrent orthopaedic injuries that should not be missed (eg, bilateral calcaneal fractures or lumbosacral spine injuries).
3. Appropriate workup begins with a thorough history and physical examination including palpation of the spine, evaluation of the contralateral foot and ankle, and close inspection of the skin to determine if there are any blanching, open wounds, or skin threatening such as in tongue-type fractures.
4. Three-view radiographs of the foot and ankle are necessary for proper evaluation. Advanced imaging in the form of CT is often required for fracture assessment and surgical planning.

5. Initial management of calcaneus fractures includes immobilization in a well-padded Jones splint, rigorous elevation, and monitoring of the skin.
6. Optimal treatment is based on fracture morphology—amount of articular and fragment displacement, soft-tissue status, and patient factors such as medical comorbidities and smoking status.
7. Surgical fixation is best performed when soft-tissue swelling has resolved (eg, positive wrinkle test), although earlier surgery using minimally invasive approaches has been demonstrated to be relatively safe.
8. Hindfoot stiffness is near ubiquitous after calcaneus fracture. Subtalar joint arthritis is common after intra-articular injuries, although less so if patients undergo surgical treatment.
9. Lateral extensile approach for calcaneal fractures has high risk of wound complications.
10. Restoration of posterior facet height can reduce risk loss of talar declination and anterior ankle impingement.

References

1. Grotz MR, Allami MK, Harwood P, Pape HC, Krettek C, Giannoudis PV: Open pelvic fractures: Epidemiology, current concepts of management and outcome. *Injury* 2005;36(1):1-13.
2. Shlamovitz GZ, Mower WR, Bergman J, et al: How (un)useful is the pelvic ring stability examination in diagnosing mechanically unstable pelvic fractures in blunt trauma patients? *J Trauma* 2009;66(3):815-820.
3. Bruce B, Reilly M, Sims S: OTA highlight paper predicting future displacement of nonoperatively managed lateral compression sacral fractures: Can it be done? *J Orthop Trauma* 2011;25(9):523-527.
4. Gaski GE, Manson TT, Castillo RC, Slobogean GP, O'Toole RV: Nonoperative treatment of intermediate severity lateral compression type 1 pelvic ring injuries with minimally displaced complete sacral fracture. *J Orthop Trauma* 2014;28(12):674-680.
5. Dwyer EP, Moed BR: Venous thromboembolism after hospital discharge in pelvic and acetabular fracture patients treated operatively. *J Orthop Surg (Hong Kong)* 2019;27(1):2309499019832815.
6. Kokubo Y, Oki H, Sugita D, et al: Functional outcome of patients with unstable pelvic ring fracture. *J Orthop Surg (Hong Kong)* 2017;25(1):2309499016684322.
7. Veronese N, Maggi S: Epidemiology and social costs of hip fracture. *Injury* 2018;49(8):1458-1460.

8. Papadimitriou N, Tsilidis KK, Orfanos P, et al: Burden of hip fracture using disability-adjusted life-years: A pooled analysis of prospective cohorts in the CHANCES consortium. *Lancet Public Health* 2017;2(5):e239-e246.

9. Hefley FG Jr, Nelson CL, Puskarich-May CL: Effect of delayed admission to the hospital on the preoperative prevalence of deep-vein thrombosis associated with fractures about the hip. *J Bone Joint Surg Am* 1996;78(4):581-583.

10. Zahn HR, Skinner JA, Porteous MJ: The preoperative prevalence of deep vein thrombosis in patients with femoral neck fractures and delayed operation. *Injury* 1999;30(9):605-607.

11. Kim SJ, Ahn J, Kim HK, Kim JH: Is magnetic resonance imaging necessary in isolated greater trochanter fracture? A systemic review and pooled analysis. *BMC Musculoskelet Disord* 2015;16:395.

12. Tay E: Hip fractures in the elderly: Operative versus nonoperative management. *Singapore Med J* 2016;57(4):178-181.

13. Taha ME, Audigé L, Siegel G, Renner N: Factors predicting secondary displacement after non-operative treatment of undisplaced femoral neck fractures. *Arch Orthop Trauma Surg* 2015;135(2):243-249.

14. Lindequist S, Törnkvist H: Quality of reduction and cortical screw support in femoral neck fractures. An analysis of 72 fractures with a new computerized measuring method. *J Orthop Trauma* 1995;9(3):215-221.

15. Shannon SF, Yuan BJ, Cross WW III, et al: Short versus long cephalomedullary nails for pertrochanteric hip fractures: A randomized prospective study. *J Orthop Trauma* 2019;33(10):480-486.

16. Dyer SM, Crotty M, Fairhall N, et al: A critical review of the long-term disability outcomes following hip fracture. *BMC Geriatr* 2016;16(1):158.

17. Honkonen SE: Indications for surgical treatment of tibial condyle fractures. *Clin Orthop Relat Res* 1994;302:199-205.

18. Gardner MJ, Yacoubian S, Geller D, et al: Prediction of soft-tissue injuries in Schatzker II tibial plateau fractures based on measurements of plain radiographs. *J Trauma* 2006;60(2):319-323.

19. Sohn HS, Yoon YC, Cho JW, Cho WT, Oh CW, Oh JK: Incidence and fracture morphology of posterolateral fragments in lateral and bicondylar tibial plateau fractures. *J Orthop Trauma* 2015;29(2):91-97.

20. Stark E, Stucken C, Trainer G, Tornetta P III: Compartment syndrome in Schatzker type VI plateau fractures and medial condylar fracture-dislocations treated with temporary external fixation. *J Orthop Trauma* 2009;23(7):502-506.

21. Marsh JL, Buckwalter J, Gelberman R, et al: Articular fractures: Does an anatomic reduction really change the result? *J Bone Joint Surg Am* 2002;84(7):1259-1271.

22. Shuler FD, Dietz MJ: Physicians' ability to manually detect isolated elevations in leg intracompartmental pressure. *J Bone Joint Surg Am* 2010;92(2):361-367.
23. Stuermer EK, Stuermer KM: Tibial shaft fracture and ankle joint injury. *J Orthop Trauma* 2008;22(2):107-112.
24. Pollak AN, Jones AL, Castillo RC, Bosse MJ, MacKenzie EJ, LEAP Study Group: The relationship between time to surgical debridement and incidence of infection after open high-energy lower extremity trauma. *J Bone Joint Surg Am* 2010;92(1):7-15.
25. Gustilo RB, Anderson JT: Prevention of infection in the treatment of one thousand and twenty-five open fractures of long bones: Retrospective and prospective analyses. *J Bone Joint Surg Am* 1976;58(4):453-458.
26. FLOW Investigators, Bhandari M, Jeray KJ, et al: A trial of wound irrigation in the initial management of open fracture wounds. *N Engl J Med* 2015;373(27):2629-2641.
27. Finkemeier CG, Schmidt AH, Kyle RF, Templeman DC, Varecka TF: A prospective, randomized study of intramedullary nails inserted with and without reaming for the treatment of open and closed fractures of the tibial shaft. *J Orthop Trauma* 2000;14(3):187-193.
28. Avilucea FR, Triantafillou K, Whiting PS, Perez EA, Mir HR: Suprapatellar intramedullary nail technique lowers rate of malalignment of distal tibia fractures. *J Orthop Trauma* 2016;30(10):557-560.
29. Keating JF, O'Brien PI, Blachut PA, Meek RN, Broekhuyse HM: Reamed interlocking intramedullary nailing of open fractures of the tibia. *Clin Orthop Relat Res* 1997;338:182-191.
30. Pfeffer GB, Easley ME, Hintermann B, Sands AK, Younger AS: *Operative Techniques: Foot and Ankle Surgery E-Book*. Elsevier Health Sciences, 2017.
31. Middleton SD, Guy P, Roffey DM, Broekhuyse HM, O'Brien PJ, Lefaivre KA: Long-term trajectory of recovery following pilon fracture fixation. *J Orthop Trauma* 2022;36(6):e250-e254.
32. Tornetta P III, Gorup J: Axial computed tomography of pilon fractures. *Clin Orthop Relat Res* 1996;(323):273-276.
33. Carter TH, Duckworth AD, Oliver WM, Molyneux SG, Amin AK, White TO: Open reduction and internal fixation of distal tibial pilon fractures. *JBJS Essent Surg Tech* 2019;9(3):e29.
34. Shah KN, Johnson JP, O'Donnell SW, Gil JA, Born CT, Hayda RA: External fixation in the emergency department for pilon and unstable ankle fractures. *J Am Acad Orthop Surg* 2019;27(12):e577-e584.
35. Hebert-Davies J, Kleweno CP, Nork SE: Contemporary strategies in pilon fixation. *J Orthop Trauma* 2020;34(suppl 1):S14-S20.
36. Kottmeier SA, Madison RD: Pilon fracture: Preventing complications. *J Am Acad Orthop Surg* 2018;26(18):640-651.

37. Marsh JL, Weigel DP, Dirschl DR: Tibial plafond fractures: How do these ankles function over time? *J Bone Joint Surg* 2003;85(2):287-295.
38. Moracia-Ochagavía I, Rodríguez-Merchán EC: Lisfranc fracture-dislocations: Current management. *EFORT Open Rev* 2019;4(7):430-444.
39. Watson TS, Shurnas PS, Denker J: Treatment of lisfranc joint injury: Current concepts. *Am Acad Orthop Surg* 2010;18(12):718-728.
40. Welck MJ, Zinchenko R, Rudge B: Lisfranc injuries. *Injury* 2015;46:536-541.
41. Stødle AH, Hvaal KH, Enger M, Brøgger H, Madsen JE, Ellingsen Husebye E: Lisfranc injuries: Incidence, mechanisms of injury and predictors of instability. *Foot Ankle Surg* 2020;26:535-540.
42. Myerson MS, Fisher RT, Burgess AR, Kenzora JE: Fracture-dislocations of the tarsometatarsal joints: End results correlated with pathology and treatment. *Foot Ankle* 1986;6:225-242.
43. Weatherford BM, Anderson JG, Bohay DR: FACS. Management of tarsometatarsal joint injuries. *J Am Acad Orthop Surg* 2017;25(7):469-479.
44. Sripanich Y, Weinberg MW, Krähenbühl N et al: Imaging in Lisfranc injury: A systematic literature review. *Skeletal Radiol* 2020;49:31-53.
45. Alcelik I, Fenton C, Hannant G, et al: A systematic review and meta-analysis of the treatment of acute Lisfranc injuries: Open reduction and internal fixation versus primary arthrodesis. *Foot Ankle Surg* 2019;26:299-307.
46. Elsoe R, Ostgaard SE, Larsen P: Population-based epidemiology of 9767 ankle fractures. *Foot Ankle Surg* 2018;24(1):34-39.
47. Egol K, Koval K, Zuckerman J: Injuries about the ankle, in *Handbook of Fractures*, ed 6. Wolters Kluwer, 2020.
48. Aiyer AA, Zachwieja EC, Lawrie CM, Kaplan JRM: Management of isolated lateral malleolus fractures. *J Am Acad Orthop Surg* 2019;27(2):50-59.
49. Asp R, Marsland D, Elliot RR: The superficial peroneal nerve: A review of its anatomy and surgical relevance. *OA Anat* 2014;2(1):6.
50. Osborn PM: Ankle fractures, in Ricci WM, Ostrum RF, eds: *Orthopaedic Knowledge Update: Trauma 5*. American Academy of Orthopaedic Surgeons, 2016, pp 563-574.
51. Sernandez H, Riehl J, Fogel J: Do early weight-bearing and range of motion affect outcomes in operatively treated ankle fractures: A systematic review and meta-analysis. *J Orthop Trauma* 2021;35(8):408-413.
52. Hsu JR, Mir H, Wally MK, Wally RB, Orthopaedic Trauma Association Musculoskeletal Pain Task Force: Clinical practice guidelines for pain management in acute musculoskeletal injury. *J Orthop Trauma* 2019;33(5):e158-e182.

53. Regan DK, Gould S, Manoli A III, Egol KA: Outcomes over a decade after a surgery for unstable ankle fractures: Functional recovery seen 1 year postoperatively does not decay with time. *J Orthop Trauma* 2016;30(7):e236-e241.
54. Russell TG, Byerly DW: *Talus fracture*, in *StatPearls [Internet]*. StatPearls Publishing, 2022. [Updated 2022 May 29]. Available at: https://www.ncbi.nlm.nih.gov/books/NBK539687/.
55. Al-Jabri T, Muthian S, Wong K, Charalambides C: Talus fractures: All I need to know. *Injury* 2021;52(11):3192-3199.
56. Aiyer A, Moore DW: *Talus Fracture (Other Than Neck)*. Orthobullets, 2021. Available at: https://www.orthobullets.com/trauma/1049/talus-fracture-other-than-neck. Accessed September 26, 2022.
57. Koehler SM: *Talus Fractures*. UpToDate, 2022. Available at: https://www.uptodate.com/contents/talus-fractures#H97922985.
58. Vosoughi AR, Fereidooni R, Shirzadi S, Zomorodian SA, Hoveidaei AH: Different patterns and characteristics of Talar injuries at two main orthopedic trauma centers in Shiraz, south of Iran. *BMC Musculoskelet Disord* 2021;22(1):609.
59. Shamrock AG, Byerly DW: *Talar neck fractures*, in *StatPearls [Internet]*. StatPearls Publishing, 2022. [Updated May 2, 2022]. Available at: https://www.ncbi.nlm.nih.gov/books/NBK542315/.
60. Schwartz AM, Runge WO, Hsu AR, Bariteau JT: Fractures of the talus: Current concepts. *Foot Ankle Orthop* 2020;5(1):2473011419900766.
61. Lee C, Brodke D, Perdue PW Jr, Patel T: Talus fractures: Evaluation and treatment. *J Am Acad Orthop Surg* 2020;28(20):e878-e887.
62. Githens M, Tangtiphaiboontana J, Carlock K, Campbell ST: Talus fractures: An update on current concepts in surgical management. *J Am Acad Orthop Surg* 2022;30(15):e1015-e1024.
63. O'Connell F, Mital MA, Rowe CR: Evaluation of modern management of fractures of the os calcis. *Clin Orthop Relat Res* 1972;83:214-223.
64. Tanke GM: Fractures of the calcaneus. A review of the literature together with some observations on methods of treatment. *Acta Chir Scand* 1982;505:1-103.
65. Bohl DD, Ondeck NT, Samuel AM, et al: Demographics, mechanisms of injury, and concurrent injuries associated with calcaneus fractures: A study of 14,516 patients in the American College of Surgeons National Trauma Data Bank. *Foot Ankle Spec* 2017;10(5):402-410.
66. Andermahr J, Helling HJ, Rehm KE, Koebke Z: The vascularization of the os calcaneum and the clinical consequences. *Clin Orthop Relat Res* 1999;363:212-218.
67. Gitajn IL, Abousayed M, Toussaint RJ, Ting B, Jin J, Kwon JY: Anatomic alignment and integrity of the sustentaculum tali in intra-articular

calcaneal fractures: Is the sustentaculum tali truly constant? *J Bone Joint Surg Am* 2014;96(12):1000-1005.
68. Berberian W, Sood A, Karanfilian B, Najarian R, Lin S, Liporace F: Displacement of the sustentacular fragment in intra-articular calcaneal fractures. *J Bone Joint Surg Am* 2013;95(11):995-1000.
69. Essex-Lopresti P: The mechanism, reduction technique, and results in fractures of the os calcis. *Br J Surg* 1952;39:395-419.
70. Sanders R, Fortin P, DiPasquale T, Walling A: Operative treatment in 120 displaced intra-articular calcaneal fractures. Results using a prognostic computed tomography scan classification. *Clin Orthop Relat Res* 1993;290:87-95.
71. Sayed-Noor AS, Agren PH, Wretenberg P: Interobserver reliability and intraobserver reproducibility of three radiological classification systems for intra-articular calcaneal fractures. *Foot Ankle Int* 2011;32(9):861-866.
72. Schepers T, van Lieshout EM, Ginai AZ, Mulder PG, Heetveld MJ, Patka P: Calcaneal fracture classification: A comparative study. *J Foot Ankle Surg* 2009;48(2):156-162.
73. Howells NR, Hughes AW, Jackson M, Atkins RM, Livingstone JA: Interobserver and intraobserver reliability assessment of calcaneal fracture classification systems. *J Foot Ankle Surg* 2014;53(1):47-51.
74. Rubino R, Valderrabano V, Sutter PM, Regazzoni P: Prognostic value of four classifications of calcaneal fractures. *Foot Ankle Int* 2009;30(3):229-238.
75. Sengodan VC, Amruth KH, Karthikeyan: Bohler's and Gissane angles in the Indian population. *J Clin Imaging Sci* 2012;2:77.
76. Willmott H, Stanton J, Southgate C: Böhler's angle—what is normal in the uninjured British population? *Foot Ankle Surg* 2012;18(3):187-189.
77. Khoshhal KI, Ibrahim AF, Al-Nakshabandi NA, Zamzam MM, Al-Boukai AA, Zamzami MM: Böhler's and Gissane's angles of the calcaneus in the Saudi population. *Saudi Med J* 2004;25(12):1967-1970.
78. Kim DH, Berkowitz MJ: Double density sign variant in fracture-dislocation of the calcaneus: Clinical tip. *Foot Ankle Int* 2012;33(6):524-525.
79. Adler SJ, Vannier MW, Gilula LA: Three-dimensional computed tomography of the foot: Optimizing the image. *Comput Med Imaging Graph* 1988;12:59-66.
80. Vannier MW, Hildebolt CF, Gilula LA, et al: Calcaneal and pelvic fractures: Diagnostic evaluation by three-dimensional computed tomography scans. *J Digit Imaging* 1991;4:143-152.
81. Brunner A, Heeren N, Albrecht F, Hahn M, Ulmar B, Babst R: Effect of three-dimensional computed tomography reconstructions on reliability. *Foot Ankle Int* 2012;33(9):727-733.

82. Frink M, Hildebrand F, Krettek C, Brand J, Hankemeier S: Compartment syndrome of the lower leg and foot. *Clin Orthop Relat Res* 2010;468(4):940-950.
83. Patzakis MJ, Wilkins J: Factors influencing infection rate in open fracture wounds. *Clin Orthop Relat Res* 1989;243:36-40.
84. Crowley DJ, Kanakaris NK, Giannoudis PV: Irrigation of the wounds in open fractures. *J Bone Joint Surg Br* 2007;89(5):580-585.
85. Erdmann MW, Richardson J, Templeton J: Os calcis fractures: A randomized trial comparing conservative treatment with impulse compression of the foot. *Injury* 1992;23(5):305-307.
86. Thordarson DB, Greene N, Shepherd L, Perlman M: Facilitating edema resolution with a foot pump after calcaneus fracture. *J Orthop Trauma* 1999;13(1):43-46.
87. Assous M, Bhamra MS: Should Os calcis fractures in smokers be fixed? A review of 40 patients. *Injury* 2001;32:631-632.
88. Gardner MJ, Nork SE, Barei DP, Kramer PA, Sangeorzan BJ, Benirschke SK: Secondary soft tissue compromise in tongue-type calcaneus fractures. *J Orthop Trauma* 2008;22(7):439-445.
89. Srour M, Inaba K, Okoye O, et al: Prospective evaluation of treatment of open fractures: Effect of time to irrigation and debridement. *JAMA Surg* 2015;150(4):332-336.
90. Zeiderman MR, Pu LLQ: Contemporary approach to soft-tissue reconstruction of the lower extremity after trauma. *Burns Trauma* 2021;9:tkab024.
91. Cotton F, Henderson FF: Results of fractures of the os calcis. *Am J Orthop Surg* 1916;14:290-298.
92. Omoto H, Nakamura K: Method for manual reduction of displaced intra-articular fracture of the calcaneus: Technique, indications and limitations. *Foot Ankle Int* 2001;22:874-879.
93. Böhler L: Diagnosis, pathology, and treatment of fractures of the os calcis. *J Bone Joint Surg* 1931;13:75-89.
94. Joseph NM, Benedick A, McMellen C, et al: Acute fixation of displaced intra-articular calcaneus fractures is safe using the sinus tarsi approach. *J Orthop Trauma* 2021;35(6):289-295.
95. Kwon JY, Guss D, Lin DE, et al: Effect of delay to definitive surgical fixation on wound complications in the treatment of closed, intra-articular calcaneus fractures. *Foot Ankle Int* 2015;36(5):508-517.
96. Pickle A, Benaroch TE, Guy P, Harvey EJ: Clinical outcome of pediatric calcaneal fractures treated with open reduction and internal fixation. *J Pediatr Orthop* 2004;24(2):178-180.
97. Dudda M, Kruppa C, Geßmann J, Seybold D, Schildhauer TA: Pediatric and adolescent intra-articular fractures of the calcaneus. *Orthop Rev (Pavia)* 2013;5(2):82-85.

98. Summers H, Ann Kramer P, Benirschke SK: Pediatric calcaneal fractures. *Orthop Rev (Pavia)* 2009;1(1):e9.
99. Petit CJ, Lee BM, Kasser JR, Kocher MS: Operative treatment of intraarticular calcaneal fractures in the pediatric population. *J Pediatr Orthop* 2007;27(8):856-862.
100. Gaskill T, Schweitzer K, Nunley J: Comparison of surgical outcomes of intra-articular calcaneal fractures by age. *J Bone Joint Surg Am* 2010;92(18):2884-2889.
101. Pflüger P, Zyskowski M, Greve F, Kirchhoff C, Biberthaler P, Crönlein M: Patient-reported outcome following operative and conservative treatment of calcaneal fractures: A retrospective analysis of 79 patients at short- to midterm follow-up. *Front Surg* 2021;8:620964.
102. Daws SB, Neary K, Lundeen G: Short-term radiographic outcomes of calcaneus fractures treated with 2-incision, minimally invasive approach. *Foot Ankle Int* 2019;40(9):1060-1067.
103. Davey MS, Staunton P, Lambert LA, Davey MG, Walsh JC: Evaluating short-term outcomes post-intra-articular calcaneal fracture fixation via a sinus tarsi approach in a non-exclusively selected cohort. *J Foot Ankle Surg* 2021;60(2):302-306.
104. Schindler C, Schirm A, Zdravkovic V, Potocnik P, Jost B, Toepfer A: Outcomes of intra-articular calcaneal fractures: Surgical treatment of 114 consecutive cases at a maximum care trauma center. *BMC Musculoskelet Disord* 2021;22(1):234.
105. Potter MQ, Nunley JA: Long-term functional outcomes after operative treatment for intra-articular fractures of the calcaneus. *J Bone Joint Surg Am* 2009;91(8):1854-1860.

4. I Fell and Cannot Use My Upper Extremity

Robert Z. Tashjian, MD, FAAOS
Nicole S. Schroeder, MD, FAAOS

SHOULDER INJURIES

Introduction

Upper extremity trauma is common after both isolated low-energy falls and high-energy injuries. Diagnosis and management of upper extremity trauma relies on an understanding of common injury patterns and the patients at risk for these injuries. Injuries are typically distributed by anatomic location first—shoulder, humerus, elbow, forearm, wrist, and hand. Within these anatomic regions, injuries are commonly divided into bony (fractures or fracture/dislocations) and soft-tissue injuries (ligament injuries). Age and energy level are useful in subdividing the types of common bony and soft-tissue injuries, which are then further subdivided based on history, physical examination, and imaging. It is important to review anatomy, presentation, and management of common upper extremity trauma of the arm and forearm, including pearls in both diagnosis and treatment.

Clavicle Fractures

- *Epidemiology*
  - 2% to 10% of all adult trauma
  - More common in young patients

Dr. Tashjian or an immediate family member has received royalties from Shoulder Innovations, Wright Medical Technology, Inc., and Zimmer; serves as a paid consultant to or is an employee of Cayenne Medical and Mitek; and has stock or stock options held in Conextions, Intrafuse, and Kator. Dr. Schroeder or an immediate family member serves as a paid consultant to or is an employee of Aiviva Pharmaceuticals.

- More than two-thirds midshaft
- Most patients treated without surgery; most heal without consequence
- Nonunion rate less than 1%; risk factors for poor healing including fracture displacement, age, smoking, comminution; nonunion rates reported as high as 60% if associated with these comorbidities

- *Pertinent Anatomy/Pathoanatomy*
  - S-shaped with anteromedial and posterolateral apex; tubular midportion
  - Close to brachial plexus and subclavian vessels
  - Deltoid, trapezius, and platysma overlie clavicle
  - Sternoclavicular and costoclavicular ligaments medially stabilize sternoclavicular joint; acromioclavicular and coracoclavicular ligaments (trapezoid [lateral] and conoid [medial]) stabilize the acromioclavicular joint
- *Pertinent History/Physical Examination Findings*
  - Mechanism of injury—fall on lateral shoulder
  - Evaluate skin for open wounds, full neurovascular examination
- *Relevant Imaging*
  - Standard radiographs include AP radiograph of clavicle and an AP view with 20° cephalic tilt
  - Examine radiograph for location (medial, middle, lateral)
  - Measure displacement and shortening; document Z-deformity (**Figure 1**)
- *Nonsurgical Measures*
  - Can be considered for most fractures independent of displacement and comminution
  - Sling for pain—discontinue when pain is tolerable
  - Physical therapy for range of motion and strengthening
  - Return to all activity at approximately 3 months after injury when fracture is radiographically healed and there is no tenderness at the fracture site
- *Surgical Intervention*
  - Indications—displaced, shortened fractures with high risk for nonunion (approximately 20 mm)
  - Nonunion rates can be calculated based on published series using age, sex, displacement, comminution, and smoking status as potential variables affecting the development of nonunion

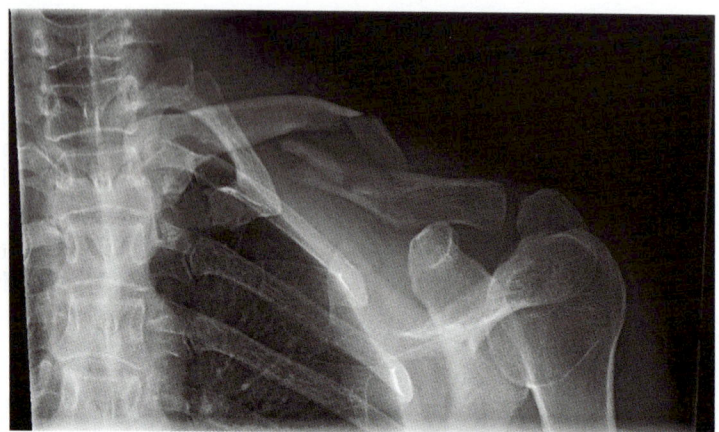

Figure 1 AP radiograph showing displaced, comminuted midshaft clavicle fracture with Z-deformity.

- Open reduction and internal fixation (ORIF)—standard method for surgical repair; performed using a plate-and-screw construct (**Figure 2**) or intramedullary nail
- Many series and meta-analyses have compared nonsurgical versus surgical treatment for midshaft clavicle fractures.
- Surgery reduces the nonunion rate, shortens the length of time to union, and potentially improves outcomes, although outcome

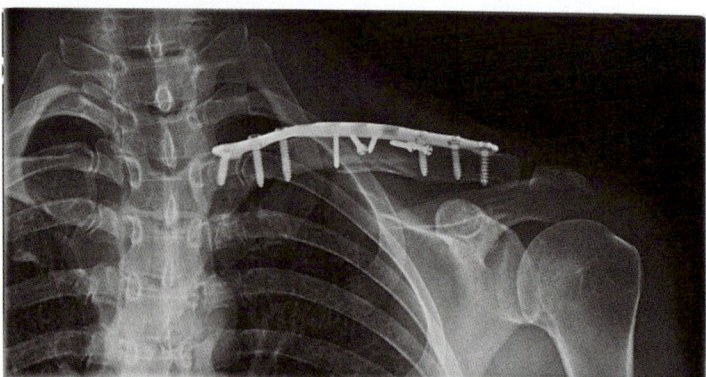

Figure 2 AP radiograph showing open reduction and internal fixation of midshaft clavicle fracture using interfragmentary lag screws and a superiorly positioned neutralization plate.

improvements in some series have not reached the minimal clinically important difference for the outcome measures.
- A meta-analysis compared surgical and nonsurgical management of midshaft clavicle fractures.
  - Time to union was 5 weeks shorter with surgical treatment.
  - The complication rate including reinterventions was higher in the surgical versus nonsurgical group, 31% versus 20%.
  - Surgical treatment provides statistically superior function over the long term although the differences do not reach clinical importance.[1]

Proximal Humerus Fractures

- *Epidemiology*
  - Third most common fracture following hip and distal radius fractures
  - 5% of all fractures
  - More common in elderly patients, although young patients can sustain these injuries due to high-energy trauma
- *Pertinent Anatomy/Pathoanatomy*
  - The proximal humerus has four parts—head, lesser and greater tuberosities, and the shaft
  - Articulates with the scapula at the glenohumeral joint
  - Supported by rotator cuff muscles attaching to the tuberosities taking origin from scapula
  - Supraspinatus, infraspinatus, and teres minor attach to the greater tuberosity and the subscapularis attaches to the lesser tuberosity
  - Suprascapular nerve innervates the supraspinatus and infraspinatus
  - Subscapular nerve innervates the subscapularis
  - The axillary nerve innervates the teres minor
    - The deltoid originates from the scapula and attaches to the humerus; the pull of the rotator cuff displaces the greater tuberosity posterior and superior and the lesser tuberosity medially, whereas the deltoid and pectoralis displace the shaft proximal and anterior.
    - The anterior and posterior humeral circumflex arteries provide most of the blood supply to the humerus, and injury during fracture can lead to osteonecrosis.

- *Pertinent History/Physical Examination Findings*
  - Mechanism of injury—fall onto the outstretched arm or a direct blow
  - Skin needs evaluation for open wounds
  - Full neurovascular examination should be performed for possible penetrating injury of the fracture into the neurovascular structures
  - The distal joints and bone of the arm should be evaluated for injury as well
- *Relevant Imaging*
  - Four radiographic views of the shoulder should be performed to evaluate fracture displacement.
  - Fracture classification is based on parts as described by Neer.
    - Displacement is considered greater than 1 cm or 45° of angulation where greater tuberosity fractures are considered displaced with greater than 0.5 cm of displacement.
    - Fractures can be classified as two-part (greater or lesser tuberosity isolated fractures, surgical neck fractures), three-part, or four-part (varus/classic or valgus) injuries.
    - Management is determined by displacement, angulation, age of the patient, and activity level.
    - CT can be helpful to determine displacement and fracture classification (**Figure 3**).
- *Nonsurgical Measures*
  - Nonsurgical treatment is considered for all nondisplaced fractures and some displaced fractures in elderly patients with low physical demands or functional goals.
    - Sling use is typically for 4 weeks, initiating motion at 2 to 3 weeks once the fracture starts to stabilize.
    - Nonsurgical management is contraindicated in fracture-dislocations.
- *Surgical Intervention*
  - Surgical treatment is considered for displaced fractures in young patients or selective displaced fractures or fracture-dislocations in elderly patients.
  - Surgical options include ORIF with locking plate constructs, intramedullary nail fixation for some surgical neck fractures, arthroscopic assisted or suture/suture anchor repair constructs for greater tuberosity fractures, and shoulder arthroplasty

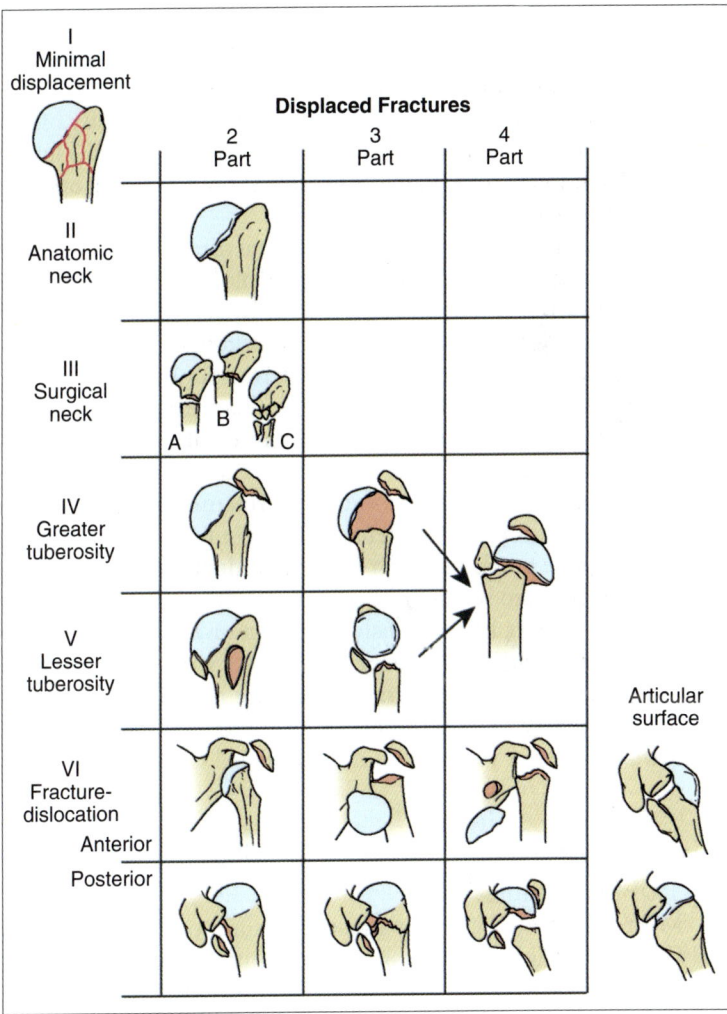

Figure 3 Diagram showing the Neer classification of proximal humerus fractures. (Reproduced from Jones CB: Proximal humeral fractures, in Boyer MI, ed: *AAOS Comprehensive Orthopaedic Review*, ed 2. American Academy of Orthopaedic Surgeons, 2014, p 295.)

(hemiarthroplasty or reverse total shoulder arthroplasty [RTSA]) for select three-part, four-part, and fracture-dislocations depending on fracture displacement, patient age, activity level, and the presence of preexisting pathology either arthritis or rotator cuff dysfunction.
- Two-part displaced (>0.5 cm) greater tuberosity fractures should be considered for ORIF with a suture/suture anchor, screw (cannulated or solid), or plate; either open or arthroscopic.
- Two-part displaced surgical neck fractures of the shoulder be considered for ORIF with either plate or intramedullary nail fixation if patients have high physical demands or are age 65 to 70 years with good bone stock.
- Displaced three-part and four-part fractures in younger patients (younger than 60 to 65 years) with severe destruction of the humeral head should be considered for hemiarthroplasty or RTSA.
- Displaced three-part and four-part fractures should be considered for RTSA in patients older than 65 to 70 years with poor bone stock but high functional demands as outcomes have shown to be superior compared with ORIF.[2] Three-part and four-part fracture-dislocations in young (younger than 60 to 65 years) higher demand patients with severe destruction of the articular surface should be managed with hemiarthroplasty, whereas similar injuries in older patients (older than 60 to 65 years) should be managed with RTSA.

Humeral Shaft Fractures

- *Epidemiology*
  - 3% of all fractures
  - Most occur in elderly patients because of falls, although younger patients can sustain the injuries because of high-energy or penetrating trauma
- *Pertinent Anatomy/Pathoanatomy*
  - The humeral shaft extends from the proximal aspect of the pectoralis major to the supracondylar ridge. There are three borders and three surfaces of the humeral shaft, including the anterolateral, anteromedial, and posterior surfaces.

Chapter 4: I Fell and Cannot Use My Upper Extremity

- The radial nerve exists from the posterior compartment into the anterior compartment through the intermuscular septum 10 to 14 cm proximal to the lateral epicondyle.
- The nerve is directly in contact with the humeral shaft for about 6.5 cm on the posterior surface of the humeral shaft within the spiral groove.
- *Pertinent History/Physical Examination Findings*
  - Secondary to low-energy falls or high-energy multitrauma
  - Osteoporosis of the humerus often a precursor to injury
  - An examination of the entire upper extremity including joints above and below as well as a neurovascular examination is required.
- *Relevant Imaging*
  - Standard two-view humeral shaft radiographs are sufficient.
  - Images of joints above and below should be performed.
  - Injuries are classified as proximal third, middle third, and distal third fractures, which assists in determining the approach for fixation if required (proximal third—anterior and anterolateral, middle third—anterolateral or posterior, distal third—posterior) (**Figure 4**).
  - Fracture location can assist in understanding the success of nonsurgical treatment—proximal third fractures are more predisposed toward nonunion and distal third fractures are more predisposed toward an inability to control the fracture alignment with nonsurgical treatment.
- *Nonsurgical Measures*
  - Most can be managed without surgery.
  - Arm is placed in coaptation splint then transitioned to fracture brace.
  - Sling is useful to assist with comfort and may be discarded after several weeks once the arm becomes less painful.
  - Range of motion of the shoulder and elbow is started as soon as pain allows therapy.
  - Fracture brace is continued until healing, which is typically 12 to 14 weeks.
  - Middle third fractures that maintain alignment in the brace (<20° sagittal deformity, <30° varus or valgus deformity, less than 2 to 3 cm of shortening) are reasonable for nonsurgical

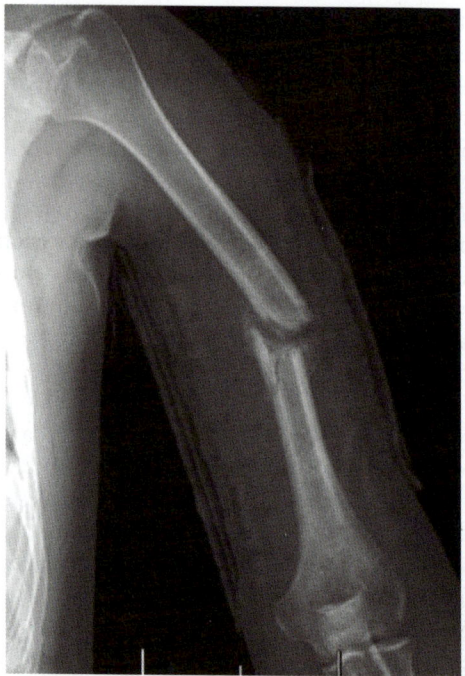

Figure 4 AP radiograph showing midshaft displaced humeral shaft fracture.

treatment and have a high rate of union (90%) and a low rate of malunion (<5%).
- Distal third fractures frequently require surgical treatment as they are difficult to maintain alignment.
- Radial nerve palsy can occur with humeral shaft fractures—10% of cases with higher incidence in distal third (Holstein-Lewis) fracture patterns. Management of radial nerve palsies should be expectant even in cases of new-onset palsy after closed reduction as long as there is not gapping on the radiographs at the fracture site.
- Relative indications for open exploration include new-onset palsy after closed reduction with gapping at the fracture site and open injuries (including gunshot wounds) requiring open reduction and fixation.

- *Surgical Intervention*
  - Surgical treatment is reserved for fractures that cannot maintain alignment with nonsurgical treatment as well as cases of multitrauma with lower extremity fractures, intra-articular extension, vascular compromise, open injuries, bilateral injuries, ipsilateral elbow or forearm fractures, and possibly segmental injuries.
  - ORIF with a long, broad dynamic compression plate with four screw holes above and four screw holes below is standard management for these injuries and is associated with high healing rates and low complication rates either through an anterolateral approach of Henry or a posterior approach depending on the location of the injury and surgeon preference (**Figure 5**).
  - ORIF has clinical results comparable to nonsurgical treatment with equivalent time to healing but improved union rates.[3]

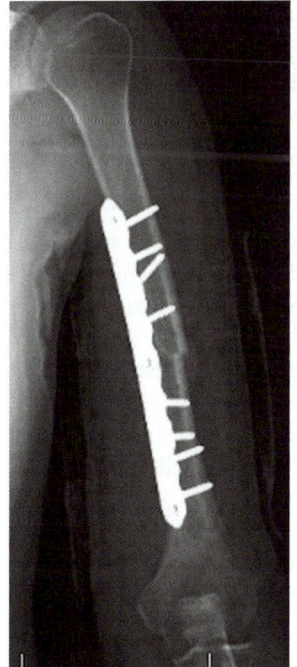

Figure 5 AP radiograph showing open reduction and internal fixation of a displaced midshaft humeral fracture with a broad 4.5-mm limited dynamic compression plate.

- Intramedullary nailing is also a reasonable approach although it has been reported to have a high rate of complications, including ipsilateral shoulder or elbow pain depending on the location of entry as well as nonunion.
- Infection rates have been reported as higher with plating versus nailing.
- Radial nerve injury rates are comparable between techniques.
- In cases of nailing, there needs to be no gapping at the fracture site, which may represent incarceration of soft-tissue and neurologic structures and during open reduction there cannot be excessive retraction on the neurologic structures.

Glenohumeral Dislocations

- *Epidemiology*
  - Anterior instability is the most common form of shoulder instability often due to a collision or fall on outstretched abducted externally rotated arm.
  - The incidence of anterior dislocations requiring closed reduction is approximately 23 of 100,000 person-years. It is three times more frequent in men and higher in younger patients.
  - Recurrent instability requiring surgery ranges between <5% and >80% depending on age, activity level, and collision or contact sports, amount of hyperlaxity, bony involvement of the humerus or glenoid, and history of prior dislocations.
- *Pertinent Anatomy/Pathoanatomy*
  - The glenohumeral joint relies on bony and soft-tissue stabilizers. The native retroversion of the glenoid provides stability.
    - Soft-tissue stabilizers include the rotator cuff, ligaments, and labrum.
    - The ligaments and labrum provide the greatest stability at end range.
    - The anterior-inferior capsule and the anterior band of the of the inferior glenohumeral ligament are the primary ligament stabilizers for anterior dislocations.
    - The labrum is the insertion site of the ligaments.
  - Instability results from labral detachment anteriorly combined with ligament stretch and/or ligament avulsion from the humerus. The labral injury may be associated with an injury to the anterior glenoid as well, creating a bony Bankart lesion.

- Impression fractures of the humeral head, Hill-Sachs lesions, are common as a result of the humeral head impacting on the glenoid during dislocation but only result in residual instability with larger sized lesions.
- *Pertinent History/Physical Examination Findings*
  - Patients present with a history of anterior shoulder instability and often pain with dislocations.
    - The history should include the mechanism of injury, which is typically a trauma in the abducted externally rotated position.
  - On physical examination, joint hypermobility should be assessed including a sulcus sign of the shoulder.
    - Anterior instability should be assessed with anterior apprehension and relocation test.
    - Anterior and posterior drawer tests as well as active compression test should be performed to evaluate the anterior, posterior, and superior labrum, respectively.
- *Relevant Imaging*
  - Standard four-view shoulder radiographs should be performed evaluating for an anterior glenoid bony Bankart injury on the axillary radiograph or anterior subluxation and a Hill-Sachs lesion on the AP radiograph or the axillary radiograph.
  - If there is any evidence of bony injury on radiograph, CT should be performed to quantify the amount of glenoid or humeral bone loss to assist in surgical decision making (**Figure 6**).
  - If surgery is considered, MRI of the shoulder should be performed to evaluate the extent of labral tearing as well as possible injury to the rotator cuff as well as humeral-based avulsions of the glenohumeral ligaments.
- *Nonsurgical Measures*
  - Initial nonsurgical treatment includes sling wear for a period of time, activity modification, and physical therapy.
    - Physical therapy is initiated at approximately 1 week to regain motion and strength, avoiding the position at risk for re-dislocation.
  - Modified activity is warranted for the first 4 to 6 weeks postdislocation to avoid contact sports and activity placing the arm at risk for re-dislocation so that there can be return to sport as tolerated.

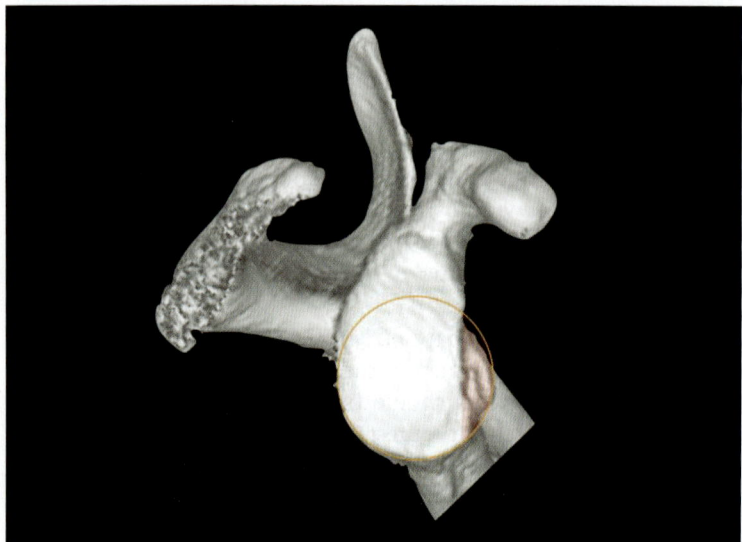

Figure 6 A three-dimensional CT scan of the glenoid; the humeral head digitally subtracted demonstrates a patient with multiple recurrences, and there is attritional bone loss of the fragment and approximately 20% of glenoid bone loss. (Reprinted from Provencher MT, Midtgaard KS, Owens BD, Tokish JM: Diagnosis and management of traumatic anterior shoulder instability. *J Am Acad Orthop Surg* 2021;29[2]:e51-e61.)

- A brace may be worn especially for in-season athletes who experience dislocation to prevent the arm from being placed into the at-risk position.
- Discussion regarding surgical intervention should include review of risks of nonsurgical management alone, which includes redislocation and potential future progressive bony, labral, and ligamentous injury that may influence the outcome of future surgical procedures versus surgical risks.
  - In patients younger than 25 years, 30% of first-time shoulder dislocations will be solitary events; between the ages 26 and 29 years this increases to 55%; between ages 30 and 33 years this increases to 70%; and between ages 34 and 40 years this increases to 80%.[4] These percentages can be useful to guide treatment.

- *Surgical Intervention*
  - Surgery is often indicated for patients with recurrent anterior shoulder instability or in cases of first-time dislocation with larger displaced bony Bankart injuries, especially when the joint is noncongruent or in specific cases of patients at high risk for recurrent instability (age younger than 20 years, contact athletes).
  - Options for surgical treatment include arthroscopic labral repair, arthroscopic labral repair plus remplissage to fill, open soft-tissue Bankart repair, or bone grafting procedures (Latarjet, iliac crest autograft, distal tibial allograft).
  - In general, indications for these surgeries are based on patient characteristics, including age and activity level, as well as anatomic variables, including extent of soft-tissue and bony injury.
  - If patients have more than 20% anterior glenoid bone loss, then a bony reconstruction procedure of the anterior glenoid is warranted, typically a Latarjet procedure.
  - More than 30% anterior glenoid bone loss often requires either iliac crest autograft or distal tibial allografting.
  - Less than 13% glenoid bone loss, a standard arthroscopic or open soft-tissue Bankart repair is often all that is required to restore stability with re-dislocation rates at 10% to 20% based on age, activity, and surgical procedure.
  - Between 13% and 20% anterior glenoid bone loss, an arthroscopic labral repair with remplissage into a medium or large-sized Hill-Sachs deformity or an open Bankart repair is often required to restore stability although some surgeons will prefer an anterior glenoid bone grafting procedure in these cases.
  - Recurrence rates for appropriately selected patients for open Bankart repair are less than 10%, which is comparable to bony reconstruction procedures although risks of bony procedures outside re-dislocation are higher including development of arthritis, prominent hardware, and neurologic injury.

Acromioclavicular Joint Separations

- *Epidemiology*
  - Most occur in young patients and result from a direct blow to the superior aspect of the adducted shoulder
  - 10% of all injuries to the shoulder girdle

- 1.8 per 100,000 individuals with 50% occurring in patients age 20 to 40 years with a 9:1 ratio of male to female patients being injured
- *Pertinent Anatomy/Pathophysiology*
  - The acromioclavicular joint is a diarthrodial joint including the distal clavicle and the medial acromion.
  - Oriented posterolateral
  - Stabilizers include the anterior and posterior acromioclavicular ligaments, the coracoclavicular ligaments including the conoid medially and the trapezoid laterally, and the deltotrapezial fascia.
  - The acromioclavicular ligaments, especially the posterosuperior capsule, resist primarily anterior and posterior translation, whereas the coracoclavicular ligaments resist superior inferior instability.
- *Pertinent History/Physical Examination Findings*
  - History of direct blow to the superior aspect of the shoulder with the arm in the adducted position
  - The skin may have abrasions.
  - There is tenderness to palpation directly over the acromioclavicular joint.
  - Deformity can be present with higher grade injuries beyond a strain (the weight of arm displaces entire shoulder girdle inferiorly; the clavicle is not superior).
  - A complete neurovascular examination and shoulder examination should be performed, looking for concomitant injuries.
- *Relevant Imaging*
  - Radiographs of the shoulder and clavicle should be performed to rule out injury.
  - Classification is based on the Rockwood classification where grade I injuries have no deformity and just tenderness, grade II injuries have less than 50% of the width of the clavicle superior translation in relation to the acromion, grade III injuries have 100% of the width of the clavicle superior translation, grade IV have posterior displacement and instability, grade V have greater than 100% superior translation, and grade VI are locked anterior dislocations under the coracoid (**Figure 7**).
  - Weighted radiographs are not required.

Chapter 4: I Fell and Cannot Use My Upper Extremity

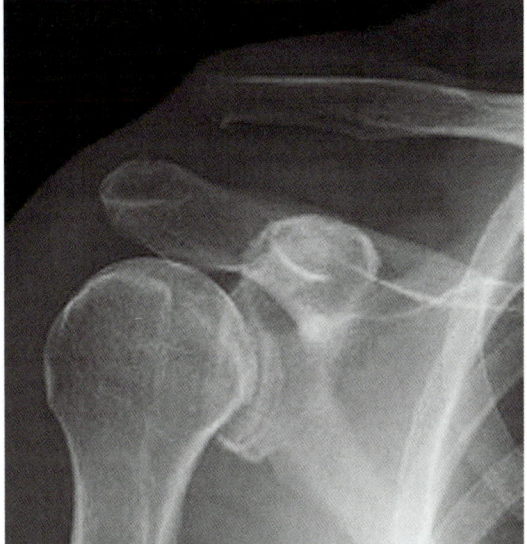

Figure 7 AP radiograph of the shoulder showing grade V acromioclavicular separation.

- *Nonsurgical Management*
  - Sling wear for 2 to 3 weeks followed by physical therapy to regain range of motion and strength
  - Avoidance of contact sports or activity where there can be direct trauma to the superior shoulder should occur for 6 weeks
  - At 6 weeks, patients are allowed to return to all activity.
  - All grade I and II injuries undergo initial nonsurgical treatment.
  - Most grade III injures should undergo nonsurgical treatment initially unless there are circumstances where the patient is of very high level of activity or sport competitively and then consideration of early repair with or without graft augmentation is reasonable.
  - Pain reduces over 2 to 3 weeks and then reevaluation of grade III injuries is the best route if there is any consideration of early surgery.
- *Surgical Treatment Intervention*
  - Surgery can be considered early for very specific grade III injuries in very high-performance athletes or those with extreme

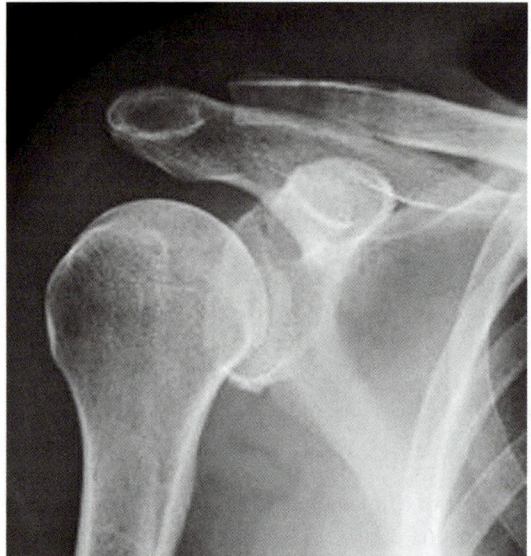

Figure 8 AP radiograph of the shoulder showing acromioclavicular joint reconstruction using hamstring allograft passed through tunnels in the clavicle and around the base of the coracoid and tied over the top of the clavicle.

demands, although most surgery is considered for grade IV, V, and VI injuries.
- Repair alone without graft augmentation using fixation between the coracoid and the clavicle can be considered if repair within 6 weeks of injuries. Otherwise, graft augmentation using either allograft or autograft is required and often should be considered even in the setting of early repair.
- Augmentation techniques vary and include fixation using interference screws or tying or sewing the graft together with going around the base of the coracoid or around the clavicle or through tunnels in the clavicle or in the coracoid. Augmentation is often backed up with suture cerclage for improved fixation (**Figure 8**).
- Acromioclavicular augmentation has been described at the same time, although it is not clear which patients would most benefit from this surgical technique.

- Borbas et al[5] performed a systematic review of repair techniques including suture fixation between the coracoid and clavicle, grafts in the same location, and the Weaver-Dunn procedure. The authors determined complication and failure rates were comparable between techniques whereas reconstruction with a graft showed superior clinical results.

Rotator Cuff Injuries

- *Epidemiology*
  - The most common cause of disability related to the shoulder
  - More than 75,000 rotator cuff repairs are performed in the United States annually.
  - Affect as many as 30% of individuals between 60 and 80 years of age and up to 50% of patients older than 80 years
  - The etiology of rotator cuff disease is unknown, although it is likely multifactorial including various intrinsic and extrinsic factors. Various factors recognized in the development of rotator cuff dysfunction include limited vascularity of the tendon, mechanical impingement on the undersurface of the acromion, and intrinsic degeneration.
- *Pertinent Anatomy/Pathoanatomy*
  - The rotator cuff consists of four muscle-tendon attachments—the supraspinatus, infraspinatus, subscapularis, and teres minor.
    - The muscles take origin from the scapula and insert onto the proximal humerus at the lesser tuberosity (subscapularis) or greater tuberosity (supraspinatus, infraspinatus, teres minor).
  - The primary role of the rotator cuff musculature is to provide dynamic stability of the glenohumeral joint through creation of a fulcrum and to provide rotational strength. The subscapularis is primarily an internal rotator; the supraspinatus assists in abduction; the infraspinatus and teres minor are primarily external rotators.
- *History and Physical Examination*
  - Patients will often describe either low-energy or high-energy mechanism of injury with either a fall on an outstretched arm or pulling or grabbing or lifting using the arm often outstretched.

- There is acute pain localized to the lateral and anterior aspect of the shoulder.
- On physical examination, resisted forward elevation in the scapular plane is often weak and painful if a supraspinatus tear is present.
  - Weakness or pain with internal or external rotation at the side would suggest a subscapularis or infraspinatus tear, respectively.
  - Often patients will have preserved elevation in small tears but with larger tears patients will have loss of active elevation.
  - Passive elevation is typically preserved.
- A neurovascular examination should be performed, especially if there is history of a concomitant shoulder dislocation.
- *Relevant Imaging*
  - Shoulder radiographs should be performed and are typically normal in the setting of a rotator cuff tear.
  - If there is concern for an acute injury based on physical examination, then MRI, ultrasonography, or CT arthrogram can be performed to evaluate the rotator cuff.
  - MRI is preferred, but if contraindicated then ultrasonography or CT arthrogram are reasonable alternatives.
    - On MRI, T2-weighted sequences are evaluated for high signal or fluid interposed between the tendon edge and the proximal humerus supporting a torn tendon (**Figure 9**).
    - The subscapularis is best visualized on the axial and sagittal sequences, whereas the supraspinatus and infraspinatus are best visualized on the coronal and sagittal images.
- *Nonsurgical Measures*
  - Nonsurgical treatment should be performed if there are no signs of full-thickness rotator cuff tear on MRI (either a rotator cuff contusion with intact tendon or a partial-thickness tear).
  - Very small full-thickness tears (<1 cm) can also be considered for nonsurgical management based on patient age, activity, and comorbidities.
  - Nonsurgical treatment consists of rest, ice, and NSAIDs followed by physical therapy for range of motion and strengthening over a 6- to 12-week period.

Chapter 4: I Fell and Cannot Use My Upper Extremity

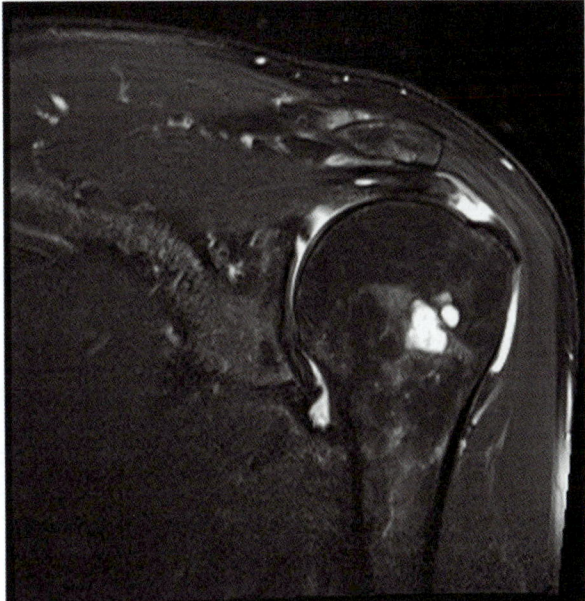

Figure 9 Coronal T2-weighted magnetic resonance sequence of the shoulder showing high signal fluid between the edge of the supraspinatus tendon and the footprint of the proximal humerus indicating a complete full-thickness rotator cuff tear.

- *Surgical Intervention*
  - Acute full-thickness traumatic rotator cuff tears should be considered for repair independent of patient age.
  - Long-term outcomes of repair compared with nonsurgical treatment in patients with small and medium-sized rotator cuff tears would support superior clinical outcomes for surgical repair compared with physical therapy.
    - Moosmayer et al[6] evaluated 103 patients randomized to rotator cuff repair versus physical therapy for small and medium-sized rotator cuff tears and determined superior clinical outcomes determined by the Constant score and American Shoulder and Elbow Surgeons Score and range of motion for the repair group.

- Surgical repair is typically performed arthroscopically using either single-row or double-row repair techniques. Large subscapularis tears can be fixed either open or arthroscopically with equivalent results.
- Postoperative outcomes after repair of acute full-thickness rotator cuff tears would support surgical repair within the first 3 to 4 months after the injury to maximize clinical outcome and likelihood for structural healing.

Top 10 Knowledge Drops for Your Rotation

1. Clavicle fractures managed with surgery have shorter time to union, higher complication rates, and statistically superior function over the long term. Most midshaft displaced clavicle fractures (less than 20 mm) can be managed without surgery, with the indication for surgery based on the chance for development of nonunion.
2. The proximal humerus has four parts: head, lesser and greater tuberosities, and the shaft, which determine classification (Neer).
3. Displacement of proximal humerus fractures is defined as >1 cm or 45° of angulation where greater tuberosity fractures are considered displaced with >0.5 cm of displacement.
4. RTSA is the preferred treatment for displaced, comminuted four-part fracture or fracture-dislocations of the proximal humerus in patients older than 70 years.
5. Middle third fractures of the humeral shaft that maintain alignment in the brace (<20° sagittal deformity, <30° varus or valgus deformity, less than 2 to 3 cm of shortening) are reasonable for nonsurgical treatment and have a high rate of union (90%) and a low rate of malunion (<5%).
6. Glenohumeral dislocations are most commonly anterior. Radiographs should be checked for Hill-Sachs lesions.
7. In patients younger than 25 years, 30% of first-time shoulder dislocations will be solitary events; between the ages of 26 and 29 years this increases to 55%; between ages 30 and 33 years this increases to 70%; and between ages 34 and 40 years this increases to 80%. These percentages can be useful to guide treatment.

8. Rockwood classification of acromioclavicular joint separations based on amount and location of displacement. Grade I injuries have no deformity and just tenderness, grade II injuries have less than 50% of the width of the clavicle superior translation in relation to the acromion, grade III injuries have 100% of the width of the clavicle superior translation, grade IV have posterior displacement and instability, grade V have greater than 100% superior translation, and grade VI are locked anterior dislocations under the coracoid.
9. The rotator cuff consists of four muscle-tendon attachments: the supraspinatus, infraspinatus, subscapularis, and teres minor. The subscapularis is primarily an internal rotator, the supraspinatus assists in abduction, the infraspinatus and teres minor are primarily external rotators.
10. Acute full-thickness rotator cuff tears of substantial size should be managed with early surgical repair (within 3 to 4 months) to maximize functional outcomes and healing.

ELBOW INJURIES

Distal Humerus Fractures

- *Epidemiology*
  - Constitute fractures distal to the supracondylar ridges. Anything proximal to the supracondylar ridges is considered a humeral shaft fracture.
  - Constitute 2% of all fractures affecting young males because of high-energy trauma as a result of commonly motor vehicle accidents or elderly female patients as a result of low-energy falls from ground level.
  - 90% of distal humerus fractures require surgical management as a result of the fracture.
- *Pertinent Anatomy/Pathoanatomy*
  - The elbow is a trochoginglymoid joint that allows rotation as well as flexion and extension.
    - There are two divergent medial and lateral columns with the trochlea between the articular surface to connect the columns.

- The trochlea is what creates bony stability of the distal humerus.
- *Pertinent History/Physical Examination Findings*
  - Typically low-energy falls in elderly patients or high-energy injuries in young patients are the inciting trauma.
  - Patients should be questioned about pain in the shoulder and wrist or forearm.
  - There is often gross deformity of the distal humerus.
    - Open wounds should be evaluated as the distal humeral shaft can penetrate the triceps and result in a posterior wound.
    - A neurologic examination and vascular examination are required as these injuries may have associated injuries.
    - Open fractures need early antibiotic management and urgent irrigation and débridement in the operating room.
- *Relevant Imaging*
  - Elbow radiographs should be performed to evaluate distal humerus fractures.
  - Injuries are classified as supracondylar (no extension into the joint) with a transverse fracture at the level of the coronoid fossa or just distal in low supracondylar injuries or intercondylar with extension into the joint.
    - They can be further classified as partial articular where only one column is involved or complete articular with the entire distal humerus separated from the humeral shaft.
    - The articular segment may be noncomminuted with a simple split or have higher levels of comminution.
  - The most common classification system is the AO classification with A type fractures being extra-articular, B type partial articular, and C type complete articular (**Figure 10**). The incidence is approximately 40% extra-articular, 25% partial articular, and 35% complete articular with approximately 7% being open. Elderly patients have a higher likelihood of open injuries and type C injuries.
  - CT can be helpful to define the fracture fragments and injury pattern if ORIF is determined to be the treatment.
- *Nonsurgical Measures*
  - Nonsurgical management does not have a significant role in management except in completely nondisplaced injuries.
    - In these injuries, the arm should be splinted for approximately 2 to 3 weeks and then assessed for range of motion.

Chapter 4: I Fell and Cannot Use My Upper Extremity

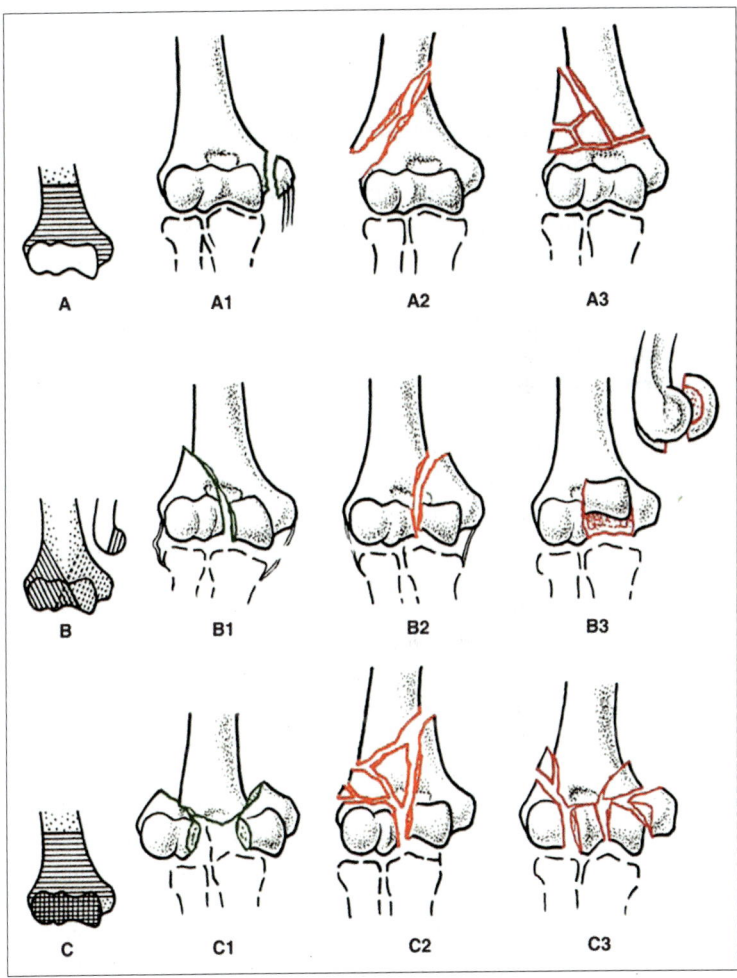

Figure 10 Illustrated AO/OTA classification of distal humerus fractures: type A, extra-articular; type B, partial articular; and type C, complete articular. Each type has further subdivisions based on the increasing complexity of the fracture pattern. (Adapted from Müller ME, Allgöwer M, Schneider R, Willenegger H, Perren SM: *Manual of Internal Fixation: Techniques Recommended by the AO-ASIF Group*, ed 3. Springer-Verlag, 1991, reproduced with permission of SNCSC.)

- Passive range of motion should be started but between range of motion sessions the arm kept in a sling. At 6 weeks post-injury, the sling may be discontinued.
- Active and active assisted lifting is allowed with expectation of healing by 10 to 12 weeks.
- Displaced fractures in unhealthy elderly patients who cannot undergo surgery is a reasonable treatment with the understanding that in general outcomes will be modest regarding motion, function, and healing with a nonunion risk over 40%.
- *Surgical Intervention*
  - Most displaced fractures require surgical treatment.
  - Surgery includes either ORIF using plate and screw fixation or a total elbow arthroplasty.
    - Indications for total elbow arthroplasty are complete distal humerus fractures with moderate to severe articular comminution in patients older than 65 to 70 years with low physical demands. Otherwise, surgical fixation of the fracture should be attempted.
  - The posterior approach is the standard approach for either total elbow arthroplasty or fixation.
    - Posterior approach can be performed with either a triceps-sparing approach or olecranon osteotomy depending on the severity of the comminution of the articular surface.
    - Most total elbow arthroplasties can be performed with a triceps on approach with condyle excision.
  - ORIF uses basic principles of compression plating using 3.5-mm limited dynamic compression plates or reconstruction plates positioned either medially and posterolaterally or direct medially and direct laterally.
    - The ulnar nerve needs to be managed during treatment and consideration of either transposition anteriorly or in situ positioning is reasonable depending on surgeon discretion.
    - Patients are started on early passive and active assisted range of motion to prevent stiffness as the construct will allow this type of stress.
    - Outcomes of ORIF are reasonable, with patients achieving a functional range of motion although complication rates are approximately 20% to 30% including stiffness, nonunion,

hardware prominence, development of posttraumatic arthritis, and ulnar neuritis.
- Dehghan et al[7] reported long-term outcomes comparing total elbow arthroplasty versus ORIF for comminuted intra-articular distal humerus fractures in patients older than 65 years. At 12.5-year follow-up, there was no statistical difference in revision surgery rates although 12% of total elbow arthroplasties required revision compared with 27% of patients who underwent ORIF. There are no differences in clinical outcomes with 90% survivorship at 15 years for total elbow arthroplasty and 70% survivorship of ORIF at 15 years.

Proximal Radius Fractures

- *Epidemiology*
  - Radial head and neck fractures typically occur after a fall on an outstretched arm.
  - Account for up to 4% of all fractures and 30% of all elbow fractures
  - Frequently associated with a dislocation of the elbow although can be in isolation
- *Pertinent Anatomy/Pathoanatomy*
  - The radial head articulates with the capitellum of the distal humerus and the proximal ulna at the lesser sigmoid notch.
  - The radial head is an important stabilizer for valgus stability as well as longitudinal stability; therefore, it is important to either repair or replace the radial head in the setting of ligament injury if it is present.
  - The radiocapitellar articulation accounts for 60% of the load transfer across the elbow.
  - There is a 45° arc of the proximal radius that does not articulate with the proximal ulna and is considered the safe zone for placement of hardware in the setting of radial head ORIF.
- *Pertinent History/Physical Examination Findings*
  - Patients will report a fall on an outstretched hand or a direct blow.
  - The patient can dislocate the elbow at the same time.
  - Often there is pain and swelling at the level of the elbow with reduced range of motion.

- On examination, bruising is often present laterally about the elbow with reduction in motion of both flexion and extension and supination and pronation.
  - In the setting of displaced fractures, understanding if there is a bony block to rotation will be important in treatment decision making.
  - Aspirating the hematoma and injection of local anesthesia can be performed to determine if there is a bony block of rotation.
  - The wrist and hand and forearm should be evaluated for tenderness and the distal radioulnar joint should be assessed for instability as isolated radial head fractures may be associated with longitudinal forearm injuries associated with interosseous membrane injuries.
  - A full neurovascular examination is required as well.
- *Relevant Imaging*
  - Radiographs of the elbow should be performed to evaluate the fracture pattern of the radial head fracture and determine if this is a complete or partial injury (is there a combination of a head and neck injury) and how many pieces of the head are involved and how comminuted.
  - CT can be useful to further evaluate the complexity of the injury to determine the overall number of pieces.
  - The Mason classification can be used with type I fractures with minimal displacement less than 2 mm with no block of rotation, type II fractures have displacement greater than 2 mm and possible mechanical block of rotation, type III fractures are severely comminuted with a discrete block of motion, and type IV injuries are associated with a dislocation.
- *Nonsurgical Measures*
  - Mason type I fractures can be managed without surgery with a simple sling.
    - The goal of treatment is early mobilization to prevent stiffness.
    - The sling can be used for 1 week for pain control but should be discarded as soon as possible.
    - Early range of motion, both active and passive, should be initiated with limitation of heavy lifting for approximately 4 to 6 weeks after the injury to allow healing.

- At 6 weeks after injury, the fracture will be healed and unrestricted activity is allowed.
- Displaced partial articular Mason type II fractures can also be considered for nonsurgical treatment and at this point there is limited consensus.
  - If there is a block of rotation, then surgical intervention should be performed.
  - Similarly, if there is associated elbow instability resulting in a subluxated ulnohumeral joint, then surgery should be performed.
  - Otherwise, there is no current agreement on displaced stable partial articular fractures even with displacement over 2 mm. Therefore, intervention is at the discretion of the surgeon.
- *Surgical Intervention*
  - Surgical treatment is typically reserved for Mason type III injuries with three options: resection, ORIF, and metal radial head arthroplasty.
    - Resection can be considered for comminuted fractures in elderly patients with no evidence of a wrist or forearm injury and no evidence of elbow ligament injury.
    - Most patients will either undergo ORIF or radial head arthroplasty.
      - Arthroplasty should be considered as an initial treatment for any fracture with greater than three articular pieces as ORIF in these injuries results in more unsatisfactory outcomes compared with injuries with two or three pieces.
      - If stable fixation cannot be achieved intraoperatively, then metal radial head arthroplasty should be performed.
  - Sun et al[8] performed a meta-analysis comparing ORIF and radial head arthroplasty for comminuted radial head fractures and determined arthroplasty had higher satisfaction rate, lower incidence of nonunion, better functional outcome scores, and shorter surgical times.
    - The study authors concluded that arthroplasty had better outcomes than ORIF with medium-term follow-up although longer term studies are required to determine outcome of arthroplasty.

- If surgical treatment is considered, either arthroplasty or ORIF, a lateral elbow approach with extensor digitorum communis split is the preferred technique.
  - Either buried or headless compression screws or a small plate can be used during ORIF taking care to have hardware only exposed in the safe zone of the proximal radius.
- If arthroplasty is considered, avoidance of overstuffing by aligning the articular surface of the radial head implant with the lesser sigmoid notch is recommended as too large an implant can lead to flexion loss as well as pain and erosion of the capitellum requiring early revision.

Proximal Ulna Fractures

- *Epidemiology*
  - Occur most commonly from low-velocity, direct, or indirect trauma to the elbow.
  - 21% of all proximal forearm fractures are proximal ulna fractures.
  - A coronoid tip fracture occurs following valgus stress, forcing the coronoid under the trochlea, and can suggest a dislocation with spontaneous reduction.
  - Direct trauma to the olecranon can result in comminuted fractures, whereas indirect trauma leading to contraction of the triceps can result in transverse olecranon fracture patterns.
- *Pertinent Anatomy/Pathoanatomy*
  - The proximal ulna consists of the olecranon process posteriorly, the coronoid process anteriorly that prevents posterior axial translation of the ulna on the humerus, and the lesser sigmoid notch that articulates with the proximal radius.
    - The olecranon prevents anterior displacement of the ulna relative to the distal humerus.
    - The triceps inserts onto the dorsal aspect of the proximal ulna and the medial and lateral collateral ligaments attach the sublime tubercle and supinator crest of the proximal ulna, respectively.
- *Pertinent History/Physical Examination Findings*
  - Patients will report a direct blow to the dorsal elbow or a fall on an outstretched arm with an eccentric contraction of the triceps or a subluxation of the elbow.

- Examination of the skin should be performed to evaluate open injuries.
  - An extension lag is often present with olecranon fractures.
  - A careful neurovascular examination is warranted as well as examination of the forearm and wrist.
- *Relevant Imaging*
  - AP and lateral radiographs should be obtained of the elbow and the wrist.
  - Olecranon fractures can be considered nondisplaced or displaced (Mayo type I), displaced without elbow instability (Mayo type II), or displaced with elbow instability (Mayo type III).
  - Coronoid fractures can be classified by the Regan and Morrey classification as avulsion fractures of the tip (type I), involving <50% of the coronoid height (type II), and involving >50% of the coronoid height (type III) (**Figure 11**).
- *Nonsurgical Measures*
  - Nonsurgical treatment can be considered for isolated coronoid fractures or nondisplaced olecranon fractures.
  - A short period of immobilization for a few weeks followed by progressive passive range-of-motion exercises for several weeks with a sling to protect the arm between exercises.
  - Fractures at 6 weeks will typically allow active range of motion and then should be followed until bony union.

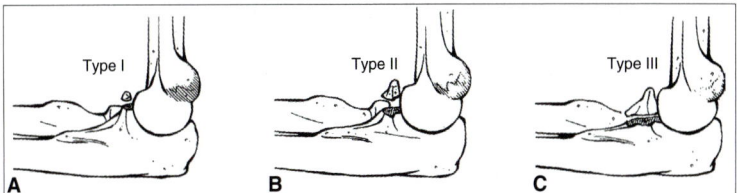

Figure 11 Diagram of elbow from the medial view. Regan-Morrey classification of fractures of the coronoid process. **A**, Type I is a simple avulsion. **B**, Type II demonstrates a single or comminuted portion involving approximately 50% of the coronoid process. **C**, Type III is a fracture involving >50% of the articulation. (Reproduced with permission from Cohen MS: Fractures of the coronoid process. *Hand Clin* 2004;20[4]:443-453.)

- *Surgical Intervention*
  - Displaced olecranon fractures should be managed with ORIF with either a tension band construct from a posterior approach or plate fixation in noncomminuted fractures.
  - In comminuted fractures, ORIF with interfragmentary screws and posterior plate fixation is required. In very proximal olecranon fractures of the tip only in elderly patients, excision of the fragment and repair of the triceps tendon can be considered using high-strength suture.
  - Coronoid fracture fixation should be considered in fractures involving more than the tip.
    - CT should be performed to determine if the anteromedial facet of the coronoid is involved. In the setting of displaced anteromedial facet or basilar fractures of the coronoid with instability, ORIF is required to prevent early progressive arthritic changes to the ulnohumeral joint.
    - A medial approach is required for repair often using small locking or buttress plates.
  - Duckworth et al[9] performed a prospective randomized trial comparing tension band and plate fixation for olecranon fractures and determined that among active patients with simple, isolated displaced olecranon fractures that there was no difference in patient-reported outcomes at 1 year postoperatively.
    - Complication rate was higher among the tension band group because of hardware removal, but more serious complications of infection and need for revision ORIF occurred only in the plate fixation group.

Simple Elbow Dislocation

- *Epidemiology*
  - Accounts for 10% to 20% of all elbow injuries and is only second to shoulder dislocations in terms of most frequent injury
  - Most commonly occurs after a fall on an outstretched hand
  - Most injuries are posterior or posterolateral and can be associated with radial head or coronoid fractures, and if so, they are no longer simple dislocations but rather considered complex dislocations.

- *Pertinent Anatomy/Pathoanatomy*
  - Elbow stability is provided by bony and soft-tissue structures.
    - The medial and lateral collateral ligament (LCL) complexes are primary stabilizers of the elbow.
      - The primary ligamentous restraint to posterolateral rotatory instability is the lateral ulnar collateral ligament, which is a portion of the LCL complex.
      - The anterior capsule also provides stability and is progressively injured during simple dislocation events.
      - The bony articulation providing stability include the olecranon and coronoid process as well as the shape of the distal humerus, specifically of the trochlea.
  - The radial head also provides bony stability to posterolateral rotatory instability.
  - The posterolateral muscles, including the anconeus and extensor carpi ulnaris, are muscular stabilizers to posterolateral rotatory instability.
  - During a simple dislocation, disruption of stabilizers typically starts laterally and then progresses medially to include the anterior capsule and finally the medial collateral ligament (MCL) complex. There are some data supporting the opposite theory. Disruption of stabilizers typically start laterally and then progress medially involving the anterior capsule and finally the MCL complex during a simple dislocation, although there are some data supporting the opposite findings (**Figure 12**).

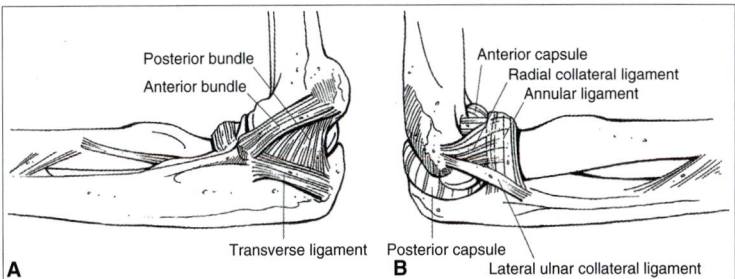

Figure 12 Diagram of the elbow from the medial (**A**) and lateral (**B**) views. Structure of the medial collateral ligament complex (**A**) and the lateral collateral ligament complex (**B**). (Reproduced from Tashjian RZ, Katarincic JA: Complex elbow instability. *J Am Acad Orthop Surg* 2006;14[5]:278-286.)

- Luokkala et al[10] studied 17 patients with simple elbow dislocations in whom MRI was performed and identified anterior capsule tears in 12, MCL injuries in 10, and LCL injuries in 9. These data would support that no single mechanism-related soft-tissue injury pattern is present, rather there are different grades of soft-tissue injuries.
- *Pertinent History/Physical Examination Findings*
  - Patients will present with a history of a fall on an outstretched hand.
  - Patients will have a history of acute injury although in patients with prior dislocations the energy required for dislocation is typically less.
  - On examination, patients will have soft-tissue swelling and deformity of the elbow.
    - A full neurovascular examination is required as well as an evaluation of the forearm and wrist for tenderness or instability to rule out a longitudinal injury to the forearm.
- *Relevant Imaging*
  - Radiographs of the elbow and wrist should be performed.
  - The elbow is typically dislocated posterolaterally with the distal humerus translated over the coronoid process with the olecranon located lateral to the trochlea on the AP radiograph.
  - Radiographs should be reviewed for concomitant radial head or coronoid process fractures that would support a complex dislocation.
    - Small coronoid tip avulsion fractures can be managed as a simple dislocation, although larger coronoid injuries or radial head fractures need to be considered in the context of complex elbow instability.
- *Nonsurgical Measures*
  - Nonsurgical treatment consists of acute reduction of the dislocation.
    - Intravenous medication is typically given for pain relief and an intra-articular lidocaine injection can also be used for anesthesia.
    - The reduction maneuver includes correction of the medial or lateral displacement followed by traction on the forearm.
      - Pressure is then placed posteriorly on the olecranon to bring it distally and anteriorly around the trochlea.

- After reduction, the elbow is taken through a range of motion to assess stability. If the arm is able to be brought into extension in neutral rotation without a dislocation, then the elbow is considered stable.
- If there is a redislocation with extension, then consideration of progressive bracing with limitation of extension over weeks can be considered versus surgical repair of the LCL.
  - If the elbow is stable with full extension, the elbow is splinted in 90° of elbow flexion and neutral rotation, and then is allowed progressive range of motion at 1 to 2 weeks with return to activity as tolerated.
- Postreduction radiographs should confirm a concentric ulnohumeral and radiocapitellar articulation. Repeat radiographs should be performed 2 to 4 days after dislocation to confirm reduction and no recurrent instability.
- *Surgical Intervention*
  - Surgical treatment is relatively uncommon, less than 1% to 2% of cases.
  - Reserved for patients with persistent instability after closed reduction with redislocation in extension
  - Indicated definitively when stability cannot be maintained without 50° or more of elbow flexion
    - In cases where the elbow remains stable only with some elbow flexion up to 50°, it is an alternative to progressive extension block bracing over 3 to 6 weeks.
  - Considered for patients where a concentric reduction cannot be maintained on postreduction radiographs
  - In the setting of persistent instability, articular cartilage or periarticular injuries must be considered as a reason for the persistent instability and MRI can be useful in the diagnosis before surgery.
  - If surgery is required, most commonly repair of the LCL complex and the injured extensor muscle mechanism is required.
  - If persistent instability occurs despite lateral repair, then repair of the MCL complex and the flexor/pronator muscle group can be considered.
  - If the patient is still experiencing instability, then static external fixation in 90° of elbow flexion should be considered.

Terrible Triad Injuries

- *Epidemiology*
  - Elbow dislocations are categorized as simple (no associated fracture) and complex (associated fracture).
  - Terrible triad injuries refer to complex elbow dislocations that include posterolateral elbow dislocation, a radial head or neck fracture, and a coronoid process fracture.
    - They are characterized by historically poor outcomes, secondary to persistent instability, stiffness, and arthrosis.
  - Nonsurgical management has a limited role in the management of terrible triad injuries.
  - Surgical treatment using a standard protocol of coronoid fracture fixation, if possible, radial head fracture fixation or replacement, and lateral ligamentous repair can result in predictable results.
- *Pertinent Anatomy/Pathoanatomy*
  - The primary stabilizing components of the elbow involved with terrible triad injuries include the radial head, the coronoid, the ligamentous structures (the lateral and medial collateral ligaments), and the common extensor mechanism.
  - The coronoid process is an important anterior and varus stabilizer to the ulnohumeral joint.
    - The coronoid process fracture in this type of injury is typically simple, transverse, and small; average height is 35% of total coronoid height.
    - Based on biomechanical data on the restoration of joint stability, most should be repaired.
    - The coronoid fragment always has some anterior capsule attached, which can be useful for soft-tissue repair of the fracture.
  - The radial head is an important secondary valgus stabilizer.
    - It provides approximately 30% of valgus stability with intact medial ligaments.
    - The radial head also is a primary restraint to posterolateral rotatory instability.
    - Complete restoration of the radial head articular surface, with repair or replacement, is required to restore elbow stability in terrible triad injuries.
  - The LCL is always injured in a terrible triad injury and usually is avulsed off the lateral epicondyle with a portion of the extensor muscles.

- The LCL complex is the primary restraint to posterolateral rotatory instability of the elbow; it prevents external rotation of the radius and ulna relative to the humerus.
- The MCL complex can sometimes be injured in terrible triad injuries, although excellent outcomes can be obtained without MCL repair, if all articular fractures and the LCL are repaired or reconstructed. MCL repair may be performed in rare cases in which stability cannot be achieved (**Figure 12**).
- *Pertinent History/Physical Examination Findings*
  - A patient's history typically includes a fall on an outstretched arm.
  - The dislocation can result from both high-energy and low-energy injuries.
  - On physical examination there is typically swelling, ecchymosis, and deformity.
    - A complete neurovascular examination needs to be performed.
    - Evaluation of the forearm and wrist for tenderness and instability needs to be performed to rule out a longitudinal forearm injury.
- *Relevant Imaging*
  - AP and lateral radiographs of the elbow prereduction and postreduction should be obtained.
  - Radiographs should be scrutinized for associated fractures of the capitellum and trochlea. PA and lateral wrist and forearm radiographs should be performed to rule out a longitudinal injury.
  - Advanced imaging is performed routinely, specifically CT with three-dimensional reconstruction to further classify the proximal radius and coronoid fractures.
  - By definition, a terrible triad injury must include a posterolateral elbow dislocation, with fractures of the coronoid and the radial head.
- *Nonsurgical Measures*
  - Most patients require surgical treatment.
  - Only those patients who, after reduction, have congruent ulnohumeral and radiohumeral articulations, have nondisplaced radial head or neck fractures, and whose elbow remains stable through a full range of elbow flexion/extension motion in neutral rotation can be treated nonsurgically.
  - Management includes 1 week of immobilization, followed by progressive range of motion. Serial radiographs should be

performed at short intervals to confirm fracture healing and the maintenance of a stable reduction.
- Najd Mazhar et al[11] evaluated patients treated nonsurgically for terrible triad injuries at average follow-up of greater than 2 years.
  - The study authors evaluated 10 patients who had a congruent joint after closed reduction, no indication for radial head or coronoid fracture fixation, no block to rotation, and a stable joint up to 45° of extension that underwent nonsurgical treatment.
  - The study authors reported excellent range of motion and functional outcomes supporting that select terrible triad injuries can be managed without surgery.
- *Surgical Intervention*
  - A systematic approach should be applied, including repair or replacement of substantial radial head fractures, coronoid fracture fixation, and LCL repair, followed by additional procedures (MCL/flexor pronator repair, dynamic or static external fixation) only if stability is not obtained.
  - In terms of surgical approach, two primary incisions: lateral (with an additional medial approach if required) or posterior can be used.
    - The deep approach to the elbow is through the lateral extensor muscles, through the Kocher interval (between the extensor carpi ulnaris and the anconeus) or through an extensor digitorum communis (EDC) split.
    - Distal extension of the EDC split may injure the posterior interosseous nerve, and the distal extension of the Kocher interval may injure the LCL.
    - If the Kocher interval is used, the Kaplan interval (the extensor carpi radialis longus and the common extensor) also can be used to increase access to the anterior joint and the coronoid process.
  - Surgical management of radial head fractures in terrible triad injuries includes fragment excision, ORIF, or radial head arthroplasty.
    - Radial head fractures should be repaired or replaced unless they involve less than 25% of the articular surface and are not critical to elbow stability. The radial head should never be resected and left without replacement in a repair of a terrible triad injury.
    - Fixation of the proximal radius should be considered in radial neck fractures with limited neck comminution or in partial articular fractures with a single piece that is not comminuted (more than one piece increases the risk for failure).

- Radial head arthroplasty is indicated in patients with comminuted fractures, surgical neck fractures with substantial neck comminution, or partial radial head fractures with two or more pieces; if some neck comminution exists, two-thirds of the shaft diameter may be used to support the prosthesis.
- Radial head excision is contraindicated in terrible triad injuries with high rates of recurrent instability, progressive arthrosis, and pain.
- Most coronoid fractures should be fixed, with the possible exclusion of very small (<10% height) pieces.
  - Most fractures can be repaired with a suture-grasping technique fixed through bone tunnels tied over the posterior aspect of the proximal ulna.
  - Larger coronoid fractures typically need fixation through a medial approach.
  - Access to the medial coronoid is best performed between the two heads of the flexor carpi ulnaris. Fixation can be performed with a 2.0 or 2.4 mm T-shaped or L-shaped plate.
- The LCL complex must be repaired after fixation of the coronoid and radial head fixation or arthroplasty; repair can be accomplished using bone tunnels or suture anchors. The elbow should be moved through a full range of flexion and extension in neutral rotation under fluoroscopy.
- If the ulnohumeral joint is persistently unstable (dislocating in extension), then further measures should be performed to restore stability.
  - If instability persists, then the MCL, along with the flexor/pronators should be repaired.
  - If instability still persists, then static or dynamic external fixation should be used. External fixation of the elbow can be used when repair of the bony injuries and the lateral and medial ligament complexes do not restore stability. This is usually an intraoperative decision based on stability during range of motion assessed fluoroscopically.
  - Slight persistent ulnohumeral widening seen on the lateral radiograph can be monitored postoperatively; residual widening often results from incompetent forearm flexors, which should be managed with active flexor exercises and the avoidance of varus stress.

Top 10 Knowledge Drops for Your Rotation

1. Distal humerus fractures are classified as supracondylar (no extension into the joint) with a transverse fracture at the level of the coronoid fossa or just distal in low supracondylar injuries or intercondylar with extension into the joint.
2. Displaced intra-articular distal humerus fractures require ORIF using a combination of parallel distal humeral plates or a medial plate combined with a posterolateral plate.
3. The radial head is an important stabilizer for valgus stability as well as longitudinal stability; therefore, it is important to either repair or replace the radial head in the setting of ligament injury if it is present.
4. The Mason classification can be used for proximal radius fractures.
5. Coronoid fractures can be classified by the Regan and Morrey classification as avulsion fractures of the tip (type I), involving less than 50% of the coronoid height (type II) and involving greater than 50% of the coronoid height (type III).
6. Simple elbow dislocations are most commonly posterior or posterolateral.
7. The primary ligamentous restraint to posterolateral rotatory instability is the lateral ulnar collateral ligament.
8. Terrible triad injuries are defined as complex elbow dislocations that include posterolateral elbow dislocation, a radial head or neck fracture, and a coronoid process fracture and require surgical fixation.
9. In terrible triad injuries, a systematic approach should be applied, including repair or replacement of substantial radial head fractures, coronoid fracture fixation, and LCL repair, followed by additional procedures (MCL/flexor pronator repair, dynamic or static external fixation) only if stability is not obtained.
10. In simple elbow dislocations, the reduction maneuver includes correction of the medial or lateral displacement followed by traction on the forearm. Pressure is then placed posteriorly on the olecranon to bring it distally and anteriorly around the trochlea. Postreduction radiographs should confirm reduction and then repeat radiographs should be performed 2 to 4 days after dislocation to confirm maintained reduction and no recurrent instability.

Chapter 4: I Fell and Cannot Use My Upper Extremity

FOREARM, DISTAL RADIUS, AND DISTAL RADIOULNAR JOINT INJURIES

Adult Forearm Fractures

- *Epidemiology*
  - Fractures of the forearm include fractures of either the radius and ulna alone or both bones, commonly referred to as a both-bone forearm fracture.
  - These fractures have a bimodal distribution, with forearm fractures in young males typically from high-energy trauma and fractures in elderly females due to low-energy falls resulting in trauma.
  - Fracture-dislocations of the forearm can occur with an ulnar shaft fracture and radial head dislocation (Monteggia) or a radial shaft fracture with distal ulnar dislocation (Galeazzi).
    - Galeazzi fractures account for 7% of all forearm fractures.
    - Monteggia fractures are more common in children but can be part of a more complex injury pattern in adults. These fracture patterns are often called fractures of necessity because they require surgical intervention in the adult population.
- *Pertinent Anatomy/Pathoanatomy*
  - The forearm bones consist of the radius and ulna. The axis of rotation of the forearm runs through radial head proximally and the ulnar fovea distally with the distal radius rotating around the distal ulna with pronosupination.
  - The radius and ulna are stabilized by three groups of ligamentous structures: the annular ligament proximally, the interosseous membrane, and the triangular fibrocartilage complex distally.
  - The interosseous membrane is responsible for dispersing axial load force to the forearm, 60% to the radiocapitellar joint and 40% to the ulnohumeral joint.
    - The central band is the key portion of interosseous membrane in addition to the distal oblique bundle.
- *Pertinent History/Physical Examination Findings*
  - Forearm fractures can lead to a significant amount of soft-tissue swelling and deformity in the forearm.

- Assessment of soft tissues must include evaluation for deformity, wounds indicative of an open fracture, and evaluation of forearm compartments.
- A thorough neurovascular examination includes documentation of a sensory examination in the median, ulnar, and radial distributions; motor examination for the anterior interosseous, median, ulnar, and posterior interosseous nerves; and radial and ulnar pulses.
- Compartment syndrome should be considered if any of the following symptoms are noted: increased turgor/tenseness in the volar or dorsal forearm; decreased sensation or numbness in any nerve distribution; pain with passive finger or wrist motion, particularly extension of digits; and decreased or absent radial or ulnar pulse.
- Compartment syndrome is considered a clinical diagnosis; however, if there is any further question of diagnosis, forearm compartment pressures can be measured.
- *Relevant Imaging*
  - Imaging of the forearm includes AP and lateral views.
    - Imaging of additional joint above (elbow) and below (wrist) should assess for associated dislocations.
- *Nonsurgical Measures*
  - In the adult, nonsurgical management is rare and isolated to nondisplaced or minimally displaced fractures, or those patients who were not surgical candidates.
    - Functional bracing or Muenster casting may be used for 6 to 8 weeks, followed by weight bearing and range-of-motion exercises.
- *Surgical Intervention*
  - ORIF is the mainstay of treatment for adult radial, ulnar shaft, and both-bone forearm fractures.
    - For both-bone forearm fracture, two separate incisions are used over either bone to prevent an increased incidence of synostosis.
    - 3.5-mm dynamic compression plating with six cortices of fixation on either side is used for fracture stabilization.
  - Most fractures require 6 weeks of no weight bearing, but early range of motion is encouraged. In the setting of a radial shaft fracture, the distal radioulnar joint (DRUJ) is assessed

for stability after the plate is applied. If the DRUJ is noted to be unstable, as in the setting of a Galeazzi fracture, the soft-tissue injury is either fixed primarily by open repair of the triangular fibrocartilaginous complex, or the joint is pinned using Kirschner wires across the distal ulna and radius.
- One study demonstrated that stability of the radial shaft fracture is dependent on the distance of the fracture from the distal radius articular surface. The incidence of DRUJ instability is 55% in fractures less than 7.5 cm from the articular surface, whereas instability is 6% in those fractures more than 7.5 cm from the joint.[12]

Distal Radius Fractures

- *Epidemiology*
  - Distal radius and ulna fractures are the most common upper extremity fracture, accounting for approximately 17.5% of fractures in adults.
  - There is a bimodal distribution pattern, with the highest rates in patients younger than 18 years and those older than 65 years. Risk factors include osteoporosis and distal radius fractures are a predictor of subsequent fragility fractures.
- *Pertinent Anatomy/Pathoanatomy*
  - The distal radius accounts for 80% of the load borne through the wrist and has three main articular facets—scaphoid, lunate, and sigmoid notch.
  - The radius is divided into three structural columns, radial, intermediate (lunate facet), and ulnar. Classification systems can be based on fracture pattern, joint involvement, or mechanism of injury.
  - Various eponyms have been assigned to classic fracture patterns, most commonly the Colles fracture (low-energy, extra-articular, dorsally displaced).
- *Pertinent History/Physical Examination Findings*
  - The classic presentation of a distal radius fracture is the fall on the outstretched hand. Patients typically present with wrist swelling with or without a deformity.
  - In higher energy injuries such as motor vehicle accidents or a fall from height, additional injuries must be ruled out.

- Assessment of soft tissues must include evaluation for deformity and wounds indicative of an open fracture (often seen over the ulnar wrist).
  - A thorough neurovascular examination includes documentation of a sensory examination in the median, ulnar, and radial distributions; motor examination for the anterior interosseous, median, ulnar, and posterior interosseous nerves; and radial and ulnar pulses.
- Acute carpal tunnel syndrome presents and progressive numbness in the median nerve distribution may be seen in up to 30% of high-energy fractures.
- *Relevant Imaging*
  - AP, lateral, and oblique radiographs of the wrist are required for adequate evaluation of a distal radius fracture.
    - AP images are assessed for intra-articular gap or step-off, radial height, and radial inclination. Standard radial height is approximately 10 to 12 mm and radial inclination is 23°.
    - The lateral image is reviewed for radiocarpal incongruity and articular tilt. The standard volar tilt is 11°. Additional imaging studies may be obtained, including a 10° lateral tilt radiograph (teardrop angle view).
    - Typically, shortening of up to 5 mm, articular displacement of up to 2 mm, and neutral tilt is acceptable; however, a more anatomic reduction is typically recommended in younger, active patients, with shortening less than 3 mm, neutral tilt, and less than 2 mm of displacement.
  - Advanced imaging modalities including CT and MRI are often used to assess intra-articular congruity and associated ligamentous injuries, such as scapholunate ligament tears.
- *Nonsurgical Measures*
  - Nonsurgical management is recommended for nondisplaced or minimally displaced fractures, or when an adequate reduction is achieved and maintained at serial follow-up imaging.
  - A patient remains non–weight bearing in a short arm cast for a total of 6 weeks. If a fracture required a reduction to improve alignment, serial radiographs are followed for up to 3 to 4 weeks to ensure adequate alignment. At the 6-week mark, wrist range of motion and weight bearing are initiated.

Chapter 4: I Fell and Cannot Use My Upper Extremity

- *Surgical Intervention*
  - Several considerations go into the management of the fracture, including patient health, activity level, patient satisfaction, and radiographic parameters.
  - Surgery has been shown to provide a slightly earlier return to function and better functional outcomes in the early postoperative period.
  - Fractures that are deemed unstable require surgical intervention to restore anatomy. Instability, albeit poorly defined, is defined as the inability of a fracture to hold a reduction.
    - Most fractures are defined as unstable if there is dorsal angulation greater than 5°, intra-articular step-off greater than 2 mm, radial shortening greater than 5 mm, or articular margin fractures.
  - Currently, most fractures are fixed with a volar locking plate through a transflexor carpi radialis approach. However, fragment-specific fixation, Kirschner wires, external fixation, and spanning dorsal plates are other options that can be used for specific fracture patterns.

Top 10 Knowledge Drops for Your Rotation

1. Galeazzi fractures are radial shaft fractures with associated DRUJ dislocations.
2. The incidence of DRUJ instability is significantly higher in fractures closer to articular surface (55% in fractures less than 7.5 cm versus 6% in those more than 7.5 cm from the joint).
3. Monteggia fractures are ulnar shaft fractures with associated radial head dislocation.
4. Standard radiographic parameters for distal radius fractures: PA: radial inclination 23°, radial height 10 to 12 mm; lateral: 11° volar tilt.
5. Unstable distal radius fractures are typically those with dorsal angulation greater than 5°, intra-articular step-off greater than 2 mm, radial shortening greater than 5 mm, or articular margin fractures.
6. The inability of a proximal pole scaphoid fractures to maintain a reduction is related to age.
7. DRUJ instability is suspected when there is an associated displaced, ulnar styloid base fracture.

8. Wrist radiographs show widening of the DRUJ on the PA view and either dorsal (more common) or volar translation of the ulna relative to the radius on the lateral.
9. To assess for a true lateral radiograph of the wrist, look for the scaphoid pisiform capitate relationship. The pisiform should overlap the volar aspects of both the scaphoid and capitate on a lateral radiograph.
10. Most distal radius fractures are fixed with a volar locking plate through a transflexor carpi radialis approach if they require surgical fixation. However, fragment-specific fixation, Kirschner wires, external fixation, and spanning dorsal plates are other options that can be used for specific fracture patterns.

WRIST AND HAND INJURIES

Perilunate Injuries

- *Epidemiology*
  - Perilunate dislocations and fracture-dislocations are rare high-energy injuries that make up less than 10% of all wrist injuries.
  - These injuries can be either ligamentous (lesser arc), bony (greater arc), or both.
  - Mayfield originally classified these injuries based on pattern of injury, with energy travelling from the radial side to the ulnar wrist in predictable pattern: stage I: scapholunate dissociation, scapholunate ligament tear; stage II: stage I + lunocapitate disruption; stage III: stage II + lunotriquetral destruction (typically dorsal perilunate); stage IV: lunate is dislocated from fossa, typically volarly.
  - The dorsal, transscaphoid perilunate fracture-dislocation is the most common pattern.
- *Pertinent Anatomy/Pathoanatomy*
  - The wrist is composed of the proximal and distal carpal rows.
  - The scapholunate interosseous ligament and the lunotriquetral interosseous ligament run between the named bones and act as the primary stabilizers of the proximal carpal row.
- *Pertinent History/Physical Examination Findings*
  - Patients present with acute wrist swelling and pain and may have numbness in the median nerve distribution.

- The hand must be examined for open wounds indicating an open dislocation or fracture-dislocation.
- Because concomitant ipsilateral injuries are common in high-energy injuries such as this, a thorough examination of the elbow and shoulder is warranted.
- These injuries can be missed on initial presentation up to 25% of the time.
- *Relevant Imaging*
  - AP, lateral, and oblique views of the wrist are obtained. Images should be scrutinized for carpal or wrist fractures.
    - On the PA view, abnormal widening of the scapholunate interval greater than 3 mm (Terry Thomas sign) can be indicative of a scapholunate ligament injury.
    - A loss of collinearity of the carpal arcs (Gilula lines) signals carpal instability or injury (**Figure 13**). The lunate may appear triangular, rather than trapezoidal, because of rotation. The lateral view may show the perilunate or lunate injury, where there is loss of collinearity of the radius, lunate, and capitate. In the setting of a greater arc injury, CT is often used to delineate fracture patterns.

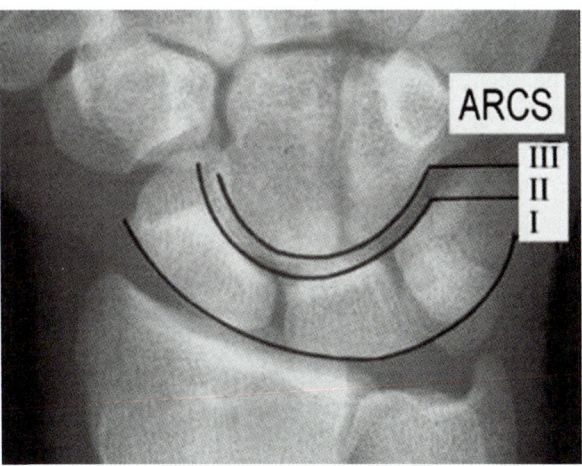

Figure 13 AP wrist radiograph showing Gilula arcs. (Reprinted with permission from Peh WCG, Gilula LA: Normal disruption of carpal arcs. *J Hand Surg* 1996;21[4]:561-566.)

- *Nonsurgical Measures*
  - Nonsurgical treatment is limited, and often reserved for the medically unstable patient.
  - All acute perilunate injuries require emergent reduction to avoid median nerve dysfunction. Reduction is typically performed under conscious sedation in the emergency department.
  - If reduction is obtained and nerve symptoms resolve, surgery can be delayed a few days until swelling improves.
- *Surgical Intervention*
  - Surgical repair is the mainstay of treatment of patients with perilunate injuries because nonsurgical management only has poor to fair outcomes.
  - If acute carpal tunnel is diagnosed, emergent decompression of the median nerve is required.
  - An extended volar carpal tunnel approach is performed.
    - If there is a volar lunate dislocation, the lunate can be reduced and the volar capsular rent repaired at the same time.
  - A dorsal approach is then performed with a scapholunate ligament repair and possible lunotriquetral ligament repair.
    - If there is an associated distal radius or carpal fracture, they are addressed at this time with ORIF.
  - The wrist is pinned for 6 to 8 weeks and a cast placed to allow for ligamentous healing. Once the pins are removed, wrist range of motion is initiated. Weight bearing is allowed once fractures are healed.

Scaphoid Fractures

- *Epidemiology*
  - Scaphoid fractures are the most common carpal fracture, accounting for 15% of all acute wrist injuries and are more common in men than women.
- *Pertinent Anatomy/Pathoanatomy*
  - More than 75% of the scaphoid bone is covered by articular cartilage.
  - The major blood supply is the dorsal carpal branch of the radial artery, which enters at the dorsal waist and provides vascularity to most of the scaphoid via retrograde flow.

- Scaphoid fractures are most often classified by anatomic location, with waist fractures being the most common (65%).
  - Proximal pole fractures account for 25% and have a high incidence of avascular nonunion because of poor blood supply.
- *Pertinent History/Physical Examination Findings*
  - Patients typically present after a fall onto an outstretched hand with varying levels of pain at the wrist.
  - Visible deformity is rare in the setting of an isolated scaphoid fracture.
  - Provocative maneuvers include tenderness over the anatomic snuffbox, scaphoid tubercle tenderness, and pain with axial load of the scaphoid through the first ray.
- *Relevant Imaging*
  - When a scaphoid fracture is suspected, three views of the wrist (AP, lateral, and oblique) and a scaphoid view are recommended.
  - The scaphoid view places the wrist in slight extension and ulnar deviation, which extends the scaphoid and allows better fracture visualization.
    - Radiographs may be negative at time of injury; however, if there is a high index of suspicion, they should be repeated in approximately 14 days.
  - MRI is more sensitive in diagnosis of occult fractures.
- *Nonsurgical Measures*
  - Minimally displaced (less than 1 mm) and nondisplaced distal pole and scaphoid waist fractures can be managed with a cast.
  - Although historically all nonsurgically minimally displaced scaphoid fractures were managed with thumb spica casting, more recent data suggest short arm casts show higher union rates at 10 weeks.
- *Surgical Intervention*
  - Displaced scaphoid fracture are often fixed with mini-open screw fixation via either a volar (waist, distal pole) or dorsal (waist, proximal pole) approach.
  - The volar approach is best used in the setting of a humpback deformity or when structural bone grafting is required.
  - Ideal fixation requires central axis placement of the cannulated screw to allow for longest construct length and rigidity.

Top 10 Knowledge Drops for Your Rotation

1. The Mayfield classification (stages I-IV) of perilunate injuries is based on pattern of injury starting from radial side.
2. Perilunate injuries are also classified as lesser arc (ligamentous injury) and greater arc (through bone/fracture).
3. Dorsal transscaphoid perilunate fracture-dislocations are the most common pattern.
4. For perilunate injuries, clenched fist AP view will assess for scapholunate ligament widening.
5. Scaphoid fractures are the most common carpal fracture.
6. The blood supply to the scaphoid is retrograde, so the proximal pole fractures are at high risk of osteonecrosis.
7. The scaphoid view places the wrist in slight extension and ulnar deviation, which extends the scaphoid and allows better fracture visualization.
8. Surgical fixation is limited to scaphoid fractures that are displaced (greater than 1 mm), comminuted, proximal pole, and those associated with perilunate injuries.
9. Provocative maneuvers to diagnose a scapoid fracture include tenderness over the anatomic snuffbox, scaphoid tubercle tenderness, and pain with axial load of the scaphoid through the first ray.
10. Minimally displaced (less than 1 mm) and nondisplaced distal scaphoid pole and scaphoid waist fractures can be managed with a cast.

HAND FRACTURES

Metacarpal and Phalangeal Fractures

- *Epidemiology*
  - Metacarpal and phalangeal fractures are extremely common.
  - Phalangeal fractures are the most common fracture in the entire skeleton and account for 10% of all fractures.
  - The incidence of phalanx fractures is approximately 0.012% of people per year in the United States.[13] Metacarpal fractures are the most common fractures in males in the second and third decades of life and typically occur from a fall or a direct blow. They are the second most common injury seen in the emergency department.

- Distal phalangeal fractures are most common and have associated nail bed injuries.
- Most metacarpal fractures are isolated injuries, which are simple, closed, and stable.
- *Pertinent Anatomy/Pathoanatomy*
  - The thumb has two phalanges whereas the remaining digits have three each.
  - The flexors and extensors of the fingers insert on the middle and distal phalanges and may be disrupted with fractures.
  - The metacarpals form the transverse and longitudinal arches of the hand and stabilized distally by the deep transverse intermetacarpal ligament and proximally by the interosseous ligaments.
  - The ligamentous structures at the carpometacarpal joints of the index and long finger are more rigid than that of the ring and small fingers.
- *Pertinent History/Physical Examination Findings*
  - Mechanism of injury typically involves a fall, crush or sports injury, or a direct impact.
  - Patients will often note pain, deformity, swelling, limited range of motion, or instability at the injury site. Given the close proximity of the bone to the skin, it is important to assess for laceration that may indicate an open fracture.
  - Rotational alignment of the digits is best assessed with finger flexion.
    - In the setting of a metacarpal fracture, there may be loss of knuckle contour due to swelling, fracture angulation, and shortening.
    - Additionally, there may be a bony prominence more proximal due to angulation.
    - Active motion may be limited by pain and therefore a local anesthetic can be used to assist once a sensory examination is complete. With a composite fist, all digits should point toward the scaphoid tubercle. If there is any concern, the contralateral hand should be assessed as well.
- *Relevant Imaging*
  - It is critical that imaging be obtained of the appropriate digit to best assess a fracture and determine management.
    - AP, lateral, and oblique hand views are ordered for suspected injuries to metacarpal region, whereas dedicated finger

radiographs should be assessed when a phalangeal fracture or dislocation is suspected.
- Overlapping digits on a lateral or oblique radiograph can obscure fracture patterns and misinform management.
- Radiographs should be assessed for angulation, fracture shortening, and rotational malalignment. Most commonly, metacarpal fractures have apex dorsal angulation.
- Both metacarpal and phalanx fractures are classified using a descriptive pattern noting location, angulation, and displacement. Location along the bone includes condyle (head), neck, shaft, and base.
- *Nonsurgical Measures*
  - Nonsurgical treatment is appropriate for simple, closed, stable fracture patterns.
    - This includes nondisplaced or minimally displaced fractures without clinical evidence of rotation.
    - Extra-articular fractures of the phalanges and metacarpals often do not require surgical intervention.
    - As long as clinical malrotation is not evident, certain degrees of angular and rotational deformity are well tolerated.
    - In the absence of rotation, extra-articular fractures with less than 10° of angulation and less than 2 mm of shortening are managed nonsurgically.
  - If the fracture is stable, treatment may include buddy-tapping to an adjacent digit and early protected range-of-motion exercises. If there is a concern for stability, a cast is used for approximately 4 weeks followed by early motion.
- *Surgical Intervention*
  - General surgical indications for metacarpal and phalangeal fractures include open fractures, intra-articular involvement, rotational malalignment, significant displacement, and multiple fractures.
  - The clearest indication for surgery is clinically significant scissoring or rotational malalignment when making a fist.
    - Each degree of rotation at the metacarpal results in 5° of rotation at the fingertip, leading to 1.5 cm of digital overlap in the closed fist.
    - Metacarpal shortening of 2 mm leads to 7° of extensor lag.
    - If the fingers are unable to retropulse past the neutral position, it is difficult to get the digit out of the palm.

- Because the MCP joint typically hyperextends approximately 20°, shortening of up to 6 mm is tolerated.
- Surgical indications for metacarpal fractures are listed in **Table 1**.
- Fixation methods typically include either percutaneous pinning or open reduction and fixation with screws, plates, or wires. If open fixation is performed, early mobilization is required to prevent adhesions.
- Specific phalanx fractures
  - Mallet fractures
    - Intra-articular fractures of the base of the distal phalanx at site of terminal extensor tendon insertion. It is critical

TABLE 1 Surgical Indications for Metacarpal Fractures[a]

General Indications
Open fractures
Multiple, displaced fractures (relative)
Polytrauma (relative)
Clinical rotational deformity >5°
Segmental loss
Intra-articular step-off
Metacarpal Head
Articular step-off >1 mm
Comminution
>25% involvement of articular surface
Epiphyseal injuries
Metacarpal Neck
Index and Long: >20° angulation, scissoring
Ring: >30° angulation, scissoring
Little: >40°-70° angulation, scissoring
Metacarpal Shaft
Shortening >6 mm
Angulation >15° index, long; >20° ring, little
Rotational deformity >5°
Metacarpal Base
Associated dislocation
Fourth and fifth: Intra-articular involvement with step-off >1 mm; fracture-dislocation with residual subluxation after reduction

[a]Fixation methods typically include either percutaneous pinning or open reduction and fixation with screws, plates, or wires. If open fixation is performed, early mobilization is required to prevent adhesions.

to address joint congruity on a lateral radiograph. If the fracture involves more than 40% of the articular surface or there is volar subluxation of the distal phalanx, surgical intervention is considered.
- Proximal phalanx base fractures
  - Often seen following low-energy falls in elderly patients. PA radiograph may appear normal but lateral radiograph often shows apex volar dorsal angulation. Surgery is considered with greater than 30° to 40° of angulation.
- Specific metacarpal fractures
  - Bennett fracture
    - Base of thumb intra-articular metacarpal fracture. Typically unstable fracture as the deforming forces (primarily the abductor pollicis longus) displaces the metacarpal shaft proximally. Comminuted variant is the Rolando fracture.
  - Boxer's fracture
    - Fracture of the neck of the fifth metacarpal fracture. This fracture can be displaced up to 40° to 70° on lateral radiograph before surgical intervention is considered. Reduction is performed by the Jahss maneuver.
  - Base of fifth metacarpal fractures
    - Often associated with hamate fractures and can see fourth or fifth carpometacarpal joint dislocations with this fracture pattern. It is critical to assess lateral radiograph to assess that joint is reduced.

Top 10 Knowledge Drops for Your Rotation

1. Imaging for hand fractures include hand radiographs for metacarpals, and finger radiographs for phalanx fractures.
2. Fracture-dislocations of the proximal interphalangeal joint are often missed on hand radiographs given inadequate laterals of fingers.
3. Each degree of rotation at the metacarpal results in 5° of rotation at the fingertip, leading to 1.5 cm of digital overlap in the closed fist. Metacarpal shortening of 2 mm leads to 7° of extensor lag.
4. Phalangeal fractures are the most common fracture in the entire skeleton and account for 10% of all fractures.

5. Distal phalangeal fractures are most common and have associated nail bed injuries.
6. Rotational alignment of the digits is best assessed with finger flexion.
7. In the absence of rotation, extra-articular fractures of the phalanges or metacarpals with less than 10° of angulation and less than 2 mm of shortening are managed nonsurgically.
8. Surgical indications for metacarpal and phalangeal fractures include open fractures, intra-articular involvement, rotational malalignment, significant displacement, and multiple fractures. The clearest indication for surgery is clinically significant scissoring or rotational malalignment when making a fist.
9. Boxer's fracture, or fracture of the neck of the fifth metacarpal, can be displaced up to 40° to 70° on lateral radiograph before surgical intervention is considered.
10. Bennett fracture, or base of thumb intra-articular metacarpal fracture, is typically an unstable fracture as the deforming forces (primarily the abductor pollicis longus) displaces the metacarpal shaft proximally.

References

1. Guerra E, Previtali D, Tamborini S, Filardo G, Zaffagnini S, Candrian C: Midshaft clavicle fractures surgery provides better results as compared with nonoperative treatment: A meta-analysis. *Am J Sports Med* 2019;47(14):3541-3551.
2. Fraser AN, Bjørdal J, Wagle TM, et al: Reverse shoulder arthroplasty is superior to plate fixation at 2 years for displaced proximal humeral fractures in the elderly: A multicenter randomized controlled trial. *J Bone Joint Surg Am* 2020;102(6):477-485.
3. van de Wall BJM, Ochen Y, Beeres FJP, et al: Conservative vs. operative treatment for humeral shaft fractures: A meta-analysis and systematic review of randomized clinical trials and observational studies. *J Shoulder Elbow Surg* 2020;29(7):1493-1504.
4. Hovelius L, Olofsson A, Sandstrom B, et al: Nonoperative treatment of primary anterior shoulder dislocation in patients forty years of age and younger. A prospective twenty-five-year follow-up. *J Bone Joint Surg Am* 2008;90(5):945-952.

5. Borbas P, Churchill J, Ek ET: Surgical management of chronic high-grade acromioclavicular joint dislocations: A systematic review. *J Shoulder Elbow Surg* 2019;28(10):2031-2038.
6. Moosmayer S, Lund G, Seljom US, et al: At a 10-year follow-up, tendon repair is superior to physiotherapy in the treatment of small and medium-sized rotator cuff tears. *J Bone Joint Surg Am* 2019;101(12):1050-1060.
7. Dehghan N, Furey M, Schemitsch L, et al: Long-term outcomes of total elbow arthroplasty for distal humeral fracture: Results from a prior randomized clinical trial. *J Shoulder Elbow Surg* 2019;28(11):2198-2204.
8. Sun H, Duan J, Li F: Comparison between radial head arthroplasty and open reduction and internal fixation in patients with radial head fractures (modified Mason type III and IV): A meta-analysis. *Eur J Orthop Surg Traumatol* 2016;26(3):283-291.
9. Duckworth AD, Clement ND, White TO, Court-Brown CM, McQueen MM: Plate versus tension-band wire fixation for olecranon fractures: A prospective randomized trial. *J Bone Joint Surg Am* 2017;99(15):1261-1273.
10. Luokkala T, Temperley D, Basu S, Karjalainen TV, Watts AC: Analysis of magnetic resonance imaging-confirmed soft tissue injury pattern in simple elbow dislocations. *J Shoulder Elbow Surg* 2019;28(2):341-348.
11. Najd Mazhar F, Jafari D, Mirzaei A: Evaluation of functional outcome after nonsurgical management of terrible triad injuries of the elbow. *J Shoulder Elbow Surg* 2017;26(8):1342-1347.
12. Rettig ME, Raskin KB: Galeazzi fracture-dislocation: A new treatment-oriented classification. *J Hand Surg Am* 2001;26(2):228-235.
13. Karl JW, Olson PR, Rosenwasser MP: The epidemiology of upper extremity fractures in the United States, 2009. *J Orthop Trauma* 2015;29(8):e242-e244.

5. My Shoulder Hurts—Now What?

William N. Levine, MD, FAAOS, FAOA
Julianne Munoz, MD, FAAOS

ROTATOR CUFF

Introduction

Rotator cuff pathology creates symptomatic and functional burdens in the adult population. It is the leading cause of shoulder-related visits to orthopaedic surgeons.[1] There are distinct physical examination features based on known anatomic relationships and biomechanics that help with diagnosis. Radiographic findings and classifications help quantify the magnitude and chronicity of the disease process. Patient-related factors play a significant role in treatment recommendations. There is no "one size fits all" treatment algorithm for the rotator cuff.

Epidemiology

- 54% of people older than 60 years have asymptomatic partial-thickness or full-thickness cuff tears[2]
- Cuff pathology increases significantly after age 50 years
  - 13% with asymptomatic tears after age 40 years
  - 20% with asymptomatic tears after age 50 years
  - 31% with asymptomatic tears after age 60 years[3]
- 50% increase in bilateral cuff tearing after age 66 years[4]
- High on the differential diagnosis for middle-aged to elderly patients with shoulder pain who are considering elective surgery

---

Dr. Levine or an immediate family member has received royalties from Zimmer and serves as an unpaid consultant to Zimmer. Dr. Munoz or an immediate family member is a member of a speakers' bureau or has made paid presentations on behalf of Arthrex, Inc.

Pertinent Anatomy/Pathoanatomy

- Rotator cuff constitutes four musculotendinous units surrounding the proximal humerus that elevate and rotate the shoulder (**Table 1**)
  - Subscapularis
    - Origin: subscapular fossa, anterior scapula
    - Insertion: lesser tuberosity medial to bicipital groove
    - Innervation: upper and lower subscapular nerves (posterior cord of plexus)
    - Function: adduction and internal rotation
  - Supraspinatus
    - Origin: supraspinatus fossa, superior to scapular spine
    - Insertion: superior greater tuberosity
    - Innervation: suprascapular nerve (superior trunk of plexus)
    - Function: abduction
  - Infraspinatus
    - Origin: infraspinatus fossa, inferior to scapular spine
    - Insertion: greater tuberosity, posterior to supraspinatus
      - Evidence suggests some fibers of the supraspinatus and infraspinatus intertwine along the greater tuberosity footprint[5]
    - Innervation: suprascapular nerve (superior trunk of plexus)
    - Function: external rotation primarily in neutral arm abduction
  - Teres minor
    - Origin: inferolateral aspect of scapular body, inferior to infraspinatus
    - Insertion: posterior greater tuberosity, inferior to infraspinatus

TABLE 1 Rotator Cuff Anatomy

Tendon	Innervation	Origin	Insertion	Function
Subscapularis	Upper/lower subscapular	Subscapular fossa	Lesser tuberosity	Internal rotation, adduction
Supraspinatus	Suprascapular	Supraspinatus fossa	Greater tuberosity	Abduction
Infraspinatus	Suprascapular	Infraspinatus fossa	Greater tuberosity	External rotation at neutral
Teres minor	Axillary	Inferolateral scapular body	Greater tuberosity	External rotation in abduction

- Innervation: axillary nerve (posterior cord of plexus)
- Function: external rotation primarily in arm abduction
- Rotator interval
  - Clinically relevant gap between upper border of subscapularis and anterior edge of supraspinatus
    - Contains: long head biceps, superior glenohumeral ligament, coracohumeral ligament
    - Relevant in instability and adhesive capsulitis pathologies
- Suprascapular nerve compression causes two types of cuff denervation atrophy (**Figure 1**)
  - Travels inferior to superior transverse scapular ligament at suprascapular notch
    - Compression at suprascapular notch: supraspinatus and infraspinatus atrophy
  - Then continues posteroinferiorly about scapula and around spinoglenoid notch
    - Compression at spinoglenoid notch: only infraspinatus atrophy

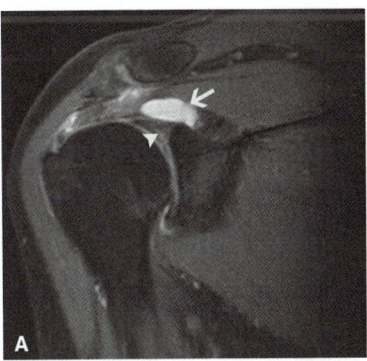
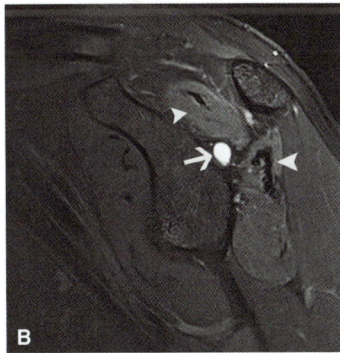

Figure 1 Magnetic resonance images demonstrating the two common sites of suprascapular nerve entrapment. **A**, Coronal T2-weighted image showing a superior labral tear (arrowhead) with parabral cyst (arrow) near the suprascapular notch. **B**, Sagittal T2-weighted image showing a parabral cyst (arrow) near the spinoglenoid notch with denervation changes seen in the supraspinatus and infraspinatus muscle bellies (arrowheads). (Reproduced with permission from Miniaci A, ed: *Disorders of the Shoulder: Sports Injuries*. Wolters Kluwer, 2013.)

- Rotator cuff tear pathology: partial thickness, full thickness, complete rupture (**Figure 2**)
  - Partial thickness: fraying and thinning of tendon
    - Bursal (superior) measured by depth
    - Articular (inferior) measured by amount of exposed footprint
    - Interstitial (intratendinous)
  - Full thickness: complete hole creating communication between bursal and intra-articular spaces

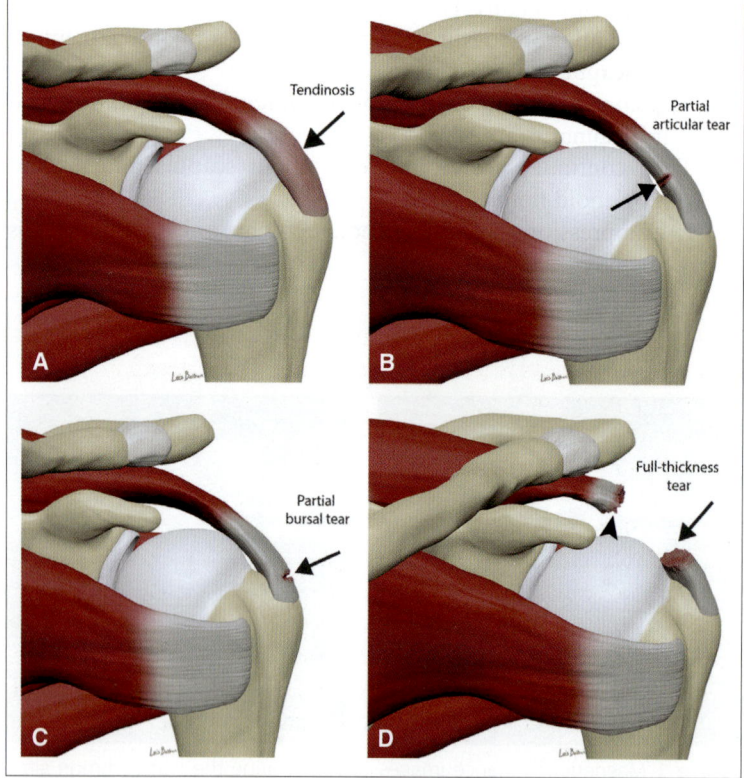

Figure 2 Rendering of various types of rotator cuff tear pathology. **A**, Tendinosis without tearing. **B**, Partial articular-sided tearing. **C**, Partial bursal-sided tearing. **D**, Full-thickness tear. Arrow shows tendon stump remaining on footprint, arrowhead shows the free edge of tear attached to muscle. (Reproduced with permission from Chew FS, ed: *Musculoskeletal Imaging: The Essentials*. Wolters Kluwer, 2018.)

- Graded by anterior-to-posterior size of hole or number of tendons involved
  - Small: one tendon and/or 1 cm or less
  - Medium: one tendon and/or 1 to 3 cm
  - Large: two tendons or 3 to 5 cm
  - Massive: two or more tendons and/or greater than 5 cm
- Complete rupture (very rare)
  - Full-thickness tear of the entire tendon anterior-to-posterior insertion

Pertinent History/Physical Examination Findings

- History: acute and chronic
  - Acute: traumatic events with forceful rotation/flexion of the shoulder
    - Dislocations after age 40 years more commonly cause cuff tearing than labral instability problems
  - Chronic: years of overuse, physical profession, overhead recreational activity
    - Pain with forward flexion, abduction, rotation
    - Weakness even more suspicious and distinguishes from impingement
- Physical examination: range of motion (ROM), strength, lag signs, pain
  - ROM: begin with active and follow with passive to distinguish from arthritis or adhesive capsulitis
    - Forward flexion, abduction, external rotation at neutral and 90° of abduction, and internal rotation at neutral and 90° of abduction
  - Strength
    - Supraspinatus: arms in 90° of abduction and in the plane of the scapula approximately 30° anterior to the plane of the body, patient upward lifts against clinician resistance
    - Infraspinatus: resisted external rotation with the arm in neutral position
    - Teres minor: resisted external rotation while at 90° of abduction
    - Subscapularis: resisted internal rotation at neutral or in 90° of abduction

- Lag signs exist for each of these testing maneuvers when the patient cannot maintain the strength-testing position for the isolated tendon
- Pain: should be used in conjunction with ROM and strength to distinguish from subacromial impingement
  - Neer sign: passive forward flexion of arm with pain after 90°
  - Neer test: impingement pain relief after injection of lidocaine into subacromial space
  - Hawkins test: passively place the arm at 90° flexion, 90° elbow flexion and examiner internally rotates the arm causing pain
  - Belly press: pain when the hand is placed on the umbilicus and the shoulder actively internally rotated
  - Liftoff test: pain or weakness with the arm placed behind the back lifting it off the sacrum

Relevant Imaging

- MRI gold standard modality to view tendon pathology but plain radiography is typically baseline for initial shoulder pain evaluation
  - Plain radiography: AP externally rotated, AP internally rotated, AP Grashey (true AP), axillary, scapular Y
  - Grashey: true AP image of the glenoid rather than the patient's body
    - Eliminates overlap of humeral head on glenoid giving a clear view of the glenohumeral joint
      - Scapula does not lie parallel to the back of the body, rather internally rotated approximately 30° to 45° to coronal plane of the body
  - Axillary: lateral projection of the joint shot up the axilla
    - Visualizes the "golf ball on golf tee" position of the humeral head on glenoid
  - Plain radiographs can demonstrate end-stage cuff tear arthropathy
    - Anterosuperior humeral head escape from glenoid
  - Can demonstrate earlier cuff disease with cystic or osteophyte changes at the greater tuberosity or subacromial spurring

- Scapular Y view can demonstrate the morphology of the acromion and subacromial spurring
  - Bigliani acromion classification
    - Type 1: flat
    - Type 2: curved
    - Type 3: hooked
- Can demonstrate alternative or concomitant disease, that is, arthritis
- MRI: T1-weighted and T2-weighted images in coronal, axial, and sagittal planes allow assessment of muscle bellies and tendon insertions
- Coronal
  - Insertion of supraspinatus and anterior fibers of infraspinatus to greater tuberosity and any retraction
  - Fanlike anterior appearance of subscapularis across the lesser tuberosity
  - Relationship of humeral head to glenoid and acromion
    - Anterosuperior escape of humeral head in cuff tear arthropathy
- Axial
  - Insertions of subscapularis, posterior infraspinatus, teres minor
  - Superior appearance of supraspinatus
  - Anterior or posterior subluxation of humeral head in glenoid
- Sagittal
  - Muscle atrophy on the medial-most cut into the scapula
    - Goutallier classification uses intramuscular atrophy
      - 0—none, 1—fat streaks, 2—more muscle than fat, 3—equal muscle to fat, 4—more fat than muscle
    - Tangent sign uses muscle bulk atrophy of supraspinatus
      - Line drawn from scapular spine to coracoid process should transect the supraspinatus muscle belly
      - When muscle belly atrophies below this line repair rate failure upward of 80%[6]
  - Can corroborate full-thickness tears from footprint
    - Cuff should appear similar to a crown attaching to tuberosities without fluid or fiber detachment

Nonsurgical Management

- Preferred first-line management of partial-thickness and many full-thickness tears as well
  - Physical therapy: cuff/deltoid strengthening and periscapular stabilization
  - Consistent NSAID course
  - Single subacromial corticosteroid injection for short-term pain/dysfunction[1]
    - Repeat injections can be considered for indefinite nonsurgical candidates
  - Limited evidence for hyaluronic acid or platelet-rich plasma[1]
    - Patients should be educated on this if incurring out-of-pocket expense

Surgical Intervention

- Indications
  - Symptomatic patients in whom the aforementioned nonsurgical management failed
  - Acute tears perform better with prompt surgery, surgical decision making advances faster here than in chronic tears if comorbidities allow[7]
  - Symptoms: pain, rotational/overhead dysfunction and weakness, lag signs
- Approaches and techniques
  - Although equivalent in the long term, arthroscopic cuff repair now dominates over open repair
    - Portals vary but standard landmarks include posterolateral border of acromion, lateral edge of acromion, coracoid process.
    - May be done in beach chair or lateral position, surgeon preference dictates
    - Viewing first takes place via posterior portal with initial intra-articular work through anterior, rotator interval portal.
    - When the arthroscope is redirected into the subacromial space, accessory lateral portals are often used for cuff manipulation, anchor placement, suturing, and repair.

- Scope repairs usually use plastic absorbable or all-thread suture anchors that are either preloaded with suture or have eyelets that previously passed sutures are loaded into.
  - Single-row and double-row repairs are clinically equivalent
    - Double row: medial row of anchors at the articular margin and a lateral row off the greater tuberosity that secure the suture limbs from the medial row (**Figure 3**)
      - Reduces the cuff tissue against the whole width of the footprint
    - Single row: one row of anchors at or near the articular margin (**Figure 4**)
      - Particularly useful for noncompliant tissue that cannot be stretched across the whole width of footprint
        - Excessive tendon repair leads to failure
      - Also useful for small tears that may only require one anchor for repair
- Cuff tear arthropathy
  - Reverse total shoulder arthroplasty (RTSA)
    - Deltopectoral approach most commonly used
      - Deltoid and pectoralis major interval

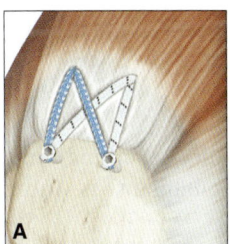
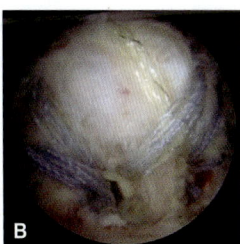
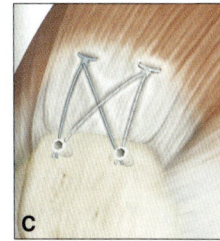

Figure 3 **A**, Rendering of a double-row repair with suture tapes and an untied medial row brought down to the lateral row. Arthroscopic image of a similar repair (**B**) with patient in beach chair position visualized from a posterolateral viewing portal. Rendering of a double-row repair (**C**) with medial row sutures tied over the top of the tendon and then brought to the lateral row. (Panels A and C reproduced with permission from Burkhart SS, Lo IK, Brady PC, Denard PJ, eds: *The Cowboy's Companion: A Trail Guide for the Arthroscopic Shoulder Surgeon*. Wolters Kluwer, 2012. Panel B courtesy of Dr. Julianne Munoz, University of Miami.)

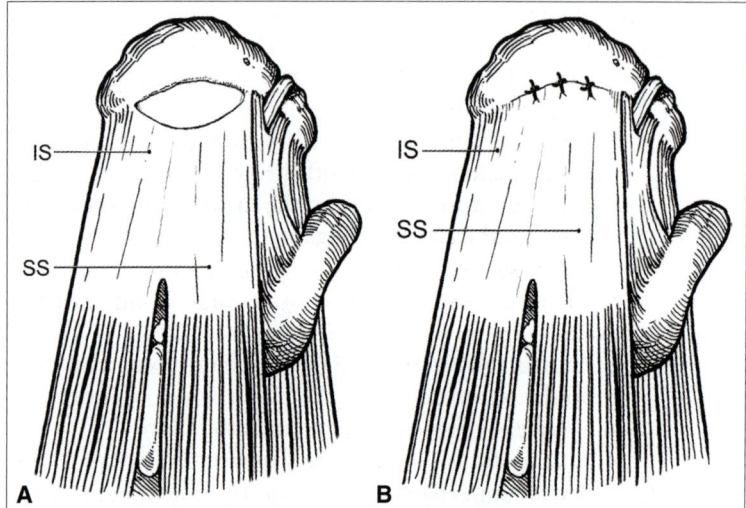

Figure 4 **A**, Illustration of a small, crescent-shaped rotator cuff tear. **B**, Illustration of a single-row repair with three anchors tied over the top of the tendon. IS = infraspinatus, SS = supraspinatus. (Reproduced with permission from Burkhart SS, Lo IK, Brady PC: *Burkhart's View of the Shoulder: A Cowboy's Guide to Advanced Shoulder Arthroscopy*. Wolters Kluwer, 2006.)

- Cephalic vein is the superficial landmark of the interval
- Conjoined tendon retracted medially
- Subscapularis peel, if it is present
  - May tag for later repair if desired
  - Not as necessary for anterior stability as in anatomic arthroplasty because the reverse implant is more constrained
  - Repair may aid in internal rotation strength if the tendon is of good quality
- Humeral osteotomy and canal/metaphyseal preparation
  - Short and long stem options now on the US market
  - Short stems save options for revision surgery down the line provided the metaphyseal bone stock supports the implant
  - Systems are designed for press-fit into the humerus with reamers and broaches
    - If bone quality or canal size precludes good press-fit, cement should be used

- Glenoid preparation
  - Glenoid surface is reamed to accommodate a baseplate
    - Glenoid baseplate systems vary significantly
      - Central peg versus screw
      - Bone ongrowth versus grafting cage options
      - All include peripheral compression or locking screws, which should be used to increase the stability of fixation
    - The baseplate-glenoid contact minimum varies with different systems and should be understood ahead of time with the chosen system
      - Older generations necessitated minimums of 80% contact, but newer arthroplasty technology can tolerate contact area as low as 60%
      - When acceptable contact is impossible to achieve with reaming, consider bone grafting or augmented baseplate options
    - Glenosphere is impacted onto the baseplate
  - Subscapularis closure if desired
  - Deltopectoral interval and skin closure
- Postoperative cuff repair management
  - Outpatient/ambulatory surgery
  - Sling immobilization and postoperative physical therapy protocols vary
    - Dependent on: tear size, tissue quality, tension on repair, considerations for patient comfort, patient reliability, surgeon preference
    - Progresses through: non–weight bearing, passive ROM, active ROM, and last, strengthening
    - Complete recovery through the rehabilitation protocol usually between 3 and 6 months depending on the aforementioned factors
  - Perioperative antibiotics to cover skin flora before incision
    - 2 g intravenous cephazolin versus weight-based vancomycin versus 900 mg clindamycin
      - Aforementioned options dependent on patient allergy profile

- Pain control
  - Regional anesthesia with peripheral nerve blocks and catheters that patients can remove at home decreases postoperative narcotic usage
  - Multimodal oral pain control regimen
    - Patients younger than 65 years
      - Tylenol 650 mg by mouth every 6 hours × 72 hours (over the counter)
      - Toradol 10 mg 1 tablet by mouth 3 times a day × 72 hours, then 1 tablet by mouth twice a day × 2 days (13 tablets)
      - Gabapentin 300 mg 1 tablet by mouth 3 times a day × 72 hours (9 tablets)
      - Oxycodone 5 mg 1 tablet by mouth every 6 hours taken as needed (20 tablets with no refills) for breakthrough pain only—maximum 4 tablets per day
    - Patients older than 65 years
      - Tylenol 650 mg by mouth every 6 hours × 72 hours (over the counter)
      - Toradol 10 mg 1 tablet by mouth 3 times a day × 72 hours, then 1 tablet by mouth twice a day × 2 days (13 tablets)
      - Gabapentin 100 mg 1 tablet by mouth 3 times a day × 72 hours (9 tablets)
      - Oxycodone 5 mg 1 tablet by mouth every 6 hours taken as needed (20 tablets with no refills) for breakthrough pain only—maximum 4 tablets per day
  - Deep vein thrombosis: rates are very low in shoulder surgery; therefore no standard prophylaxis protocol exists and many use none
- Complications
  - Most common is failure
    - Presents as inability to progress through rehabilitation, persistent or new-onset pain and/or overhead/rotational weakness
  - Stiffness
  - Anchor pullout, may result in loose body
  - Persistent pain
  - Infection, less than 1%

- Outcomes
  - Healing rates for single-row and double-row repairs vary between 70% and 80% in the literature[8]
  - Retears most commonly seen in: older patients, smokers, and those with larger tears, decreased bone mineral density, diabetes mellitus, increased tendon retraction, and atrophy
  - Patients can still do well despite retear
    - Perhaps because of concomitant subacromial decompression or other pain-relieving procedures at time of repair, that is, biceps or acromioclavicular work
- Postoperative RTSA management
  - All of the aforementioned considerations with the following additions
  - More likely to experience overnight hospital stay for 24-hour antibiotic administration and pain control
    - Many are moving to the ambulatory model, however
  - Postoperative Grashey and axillary plain radiographs should be taken either in the operating room after case completion or in the postoperative anesthesia care unit (PACU) to confirm the desired implant position and absence of dislocation or periprosthetic fracture
  - Sling and rehabilitation protocols also vary, but in general patients are safer to begin motion out of the sling and weight bearing more rapidly than patients who undergo cuff repair
    - Internal rotation behind the back is the most vulnerable position for early implant dislocation, so this should be limited in the weeks following surgery while the anterior surgical incision and soft tissues are healing
  - Complication profile is higher: stiffness, dislocation, periprosthetic fracture, scapular notching, implant loosening, persistent pain, infection (closer to 5%)
  - Outcomes: excellent pain relief in most of the patients and functional overhead motion
    - Survival rates even in younger patients (younger than 65 years) are promising
      - 99% at 2 years, 91% to 98% at 5 years, 88% at 10 years[9]
- Both cuff repair and RTSA come with distinct risk and benefit profiles and each of them is an excellent surgical option in the appropriately indicated patient

Top 10 Knowledge Drops for Your Rotation

1. Rotator cuff disease prevalence increases rapidly after age 50 years.
2. The rotator cuff is composed of the subscapularis (upper/lower subscapular nerve), supraspinatus (suprascapular nerve), infraspinatus (suprascapular nerve), and teres minor (axillary nerve).
3. Suprascapular nerve compression: superior scapular notch causes supraspinatus and infraspinatus weakness; spinoglenoid notch causes only infraspinatus weakness.
4. Full-thickness cuff tear size is as follows: small—less than 1 cm, one tendon; medium—1 to 3 cm, one tendon; large—3 to 5 cm, two tendons; massive—greater than 5 cm, three or four tendons.
5. Dislocation after age 40 years will more commonly cause rotator cuff tear than labral pathology.
6. Belly press and liftoff tests signal subscapularis pathology.
7. Coronal MRI shows supraspinatus/infraspinatus tearing; axial MRI shows subscapularis tearing; sagittal MRI shows atrophy.
8. Rotator cuff repair failure increases with age, tear size, tendon retraction, muscle atrophy, decreased bone mineral density, and in patients who are smokers and those with diabetes mellitus.
9. There are no long-term clinical differences between open versus scope or single-row versus double-row rotator cuff repairs.
10. RTSA is a surgical treatment of choice for end-stage rotator cuff disease, cuff tear arthropathy.

INSTABILITY

Introduction

Shoulder instability is one of the main shoulder complaints in the emergency department and clinic settings. Initial traumatic instability can beget chronic instability, and patients can present to the clinician at any point along the spectrum. The clinician must know the signs, symptoms, and radiologic findings suggestive of instability and be well aware of particular at-risk populations that achieve better outcomes with surgical management versus those that do quite well with nonsurgical care.

Epidemiology

- Anterior instability
  - 0.08 per 1,000 person-years in rural US communities[10]
  - 0.17 to 0.24 per 100 person-years in European urban setting[11]
  - Tenfold higher in US military personnel, 1.69 per 1,000 person-years[12]
- Posterior instability
  - 4.64 per 100,000 person-years[13]
- Multidirectional instability (MDI)
  - Difficult to pinpoint exact incidence in the literature
  - Most common in younger, female patients

Pertinent Anatomy/Pathoanatomy

- Requires coordinated static and dynamic soft-tissue stabilizers to the glenohumeral joint
  - Static stabilizers (**Table 2**)
    - Labrum—fibrocartilaginous ring around the glenoid
      - Increases concavity-compression mechanism that keeps humeral head reduced into the glenoid
    - Joint capsule and glenohumeral ligaments (GHL) (**Figure 5**)
      - Anterior capsule and superior GHL
        - Prevent anterior translation with arm at neutral
      - Anterior capsule and middle GHL
        - Prevent anterior translation with arm in 45° of abduction
      - Anterior capsule and anteroinferior GHL
        - Prevent anterior translation with arm in 90° of abduction
      - Posterior capsule and posteroinferior GHL
        - Prevents posterior translation particularly in forward flexion and internal rotation
        - American football lineman blocking position

TABLE 2 Static Glenohumeral Stabilizers

Ligament	Constraint Provided
Superior glenohumeral	Anterior: arm in neutral abduction
Middle glenohumeral	Anterior: arm in 45° of abduction
Anterior inferior glenohumeral	Anterior: arm in 90° of abduction
Posterior inferior glenohumeral	Posterior: arm in forward flexion and internal rotation

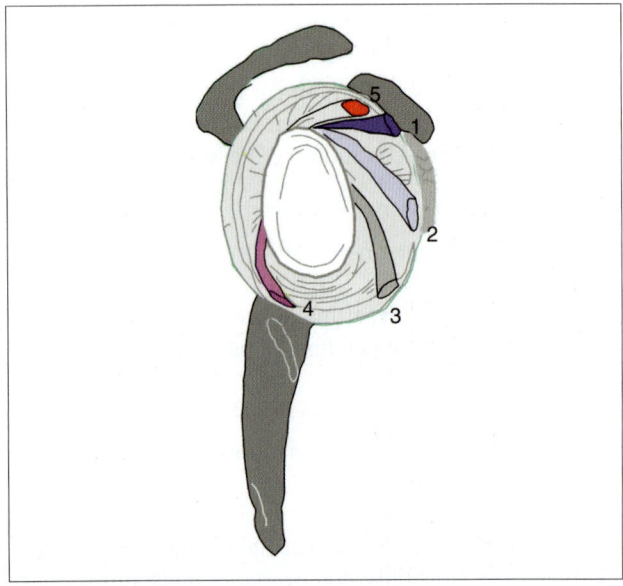

Figure 5 Schematic drawing showing the glenohumeral ligaments of a right shoulder. 1 = superior glenohumeral ligament, 2 = middle glenohumeral ligament, 3 = anterior band of inferior glenohumeral ligament, 4 = posterior band of inferior glenohumeral ligament, 5 = long head of the biceps tendon. (Reproduced with permission from Debski RE, Takeuchi S, Mattar LT: Anatomy and function of the shoulder structures, in Nicholson GP, ed: *Orthopaedic Knowledge Update®: Shoulder and Elbow 5*. American Academy of Orthopaedic Surgeons, 2020, p 3.)

- Dynamic stabilizers
  - Rotator cuff tendons
    - Increase concavity-compression mechanism to keep head centered when tensioned in a coordinated fashion
- Anterior instability
  - Initial instability event can produce anterior damages that beget further instability
    - Anteroinferior labral tear (Bankart lesion)
    - Anteroinferior glenoid rim fracture (bony Bankart lesion)
    - Posterior humeral head impaction fracture (Hill-Sachs lesion)
      - Occurs when humeral head slams against anterior glenoid during the dislocation event

- Inferior glenohumeral ligament, middle glenohumeral ligament, superior glenohumeral ligament tearing from the glenoid
- Humeral avulsion of glenohumeral ligament
  - GHL tearing from the humeral side
- Superior rotator cuff tears (supraspinatus and infraspinatus tears), subscapularis tears, and greater tuberosity fractures
  - Patients older than 40 years at higher risk
- Posterior instability
  - Posterior labral tear
  - Posterior glenoid rim fracture
  - Anterior humeral head impaction fractures
  - Posterior inferior glenohumeral ligament damage
- MDI
  - Generalized ligamentous laxity

Pertinent History/Physical Examination Findings

- History may present as acute traumatic, chronic/repetitive microtraumatic, MDI, and voluntary
  - Trauma (dislocation and subluxation) history should include the following elements:
    - Pain and anxiety of dislocating (apprehension) in vulnerable positions
    - Circumstances of dislocation (traumatic versus daily activity)
    - Number of dislocation events
    - Age at first dislocation
    - Type and competitive level of any relevant sports
    - Self-reduction versus reduction by a health care professional
- Physical examination
  - Active ROM followed by passive ROM in forward flexion, abduction, external rotation at neutral and 90° of abduction, and internal rotation at neutral and 90° of abduction
- Instability examination maneuvers to target the aforementioned pathology
  - Anterior apprehension and Jobe relocation testing
    - Patient supine to stabilize scapula as examiner slowly abducts arm to 90° and externally rotates to patient tolerance
      - Creates a subluxation event and patient will complain of pain or anxiety that the shoulder will dislocate (apprehension)

- Clinician then places a posterior force on the humeral head to reduce it back into the glenoid (Jobe relocation)
  - Patient should experience relief of pain/apprehension
- Posterior instability
  - Jerk test
    - Patient seated while clinician stabilizes scapula with one hand. The clinician's other hand places patient arm in 90° of abduction and 90° of internal rotation, then creates a horizontal adduction motion on the arm across the patient's body. Pain or clunk signals positive examination
  - Kim test
    - Patient seated with arm in 90° of abduction while clinician holds elbow and lateral upper arm while applying an axial load into the glenoid, then forward flexes 45° with a posteroinferior force toward the glenoid. Pain or clunk signals positive examination
- Load and shift test (appropriate for all instability)
  - Patient seated with clinician's hand stabilizing scapula, or supine
  - When patient supine, the clinician abducts and flexes the arm 20° and axially loads the humeral head into the glenoid, then creates anterior and posterior translational forces to determine the amount of translation
    - Grade 1—normal, 50% translation
    - Grade 2—abnormal, humeral head perches on glenoid
    - Grade 3—abnormal, humeral head dislocates
    - Examination often most reliable under general anesthesia before surgery because awake patients often guard against the examination
- Beighton score (particularly useful for MDI and voluntary dislocators)
  - Assessment of generalized ligamentous laxity
  - Score totals 9, less than and equal to 4 is normal for all of the various thresholds that exist
    - Passive small finger dorsiflexion—1 point each (2)
    - Passive apposition of thumb to volar forearm—1 point each (2)

- Elbow hyperextension—1 point each (2)
- Knee hyperextension—1 point each (2)
- Palms flat on floor during forward flexion at the waist with knees extended—1 point
- Inferior sulcus sign (useful for ligamentous laxity and inferior instability)
  - Patient seated as clinician pulls downward axial traction on the arm and observes any sulcus formed between the lateral acromion and humeral head or a pain or clunk

Relevant Imaging

- Plain radiographs
  - AP external rotation, AP internal rotation, Grashey (true AP), axillary, scapular Y views
    - Assess for reduced glenohumeral joint on the axillary
      - Posterior dislocations still commonly missed in the emergency department setting if only AP radiographs obtained
        - Classic lightbulb sign on an AP plain radiograph with an internally rotated shoulder on examination should immediately raise suspicion for posterior dislocation. Axillary view will confirm diagnosis and must always be obtained for patients with acute, traumatic instability in the emergency department
    - Scrutinize the glenoid rim for fracture or attritional insufficiency
    - Take note of Hill-Sachs lesions along the humeral head
- MRI
  - Mainstay of soft-tissue evaluation for capsulolabral injury
  - Magnetic resonance arthrogram can increase sensitivity (**Figure 6**)
    - Dye injected into glenohumeral joint before imaging
  - Axial cuts
    - Visualize anterior and posterior capsulolabral attachments to glenoid
    - Glenoid fractures or attritional loss evident
    - Hill-Sachs and reverse Hill-Sachs lesions apparent

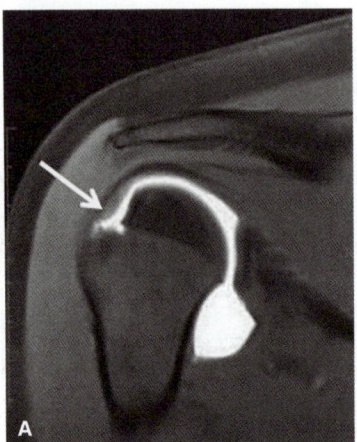 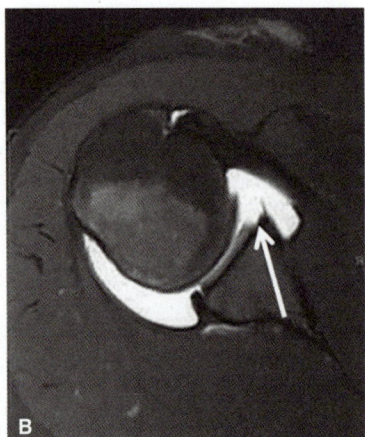

Figure 6 Magnetic resonance arthrogram of anterior shoulder instability injury. Coronal image (**A**) showing superior Hill-Sachs humeral head compression fracture and axial image (**B**) demonstrating the soft-tissue Bankart tear and chondral lesion. (Reproduced with permission from Chhabra A, Soldatos T, eds: *Musculoskeletal MRI Structured Evaluation*. Wolters Kluwer, 2014.)

- Coronal cuts
  - Demonstrate humeral avulsion of glenohumeral ligament lesions well
    - Seen as soft-tissue structures from the glenoid floating in the dye or synovial fluid extravasating from ruptured humeral capsuloligamentous attachment site
  - Superior labral pathology well visualized
- Sagittal cuts
  - May demonstrate gaps or fluid leakage between labrum and glenoid
  - May visualize glenoid fracture or attritional loss from en face view
- CT
  - Should be used when radiography or MRI demonstrates glenoid fracture or attritional bone loss or in any failed prior instability repair
    - Thin-cut, 2-mm scan because 3 and 4 mm of glenoid loss can amount to a significant percentage of the total surface area of joint

- Three-dimensional reconstructions with humeral head subtraction can provide a better image for injury measurement and surgical planning

Nonsurgical Management

- Dependent on symptoms and risks for redislocation
  - Older patients with traumatic instability have lower redislocation risk (assuming no acute cuff tearing)
    - Nonsurgical management very reasonable in this group
  - Patients younger than 40 years, particularly those in their second decade, have much higher redislocation risk even after first traumatic dislocation
    - Nonsurgical management should be used cautiously in this group and must be monitored closely if chosen
      - Continued instability should prompt a move toward surgical care
    - In-season athletes may attempt bracing treatment to delay surgical management, but close monitoring for continued instability should signal move toward surgery
  - MDI and voluntary dislocators
    - Always benefit from consistent, prolonged nonsurgical care with physical therapy regimen directed at strengthening the dynamic stabilizers to overcome generalized ligamentous laxity and muscular imbalances
      - This group has notoriously unreliable surgical outcomes and therefore stand to benefit the most from nonsurgical therapy
      - Should be used for 9 to 12 months before surgical consideration
- Nonsurgical care plan
  - Physical therapy aimed at strengthening and coordinating dynamic stabilizers of glenohumeral joint (rotator cuff and periscapular muscles)
    - Optimizes concavity-compression mechanism
  - Pain relief
    - NSAID
    - Intra-articular corticosteroid injection, if nonsurgical management is the ultimate goal

Surgical Intervention

- Indications
  - Determined by risk of recurrent dislocation, functional limitations/symptoms, efficacy of any nonsurgical care given
  - Repeat instability can beget further instability—causing damage that predisposes to glenohumeral arthritis
  - Risks for recurrent dislocation
    - Age
      - Younger than 20 years—+90%
      - Each decade thereafter approximately 10% to 15% decrease in risk until fifth decade where cuff injuries become more common than recurrent dislocation[14]
  - Contact sports
  - Higher levels of competitive athletic play
  - Acute bony fracture, significant chronic bone loss
  - Therefore, young, athletes in high levels of contact athletic play should be given high consideration for early surgical management
- Surgical options
  - Soft-tissue (capsulolabral) repair
    - Arthroscopic
      - Reasonable option for acute, subacute soft-tissue trauma without or less than 13% to 15% glenoid bone loss
      - Wide surgeon variability in positioning (beach chair versus lateral decubitus) and technique
        - Typically, anterior and posterior portals used for viewing and anchor/suture work (**Figure 7**)
        - Ultimate goal to reestablish contact between capsulolabral complex and glenoid rim
          - Must re-create the inferior capsulolabral sling that stabilizes the humeral head
            - Achieved by advancing the soft tissues somewhat superiorly, no more than 1 cm advancement to avoid excessive stiffness
        - Commonly used instrumentation
          - Suture, suture tapes, suture links/loops
          - Suture anchors (preloaded with suture, eyelets to dunk previously passed suture, knotless mechanisms)
          - Suture lassos, biting suture passers

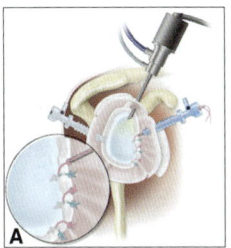 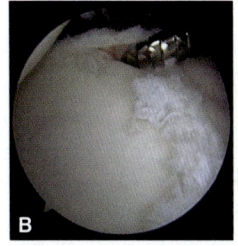 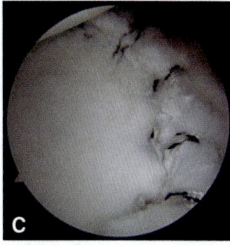

Figure 7 **A**, Schematic of arthroscopic labral repair with the camera viewing from anterosuperior portal and work occurring through the anteroinferior and posterior portals. Arthroscopic images of a right shoulder Bankart repair in lateral position viewing from an anterosuperior portal with a rasp instrument (**B**) demonstrating the inferior aspect of the tear and the final suture anchor repair (**C**). (Panel A reproduced with permission from Snyder SJ, Bahk M, Burns J, Getelman M, Karzel R, Auerbach DM, eds: *Shoulder Arthroscopy*, ed 3. Wolters Kluwer, 2014. Panels B and C courtesy of Dr. Julianne Munoz, University of Miami.)

- Each torn quadrant should be secured with three suture anchors
  - Essentially one anchor per hour on clock face of the glenoid
- Open capsulolabral repair
  - Relevant in multiple settings
    - Data show decreased failure rate compared with arthroscopic repair in young, competitive, contact athletes[15]
    - Also useful in revision scenarios from failed arthroscopic repair without bone loss
  - Technique
    - Limited deltopectoral approach
    - Subscapularis and capsular complex dissected off lesser tuberosity and proximal humerus
    - Labral repair performed in manner equivalent to arthroscopic
    - Capsular complex and/or subscapularis can be advanced and tightened on closure for additional stability
    - Additional scarring of open repair may also account for added stability seen in the young, high-contact group

- Bony stabilization procedures
  - Critical glenoid bone loss value still debated
    - Minimum end 13.5% and almost universally agreed on by 20%
    - Soft-tissue repairs have significantly higher failure rates and worse outcome scores[16]
  - Latarjet coracoid transfer (**Figure 8**)
    - Good option for up to 20% to 25% bone loss
    - Medialized incision for a deltopectoral approach
    - Subscapularis split horizontally to gain access to capsule
    - Capsule opened in a variety of ways (split, L-shaped, or T-shaped capsulotomies)
    - Coracoid resected just distal to the coracoclavicular ligaments
    - Transferred to the anterior glenoid rim with the inferior aspect lining up with the 5 to 5:30 clock-face position (right shoulder)
    - Stabilized with two compressive screws

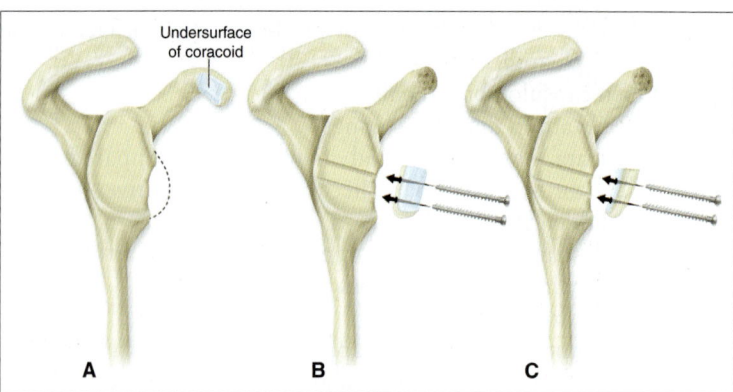

Figure 8 **A**, Schematic of classic and congruent-arc Latarjet techniques. The congruent-arc technique (**B**) places the inferolateral smooth surface of the coracoid parallel to the glenoid surface by rotating the graft 90°. **C**, The classic Latarjet technique places that inferolateral smooth surface down on the glenoid neck, providing a wider area for screw fixation. (Reproduced with permission from Snyder SJ, Bahk M, Burns J, Getelman M, Karzel R, Auerbach DM, eds: *Shoulder Arthroscopy*, ed 3. Wolters Kluwer, 2014.)

- Conjoin tendon brought along with the bone graft to add a soft-tissue sling of stability to the construct
- Capsular closure varies by surgeon preference, but subscapularis split sutured closed
- Other autograft and allograft options
  - When bone loss increases past 25%, the coracoid typically not large enough to overcome the deficit
    - Iliac crest autograft or allograft
    - Distal tibial plafond osteochondral allograft
      - Tibial plafond radius of curvature closely resembles that of glenoid[17]
      - Added benefit of a chondral surface for joint space
  - Techniques are all similar to the Latarjet procedure
- Postoperative management
  - Outpatient/ambulatory surgery
  - Sling immobilization and postoperative physical therapy protocols vary
    - Sling immobilization typically from 2 to 6 weeks depending on size of repair and/or bone healing considerations
    - Progresses through: non–weight bearing, passive ROM, active ROM, and last, strengthening
      - Non–weight bearing is generally universal until the 12-week mark
      - External rotation, particularly in abduction, advances in protected fashion throughout the rehabilitation for anterior instability as this is the position of dislocation
        - External rotation begins with arm at neutral and then progressive degrees of abduction as the weeks advance in the protocol
    - Complete recovery through the rehabilitation protocol usually between 3 and 6 months depending on the aforementioned factors
      - Sport-specific training in therapy may occur once strengthening progresses, usually not until the 4- to 6-month range
  - Perioperative antibiotics to cover skin flora before incision
    - 2 g intravenous cephazolin versus weight-based vancomycin versus 900 mg clindamycin
      - Aforementioned options dependent on patient allergy profile

- Pain control
  - Regional anesthesia with peripheral nerve blocks and catheters that patients can remove at home decreases postoperative narcotic usage
  - Multimodal oral pain control regimen
    - Tylenol 650 mg by mouth every 6 hours × 72 hours (over the counter)
    - Toradol 10 mg 1 tablet by mouth 3 times a day × 72 hours, then 1 tablet by mouth twice a day × 2 days (13 tablets)
    - Gabapentin 300 mg 1 tablet by mouth 3 times a day × 72 hours (9 tablets)
    - Oxycodone 5 mg 1 tablet by mouth every 6 hours taken as needed (20 tablets with no refills) for breakthrough pain only—maximum 4 tablets per day
  - Deep vein thrombosis: rates are very low in shoulder surgery; therefore, no standard prophylaxis protocol exists and many use none
  - Imaging
    - Intraoperative portable or postoperative plain radiographs in bony stabilization procedures to confirm graft and hardware position and absence of subluxated/dislocated humeral head
- Complications
  - Most common are failure and stiffness
    - Failure presents as inability to progress through rehabilitation, persistent or new-onset pain, popping, or repeat dislocation/subluxation events
      - Consider magnetic resonance arthrogram when failure suspected in soft-tissue cases
      - Repeat plain radiographs at follow-ups for patients with bony stabilization to confirm graft incorporation
        - Rule out graft migration, resorption, screw cutout
        - Axillary view particularly helpful for this evaluation
  - Anchor pullout, may result in loose body
  - Persistent pain
  - Infection, less than 1%

- Outcomes
  - Bankart repair versus Latarjet procedure
    - Repeat dislocation rates of 15.1% versus 7.7%, respectively, at long-term follow-up[18]
    - Highlights the needs for correct patient selection for soft-tissue versus bony procedures
  - Tibial plafond osteochondral allograft
    - Equivalent recurrence rates to Latarjet procedure in the patient group with advanced bone loss greater than 20% to 25%[19]
  - Outcomes for all of these procedures are very promising, but patient selection based on the observed pathology and specific functional demands are key to surgical success and recurrence rates

Top 10 Knowledge Drops for Your Rotation

1. Labrum and glenohumeral ligaments provide static glenohumeral stability, and the cuff is dynamic.
2. Anterior dislocations often cause Bankart lesions at the anteroinferior labrum and Hill-Sachs lesions in the posterosuperior humeral head.
3. Age older than 40 years is a risk factor for cuff tears and greater tuberosity fractures after dislocation.
4. Age at first dislocation, number of dislocations, type, and competition level of sport are key factors to determining recurrence risk.
5. Load and shift, anterior apprehension test, and Jobe relocation test examine anterior instability. Load and shift, Kim, and jerk tests aid in posterior instability diagnosis.
6. MRI is the gold standard modality for evaluating soft-tissue instability pathology.
7. CT is used to evaluate acute fracture or chronic attritional glenoid bone loss.
8. MDI should be managed nonsurgically with consistent physical therapy efforts for 12+ months.
9. There are roles for both arthroscopic and open labral repair.
10. Bone loss of 20% or higher requires a bone transfer or graft procedure.

ADHESIVE CAPSULITIS

Introduction

Adhesive capsulitis, also referred to as frozen shoulder, is a condition marked by severe pain and inflammation leading to contracture and range of motion loss. The key features that differentiate it from other diagnoses are the symmetric loss of passive and active ROM in shoulders that have no arthritis and normal radiographs.

Epidemiology

- Prevalence of 2% to 5%[20]
- Women and patients with diabetes more commonly affected
- Type 2 diabetes is also a risk factor
- Other risk factors
  - Hyperthyroidism
  - Previous shoulder, breast, or cervical spine surgery
- Etiology remains unclear

Pertinent Anatomy/Pathoanatomy

- Inflammatory contracture of the shoulder capsule
- Biopsy of the capsule demonstrates chronic inflammatory infiltrate, absence of synovial lining, and moderate to extensive subsynovial fibrosis[21]
- In global adhesive capsulitis, all capsular structures are involved
  - Rotator interval
  - Anterior capsule
  - Posterior capsule
- Rotator cuff muscles and tendons, biceps tendon typically are not involved
- It is rare to have a full-thickness rotator cuff tear and adhesive capsulitis concurrently (it can occur, but rarely)

Pertinent History/Physical Examination Findings

- History
  - Patients will relate atraumatic onset of shoulder pain (often begins as bursitis)

- Patients will recall increasing pain over a period of time (can be relatively acute) with a concurrent decreased range of motion (it is the decreased range of motion that often causes them to finally seek medical attention)
- Patients will note the inability to reach the back pocket, use the arm for toileting, reach the bra, wash the opposite axilla, etc
- Physical examination
  - Pearl: must place any patient who demonstrates any decreased range of motion in the upright position immediately into the supine position and reexamine
  - Patients will compensate with scapulothoracic motion, move their whole body, etc (the clinician can be fooled if the patient is not in the supine position)
  - Hallmark of adhesive capsulitis is the symmetric loss of active and passive range of motion. In other words, sometimes patients will stop raising their arm in forward elevation because of pain but passively the clinician can fully raise the arm—this is not adhesive capsulitis
  - The rotator cuff examination is typically normal with respect to strength
  - Impingement tests (Neer and Hawkins) are not applicable in patients with adhesive capsulitis—these tests rely on full, unimpeded range of motion and would be positive in the face of a frozen shoulder because all movement in those ranges hurts due to the restricted motion

Relevant Imaging

- Standard three-view radiograph series is critically important—true AP (Grashey view), outlet view, and axillary view.
- Diagnoses to rule out
  - Posterior dislocation (missed still in North America up to 60% of the time because of failure to obtain axillary radiograph). Key to this diagnosis is fixed internal rotation (light bulb sign on true AP) and inability to externally rotate even beyond neutral.
  - Glenohumeral osteoarthritis: patients with glenohumeral degenerative joint disease can have profound loss of motion as well, but this is a completely different diagnosis compared with adhesive capsulitis.

- CT is not routinely necessary for this diagnosis.
- MRI is not routinely necessary for this diagnosis.
- Many patients will be referred already having had MRI ordered by their primary care physician, but unless there is suspicion of a concurrent rotator cuff tear (weakness on examination, proximal migration of the humerus on plain radiographs, etc), MRI need not be ordered in most cases.

Nonsurgical Management

- Approximately 90% of patients with adhesive capsulitis are successfully treated without surgery.[22]
- Typical treatment program for initial evaluation:
  - Confirm diagnosis from history, examination, and plain radiographs.
  - Start physical therapy program 3 times per week for 6 weeks.
  - Ask patient to bring family member (whenever possible) to physical therapy session so they can be properly instructed on how to assist with the home stretching exercise program.
  - Have patient buy-in to home stretching program—must be done daily in addition to the thrice-weekly physical therapy program.
  - NSAID prescription—help to decrease inflammation and allow physical therapist, patient, and family member to break up the scar tissue necessary to heal the frozen shoulder.
- Patient returns in 6 weeks following initial treatment plan (physical therapy, home stretching, and NSAIDs).
  - If patient is no better or only marginally better, typically proceed with ultrasound-guided glenohumeral cortisone injection (cocktail including 4 mL 1% lidocaine, 4 mL 0.5% bupivacaine, and 2 mL triamcinolone). Many doctors/surgeons use a much smaller amount, which can lead to failure of the injection.

Surgical Intervention

- Indications
  - Indications for surgery include failure to respond to the aforementioned nonsurgical algorithm—6 months is typically considered appropriate time if the patient has been completely compliant

- One study showed that risk factors for predicting failure of nonsurgical management included those patients who did not respond positively (or regressed) 4 months into the treatment plan[22]
- Key findings on history
  - Pain
  - Loss of range of motion
- Key findings on examination
  - Symmetric loss of active and passive motion
  - Examine the patient in the supine position to confirm
- Technique
  - Ambulatory surgery
  - Interscalene anesthetic block (do not typically use general anesthesia)
  - Applied anatomy/approach
    - Beach chair position
    - Standard posterior portal (approximately 2 cm distal and approximately 1 cm medial to posterolateral acromion)
    - Must be careful to avoid transhumeral placement of arthroscope when attempting to enter the contracted frozen shoulder; aim a little higher than normal to try and place scope in the upper one-third of the joint; risk is going to proximal and entering the subacromial space
  - Surgical keys
    - Methodical ablation of the capsular contracture
      - Start with the rotator interval release—protect the labrum, articular cartilage, subscapularis, and biceps tendons
        - Coracohumeral and superior glenohumeral ligament release
        - Keys to complete release
          - Humerus will lateralize
          - Visualize the coracoacromial ligament, coracoid, and strap muscles from the glenohumeral joint (not typical to see these structures from the glenohumeral joint)
      - Anterior capsular release
        - Middle glenohumeral ligament and inferior glenohumeral ligament release
        - Protect subscapularis tendon

- Be cautious regarding axillary nerve
- Use cautery to approximately 5-o'clock position (right shoulder) and then stop because nerve is very close in frozen shoulder
- Perform gentle manipulation under anesthesia
    - Remove arthroscope from shoulder
    - Take arm out of extremity holder
    - Short lever arm
    - Forward elevation first—should hear and feel pops as final inferior capsular contracture is released
    - External rotation second—there may or may not be any adhesions left, but the resultant forward elevation and external rotation should be tension-free at this point
    - Place scope back in from posterior portal and the anteroinferior release will extend where cautery was stopped at 5-o'clock position into the inferior pouch—it extends like a zipper opening up
    - Keys to complete release
        - Complete visualization of subscapularis tendon
- Posterior capsular release
    - Place switching stick into anterior cannula and place scope anteriorly
    - Find anterosuperior release just anterior to biceps tendon/labrum
    - Continue release from anterosuperior capsule posteriorly all the way to the posterior portal—do not injure superior labrum or rotator cuff; re-create normal space between superior labrum and cuff
    - Keys to complete release
        - Visualization of infraspinatus muscle fibers
- Postoperative orders
    - Must obtain radiographs in the PACU (can be a source of postoperative litigation if patient experiences a dislocation following extensive release and there is no radiographic evidence that the joint was reduced)
    - Must rule out proximal humerus fracture
    - Show the patient their range of motion in the PACU (full range of motion); their range of motion can be videoed with

the patient's own phone so they can refer back to it when they are home
- Physical therapy
  - Do not proceed with this surgery if the patient does not have postoperative physical therapy sessions scheduled (minimum of 3 times per week)
  - Tell the patient to wear a sling only as they leave the hospital, but as soon as interscalene block wears off they should be out of the sling at all times
- Postoperative pain protocol
  - Multimodal analgesia (patients younger than 65 years)
    - Tylenol 650 mg by mouth every 6 hours × 72 hours (over the counter)
    - Toradol 10 mg 1 tablet by mouth 3 times a day × 72 hours, then 1 tablet by mouth twice a day × 2 days (13 tablets)
    - Gabapentin 300 mg 1 tablet by mouth 3 times a day × 72 hours (9 tablets)
    - Oxycodone 5 mg 1 tablet by mouth every 6 hours taken as needed (20 tablets with no refills) for breakthrough pain only—maximum 4 tablets per day
  - Multimodal analgesia (patients older than 65 years)
    - Tylenol 650 mg by mouth every 6 hours × 72 hours (over the counter)
    - Toradol 10 mg 1 tablet by mouth 3 times per day × 72 hours, then 1 tablet by mouth twice a day × 2 days (13 tablets)
    - Gabapentin 100 mg 1 tablet by mouth 3 times per day × 72 hours (9 tablets)
    - Oxycodone 5 mg 1 tablet by mouth every 6 hours taken as needed (20 tablets with no refills) for breakthrough pain only—maximum 4 tablets per day
- Pearls and pitfalls
  - Must have tension-free range of motion
  - More motion will not be achieved after surgery but the patient can certainly lose motion, with pain, difficulty complying with home exercises, delay in going to physical therapy as contributing factors
  - Must obtain radiographs in PACU

- Potential complications
  - Proximal humerus fracture
  - Shoulder dislocation
  - Subscapularis avulsion
- Outcomes
  - A recent systematic review showed that surgical treatment was most effective method to increasing range of motion[23]

Top 10 Knowledge Drops for Your Rotation

1. History—look for comorbidities, especially diabetes mellitus
2. Examination—global loss of motion
3. Examination—examine in supine position to avoid being fooled
4. Examination—active motion loss = passive motion loss
5. Examination—do not be fooled by locked posterior dislocation or glenohumeral arthritis
6. Imaging studies—must have 90° orthogonal radiographs to rule out missed posterior dislocation
7. Nonsurgical management—successful in approximately 90% of patients
8. Nonsurgical management—physical therapy, home exercises, and cortisone injections when necessary
9. Surgery
   a. Very successful when necessary
   b. Meticulous excision/release of global contracture
   c. Must obtain PACU radiographs to rule out fracture or dislocation
10. Must have willing and able patient who can comply with postoperative rehabilitation protocol to maximize success

GLENOHUMERAL OSTEOARTHRITIS

Introduction

Symptomatic glenohumeral osteoarthritis is characterized by pain, loss of motion, and progressive loss of shoulder function. Radiographic changes include joint space narrowing and obliteration, subchondral sclerosis, cysts, and osteophyte formation.

Epidemiology

- Primary and secondary
- Primary
  - Large age range but often differentiated into younger than 50 years and older than 50 years
  - No known cause for the arthritis
  - Unclear what the true incidence and prevalence are
- Secondary
  - Posttraumatic
  - Postinflammatory/postinfectious
  - Postoperative[24]
  - Sequelae of osteonecrosis
- Etiology remains unclear

Pertinent Anatomy/Pathoanatomy

- Erosion of articular cartilage
- Continued progression to loss of posterior glenoid bone (increased retroversion)
- Development of capsular contracture and progressive loss of motion
- Typically not associated with rotator cuff tearing
- Strength well preserved

Pertinent History/Physical Examination Findings

- History
  - No pain at rest (especially in early stages)
  - Pain with activities—especially with reaching overhead, cross-body, or behind the back
  - Pain at night
  - Insidious onset—not typically a one-time traumatic event
- Physical examination
  - Pearl: similar to adhesive capsulitis examination—must place any patient who demonstrates any decreased range of motion in the upright position immediately into the supine position and reexamine
  - Patients will compensate with scapulothoracic motion, move their entire body, etc (the clinician can be fooled if the patient is not in the supine position)

- Hallmark of osteoarthritis is the loss of internal rotation
- Crepitus and grinding with examination—often painful for the patient
- The rotator cuff examination is normal with respect to strength
- Impingement tests (Neer and Hawkins) are not applicable in patients with osteoarthritis—these tests rely on full, unimpeded range of motion and of course would be positive in the face of arthritis because any motion in those ranges hurt through the restricted motion

Relevant Imaging

- Standard three-view radiograph series is critically important—true AP (Grashey view), outlet view, and axillary view (**Figure 9**)
- Radiographic hallmarks of osteoarthritis (**Figures 10** and **11**)
  - Loss of joint space (asymmetric more common in degenerative arthritis [posterior] versus symmetric in inflammatory arthritis)
  - Osteophyte formation
  - Subchondral sclerosis
  - Subchondral cyst formation
- Diagnoses to rule out
  - Posterior dislocation (missed still in North America up to 60% of the time because of failure to obtain axillary radiograph). Key to this diagnosis is fixed internal rotation (light bulb sign on true AP view) and inability to externally rotate even beyond neutral

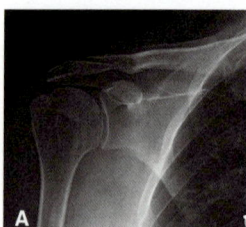
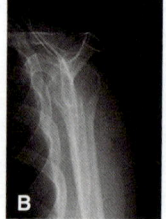
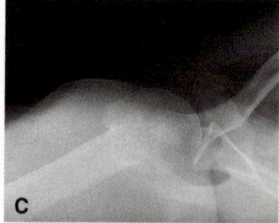

Figure 9 **A**, True AP (Grashey view) of a normal glenohumeral joint demonstrating appropriate joint space preservation between the humeral head and the glenoid. **B**, Outlet view from the same patient. **C**, Axillary lateral view from the same patient. Note normal "golf ball on golf tee" appearance. (Courtesy of Dr. William Levine, Columbia Orthopedics.)

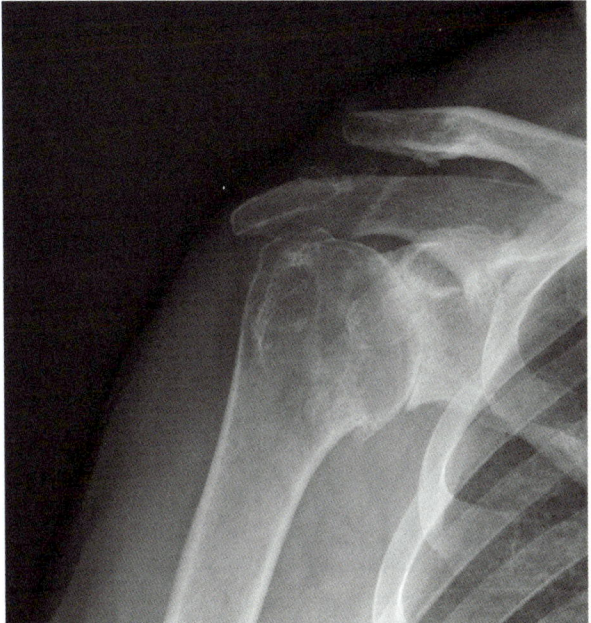

Figure 10 True AP radiographic view from a 70-year-old man with rheumatic heart disease with end-stage osteoarthritis of the right shoulder. Note the complete obliteration of the joint space, subchondral sclerosis, and osteophyte formation. (Courtesy of Dr. William Levine, Columbia Orthopedics.)

- Rotator cuff tear arthropathy—patient will have degenerative joint disease in addition to massive rotator cuff tear with resultant proximal humeral migration
- CT is not routinely necessary for this diagnosis but is used for preoperative planning
- MRI is not routinely necessary for this diagnosis
- Many patients will be referred already having had MRI ordered by their primary care physician, but unless there is suspicion of a concurrent rotator cuff tear (weakness on examination, proximal migration of the humerus on plain radiographs, etc), MRI need not be ordered in most cases. Fewer than 5% of patients with glenohumeral osteoarthritis have concurrent rotator cuff tears.

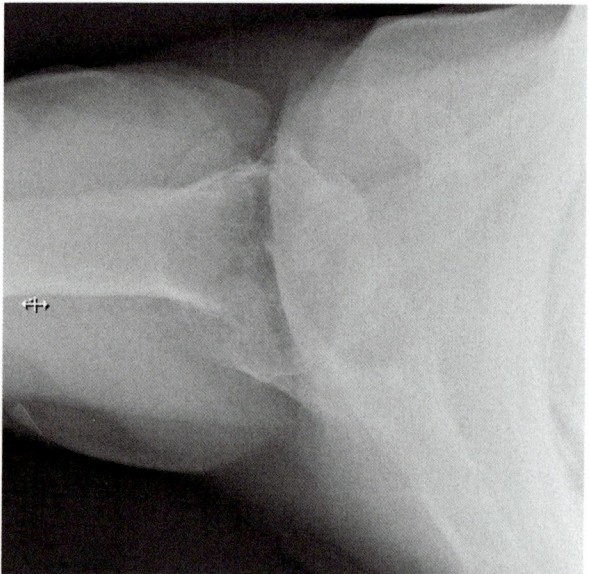

Figure 11 Axillary lateral radiograph from the same patient described in Figure 10. Note the complete joint space obliteration and the posterior glenoid erosion. (Courtesy of Dr. William Levine, Columbia Orthopedics.)

- Walch classification[25] (113 shoulders studied using CT) (**Figure 12**)
  - Type A—concentric wear of the glenoid with centered humeral head (59%)
  - Type B—eccentric wear with posterior glenoid erosion and posterior humeral head subluxation (32%)
  - Type C—glenoid retroversion greater than 25° (9%)

Nonsurgical Management

- Early arthritis can be managed with NSAIDs, physical therapy, home exercises, activity modification.
- Injections should be used with caution with growing evidence that there is an associated increased risk of infection following shoulder arthroplasty in patients who have had previous injections.
- Current recommendation is to delay shoulder arthroplasty 3 months from the time of most recent glenohumeral injection.[26]

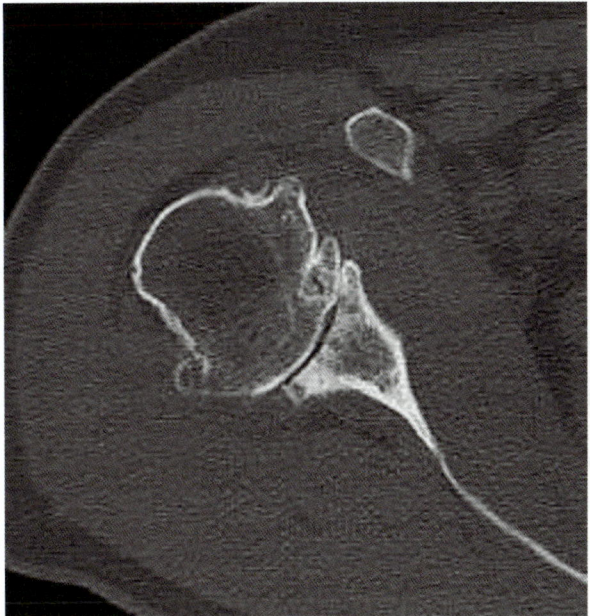

Figure 12 Axial CT scan from same patient described in Figure 10 showing posterior erosion (B2 glenoid) and end-stage arthritis. (Courtesy of Dr. William Levine, Columbia Orthopedics.)

- Typical treatment program for initial evaluation
  - Confirm diagnosis from history, examination, and plain radiographs.
  - Start physical therapy program twice per week for 6 weeks.
  - Physical therapy can aggravate symptoms, so it is important to inform patient and make sure they stop physical therapy if they experience increased symptoms.
  - NSAID prescription—help to decrease inflammation and pain.
  - Try to limit or avoid glenohumeral injections.

Surgical Intervention

- Indications
  - Indications for surgery include failure to respond to the nonsurgical algorithm
  - Progressive loss of motion with correlating decreased function and increased pain

- Patients will tell you when they are ready for surgery—you do not have to tell them
- Key findings on history
  - Progressive increase in pain (can't live with symptoms any longer)
  - Progressive loss of range of motion
- Key findings on examination
  - Symmetric loss of active and passive motion
  - Examine the patient in the supine position to confirm
  - Crepitus/grinding with attempts to range the shoulder
- Technique
  - Ambulatory or 23-hour-stay surgery (approximately 70% ambulatory now)
  - Interscalene anesthetic block (+/− general anesthesia—this is patient and anesthesiologist specific)
  - Applied anatomy/approach
    - Beach chair position
    - Standard deltopectoral approach
      - Identify cephalic vein
      - Deltoid lateral, pectoralis major medial
    - Identify coracoid process (lighthouse of the shoulder)
      - Neurovascular structures are primarily medial to coracoid
    - Subscapularis management—discussed later
    - Glenoid exposure—discussed later
    - Subscapularis repair/closure
  - Surgical keys
    - Access to the glenohumeral joint—three common options
      - Lesser tuberosity osteotomy
      - Subscapularis peel
      - Subscapularis tenotomy
    - Release the subscapularis and capsule off the humerus to allow dislocation of the humerus into the surgical field
    - Humeral head osteotomy (for most of the systems, the humeral head is removed; for a few systems, the humeral head is not resected but instead reshaped to accommodate the specific humeral prosthesis)
    - For short and standard-stem prostheses: mill the intramedullary canal to fit the prosthesis, then trial and place head

- For stemless devices: prepare the metaphysis to accept the metaphyseal component, then trial and place head
- Glenoid exposure (**Figure 13**)
  - The soft-tissue releases necessary to dislocate the humerus assist with having appropriate access to the glenoid
  - Fukuda retractor placed posteriorly to protect the humerus and move it out of the way
  - 90° Bankart retractor placed anteriorly and secured to the drapes with a clamp to minimize assistants
  - Large Hohmann retractor placed superiorly to give excellent and reproducible exposure to the glenoid every time
- Glenoid preparation
  - Reaming is critical to have the glenoid bone match the back-side of whichever glenoid implant is being used—goal is to achieve at least 90% contact

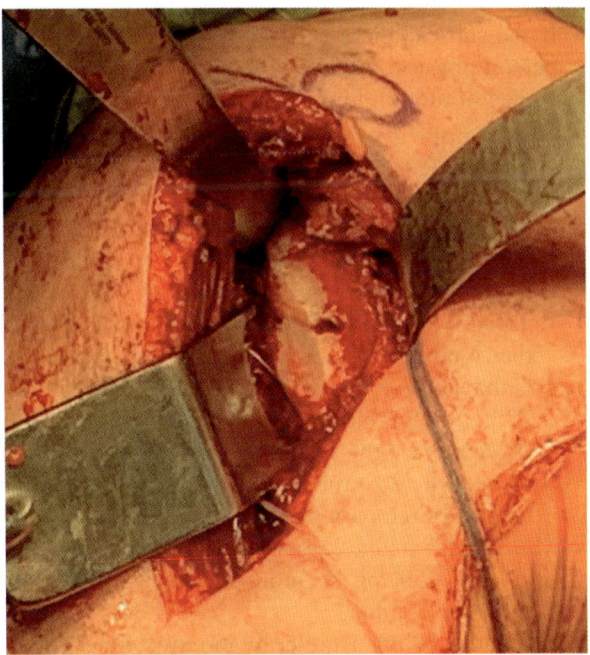

Figure 13 Intraoperative view of glenoid with posterior erosion. (Courtesy of Dr. William Levine, Columbia Orthopedics.)

- If contact is less than 90% may have to ream more, use bone graft, or use an augmented glenoid component
- If contact is severely compromised, may need to consider using reverse total shoulder arthroplasty (TSA) as opposed to anatomic total shoulder
- Subscapularis repair
  - Critical to success of anatomic TSA
  - Lesser tuberosity osteotomy advocates believe stronger and better due to bone-to-bone healing
  - A recent randomized controlled trial did not show superiority, however, and determined that it is ultimately dealer's choice on which technique surgeons use[27]
- Postoperative orders
  - Must obtain radiographs in the PACU (true AP and axillary views to confirm appropriate prosthesis placement, no evidence of dislocation, etc) (**Figures 14** and **15**)
  - Physical therapy
    - If the subscapularis is of good integrity, then formal, in-person physical therapy will begin the day after surgery
    - Range of motion limitations determined by intraoperative findings—quality of tendon, quality of repair—subscapularis integrity is critical to ultimate success of anatomic TSA
  - Postoperative pain protocol
    - Multimodal analgesia (patients younger than 65 years)
      - Tylenol 650 mg by mouth every 6 hours × 72 hours (over the counter)
      - Toradol 10 mg 1 tablet by mouth 3 times a day × 72 hours, then 1 tablet by mouth twice a day × 2 days (13 tablets)
      - Gabapentin 300 mg 1 tablet by mouth 3 times a day × 72 hours (9 tablets)
      - Oxycodone 5 mg 1 tablet by mouth every 6 hours taken as needed (20 tablets with no refills) to be taken for breakthrough pain only—maximum 4 tablets per day
    - Multimodal analgesia (patients older than 65 years)
      - Tylenol 650 mg by mouth every 6 hours × 72 hours (over the counter)
      - Toradol 10 mg 1 tablet by mouth 3 times per day × 72 hours, then 1 tablet by mouth twice a day × 2 days (13 tablets)

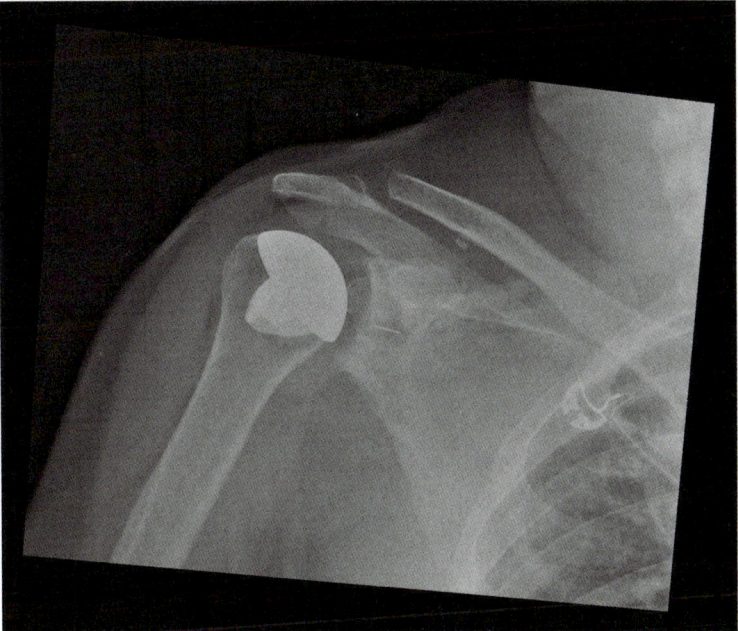

Figure 14 Postoperative anesthesia care unit true AP radiograph demonstrating anatomic positioning of the stemless total shoulder arthroplasty (same patient from Figure 13). (Courtesy of Dr. William Levine, Columbia Orthopedics.)

- Gabapentin 100 mg 1 tablet by mouth 3 times a day × 72 hours (9 tablets)
- Oxycodone 5 mg 1 tablet by mouth every 6 hours taken as needed (20 tablets with no refills) for breakthrough pain only—maximum 4 tablets per day
• Pearls and pitfalls
  • Nonsurgical management of glenohumeral osteoarthritis not particularly successful
  • Avoid glenohumeral injections if at all possible
  • When patients are ready, anatomic TSA has an extremely successful track record of success
  • Subscapularis integrity critical to success of anatomic TSA
  • If subscapularis fails, may need to convert to reverse TSA

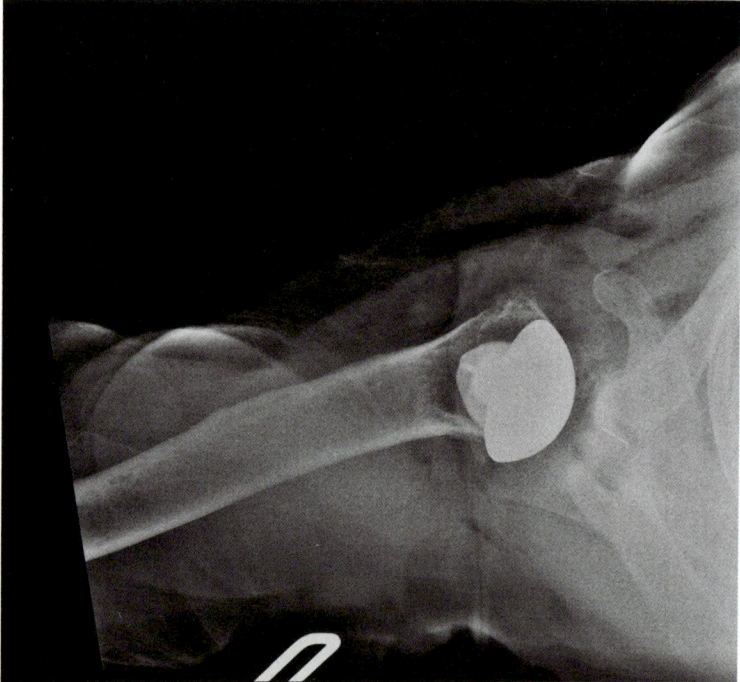

Figure 15 Postoperative anesthesia care unit axillary radiograph demonstrating anatomic position of the stemless total shoulder arthroplasty (note the metal marker in the polyethylene glenoid component for tracking purposes). (Courtesy of Dr. William Levine, Columbia Orthopedics.)

- Patients must be informed that they have the harder part of the postoperative rehabilitation protocol—if they do not perform their daily exercises they can have a compromised outcome.
- Outcomes
  - Recent American Academy of Orthopaedic Surgeons clinical practice guidelines show strong support recommending total shoulder arthroplasty over hemiarthroplasty for the management of glenohumeral osteoarthritis in most patients.[28]

Top 10 Knowledge Drops for Your Rotation

1. History—progressive increased pain with insidious onset
2. Examination—global loss of motion
3. Examination—examine in supine position to avoid being fooled
4. Examination—active motion loss = passive motion loss
5. Examination—crepitus and grinding that is often painful and audible
6. Imaging studies—evaluate for type of glenoid (Walch classification)
7. Nonsurgical management—not particularly successful but worth trying in milder early stages of degenerative joint disease
8. Nonsurgical management—Physical therapy: do not send patients with advanced degenerative joint disease for physical therapy—will often exacerbate the underlying symptoms
9. Surgery
   a. Tremendously positive outcomes for patients who undergo shoulder arthroplasty
   b. 97% patient satisfaction in one meta-analysis[29]
10. Must have willing and able patient who can comply with postoperative rehabilitation protocol to maximize success

References

1. Weber S, Chahal J: AAOS clinical practice guideline summary: Management of rotator cuff injuries. *J Am Acad Orthop Surg* 2020;28:e193-e201.
2. Sher JS, Uribe JW, Posada A, Murphy BJ, Zlatkin MB: Abnormal findings on magnetic resonance images of asymptomatic shoulders. *J Bone Joint Surg Am* 1995;77:10-15.
3. Tempelhof S, Rupp S, Seil R: Age-related prevalence of rotator cuff tears in asymptomatic shoulders. *J Shoulder Elbow Surg* 1999;8(4):296-299.
4. Yamaguchi K, Ditsios K, Middleton W, Hildebolt C, Galatz L, Teefery S: The demographic and morphological features of rotator cuff disease: A comparision of asymptomatic and symptomatic shoulders. *J Bone Joint Surg Am* 2006;88(8):1699-1704.

5. Mochizuki T, Sugaya H, Uomizu M, et al: Humeral insertion of the supraspinatus and infraspinatus. New anatomical findings regarding the footprint of the rotator cuff. *J Bone Joint Surg* 2009;91(suppl 2, pt 1):1-7.
6. Kissenberth M, Rulewicz G, Hamilton S, Bruch H, Hawkins R: A positive tangent sign predicts the repairability of rotator cuff tears. *J Shoulder Elbow Surg* 2014;23(7):1023-1027.
7. Duncan N, Booker S, Gooding B, Geoghegan J, Wallace W, Manning P: Surgery within 6 months of an acute rotator cuff tear significantly improves outcome. *J Shoulder Elbow Surg* 2015;24(12):1876-1880.
8. Bedeir Y, Jimenez A, Grawe B: Recurrent tears of the rotator cuff: Effect of repair technique and management options. *Orthop Rev (Pavia)* 2018;10(2):7593.
9. Goldenberg B, Samuelsen B, Spratt J, Dornan G, Millett P: Complications and implant survivorship following primary reverse total shoulder arthroplasty in patients younger than 65 years: A systematic review. *J Shoulder Elbow Surg* 2020;29(8):1703-1711.
10. Krøner K, Lind T, Jensen J: The epidemiology of shoulder dislocations. *Arch Orthop Trauma Surg* 1989;108:288-290.
11. Nordqvist A, Petersson CJ: Incidence and causes of shoulder girdle injuries in an urban population. *J Shoulder Elbow Surg* 1995;4(2):107-112.
12. Waterman B, Owens B, Tokish J: Anterior shoulder instability in the military athlete. *Sports Health* 2016;8(6):514-519.
13. Woodmass J, Lee J, Wu I, et al: Incidence of posterior shoulder instability and trends in surgical reconstruction: A 22-year population-based study. *J Shoulder Elbow Surg* 2019;28(4):611-616.
14. Spang J, Mazzocca A, Arciero R: The unstable shoulder, in Boyer M, ed: *AAOS Comprehensive Orthopaedic Review 2*. American Academy of Orthopaedic Surgeons, 2014, p 932.
15. Balg F, Boileau P: The instability severity index score. A simple pre--operative score to select patients for arthroscopic or open shoulder stabilisation. *J Bone Joint Surg Br* 2007;89(11):1470-1477.
16. Shaha J, Cook J, Song D, et al: Redefining "critical" bone loss in shoulder instability: Functional outcomes worsen with "subcritical" bone loss. *Am J Sports Med* 2015;43(7):1719-1725.
17. Provencher MT, Ghodadra N, LeClere L, et al: Anatomic osteochondral glenoid reconstruction for recurrent glenohumeral instability with glenoid deficiency using a distal tibia allograft. *Arthroscopy* 2009;25(4):446-452.
18. Rollick N, Ono Y, Kurji H, et al: Long-term outcomes of the Bankart and Latarjet repairs: A systematic review. *Open Access J Sports Med* 2017;8:97-105.

19. Frank R, Romeo A, Richarson C, et al: Outcomes of Latarjet vs. distal tibia allograft for anterior shoulder instability repair: A matched cohort analysis. *Am J Sports Med* 2018;46(5):1030-1038.
20. Lewis J: Frozen shoulder contracture syndrome – Aetiology, diagnosis and management. *Man Ther* 2015;20:2-9.
21. Neviaser J: Adheisve capsulitis of the shoulder. *J Bone Joint Surg* 1945;27:211-222.
22. Levine WN, Kashyap CP, Bak SF, Ahmad CS, Blaine TA, Bigliani LU: Nonoperative management of idiopathic adhesive capsulitis. *J Shoulder Elbow Surg* 2007;16:569-573.
23. Forsythe B, Lavoie-Gagne O, Patel BH, et al: Efficacy of arthroscopic surgery in the management of adhesive capsulitis: A systematic review and network meta-analysis of randomized controlled trials. *Arthroscopy* 2020;37(7):2281-2297.
24. Kruckeberg B, Leland DP, Bernard CD, et al: Incidence of and risk factors for glenohumeral osteoarthritis after anterior shoulder instability a US population-based study with average 15-year follow-up. *Orthop J Sports Med* 2020;8(11):2325967120962515.
25. Walch G, Badet R, Boulahia A, Khoury A: Morphologic study of the glenoid in primary glenohumeral osteoarthritis. *J Arthroplasty* 1999;14:756-760.
26. Werner BC, Cancienne JM, Burrus MT, Griffin JW, Gwathmey FW, Brockmeier SF: The timing of elective shoulder surgery after shoulder injection affects postoperative infection risk in Medicare patients. *J Shoulder Elbow Surg* 2016;25(3):390-397.
27. Levine WN, Munoz J, Hsu S, et al: Subscapularis tenotomy versus lesser tuberosity osteotomy during total shoulder arthroplasty for primary osteoarthritis: A prospective, randomized controlled trial. *J Shoulder Elbow Surg* 2019;28(3):407-414.
28. Khazzam M, Gee A, Pearl M: Management of glenohumeral osteoarthritis. *J Am Acad Orthop Surg* 2020;28(19):781-789.
29. Radnay CS, Setter KJ, Chambers L, Levine WN, Bigliani LU, Ahmad CS: Total shoulder replacement compared with humeral head replacement for the treatment of primary glenohumeral osteoarthritis: A systematic review. *J Shoulder Elbow Surg* 2007;16:396-402.

6

My Elbow Hurts

Charles M. Jobin, MD, FAAOS
Charles Cassidy, MD, FAAOS

Introduction

Elbow pain is a common musculoskeletal complaint of adults. Elbow tendinitis is the most common cause for why people complain, "my elbow hurts." Elbow tendinitis affects both the lateral and medial elbow but other disorders such as compressive neuropathy of the ulnar nerve at the cubital tunnel and distal biceps tendon injuries are also common disorders of the elbow.

LATERAL EPICONDYLITIS

Lateral epicondylitis is an overuse injury involving repetitive overloading at the origin of common extensor tendons at the lateral epicondyle. This leads to tendinosis and a dysplasia of tissue at the tendinous origin of extensor carpi radialis brevis (ECRB).

Dr. Jobin or an immediate family member is a member of a speakers' bureau or has made paid presentations on behalf of Acumed, LLC, Biomet, and Zimmer; serves as a paid consultant to or is an employee of Acumed, LLC, Biomet, DePuy, a Johnson & Johnson Company, Integra Lifesciences, Smith & Nephew, and Zimmer; has received research or institutional support from Acumed, LLC; and serves as a board member, owner, officer, or committee member of the American Board of Orthopaedic Surgery, Inc. and the American Shoulder and Elbow Surgeons. Dr. Cassidy or an immediate family member serves as a paid consultant to or is an employee of AM Surgical and serves as an unpaid consultant to Synthes.

Epidemiology

- Most common cause of elbow pain in patients who present with elbow symptoms
  - Affects 1% to 3% of adults annually
  - More common in the dominant arm
  - Most common in patients between ages 35 and 50 years[1]
  - Men and women equally affected, and condition is independent of ethnicity [2]
- Although lateral epicondylitis is commonly referred to as tennis elbow, only 10% of affected patients actually play tennis.[3]
  - In racket sports, risk factors for lateral epicondylitis include poor swing mechanics, a heavy racket, incorrect racket grip size, and high string tension.
  - Lateral epicondylitis develops in approximately 50% of recreational tennis players at some point.
- Certain occupations may also predispose to the development of lateral epicondylitis.
  - In one study, 50% to 70% of patients reported that work was associated with the onset of symptoms.[2]
  - Industries with the highest incidence include construction, manufacturing, and wholesale/retail, likely because of their manual nature, involving repetitive activities of the wrist and elbow.[2]
    - Vibratory tools, in particular, have been implicated.
  - 10.5% of manual workers may experience elbow pain and 2.5% have a confirmed diagnosis of lateral epicondylitis.[3]
  - Consequently, lateral epicondylitis is a public health issue, causing significant economic impact because of absenteeism from work and associated health care costs.

Pertinent Anatomy/Pathoanatomy

- The common extensor origin on the lateral epicondyle of the distal humerus is the anatomic area that is affected in lateral epicondylitis.
- The extensor carpi radialis longus (ECRL) originates from the lateral supracondylar ridge, whereas the remaining muscles originate from the lateral epicondyle, including the ECRB, extensor

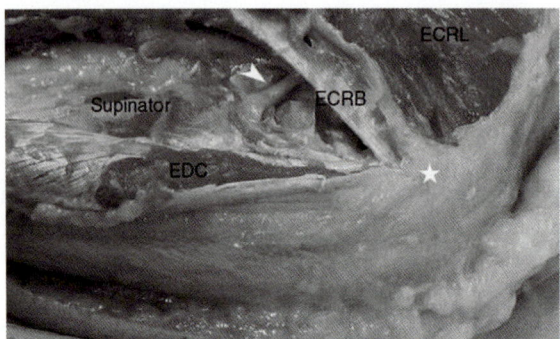

Figure 1 Cadaver photo of the location of the posterior interosseous nerve (arrowhead) crossing deep to the extensor communis radialis longus (ECRL) and extensor communis radialis brevis (ECRB), entering the supinator at the level of the radial head. The lateral epicondyle is marked with a star. The ECRB and extensor digitorum communis (EDC) have been separated to aid in visualization. (Reprinted from Calfee RP, Patel A, DaSilva MF, et al: Management of lateral epicondylitis: Current concepts. *J Am Acad Orthop Surg* 2008;16[1]:19-29.)

digitorum communis, extensor digiti minimi, extensor carpi ulnaris, and anconeus (**Figure 1**).
- The lateral ulnar collateral ligament (LUCL) also originates from the lateral epicondyle and traverses posterolaterally and around the radial head to the ulnar supinator crest.
- The nerves that are in this area include the posterior interosseous nerve (PIN), which enters a split in the supinator muscle (arcade of Frohse) just distal to the radial head.
  - Compression of the PIN can lead to radial tunnel syndrome, which is a diagnosis of exclusion and may coexist with lateral epicondylitis.
- The pathophysiology of lateral epicondylitis includes overuse of the ECRB.
  - With grip, the ECRB is instrumental in stabilizing the wrist to allow the digits to function effectively.
  - Overuse is precipitated by repetitive wrist extension and forearm pronation.
  - The condition is therefore common in tennis players, especially during backhand swings where the wrist extensors

are overloaded, firing eccentrically, and receive the vibratory impact during ball strike.
- The pathoanatomy of lateral epicondylitis may begin as a microtear of the origin of ECRB.
  - In a small number of cases (10%), the condition can involve microtears of ECRL and/or extensor carpi ulnaris.
  - The classic histologic finding of the affected tissue is angiofibroblastic hyperplasia, which includes fibroblast hypertrophy, disorganized collagen, vascular hyperplasia,[4] and a tendinosis-like microstructure.

Pertinent History/Physical Examination Findings

- The pertinent history of lateral epicondylitis includes lateral elbow pain worse with activity that does not resolve over a few weeks and started with a minor injury or seemingly benign activity such as yard work, sport activity, or manual labor.
  - Commonly there is associated loss of grip strength.
  - Pain may occasionally radiate down the dorsal forearm.
- The physical examination findings include point tenderness at or near the ECRB origin, typically no more than 0 to 2 cm distal to the bony lateral epicondyle.
  - Provocative tests include pain on resisted wrist extension exacerbated by elbow extension, and pain with full passive stretch of the ECRB by extending and pronating the elbow with the wrist maximally flexed.
  - Grip strength may be diminished, and the finding is accentuated by having the patient grip the dynamometer while the elbow is extended.
  - A careful nerve examination should also be performed to exclude concomitant entrapment neuropathy of the radial, ulnar, and median nerves at the elbow.
  - The classic findings of radial tunnel syndrome include tenderness over the PIN 3 to 5 cm distal to the lateral epicondyle, pain on resisted supination, and pain on resisted long finger extension.
- Differential diagnosis includes elbow plica syndrome, posterolateral rotatory instability and radial tunnel syndrome, occult fracture of the radial head/neck, radiocapitellar arthritis, capitellar osteochondritis dissecans, biceps or triceps tendinitis, and cervical radiculopathy.

Relevant Imaging
- Radiography
  - Approximately 47% of patients with lateral epicondylitis have calcifications adjacent to the lateral epicondyle on radiographs,[5] although presence of calcifications does not appear to be related to the timing of clinical presentation.[2]
  - Radiographs also should be used to exclude other common causes of elbow symptoms such as early arthritis with osteophytes, loose bodies, joint space narrowing, fracture, or other bony lesions.
- Magnetic resonance imaging
  - Noncontrast MRI is not necessary for diagnosis of lateral epicondylitis but helps rule out concomitant intra-articular pathology or other diagnosis.
  - MRI often shows increased signal at the ECRB tendon origin, thickening and edema of the ECRB tendon, or a partial articular surface tear of the ECRB origin; bony edema at the lateral epicondyle is rare.
  - Interestingly, one study demonstrated that there is an inverse relationship between the degree of tendinopathy and reported pain. In other words, the pain is often worse with partial ECRB tears than with complete tears.
- Ultrasonography
  - Less expensive but requires an experienced operator and evaluator.
  - Ultrasonography findings of lateral epicondylitis include structural changes affecting the extensor tendons, such as thickening, thinning, hypoechoic areas, and tendon tears, bone irregularity, and calcific deposits.
  - Neovascularization can also be assessed by color Doppler.

Nonsurgical Measures
- Mainstay of treatment for lateral epicondylitis; almost 95% of patients fully recover without surgery by 6 months
  - Currently no accepted standardized treatment regimen
  - Very few studies have compared outcomes with and without treatment, so remains unclear whether favorable outcomes should be attributed to the nonsurgical treatment used or to the natural history of the disorder[3]

- Reasonable to initially try rest and avoidance of provocative activities
- For tennis players, trials of a larger racket grip size, use of a slower playing surface, more flexible racket, lower string tension, and evaluation of technique may be important components of nonsurgical treatment
- Physical therapy: stretching, eccentric muscle strengthening, and joint mobilization
  - Deep friction massage is often used in physical therapy programs but has not been found to be helpful.[3]
  - Other modalities with limited evidence include low-frequency transcutaneous electrical nerve stimulation, ultrasonography, and pulsed magnetic wave therapies.[3]
  - Physical therapy regimens may include strengthening exercises of the scapular stabilizers and shoulder muscles, which are necessary for correct elbow function.
  - Physical therapy may be beneficial in the short term, but most studies show no advantage in the long term.[6]
- NSAIDs are often used for short-term symptomatic relief, but data are limited regarding the efficacy of NSAIDs in the treatment of lateral epicondylitis,[6] and there have been no differences found between oral and topical NSAIDs.[7]
- Injections: second-line treatment option
  - Corticosteroid injections
    - One of the most widely used treatments for lateral epicondylitis; provide substantial symptomatic relief for several weeks.
      - At 4 weeks, 92% of patients experience improved or complete pain relief.[6]
    - Can be especially useful when short-term improvements are needed—for example, in a professional tennis player in midseason.
    - Other evidence suggests that corticosteroids should be avoided, as most patients improve without corticosteroids and better long-term results are achieved without them.[7]
    - Adverse effects have been reported with long-term use of corticosteroids—patients who receive corticosteroids are better at 6 weeks, but are substantially worse at 1 year.[3]
      - Other evidence indicates short-term benefits of corticosteroids are paradoxically reversed after 6 weeks, with

high recurrence of pain at 1 year (72%) compared with only 8% recurrence in those who receive physical therapy alone.[6]
- Having more than three corticosteroid injections is the strongest predictor of surgical treatment failure in the future.[3]
- The worse long-term outcomes with corticosteroid injections have been thought to be related to weakening of the tendon or inducing iatrogenic posterolateral rotatory instability.
- Biologic injectables, including autologous blood injections (ABIs) and platelet-rich plasma (PRP) injections, are becoming more commonly used.
  - ABIs stimulate an inflammatory response, which is thought to bring in nutrients to promote healing.
    - There have been good short-term results with this modality; however, no benefit has been shown with long-term follow-up.[7]
    - Currently, ABI is recommended only for cases in which other nonsurgical modalities have failed.
  - PRP injections introduce platelets and high concentrations of growth factors that may induce a local healing response in the tendon.
    - Data are conflicting, but some reliable evidence shows that when compared with dry needling, patients treated with PRP had improved pain scores.[6]
    - PRP injections have limited adverse effects, and in both short-term and long-term follow-up they show decreased pain scores.[6]
      - May even reduce the need for surgical intervention[6]
    - Major concerns with PRP include the significant differences that exist between the available PRP systems, formulations, and techniques, and the expense that is not currently covered by most insurance.
  - When comparing injectable treatments, studies show a short-term advantage of corticosteroid injections compared with PRP injections, but PRP injections appear to be superior in the long term, with benefits lasting up to 2 years or longer.[6]
    - PRP injections have a lower risk of complications compared with corticosteroid injections.

- Simply inserting a needle may have therapeutic benefit, and dry needling of the epicondylar area has been shown to have better results than NSAIDs and forearm bracing.
- Overall, biologic therapies, including PRP and ABI, have been shown to be more efficacious than steroids in the long-term management of lateral epicondylitis and have minimal side effects.[6]
- Less commonly used nonsurgical treatments
  - Percutaneous radiofrequency treatments are performed by introducing a radiofrequency electrode percutaneously under ultrasound guidance, which ablates the pathologic tissue.
    - Good outcomes have been reported with this treatment modality.[7]
  - Extracorporeal shock wave therapy (ESWT) is performed by applying a generator of specific frequency sound waves directly onto the skin overlying the ECRB tendon, which is proposed to promote tissue healing, as well as have an analgesic effect.
    - ESWT has not been shown to be beneficial over other treatments and placebo.[6]
  - Low-level laser therapy has shown some short-term benefits when using an adequate dose and wavelength.[3,7]
  - Acupuncture has shown good outcomes on short-term follow-up, but long-term results are unclear.[7]
  - Botulinum A injections into the extensor muscles have been used as a method to reduce tension on the ECRB origin, which may be beneficial for pain relief.[7]
    - The temporary paralysis of the extensors may prevent further microtrauma to the ECRB origin, allowing the pathologic tissue to heal.
    - Effects seem to be short-lived and may cause incapacitating extensor muscle weakness.
- Bracing
  - Commonly used braces include counterforce braces with a proximal forearm strap and wrist extension splints.
    - Thought to work by reducing tension in the wrist extensor tendons and the compressive force of the forearm strap limits expansion and force generated by the extensor muscles

- There is conflicting evidence on the efficacy of bracing for lateral epicondylitis—although some studies have shown improvements in pain and grip strength.[3,6,7]
  - Prolonged use can lead to development of nerve dysfunction.
- Risk factors for failure of nonsurgical treatment include older age, obesity, smoking, manual labor, dominant arm involvement, workers' compensation, concurrent radial tunnel syndrome, multiple prior corticosteroid injection, splinting or orthopaedic surgery, use of psychoactive medications, and poor coping mechanisms.
  - Nonsurgical treatment is more likely to fail in patients with longer duration of symptoms and those with higher baseline pain levels.[2,3,6]

Surgical Intervention

- Not considered before 6 to 12 months of nonsurgical treatment
  - Should be reserved for a clear diagnosis of isolated lateral epicondylitis.
  - Often MRI is obtained to ensure no other significant intra-articular pathology.
- The three most commonly performed surgical procedures for lateral epicondylitis all involve the release of the ECRB origin, which can be accomplished via open, percutaneous, or arthroscopic methods.
  - Choice of procedure depends mainly on the comfort level of the surgeon, as there remains controversy regarding the best surgical approach.
    - No consensus regarding the best surgical technique.
    - Among newly trained orthopaedic surgeons, 85.8% of procedures for lateral epicondylitis were done with an open technique, 6.4% with a percutaneous approach, and 7.8% arthroscopically.[6]
    - Arthroscopic treatment may be preferable when other intra-articular pathologies need to be addressed at the same time, such as plica, synovitis, loose bodies, or evaluation and treatment of cartilage lesions.
  - Risk factors associated with surgical failure: older age, obesity, smoking, and prior corticosteroid injection.[3]

- Open release and débridement
  - Performed with an incision over the common extensor origin.
  - Dissection is carried down to the level of the fascia, which is then incised longitudinally between the lower border of the ECRL and common extensor tendon.
  - The lower border of the ECRL is elevated superiorly, revealing the deeper ECRB. Typically, the diseased ECRB tendon is grayish and does not have the glistening appearance of the normal white tendon.
  - The abnormal tendon is excised until more normal tendon boundaries are encountered, typically about 8 × 16 mm in area.
  - The epicondyle is decorticated and roughened to expose some marrow elements of the bone and stimulate a healing response if a repair is performed.
  - If the deep capsule is breached, it can be repaired with a simple absorbable stitch.
  - The ECRB–extensor digitorum communis interval is then repaired side to side and, if a repair to the epicondyle is performed, then an anchor may be used to secure the tendon to bone.
- Percutaneous procedure
  - Performed using topographic landmarks.
  - A stab incision is made anterior to the lateral epicondyle, at the level of the tendinous origin of the common extensors.
  - Through this incision, the scalpel is rotated superiorly, releasing the ECRB origin.
  - Care must be taken to protect the lateral ligament complex.
- Arthroscopic release and débridement
  - Advantages: excellent joint visualization and ability to address any intra-articular pathology (**Figure 2**).
  - Through a proximal medial portal, the anterior radiocapitellar joint is visualized and a lateral portal is used to resect the lateral capsule anterior to the epicondyle, with care to protect the anterior capsule where the radial nerve passes.
  - Through the capsular window, the ECRB tendon is identified and is resected form the epicondylar origin.

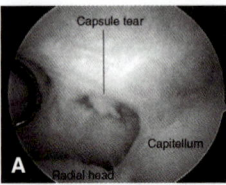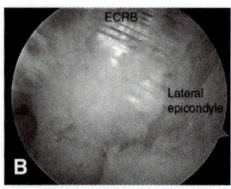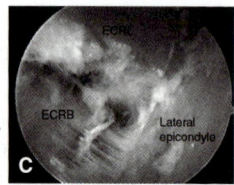

Figure 2 Arthroscopic view of a capsular tear via a medial portal in a right elbow. **A**, Initial view of the lateral capsule with a linear tear. **B**, Normal extensor carpi radialis brevis (ECRB) tendon following débridement of degenerative deep tissue. **C**, Final view of the ECRB and extensor carpi radialis longus (ECRL), with a clear distinction marking the proximal extent of débridement. (Reprinted from Calfee RP, Patel A, DaSilva MF, et al: Management of lateral epicondylitis: Current concepts. *J Am Acad Orthop Surg* 2008;16[1]:19-29.)

- Importantly, the resection of the ECRB tendon should not pass posterior to the mid-radial head to protect the LUCL from iatrogenic transection.
- The epicondyle may be decorticated with a burr or drilled with a Kirschner wire to help stimulate a healing response at the lateral epicondyle as well.
- Postoperative care
  - The elbow can be wrapped with a soft dressing or a long arm splint for comfort for 7 to 10 days and then elbow range of motion is allowed. Some surgeons also apply a wrist splint to prevent excessive activation of extensor muscles.
  - Patients are instructed not to lift more than 5 lb or engage in repetitive activities until 6 weeks postoperatively and then they are allowed to begin strengthening and full weight bearing.
  - Prophylactic preoperative antibiotics are standard if implants such as a suture anchor is placed, and some institutions will not give antibiotics for soft-tissue release surgeries without hardware.
  - No venous thromboembolism prophylaxis is required unless there is a clotting disorder.

- Pain medications include standard multimodal analgesia such as acetaminophen, NSAIDs, gabapentin, and a light-strength narcotic.
- Pearls and pitfalls
  - Iatrogenic injury to the LUCL from ECRB débridement posterior to the mid-radial head and through the LUCL fibers
    - If the LUCL is débrided, this may lead to posterolateral rotatory instability of the elbow with posterior subluxation of the radial head on the capitellum in supination and valgus stress.[8]
  - Radial nerve injury is a rare but serious complication of arthroscopic débridement and is often related to the use of suction during motorized shaver débridement.
    - Only gravity suction should be used when the shaver blades are turned off.
    - With arthroscopic treatment, all major nerves are at risk with portal creation and débridement.
    - Understanding the basics of safe elbow arthroscopy is a must during any elbow arthroscopic procedure.
  - Missed diagnosis, possibly missed radial nerve entrapment syndrome, which can be seen in up to 5% of patients with lateral epicondylitis
  - Heterotopic ossification related to excessive tissue injury around the elbow, head trauma in the postoperative period, prolonged elbow immobilization, or remaining bony debris at the surgical field.
    - Heterotopic bone risk may be reduced with thorough irrigation following bone decortication.
    - Oral indomethacin for 2 to 3 weeks postoperatively may have some protective effects against development of heterotopic ossification.
  - The overall complication rate for surgical interventions for lateral epicondylitis is low—with a complication rate of 4.3% for open procedures, 1.9% for percutaneous procedures, and 1.1% for arthroscopic procedures.[2]
    - Complication rates are similar among all the techniques, with slightly higher rates of superficial wound infections with the open technique.[9]

- Complications are potentially more severe with arthroscopic procedures because of the increased risk of nerve injury.[2]
- Outcomes of surgical treatment of lateral epicondylitis are positive but not perfect.
  - Excellent outcomes in 75% were found by Nirschl and Pettrone[4] from open débridement. They also found 97% of patients were improved from surgery, and 85% were able to fully resume their preinjury activity.
  - Although these outcomes are encouraging, a significant proportion of patients report persistent mild intermittent lateral epicondylar symptoms.[10]
  - In a long-term prospective study, 24% had persistent pain at 1 year postoperatively, decreasing to 9% at 5 years postoperatively.[11]
  - Arthroscopic débridement outcomes are almost equally encouraging but not perfect, with only 62% to 80% of patients experiencing complete elimination of lateral elbow pain.[12,13] However, arthroscopic surgery allowed patients a faster return to work at an average of 11 days.
  - A large comparative study by Szabo et al[14] followed patients for 2 years after arthroscopic, open, or percutaneous lateral epicondyle release and found no statistical difference in outcomes between the surgical techniques. They found a 6% failure rate of all combined techniques that were successfully treated with a cortisone injection. Interestingly, 44% of patients who underwent arthroscopic débridement had intra-articular pathology during arthroscopy.
  - Another retrospective comparative study[15] of open versus arthroscopic débridement found at 6 months' follow-up nearly identical outcomes, with 70% good or excellent outcomes in each group. Arthroscopic surgery allowed earlier return to work.
  - In a prospective randomized trial, percutaneous release was superior to open release in the Disabilities of the Arm, Shoulder and Hand score; patient satisfaction; and faster return to work.[16]

Top 10 Knowledge Drops for Your Rotation

1. Lateral and medial epicondylitis are not an inflammation but rather the cellular change of angiofibroblastic hyperplasia.
2. Lateral epicondylitis primarily affects the ECRB tendon origin.
3. Lateral epicondylitis may be managed with PRP injection with strong evidence of PRP efficacy.
4. For lateral epicondylitis, the best provocative test is pain on resisted wrist extension exacerbated by elbow extension.
5. Pain is often worse with partial ECRB tears than with complete tears noted on MRI.
6. Nearly 95% of patients fully recover without surgery by 6 months.
7. Having more than three corticosteroid injections is the strongest predictor of surgical treatment failure in the future.
8. All surgical treatments involve release of the ECRB origin.
9. Return to work is faster with percutaneous and arthroscopic techniques than with open surgery.
10. The LUCL is at risk with surgical débridement of the lateral epicondyle posterior to the mid-equator of the radial head.

MEDIAL EPICONDYLITIS

Medial epicondylitis is, in many ways, analogous to the much more common lateral epicondylitis. It is an overuse injury, resulting in degeneration of the tendinous origin of the flexor-pronator muscles. Histologically, the affected tissue is identical to that seen in lateral epicondylitis. Nonsurgical measures are the mainstay and the condition is usually self-limited.

Epidemiology

- Medial epicondylitis is 5 to 10 times less common than lateral epicondylitis.
  - Affects men and women equally and commonly affects the dominant extremity in 75% of cases
  - Disorder of young adults, most commonly in third to fourth decades of life[17]

- Although the condition is also known as golfer's elbow, most people with medial epicondylitis are not athletes.
- Risk factors include repetitive wrist flexion and/or forearm pronation.
  - This is commonly seen in sports with overhead throwing during ball release or racket or club swinging in forehand swings or the trailing arm in a two-handed swing that is the power arm. Thus, medial epicondylitis is common in golfers, baseball pitchers, javelin throwers, bowlers, weightlifters, and other athletes playing racquet sports such as tennis and squash.
  - Medial epicondylitis may develop from poor swing mechanics or with late ball strike when the racket head is behind the elbow at the point of ball contact.
  - Some believe the use of vibration dampeners on racket strings may reduce the incidence of medial epicondylitis.
- Occupations associated with medial epicondylitis include carpenters, construction workers, and plumbers.[18]
  - Medial epicondylitis in laborers is frequently associated with carpal tunnel syndrome, lateral epicondylitis, and/or rotator cuff tendinitis because of the nature of the overuse of the entire upper extremity.

Pertinent Anatomy/Pathoanatomy

- The diseased tissue of medial epicondylitis involves the common flexor tendons, known as the flexor-pronator mass, as they attach on the medial epicondyle.
  - They attach to the anterior aspect of the medial epicondyle more superficially than the anterior bundle of the medial collateral ligament (MCL).
  - The common flexor tendon fibers run parallel to the MCL.
  - The flexor-pronator mass includes the pronator teres, flexor carpi radialis, flexor digitorum superficialis, palmaris longus, and the flexor carpi ulnaris (FCU).
  - The FCU is innervated by the ulnar nerve, whereas the other muscles are innervated by the median nerve.
- Sports or manual labor that requires excessive flexor-pronator force may overload and strain the flexor-pronator mass, initiating

a bout of medial epicondylitis and potentially overloading the anterior band of the medial ulnar collateral ligament (MUCL).
  - The anterior band MUCL is the primary static restraint to elbow valgus force, whereas the flexor-pronator mass provides the dynamic restraint to elbow valgus force.
  - A weakened flexor-pronator mass jeopardizes the health of the MUCL when the elbow experiences repetitive and extreme valgus loads, such as in the throwing arm of baseball pitchers who experience flexor-pronator mass fatigue.
- The pathoanatomy of medial epicondylitis includes microtrauma to insertion of flexor-pronator mass tendons caused by repetitive activities.
  - This has been traditionally thought to affect the pronator teres more than the flexor carpi radialis, although all muscles of the common flexor tendon may be involved.
  - Medial epicondylitis is characterized by peritendinous inflammation, followed by histopathology angiofibroblastic hyperplasia, followed by breakdown and fibrosis with possible calcification.
- Differential diagnosis most commonly includes MCL injury in overhead throwing athletes, cubital tunnel syndrome of the ulnar nerve, fracture of the medial epicondyle, especially in adolescents with medial epicondyle apophyseal injuries, cervical radiculopathy, triceps tendinitis, and bone bruise.

Pertinent History/Physical Examination Findings

- Patients with medial epicondylitis may report a history of repetitive elbow use, gripping, or valgus stress activities.
  - Typical symptoms include insidious onset of pain over the medial epicondyle without a specific traumatic injury.
    - Medial elbow pain is described to be worse with wrist and forearm motion and worse with gripping.
    - Overhead throwers may complain of medial pain during late cocking and early acceleration during throwing, and racket sport players experience this pain during ball strike.
  - Associated cubital tunnel syndrome is fairly common, and patients may complain of numbness or tingling in ulnar digits.
  - Rarely, patients may present with a history of a recent contusion to the medial elbow initiating the epicondylitis.

- Physical examination findings include tenderness 5 to 10 mm distal and anterior to the medial epicondyle.
  - There may be soft-tissue swelling and warmth if inflammation is present.
  - The provocative tests include medial epicondyle pain with resisted forearm pronation and wrist flexion with the elbow extended.
  - It is important to examine for associated conditions such as MUCL injury that is characterized by medial elbow pain with valgus elbow loading during elbow flexion, by performing the milking maneuver and the moving valgus stress test.
  - The ulnar nerve should be examined for compressive neuropathy by performing the Tinel sign and elbow flexion-compression test; it consists of tapping over the ulnar nerve in the cubital tunnel.
    - A positive test results in the production of electric-shock–like sensations in the ulnar nerve distribution.
      - False-positive rate is approximately 36%.
    - The elbow flexion-compression test involves direct pressure over the ulnar nerve in the cubital tunnel while simultaneously holding the elbow in maximal elbow flexion and forearm pronation for 30 seconds.
      - Reproduction of numbness and tingling in the ring and little fingers is considered to be a positive result.
    - The ulnar nerve should also be palpated for ulnar subluxation over the medial epicondyle during elbow flexion.

Relevant Imaging

- Radiographs
  - AP and lateral radiographs of the elbow are usually normal, but 25% may show evidence of calcification of the common flexor tendon or MCL in cases of medial epicondylitis.[17]
  - Important for identifying degenerative joint changes such as posteromedial osteophytes or joint space narrowing
  - Stress radiography or stress ultrasonography may be used for assessing subtle valgus instability of the elbow joint.
- Ultrasonography
  - May show hypoechoic and anechoic areas of focal degeneration.

- Magnetic resonance imaging
  - Useful imaging modality in patients with unclear source of medial elbow pain and to evaluate concomitant pathology such as MUCL injury in overhead throwers, degenerative elbow changes, and loose bodies
  - May rule out rupture of flexor-pronator origin or muscle injury to the pronator teres
  - Common findings of medial epicondylitis include tendinosis, increased tendon signal on T2-weighted images, peritendinous edema.
- Nerve studies (electromyography/nerve conduction study)
  - May be beneficial if coexistent cubital tunnel syndrome exists or the diagnosis is unclear

Nonsurgical Measures

- Mainstay of treatment is nonsurgical
- First-line therapy: rest and activity modification, with an effort to avoid activities that exacerbate symptoms, including repetitive wrist flexion, forearm pronation, and valgus stress about the elbow.
  - Athletes with a concomitant MUCL injury should also refrain from throwing for 6 to 12 weeks, with particular attention to avoiding valgus stress during the 6 weeks of treatment.
  - Ice and NSAIDs for symptomatic relief
  - Splinting and bracing, including extension splinting in patients with concomitant ulnar neuritis, counterforce bracing, will limit the maximal contractile force able to be generated by the flexor-pronator mass, and kinesiology taping techniques.
    - Patients treated with counterforce bracing show improvement in pain and function in comparison with physical therapy at 6 weeks, but show no difference after 26 weeks.[19]
    - With an additional MUCL injury, a hinged elbow brace can be used to provide varus-valgus stability.
    - Caution should be taken with all splinting and bracing to avoid prolonged elbow immobilization, which can lead to joint stiffness.

- Physical therapy is also a critical component of nonsurgical management.
  - Initially passive range of motion and eccentric contraction are avoided to prevent putting excessive stress on the tendon.
  - The first goal of therapy is to return to full, painless range of motion, after which the focus turns to flexor-pronator mass stretching and, finally, eccentric strengthening.
  - All patients additionally benefit from improved shoulder range of motion, strengthening of the shoulder girdle, and scapular stabilization.
  - Finally, a main goal of therapy is reconditioning the upper limb to prevent undue stress at the elbow to prevent recurrence of symptoms.
- ESWT may be helpful in some patients.
  - Some studies have shown that patients report worse pain scores during the first 2 weeks of treatment with ESWT, but report improvement in pain at 8 weeks.[17]
  - ESWT appears to be more beneficial for patients with lateral epicondylitis.[17]
  - Acupuncture has also been shown to be helpful in some patients, although the level of evidence is low.
- Second-line therapy
  - Corticosteroid injection can be offered to reduce medial elbow discomfort. Injections have been shown to lead to acute improvement in pain for 6 weeks after injection, but show no difference compared with patients who do not receive injections at 3 months.[17]
    - High recurrence of pain and lack of benefit with corticosteroid injections at 1 year compared with observation and physical therapy[19]
    - Complications of steroid injections include skin depigmentation, tendon weakening, and ulnar nerve injury.
  - Biologic injections—including ABI and PRP—have been less studied in the treatment of medial epicondylitis.
    - Small studies show symptomatic improvements in patients in the intermediate term (12 to 26 weeks) when compared with corticosteroids.[19]

- Nonsurgical treatment has been found to be successful in more than 95% of patients.
  - However, when patients were treated with observation alone, symptoms of medial epicondylitis persist between 6 months and 2 years, so it is unclear how much additional benefit nonsurgical treatment measures have in addition to the natural history of medial epicondylitis.
  - A prolonged trial of these conservative treatments may be more appropriate in medial epicondylitis because of the less predictable success of surgical treatment compared with lateral epicondylitis.

Surgical Intervention

- Indications
  - Up to 6 months of nonsurgical management that fails to reduce symptoms to an acceptable level in a compliant patient
    - Symptoms should be severe and affecting quality of life and limiting activities of daily living and/or work.
  - Clear diagnosis of medial epicondylitis
  - Other pathologies should be ruled out or diagnosed and treated surgically at the same time, such as cubital tunnel syndrome.
- Surgical care focuses on débridement of tendinous origin of the common flexor tendon origin and reattachment of flexor-pronator group (**Figure 3**), by either a fascial splitting or Z-lengthening approach.
  - Arthroscopic management of medial epicondylitis is not commonly performed.
  - Open débridement and reattachment involves a medial approach to the elbow.
    - The medial antebrachial sensory nerves should be protected superficial to the forearm fascia.
    - The pronator teres/flexor carpi radialis interval is opened in line with its fibers.
    - The pathologic tissue has a characteristic gray milky appearance, which is distinct from that of the healthy tendon.
    - After the abnormal tendon is débrided typically the area is repaired by a side-to-side suture repair and, if necessary, with an anchor in the medial epicondyle to repair the tendon to the bone.
    - The medial epicondyle cortex should be roughened and/or drilled to enhance healing before tendon repair.

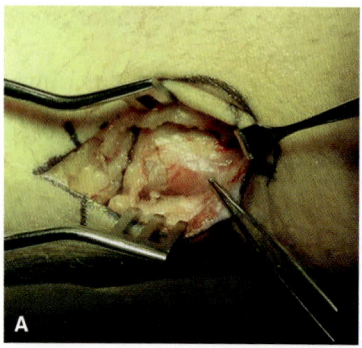
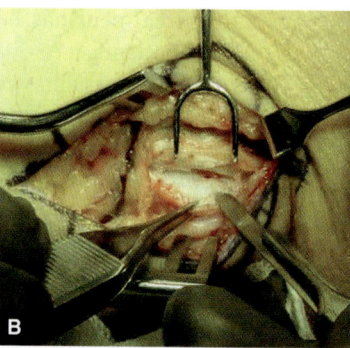
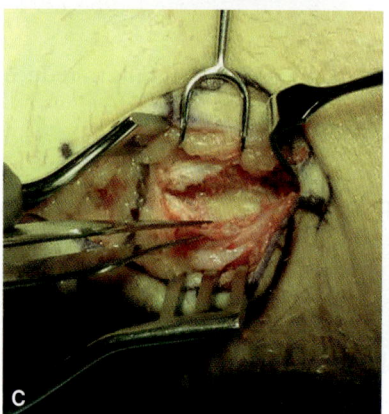
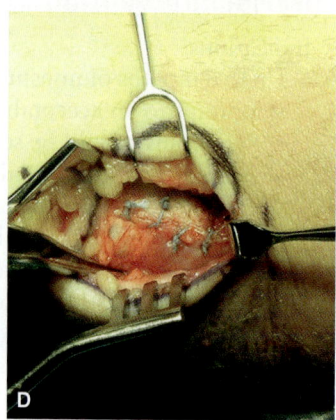

Figure 3 Intraoperative photographs of an elbow with medial epicondylitis showing the pathologic change of the intact common flexor tendon (**A**), the tendon after débridement of diseased tissue (**B**), exposure of the medial epicondyle (**C**), and side-to-side repair of the common flexor tendon (**D**). (Reprinted from Amin NH, Kumar NS, Schickendantz MS: Medial epicondylitis: Evaluation and management. *J Am Acad Orthop Surg* 2015;23[6]:348-355.)

- Concomitant cubital tunnel in situ nerve release or ulnar nerve anterior transposition can be performed in cases of associated cubital tunnel syndrome.
- Postoperative care
  - Soft dressing or elbow splint for 7 to 10 days, followed by gentle elbow motion.
  - Some surgeons prefer to immobilize the wrist with a splint to protect the repair and limit unimpeded use of the hand.

- Passive wrist extension stretching and active strengthening of volar wrist flexion is avoided for the first 3 to 4 weeks in the immediately postoperative period to offload the tendon repair and enhance tendon to bone healing.
- Strengthening is typically begun at 6 to 8 weeks and return to sport is at 3 to 6 months depending on symptoms and recovery progress.
- Pearls and pitfalls
  - Most common complication is medial antebrachial cutaneous nerve injury from traction or transection with numbness or development of a painful neuroma
    - This risk can be minimized with identification of the nerve branches superficial to the fascia and retracting them out of the surgical field.
  - Ulnar nerve injury is also possible from retraction or sharp injury if the location of the nerve is not appreciated within the FCU.
  - The median nerve may be injured if dissection is carried deep and distal into the pronator teres.
- Outcomes
  - Outcomes are good to excellent in 80% of surgically treated patients, which is less than lateral epicondylitis.
    - Outcomes are also worse when ulnar nerve symptoms are present preoperatively.
  - Surgical outcomes of open débridement and repair are mixed but generally satisfactory to excellent.
    - Vangsness and Jobe[20] reported over 95% excellent or good results, with only one patient failing to return to sport at 6-year follow-up.
    - Gabel and Morrey[21] reported on 30 elbows with medial epicondylitis and found the best results in patients no or mild concomitant ulnar neuritis.
    - Kurvers and Verhaar[22] reported approximately 70% likelihood of being symptom-free 4 years after surgery with the failures being among the patients requiring concomitant ulnar nerve decompression.
    - Gong et al[23] described a Z-lengthening of the flexor-pronator mass and, at 3-year follow-up, all patients reported improved symptoms.

Top 10 Knowledge Drops for Your Rotation

1. The incidence of medial epicondylitis is 5 to 10 times less common than that of lateral epicondylitis.
2. The histopathology of medical epicondylitis is identical to lateral epicondylitis.
3. The structures most commonly involved include the flexor carpi radialis and the lower border of the pronator teres origins.
4. Concomitant cubital tunnel syndrome is common. However, Tinel sign has a 36% false-positive rate.
5. For medial epicondylitis, the best provocative test is pain on resisted pronation and wrist flexion exacerbated by elbow extension.
6. In tennis strokes, medial epicondylitis primarily affects the forehand, whereas lateral epicondylitis affects the backhand.
7. Corticosteroid injections provide short-term relief (6 weeks), but the effect seems to be short-lived, with recurrence of symptoms in many patients by 3 months.
8. Medial epicondylitis surgery has a high failure rate in patients with concomitant cubital tunnel syndrome.
9. Surgical treatment via either a fascial split or Z-plasty in the flexor-pronator origin includes débridement of all abnormal tissue.
10. The most common surgical complication is injury to the medial antebrachial cutaneous nerve during exposure.

DISTAL BICEPS RUPTURE

Rupture of the distal biceps tendon is an injury that typically occurs in the dominant arm of men between 40 and 50 years old during eccentric contraction of the biceps while, for example, carrying furniture or attempting to catch a heavy falling object or lift a stuck window open. Risk factors for rupture are degenerative changes at the tendon attachment, decreased vascularity, and tendon impingement against the ulna from a prominent radial tuberosity. Although nonsurgical management is an option, it leaves the elbow 20% to 40% weaker in flexion and supination, respectively. Consequently, healthy active people with distal biceps tendon ruptures often benefit from early surgical repair. Multiple techniques are available to reattach the distal biceps tendon, including suture anchors, cortical buttons, and interosseous screws, but all techniques yield excellent surgical outcomes despite differences in biomechanical load testing. Complications include sensory and motor nerve injuries, heterotopic ossification, and infection. Postoperative care includes early return to motion and to activities of daily living while weight training and sport are delayed for 2 to 4 months postoperatively.

Epidemiology

- Incidence: 1.2 per 100,000 people per year
  - In the dominant arm more than 80% of the time
  - 90% of cases in men and most common in people in their 40s
    - Small percentage occur in women, who are more likely to present in their sixth decade with partial tears that usually have a degenerative etiology[24]
- Injuries usually result from excessive eccentric biceps contraction as the arm is forced from a flexed to an extended position while trying to resist this activity.
- Risk factors
  - Tobacco use is a significant risk factor.
  - Anabolic steroid use causes increased tendon stiffness, as well as increased biceps muscle strength, both of which contribute to risk of rupture.[25]
  - Others: elevated body mass index, Cushing syndrome, oral steroids, and the natural aging process[24,26]

Pertinent Anatomy/Pathoanatomy

- The distal biceps tendon inserts on the bicipital tuberosity on the proximal radius.
  - The tendon runs between the pronator teres and brachioradialis and superficial to the brachialis muscle.
  - The tuberosity provides a cam effect to increase the supination torque created by biceps contraction.
  - The tendon attachment on the tuberosity has a footprint area of 21 mm in length and 7 mm in width.[27]

- The distal biceps tendon has distinct insertions of the short head and the long head contributions.
- The short head portion of the tendon inserts more distally, and usually covers the apex of the tuberosity, making the short head the stronger elbow flexor, whereas the long head, attaching more posteriorly, further from the axis of rotation of the forearm, is the greater supinator.
- With injury, the distal biceps tendon almost always avulses from its insertion.
- The lacertus fibrosus typically originates from the distal short head of the biceps tendon and can be a tether for the tendon to prevent complete retraction when the distal biceps ruptures.
- The distal biceps tendon has three zones of vascularity.
  - Proximal zone: includes the musculotendinous junction and is supplied by branches of the brachial artery
  - Distal zone: includes the tendon insertion on the radial tuberosity and is supplied by branches of the posterior interosseous recurrent artery
  - Middle zone, considered the hypovascular zone
    - The middle zone is supplied by branches of both the brachial artery and the posterior interosseous recurrent artery, but through a thinner paratenon covering.
    - The limited vascular supply of this portion of the tendon, as well as evidence that this zone may be most likely to be impinged during forearm rotation, may contribute to impaired tendon repair, which may make this area more susceptible to rupture and injury.[24,25]
- The biceps is innervated by the musculocutaneous nerve, which travels down the arm between the biceps and the brachialis and terminates as the lateral antebrachial cutaneous nerve, supplying sensation to the volar and lateral aspect of the forearm.

Pertinent History/Physical Examination Findings

- People who sustain a distal biceps rupture complain of a painful pop in their elbow and the feeling of biceps cramping or visibly seeing their biceps ball up into their arm.

- Physical examination findings: asymmetric biceps muscle belly with proximal retraction, puckering of the skin in the antecubital fossa with retracted tears, medial elbow bruising, weakness and pain with resisted elbow flexion and forearm supination.
- Palpation of the antecubital fossa reveals an absence of a taut distal biceps tendon that can be compared with the contralateral uninjured elbow.
  - The lacertus fibrosus may remain intact and can be confused for an intact distal biceps.
  - The most reliable physical examination maneuver is the hook test.
    - It is performed with the elbow actively flexed to 90°, with the forearm supinated. The examiner uses a finger to hook around the lateral aspect of the biceps tendon.
    - With an intact biceps tendon, the finger can be hooked around the distal biceps tendon. When there is a complete distal biceps tear, the examiner's finger cannot hook around anything and the test is considered positive.
- Some patients with untreated distal biceps tears will complain of a cramping sensation with heavy use.

Relevant Imaging

- Radiographs
  - Usually normal and are useful to rule out or exclude associated bony injuries
- Magnetic resonance imaging
  - Useful to confirm the diagnosis, to rule out a partial tear or a myotendinous junction tear, and for evaluation in chronic tears
  - MRI findings of acute rupture include a retracted distal biceps tendon surrounded in seroma fluid and a bare radial tuberosity (**Figure 4**).
  - Specific arm positioning in flexion, abduction, and forearm supination allows for ideal assessment of the retracted biceps tendon and bare radial tuberosity.
- Ultrasonography may also be effective to confirm distal biceps rupture in patients who cannot undergo MRI.

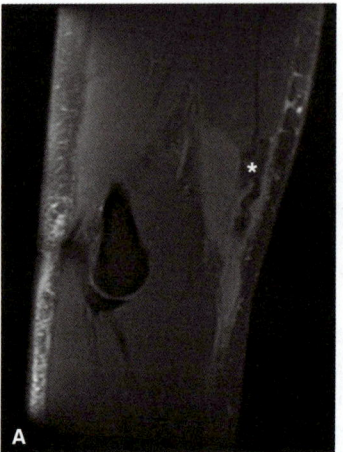 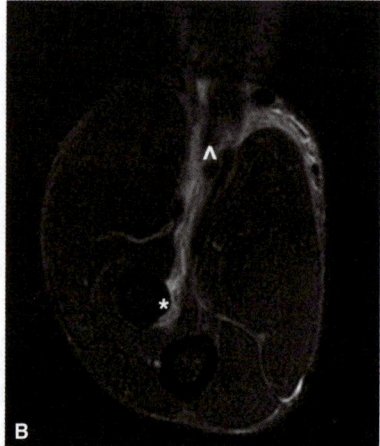

Figure 4 **A**, Sagittal T2-weighted magnetic resonance image shows distal biceps tendon rupture with retraction and the tendon (asterisk) visualized in a pocket of seroma fluid with a serpentine appearance rather than a taught straight-line appearance of a nonruptured tendon. The biceps muscle is seen proximal and confluent with the tendon confirming that torn tendon is the distal biceps tendon. **B**, T2-weighted magnetic resonance image with the tendon in flexion, abduction, and supination demonstrating the bare bicipital tuberosity (asterisk) and retracted biceps tendon proximally (arrow) with the biceps tendon sheath full of high fluid signal.

Nonsurgical Measures

- Indicated in low-demand or medically ill patients.
- Nonsurgical care typically results in painless elbow function with mild weakness and fatigability in elbow flexion of approximately 20% and supination of 40%.
  - Supination is important for tasks such as using a screwdriver, turning a doorknob, and other twisting tasks.

Surgical Intervention

- Two main surgical approaches are used for distal biceps repair: the anterior single-incision technique and the two-incision technique, which includes anterior and posterior incisions. There are benefits and drawbacks to each approach.
  - Anterior single-incision approach
    - Benefits: minimally invasive and carries less risk of radioulnar synostosis

- Drawback: associated with a higher rate of neurologic complications
  - Less invasive fixation techniques and implants have improved the safety of a single-incision approach.
- Technique
  - The interval for the anterior approach is between the brachioradialis and pronator teres.
  - The lateral antebrachial cutaneous nerve is identified as it runs in this interval near the fascial plane.
  - Deeper dissection is developed and with lateral retraction of the brachioradialis and medial retraction of the pronator teres and the median nerve and brachial artery.
  - Ligation of the recurrent branch of the radial artery increases exposure and minimizes risk of hematoma formation and may protect against heterotopic ossification.
  - The PIN is protected with forearm supination and using blunt nonlevering instruments for lateral retraction.
- Two-incision approach uses anterior incision for retrieval of the distal biceps tendon stump and for tunneling through the interosseous space and a posterior incision for tendon attachment to the radial tuberosity.
  - Technique
    - After the biceps is identified, the radial tuberosity is palpated in the interval between the pronator teres and brachioradialis, and a curved clamp containing the tendon sutures is passed through the interosseous space aiming laterally until it is palpated on the dorsal proximal forearm.
    - The posterior incision is then made over the clamp and dissection splits the extensor carpi ulnaris muscle and then splits the supinator to access the tuberosity.
    - Because this approach risks radioulnar synostosis, the ulna is not exposed.
    - Pronation of the forearm protects the PIN, which often is not visualized.

- Fixation
  - The fixation technique used is at the discretion of the surgeon, and each technique again has benefits and drawbacks.
    - Fluoroscopy is typically used to confirm appropriate positioning of hardware and confirmation of the location of the radial tuberosity (**Figure 5**).
    - Repair within 2 to 3 weeks of rupture makes finger dissection down to the radial tuberosity easy and safe.
    - The distal tendon stump is often found in a seroma and can be milked out of the wound without instrument dissection or clamping blindly.
    - The repaired distal biceps should be able to at least hold 50 N of force, which correlates with flexing the elbow against gravity.
      - The force necessary to rupture the distal biceps tendon is approximately 204 N, approximately 45 lb.

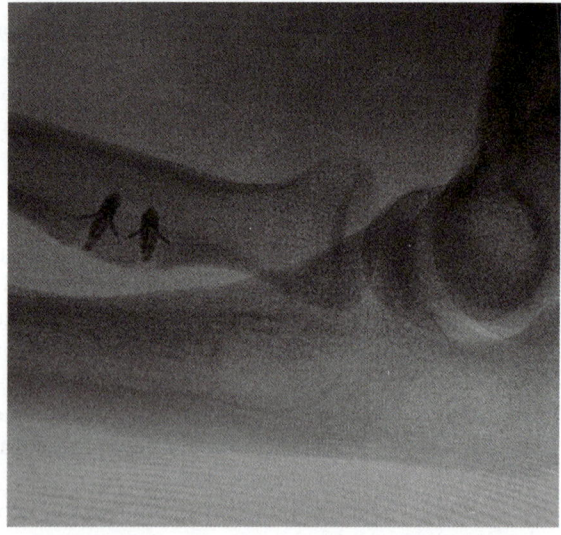

Figure 5 Intraoperative fluoroscopy confirms appropriate location and position of suture anchor hardware during distal biceps tendon repair to the radial tuberosity.

- The most basic repair technique is the bone tunnel using a two-incision approach.
  - The tuberosity is prepared with a burr to create a trough, and then transosseous tunnels are drilled into the base of this trough and the tendon dunked into the trough and secured with transosseous sutures.
- A suture anchor technique commonly uses a single-incision approach.
  - The radial tuberosity is lightly decorticated to prepare for bone-tendon healing.
  - Two suture anchors are inserted into the tuberosity toward the ulnar edge of the tuberosity and the tendon tied down to the bone using a tension slide technique after Krakow suture fixation to the tendon.
  - This repair sequence maximizes tendon-to-bone contact and surface area and effectively re-creates the footprint of the distal biceps insertion.[28]
  - The suture anchor technique does not drill thru the far cortex and therefor reduced the risk of iatrogenic PIN injury.
- An intraosseous screw technique uses a single incision, and the tendon is repaired into a bone socket in the tuberosity that will accept the caliber of the distal biceps tendon.
  - The interference screw and tendon are inserted into the socket and screwed down to repair the tendon.
  - Downsides of this technique include socket lysis over time that risk fracture, nonanatomic overreduction of the tendon into the bone, and creation of bone debris that may contribute to heterotopic ossification.
- A cortical button suspensory technique uses a metal button that is passed through a small hole in the radial tuberosity and flipped to lay flat on the dorsal aspect of the radius.
  - The tendon can either be repaired into a socket or flush with the tuberosity footprint using the tension slide technique to bring the tendon down to the bone.
  - Intraosseous buttons may also be used but are difficult to flip intramedullary within the small space of the radial tuberosity.

- Fluoroscopy should be used to confirm placement and flipped seating of the button against the bone cortex.
- The PIN is at risk for entrapment with the button and can get injured.
- It is imperative that bicortical holes be drilled perpendicular to the tuberosity with the forearm in full supination.
- Mazzocca et al[28] measured the biomechanical load to failure of these four techniques and found the button technique had the highest load to failure (440 N) compared with suture anchor (380 N), bone tunnel (310 N), and the interference screw (230 N).
  - Each of these loads to failure is beyond the force required to tear a native tendon at approximately 210 N.[29]
- Postoperative care
  - Depending on the repair technique, timing, and surgeon preference, the arm may be placed into a sling or is immobilized in a splint for 1 to 2 weeks after surgery.
  - When tears are acutely repaired without tension, a splint is not needed and early elbow range of motion is allowed, which improves patient satisfaction (**Figure 6**) and has no negative effect on healing or strength.[30]
  - Gentle flexion and extension exercises without weight or resistance may be started at that point.
  - Strengthening is begun at 6 to 8 weeks, with a return to sport or heavy activities at 3 to 5 months.
- Outcomes
  - Outcomes from surgical repair are superior to nonsurgical care for restoring elbow flexion strength, supination strength, and improving upper extremity endurance.[12]
  - The outcomes of distal biceps repair are excellent, with low rates of complications.
    - Studies with suture anchor techniques report less elbow motion loss (1° to 5°) and greater recovery of strength and endurance with return of more than 94% of isokinetic strength testing.[31,32]
  - A report using the button technique in 26 patients showed a strength recovery of 80% for flexion and 91% for supination. Two patients had heterotopic ossification but were asymptomatic.[33]

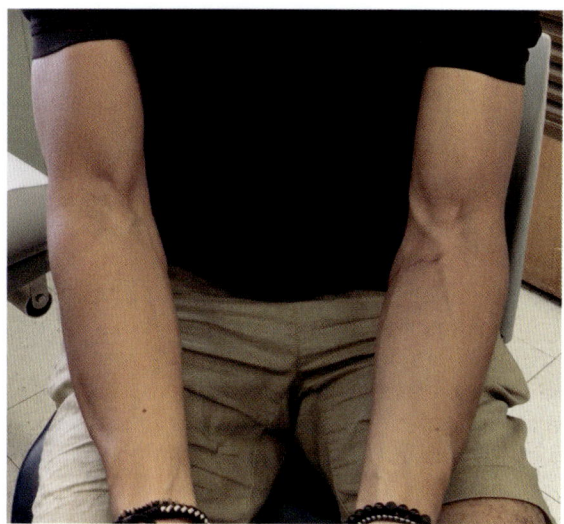

Figure 6 Clinical photograph of anterior elbows in forearm supination demonstrates left elbow distal biceps repair with restoration of biceps muscle contour, location, with a visible distal biceps tendon prominence in the antecubital fossa that nearly mirrors the uninjured contralateral right elbow.

- Comparing two-incision to single-incision techniques in a randomized controlled trial (RCT) demonstrated no significant differences in outcomes except a greater prevalence of temporary sensory neurapraxia of the lateral antebrachial cutaneous nerve in the single-incision group.[34]

Top 10 Knowledge Drops for Your Rotation

1. Distal biceps tears occur from eccentric contracture of the elbow flexors.
2. The short head inserts distally on the biceps tuberosity and has more mechanical advantage as an elbow flexor.
3. The long head inserts proximally and posteriorly on the biceps tuberosity and has more mechanical advantage as a supinator.
4. An intact lacertus fibrosus may limit proximal retraction of the ruptured distal biceps, making diagnosis more challenging.

5. The hook test, in which the examiner's finger is unable to hook the distal biceps tendon, is indicative of rupture.
6. When ordering MRI, the flexion, abduction, supination position allows for simultaneous evaluation of the distal biceps tendon and biceps tuberosity.
7. Cortical button fixation is the strongest method of reattachment of the distal biceps tendon.
8. Single-incision distal biceps repair has a higher complication rate of lateral antebrachial cutaneous nerve sensory neurapraxia than the two-incision approach.
9. The two-incision approach has a higher risk of symptomatic heterotopic ossification than the one-incision approach.
10. Untreated distal biceps rupture results in 20% loss of elbow flexion strength and 40% loss of supination strength.

ULNAR NERVE COMPRESSION

Cubital tunnel syndrome is a common compressive neuropathy of the ulnar nerve in the elbow. Symptoms include a constellation of numbness, tingling, sensory changes of the ring and little finger, and loss of dexterity. Treatment typically begins with nonsurgical modalities, extension bracing at night, and avoidance of the provocative activities. Surgery for decompression and possible anterior transposition is indicated based on severity, failure of nonsurgical care, and etiology of the compression causing the symptoms.

Epidemiology

- Cubital tunnel syndrome is a common elbow disorder with an incidence of 25 per 100,000 people per year, second to carpal tunnel syndrome as the most common compression neuropathy of the upper extremity.
- Associated conditions include cubitus varus or valgus deformities of the elbow, medial epicondylitis, elbow arthritis, trauma and instability, burns with elbow stiffness, and chronically stiff elbows that have regained motion following surgery or therapy.

Pertinent Anatomy/Pathoanatomy

- The ulnar nerve travels across the elbow in the cubital tunnel between the medial epicondyle and olecranon.
  - In the arm above the elbow, it pierces the intramuscular septum at the arcade of Struthers, which is located approximately 8 cm proximal to the medial epicondyle as it passes from the anterior to posterior compartment of the arm.
  - It then enters cubital tunnel that has a roof formed by FCU fascia and Osborne ligament that travels from the medial epicondyle to the olecranon. The floor of the cubital tunnel is formed by posterior and transverse bands of the MCL and elbow joint capsule.
- Sites of compressive entrapment of the ulnar nerve: arcade of Struthers, medial head of triceps compressing the nerve against the medial intermuscular septum, area between Osborne ligament and the MCL within the cubital tunnel, between the two heads of FCU and its investing fascial aponeurosis, and medial epicondyle itself if the ulnar nerve dynamically subluxates anteriorly with elbow flexion.
  - Anatomic variants may also contribute to nerve compression, including the anconeus epitrochlearis, which is an anomalous muscle from the medial olecranon to the medial epicondyle.
  - Alterations in the cubital tunnel may result from posttraumatic and degenerative conditions such as distal humerus malunions, medial epicondyle nonunions, osteophytes from arthritis, heterotopic ossification, ganglion cysts, and even tumors.

Pertinent History/Physical Examination Findings

- Symptoms of cubital tunnel syndrome include paresthesias of little finger and the ulnar half of ring finger and the ulnar dorsal hand.
  - An anatomic variant may also include the third web space (radial half of the ring finger and ulnar half of the long finger).
  - These symptoms typically may worsen with activities such as phone use with an excessively flexed elbow for extended periods of time, occupational or athletic activities requiring repetitive elbow flexion, sleeping with the elbow in flexion, or direct blows to the medial elbow causing contusion, such as hitting the funny bone.

- Physical examination findings classically include decreased sensation in ulnar digits and, in advanced cases, may affect motor function with interosseous atrophy, ring and little finger clawing, weakness of the flexor digitorum profundus to the ring and little fingers, and paralysis of intrinsic muscles including the adductor pollicis, deep head flexor pollicis brevis, interossei, and lumbricals 4 and 5. The result is weakness of grip and pinch.
  - Examiners should look and feel for ulnar nerve subluxation over the medial epicondyle as the elbow moves through a flexion-extension arc.
- Other physical examination signs
  - Froment sign:[35] demonstrated by compensatory thumb interphalangeal hyperflexion by flexor pollicis longus during key pinch to compensate for the loss of adduction and metacarpophalangeal flexion by adductor pollicis
  - Jeanne sign: includes compensatory thumb metacarpophalangeal hyperextension and thumb adduction by extensor pollicis longus with key pinch as this compensates for loss of interphalangeal extension and thumb adduction by adductor pollicis
  - Wartenberg sign: characterized by persistent little finger abduction and extension during attempted adduction secondary to weak third palmar interosseous and little finger lumbrical muscles
  - Masse sign: characterized by palmar arch flattening and loss of ulnar hand elevation secondary to hypothenar atrophy and decreased little finger metacarpophalangeal joint flexion
- Provocative tests
  - Tinel sign: positive when symptoms are reproduced by tapping over the cubital tunnel
  - Elbow flexion-compression test: positive when symptoms are reproduced by direct pressure over the cubital tunnel while maintaining the elbow in maximal flexion and pronation for 60 seconds

Relevant Imaging

- Radiographs
  - Typically normal but obtained to rule out concomitant pathology that may contribute to cubital tunnel syndrome such as elbow arthritis, fracture, or heterotopic bone

- Electromyography/nerve conduction velocity
  - Helpful in establishing diagnosis and prognosis as the threshold for diagnosis includes conduction velocity less than 50 m/s across elbow[35] and low amplitudes of sensory nerve action potentials and compound muscle action potentials

Nonsurgical Measures

- First line of treatment in patients with mild symptoms
  - Includes NSAIDs, activity modification (avoiding leaning on elbow or prolonged elbow flexion), and nighttime elbow extension splinting
  - Effective in half of cases
- Cubital tunnel syndrome is classified using the McGowan and Dellon classification.
  - Type 1: subjective sensory symptoms without objective loss of two-point sensibility or muscular atrophy
  - Type 2A: sensory symptoms and weakness on pinch and grip without atrophy
  - Type 2B: with sensory symptoms and atrophy and intrinsic muscle strength less than 4 out of 5
  - Type 3: profound muscular atrophy and sensory disturbance

Surgical Intervention

- Surgical care includes in situ decompression without transposition, decompression with transposition, and medial epicondylectomy in rare and selected cases.
  - In situ ulnar nerve decompression without transposition is indicated when nonsurgical management fails and before motor denervation occurs (**Figure 7**).
    - Outcomes: 80% to 90% good results when symptoms are intermittent and denervation has not yet occurred.
      - However, poor prognosis and outcomes are observed in most patients with intrinsic muscle atrophy.
      - Meta-analyses have shown similar clinical results with significantly fewer complications from in situ decompression compared with decompression with transposition.
    - Technique: Release of fascial structures over the ulnar nerve along the medial aspect of the elbow, including Osborne

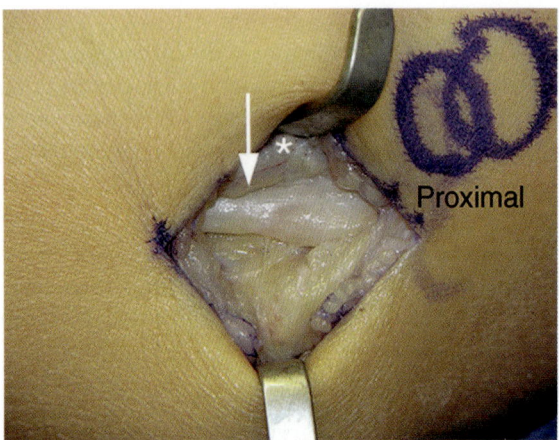

Figure 7 Intraoperative photograph showing in situ decompression of the ulnar nerve. Note the hourglass shape of the nerve (arrow) resulting from chronic compression and the reactive enlargement of the nerve proximal to the compression point. The asterisk marks the medial epicondyle. (Reprinted from Staples JR, Calfee R: Cubital tunnel syndrome: Current concepts. *J Am Acad Orthop Surg* 2017;25[10]:215e-224e.)

ligament and the superficial and deep fascia of the FCU along the course of the ulnar nerve.
- Some authors recommend releasing the fascia between the medial triceps and medial intermuscular septum, and the arcade of Struthers proximally.
- Ulnar nerve decompression and anterior transposition is indicated in patients with symptomatic subluxating nerves, those with failed in situ release, and in patients with a disrupted cubital tunnel from tumor, osteophytes, or heterotopic bone or hardware.
  - Outcomes: similar to in situ release, but there is increased risk of creating a new point of compression from the transposition.
  - Technique: Same as in situ except the transposition part of the surgery, which can be performed as a submuscular, intramuscular, or subcutaneous transposition.
    - The nerve is decompressed circumferentially to allow for transposition while trying to preserve the vessels that

run along it as well as the inferior ulnar collateral artery branch to the ulnar nerve, which is located proximal to the medial epicondyle.
- It is also important to excise the distal part of the medial intermuscular septum so that as the nerve is transposed anteriorly it does not get compressed by this bandlike structure.
- Once transposed, it can be secured with subcutaneous tissue and fat; some prefer to use an anterior fascial sling from the anterior aspect of the FCU (**Figure 8**).
- Intramuscular transposition places the nerve within or beneath the flexor-pronator mass.
• Medial epicondylectomy is rarely the preferred treatment unless other options will not work, such as in extremely thin

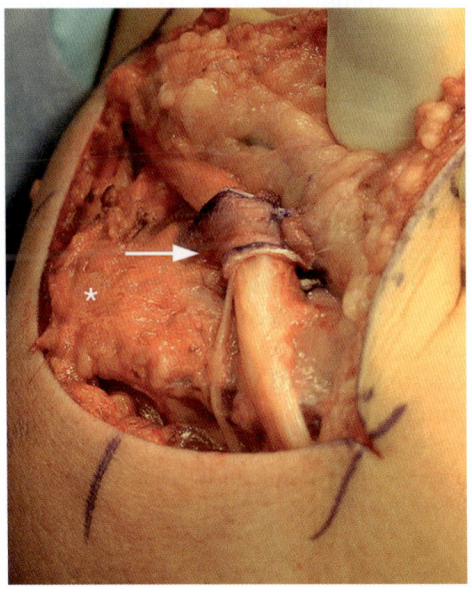

Figure 8 Intraoperative photograph showing subcutaneous transposition of the ulnar nerve. A fascial sling (arrow) is sutured to subcutaneous tissue, keeping the ulnar nerve anterior to the medial epicondyle (asterisk). (Reprinted from Staples JR, Calfee R: Cubital tunnel syndrome: Current concepts. *J Am Acad Orthop Surg* 2017;25[10]:215e-224e.)

patients with inadequate subcutaneous tissue to perform a transposition.
  - Outcomes: mixed; risk of destabilizing the medial elbow by damaging the medial ulnar collateral ligament.
  - Technique: epicondylectomy is performed with an oblique osteotomy of the medial epicondyle to preserve the MCL and allow a repair of the periosteum.
- Outcomes
  - Comparative studies have failed to demonstrate superiority of one technique over another.
    - An RCT comparing in situ decompression to submuscular transposition found that both procedures were equally effective.[36]
    - Another RCT compared in situ decompression to subcutaneous transposition and at 1 year concluded that 48% of patients who underwent simple decompression and 60% of patients who underwent anterior transposition were free of signs and symptoms of cubital tunnel syndrome.[37]
    - Another RCT of severe cubital tunnel syndrome compared in situ decompression and submuscular transposition demonstrated no difference in clinical or electrophysiologic outcomes at 4-year follow-up; approximately 50% of patients had an excellent outcomes.[38]
    - Another RCT comparing subcutaneous anterior transposition or in situ decompression found no substantial differences.[39]
    - An interesting RCT of medial epicondylectomy compared with anterior transposition demonstrated no difference between these treatments except that the satisfaction was greater in the medial epicondylectomy group.[40]
  - In situ decompression risks persistent symptoms secondary to continued nerve tension or instability of the nerve.
    - Nevertheless, two RCTs have shown equal outcomes of in situ decompression and decompression with transposition.[36,37]
    - In the case of a dynamically unstable ulnar nerve that subluxates onto or over the medial epicondyle during elbow flexion, most surgeons recommend transposition or epicondylectomy despite most randomized controlled series

showing that nerve stability during in situ release did not affect outcomes.
- Complications include incomplete symptom relief, particularly in cases of advanced cubital tunnel syndrome with atrophy or inadequate decompression.
  - Other complications include recurrence of cubital tunnel symptoms secondary to perineural scarring or nerve tethering at the intermuscular septum or FCU fascia.
    - There is a higher rate of recurrence for cubital tunnel release than after carpal tunnel release.
  - Other complications include direct nerve injury with neuroma formation, or iatrogenic injury to a branch of the medial antebrachial cutaneous nerve may cause persistent posteromedial elbow paresthesias.

Top 10 Knowledge Drops for Your Rotation

1. Cubital tunnel syndrome is known as cellphone elbow because it may be provoked by prolonged elbow flexion.
2. The arcade of Struthers is located approximately 8 cm proximal to the medial epicondyle.
3. The floor of the cubital tunnel is the posterior band of the MCL.
4. Wartenberg sign is the inability to adduct the little finger.
5. The anconeus epitrochlearis, an anomalous muscle originating from the medial epicondyle and inserting on the olecranon, may be a cause of cubital tunnel syndrome.
6. The gold standard confirmatory test is a nerve conduction study (nerve conduction velocity/electromyography), demonstrating focal conduction slowing at the elbow.
7. Motor weakness and muscle atrophy are poor prognostic factors for cubital tunnel surgery.
8. With some exceptions, there is no clear benefit to anterior transposition during cubital tunnel release.
9. Intraoperatively, if the ulnar nerve subluxates after decompression, the most commonly performed next step is anterior transposition. Another option is medial epicondylectomy.
10. Anterior transposition includes excision of the distal portion of the medial intermuscular septum.

Acknowledgment

The authors thank Anna Michalowski, BS, for her contributions during manuscript preparation.

References

1. Aben A, De Wilde L, Hollevoet N, et al: Tennis elbow: Associated psychological factors. *J Shoulder Elbow Surg* 2018;27(3):387-392.
2. Keijsers R, de Vos RJ, Kuijer PPF, van den Bekerom MP, van der Woude HJ, Eygendaal D: Tennis elbow. *Shoulder Elbow* 2019;11(5):384-392.
3. Lenoir H, Mares O, Carlier Y: Management of lateral epicondylitis. *Orthop Traumatol Surg Res* 2019;105(8 suppl):S241-S246.
4. Nirschl RP, Pettrone FA: Tennis elbow. The surgical treatment of lateral epicondylitis. *J Bone Joint Surg Am* 1979;61(6A):832-839.
5. Shillito M, Soong M, Martin N: Radiographic and clinical analysis of lateral epicondylitis. *J Hand Surg Am* 2017;42(6):436-442.
6. Lai WC, Erickson BJ, Mlynarek RA, Wang D: Chronic lateral epicondylitis: Challenges and solutions. *Open Access J Sports Med* 2018;9:243-251.
7. Vaquero-Picado A, Barco R, Antuña SA: Lateral epicondylitis of the elbow. *EFORT Open Rev* 2016;1(11):391-397.
8. Calfee RP, Patel A, DaSilva MF, Akelman E: Management of lateral epicondylitis: Current concepts. *J Am Acad Orthop Surg* 2008;16(1):19-29.
9. Pierce TP, Issa K, Gilbert BT, et al: A systematic review of tennis elbow surgery: Open versus arthroscopic versus percutaneous release of the common extensor origin. *Arthroscopy* 2017;33(6):1260-1268.e2.
10. Rosenberg N, Henderson I: Surgical treatment of resistant lateral epicondylitis. Follow-up study of 19 patients after excision, release and repair of proximal common extensor tendon origin. *Arch Orthop Trauma Surg* 2002;122(9-10):514-517.
11. Verhaar J, Walenkamp G, Kester A, van Mameren H, van der Linden T: Lateral extensor release for tennis elbow. A prospective long-term follow-up study. *J Bone Joint Surg Am* 1993;75(7):1034-1043.
12. Baker CL Jr, Murphy KP, Gottlob CA, Curd DT: Arthroscopic classification and treatment of lateral epicondylitis: Two-year clinical results. *J Shoulder Elbow Surg* 2000;9(6):475-482.
13. Mullett H, Sprague M, Brown G, Hausman M: Arthroscopic treatment of lateral epicondylitis: Clinical and cadaveric studies. *Clin Orthop Relat Res* 2005;439:123-128.
14. Szabo SJ, Savoie FH III, Field LD, Ramsey JR, Hosemann CD: Tendinosis of the extensor carpi radialis brevis: An evaluation of three methods of operative treatment. *J Shoulder Elbow Surg* 2006;15(6):721-727.

15. Peart RE, Strickler SS, Schweitzer KM Jr: Lateral epicondylitis: A comparative study of open and arthroscopic lateral release. *Am J Orthop (Belle Mead NJ)* 2004;33(11):565-567.
16. Dunkow PD, Jatti M, Muddu BN: A comparison of open and percutaneous techniques in the surgical treatment of tennis elbow. *J Bone Joint Surg Br* 2004;86(5):701-704.
17. Amin NH, Kumar NS, Schickendantz MS: Medial epicondylitis: Evaluation and management. *J Am Acad Orthop Surg* 2015;23(6):348-355.
18. Barco R, Antuña SA: Medial elbow pain. *EFORT Open Rev* 2017;2(8):362-371.
19. Zahn KV, Byerly DW: Medial epicondyle injection, in: *StatPearls* [Internet]. StatPearls Publishing, 2020.
20. Vangsness CT Jr, Jobe FW: Surgical treatment of medial epicondylitis. Results in 35 elbows. *J Bone Joint Surg Br* 1991;73(3):409-411.
21. Gabel GT, Morrey BF: Operative treatment of medial epicondylitis. Influence of concomitant ulnar neuropathy at the elbow. *J Bone Joint Surg Am* 1995;77(7):1065-1069.
22. Kurvers H, Verhaar J: The results of operative treatment of medial epicondylitis. *J Bone Joint Surg Am* 1995;77(9):1374-1379.
23. Gong HS, Chung MS, Kang ES, Oh JH, Lee YH, Baek GH: Musculofascial lengthening for the treatment of patients with medial epicondylitis and coexistent ulnar neuropathy. *J Bone Joint Surg Br* 2010;92(6):823-827.
24. Holt J, Preston G, Heindel K, Preston H, Hill G: Diagnosis and management strategies for distal biceps rupture. *Orthopedics* 2019;42(6):e492-e501.
25. Savin DD, Watson J, Youderian AR, et al: Surgical management of acute distal biceps tendon ruptures. *J Bone Joint Surg Am* 2017;99(9):785-796.
26. Tjoumakaris FP, Bradley JP: Distal biceps injuries. *Clin Sports Med* 2020;39(3):661-672.
27. Sutton KM, Dodds SD, Ahmad CS, Sethi PM: Surgical treatment of distal biceps rupture. *J Am Acad Orthop Surg* 2010;18(3):139-148.
28. Mazzocca AD, Burton KJ, Romeo AA, Santangelo S, Adams DA, Arciero RA: Biomechanical evaluation of 4 techniques of distal biceps brachii tendon repair. *Am J Sports Med* 2007;35(2):252-258.
29. Jobin CM, Kippe MA, Gardner TR, Levine WN, Ahmad CS: Distal biceps tendon repair: A cadaveric analysis of suture anchor and interference screw restoration of the anatomic footprint. *Am J Sports Med* 2009;37(11):2214-2221.
30. Bain GI, Prem H, Heptinstall RJ, Verhellen R, Paix D: Repair of distal biceps tendon rupture: A new technique using the Endobutton. *J Shoulder Elbow Surg* 2000;9(2):120-126.

31. Balabaud L, Ruiz C, Nonnenmacher J, Seynaeve P, Kehr P, Kehr E: Repair of distal biceps tendon ruptures using a suture anchor and an anterior approach. *J Hand Surg Br* 2004;29(2):178-182.

32. Weinstein DM, Ciccone WJ II, Buckler MC, Balthrop PM, Busey TD, Elias JJ: Elbow function after repair of the distal biceps brachii tendon with a two-incision approach. *J Shoulder Elbow Surg* 2008;17(1 suppl):82S-86S.

33. Peeters T, Ching-Soon NG, Jansen N, Sneyers C, Declercq G, Verstreken F: Functional outcome after repair of distal biceps tendon ruptures using the endobutton technique. *J Shoulder Elbow Surg* 2009;18(2):283-287.

34. Grewal R, Athwal GS, MacDermid JC: Single versus double-incision technique for the repair of acute distal biceps tendon ruptures: A randomized clinical trial. *J Bone Joint Surg Am* 2012;94(13):1166-1174.

35. Staples JR, Calfee R: Cubital tunnel syndrome: current concepts. *J Am Acad Orthop Surg* 2017;25(10):215e-224e.

36. Biggs M, Curtis JA: Randomized, prospective study comparing ulnar neurolysis in situ with submuscular transposition. *Neurosurgery* 2006;58(2):296-304.

37. Bartels RH, Verhagen WI, van der Wilt GJ, Meulstee J, van Rossum LG, Grotenhuis JA: Prospective randomized controlled study comparing simple decompression versus anterior subcutaneous transposition for idiopathic neuropathy of the ulnar nerve at the elbow: Part 1. *Neurosurgery* 2005;56(3):522-530.

38. Gervasio O, Gambardella G, Zaccone C, Branca D: Simple decompression versus anterior submuscular transposition of the ulnar nerve in severe cubital tunnel syndrome: A prospective randomized study. *Neurosurgery* 2005;56(1):108-117.

39. Nabhan A, Ahlhelm F, Kelm J, Reith W, Schwerdtfeger K, Steudel WI: Simple decompression or subcutaneous anterior transposition of the ulnar nerve for cubital tunnel syndrome. *J Hand Surg Br* 2005;30(5):521-524.

40. Geutjens GG, Langstaff RJ, Smith NJ, Jefferson D, Howell CJ, Barton NJ: Medial epicondylectomy or ulnar-nerve transposition for ulnar neuropathy at the elbow? *J Bone Joint Surg Br* 1996;78(5):777-779.

# 7

My Hand Hurts

Dawn M. LaPorte, MD, FAAOS
Seth D. Dodds, MD, FAAOS

Introduction

Four classic hand surgery pathologies are described, answering the question, Why does my hand hurt? These four problems range in their anatomic focus and etiology. One of the most fulfilling aspects of hand surgery is the ability to treat conditions related to the entire musculoskeletal system. In general, orthopaedics tends to focus on bones and joints. However, in the adventurous realm of hand surgery, the conditions to be treated range from the foundation of the bone, to the moving articulation, to the ligaments that maintain stability, to the muscles and tendons that power the joints, to the blood vessels that provide hand vascularity, to the nerves that supply motor and sensory function, and finally to the skin that envelops the hand in its composite.

CARPAL TUNNEL SYNDROME

Epidemiology

- Most common compression neuropathy; affects 3% to 8% of adults in the general population
- Caused by increased pressure within the carpal tunnel, resulting in compression of the median nerve and characterized by pain

---

Dr. LaPorte or an immediate family member serves as a board member, owner, officer, or committee member of ACGME - Orthopaedic RRC, American Orthopaedic Association, American Society for Surgery of the Hand, and Ruth Jackson Orthopaedic Society. Neither Dr. Dodds nor any immediate family member has received anything of value from or has stock or stock options held in a commercial company or institution related directly or indirectly to the subject of this chapter.

and paresthesias on the palmar-radial aspect of the hand, often worse at night
- The cause is not typically identified; however, carpal tunnel syndrome (CTS) has been associated with trauma, repetitive motion, and different medical conditions.
- Risk factors for CTS:[1]
  - Seen more in females than males (3:1 ratio)
  - Diabetes (odds ratio, 1.9)
  - Thyroid disorders
  - Pregnancy
  - Alcoholism
  - Inflammatory arthritis
  - Obesity
  - Repetitive activities
  - Mucopolysaccharidoses
- CTS is frequently bilateral (16% to 87%).

Pertinent Anatomy/Pathoanatomy

- Nerve roots C5 to T1 contribute to the median nerve, but C5 input is not consistent.
  - The median nerve arises from the medial and lateral cords of the brachial plexus. It runs lateral to the brachial artery and superficial to the brachialis and deep to the biceps in the arm and crosses anterior to the brachial artery and then progresses into the forearm medial to the artery. It lies medial to the brachial artery at the antecubital fossa and both lie medial to the biceps tendon. It then enters the forearm between the ulnar and the humeral head of the pronator teres and, distally, passes deep to the flexor digitorum superficialis (FDS) at its proximal arch and travels between the FDS and the flexor digitorum profundus (FDP).
  - The anterior interosseous nerve arises from the median nerve just distal to the arch of the FDS and the palmar cutaneous branch of the median nerve branches from the main nerve 5 to 7 cm proximal to the volar wrist crease. The median nerve passes between the flexor carpi radialis and the FDS at the distal forearm before entering the carpal tunnel. The recurrent motor branch typically branches radial to the median nerve through the carpal tunnel to supply the thenar muscles. Distal

to the carpal tunnel, the median nerve branches into digital nerves to supply sensation to the thumb, index, long, and the radial ring finger.
- The borders of the carpal tunnel include the transverse carpal ligament volarly, the carpal bones dorsally, the hook of the hamate and triquetrum ulnarly, and the scaphoid tubercle and trapezium radially.
- Ten structures pass through the carpal canal—nine flexor tendons and the median nerve (**Figure 1**). The tendons are the FDS to the index through the little finger, the FDP to the index through the little finger, and the flexor pollicis longus.
- Increased pressure on the median nerve is caused by decreased space in the carpal canal, which can be secondary to bony anatomy, for example, a fracture, flexor tenosynovitis. Increased pressure on the nerve results in decreased perfusion and in turn compromised function of the nerve.
- The recurrent motor branch is the only motor branch to arise from the median nerve at the level of the carpal canal. It innervates the thenar muscles, including the abductor pollicis brevis (APB), which provides thumb opposition.

Pertinent History/Physical Examination Findings

- Typical complaints: numbness and/or tingling in a median nerve distribution, frequently worse at night.
  - Patients may awaken at night with pain and/or numbness and feel as if they have to shake out their hand(s) (flick sign has 90% sensitivity/specificity).
  - Patients may complain of weakness or dropping objects or difficulty with fine motor tasks.
- Diagnosis is frequently made through a comprehensive history and examination and may be confirmed with electrodiagnostic testing.
- Typical examination findings
  - Subjective diminished light touch sensation in the thumb, index, and long, and radial half of the ring finger
  - Diminished two-point discrimination
  - Positive Tinel test (**Figure 2**)—paresthesias in a median nerve distribution after tapping over the median nerve at the wrist (sensitivity 38% to 100%, specificity 55% to 100%)

Chapter 7: My Hand Hurts

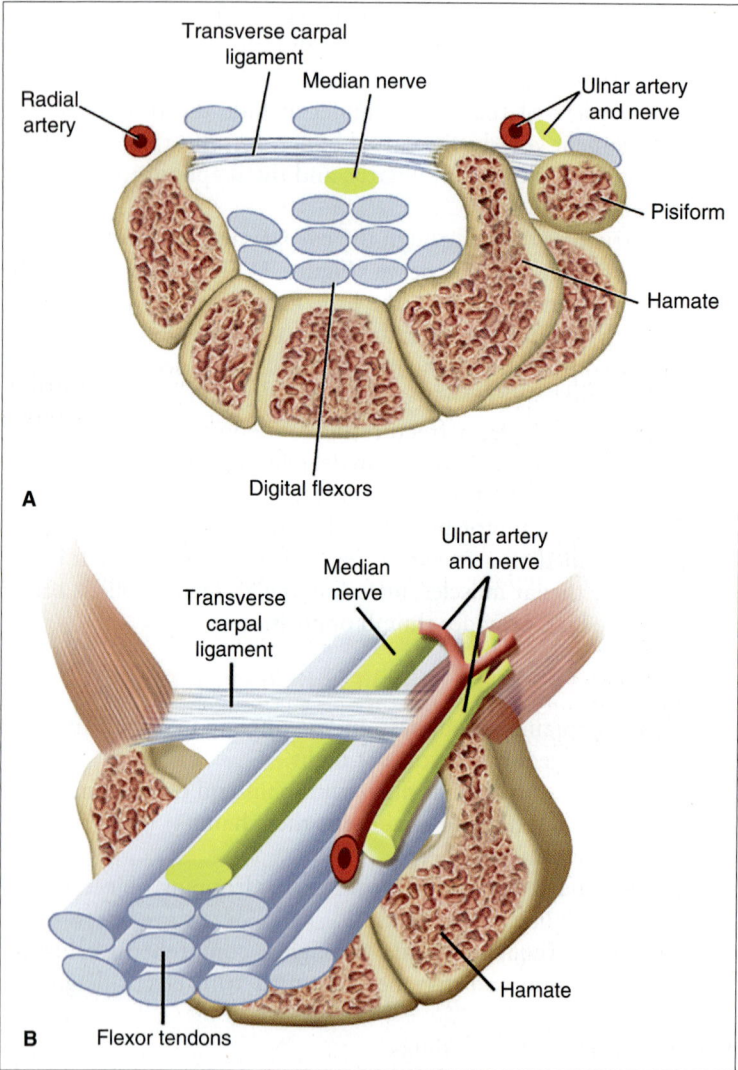

Figure 1 **A**, Anatomic drawing of the carpal tunnel. **B**, Cross-section of the carpal tunnel with the ulnar artery and nerve superficial to the transverse carpal ligament. (Reproduced with permission from Wiesel SW, Albert T: *Operative Techniques in Orthopaedic Surgery*, ed 3. Wolters Kluwer, 2021, Part 6, Figure 60.1.)

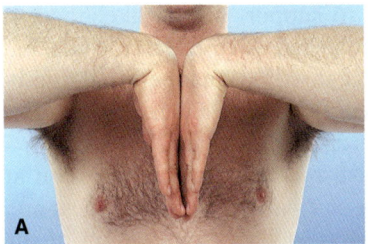
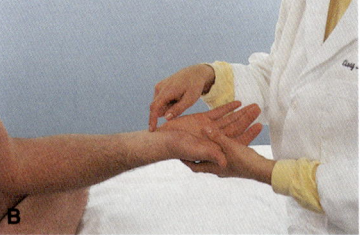

Figure 2 Clinical photographs show the Phalen test (**A**) and the Tinel test (**B**). © B. Proud.

- Positive Phalen test—paresthesias in a median nerve distribution after holding the wrist hyperflexed for 30 seconds (note: maintain the elbow in full extension so as not to confound with compression of the ulnar nerve) (sensitivity 42% to 85%, specificity 54% to 98%)[2]
- Positive Durkan test—paresthesias in a median nerve distribution after holding pressure for 30 seconds over the carpal tunnel
  - Durkan compression test has been shown to have the highest sensitivity for CTS (83% to 89%).[3]
- More advanced cases: atrophy of the thenar muscles and weakness in opposition of the thumb, tested by assessing strength against resisted opposition (**Figure 3**)

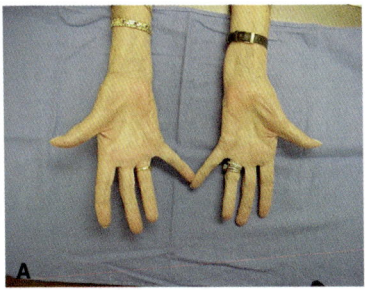
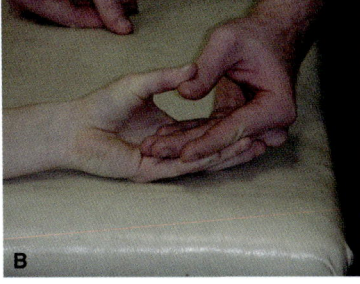

Figure 3 **A**, Clinical photograph from a 72-year-old woman with thenar atrophy associated with advanced carpal tunnel syndrome. **B**, Clinical photograph shows testing thumb opposition (abductor pollicis brevis) strength against resistance.

- The CTS-6 is a validated scale to support a high likelihood of CTS and can also measure responsiveness to release; it is based on symptoms in the median nerve distribution, nocturnal numbness, thenar atrophy or weakness, positive Phalen test, positive Tinel sign, and loss of two-point discrimination.[4]
- Patients may have a double crush syndrome or compression at multiple levels, and examination of a patient with numbness and tingling in the hand should always include examination of the cervical spine.
  - Differential diagnosis includes cervical radiculopathy, thoracic outlet syndrome, pronator syndrome, and polyneuropathy.

Relevant Imaging

- Ultrasonography can be used for diagnosis of CTS.
  - Typically the cross-sectional area of the median nerve is measured at the proximal carpal tunnel.
- Gold standard for diagnosis: nerve conduction study and electromyogram (EMG)
  - Electrodiagnostic studies are typically performed by a neurologist or physiatrist and measure sensory and motor conduction in addition to the EMG.
  - Prolonged sensory and or motor latency indicates a loss of myelin, and EMG changes (in the APB for CTS) indicate axonal loss.
  - Electrodiagnostic studies can confirm the presence and severity of compression as well as the level or levels of compression and which nerve or nerves are affected.

Nonsurgical Measures

- The first line of treatment for CTS is a cock-up wrist splint to be worn while sleeping.
  - The goal is to prevent flexion of the wrist at night and therefore decrease pressure on the median nerve.
- If a patient has persistent symptoms despite nighttime splinting for at least 1 month, a trial of corticosteroid injection at the carpal canal may be considered. The injection can be both diagnostic and therapeutic.
  - Up to 80% of patients have improvement initially with corticosteroid injection; however, only 20% to 31% have persistent relief at 1 year.

- If a patient has relief with corticosteroid injection but then symptoms recur, they should have an excellent prognosis with surgical carpal tunnel release (CTR).
- CTS in pregnancy will usually resolve after delivery.
  - Initial treatment is with nighttime splinting. Corticosteroid injection is considered safe during pregnancy and is recommended if splinting does not resolve symptoms.
  - CTR is not frequently necessary in pregnancy but can be considered (with local anesthesia) if symptoms persist despite nonsurgical measures.

Surgical Intervention

- Indications
  - Patients who have persistent symptoms despite nonsurgical measures—nighttime splinting plus or minus corticosteroid injection—are candidates for CTR.
  - Patients who present initially with weakness or thenar atrophy or who have EMG changes should be encouraged to pursue CTR directly to prevent progression of motor loss.
- Techniques
  - CTR surgery can be performed as an open or endoscopic procedure.
    - The literature shows that long-term results are comparable between open and endoscopic procedures. There is a slightly increased risk of nerve injury with endoscopic CTR and an earlier return to work with the endoscopic release. The decision between open or endoscopic surgery is frequently based on surgeon preference or experience.
  - Open CTR
    - The surgery is performed under tourniquet, typically with local anesthesia plus or minus sedation, but can be performed wide awake with local anesthesia and no tourniquet.
      - A longitudinal incision is marked in the palm in line with the ring digit extending distally from the Kaplan cardinal line to proximally 5 mm distal to the distal wrist crease (**Figure 4**).
      - Make an incision through the skin and carry it through the palmar fascia (longitudinal running fibers), exposing the transverse carpal ligament (transverse running fibers).

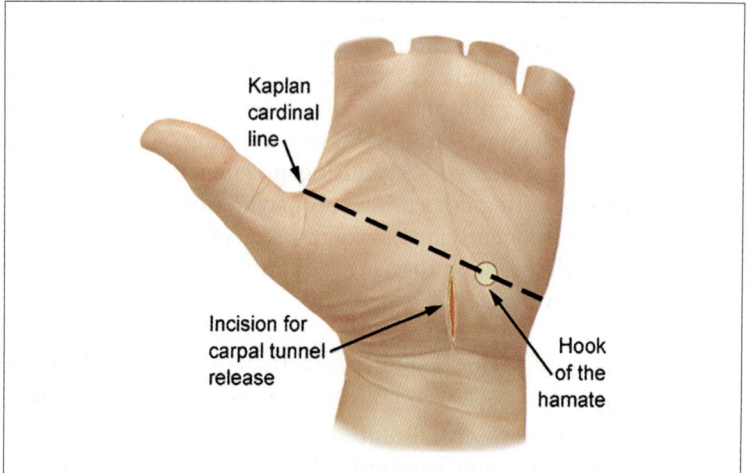

Figure 4 Schematic drawing shows the incision for open carpal tunnel release. The Kaplan cardinal line is used as a guide for the distal aspect of the incision. The incision is in line with the radial aspect of the ring finger and is made just radial to the hook of the hamate. (Reproduced with permission from Hunt TR, Wiesel SW: *Operative Techniques in Hand, Wrist, and Forearm Surgery*. Wolters Kluwer, 2010, Technique Figure 107.3.)

- Palpate the hook of the hamate, which is the ulnar border of the transverse carpal ligament.
- The transverse carpal ligament is split in a longitudinal fashion just radial to the hook of the hamate, taking care to prevent injury to the underlying median nerve.
  - Releasing the transverse carpal ligament at its more ulnar aspect decreases the risk of injury to the recurrent motor branch in the rare incidence of a transligamentous branch.
- The ligament should be split distally to the level of the sentinel fat (indicating the vascular arch) and proximally under direct visualization.
  - The most proximal aspect of the transverse carpal ligament as well as the distal aspect of the antebrachial

fascia can be split with dissecting scissors under direct visualization; the tips should be pointed ulnarly to avoid injury to the palmar cutaneous branch of the median nerve.
- Postoperative orders
  - The patient does not bear weight on their hand and ideally does no lifting beyond a cup of coffee for 2 weeks.
    - The patient returns at 2 weeks for a wound check, sutures are removed, and the patient can gradually resume activity.
    - A small number of pills (approximately 5) of tramadol or Tylenol #3 may be given, though most patients will do well solely with over-the-counter medication, acetaminophen or ibuprofen.
  - Anatomic variants such as a transligamentous recurrent motor branch may put the nerve at risk during surgical release. In the initial postoperative period, watch for signs of infection.
    - Patients who have pain or nighttime waking preoperatively will often have relief of those symptoms shortly after surgery.
    - The numbness and paresthesias can gradually improve over the course of 1 year.
  - The most common reason for persistent symptoms after CTR is an incomplete release. Other possible causes for persistent symptoms include double crush and incorrect diagnosis.
- Endoscopic CTR (**Figure 5**)
  - Endoscopic CTR uses a thin tube device with a camera attached (endoscope) guided through a small transverse incision in the wrist.
  - The endoscope allows the surgeon to directly see the internal structures of the wrist, including the transverse carpal ligament, without opening the area with a standard longer incision.
  - The device contains both the camera and the cutting tool and, during endoscopic CTR, the transverse carpal ligament is cut, releasing pressure on the median nerve.

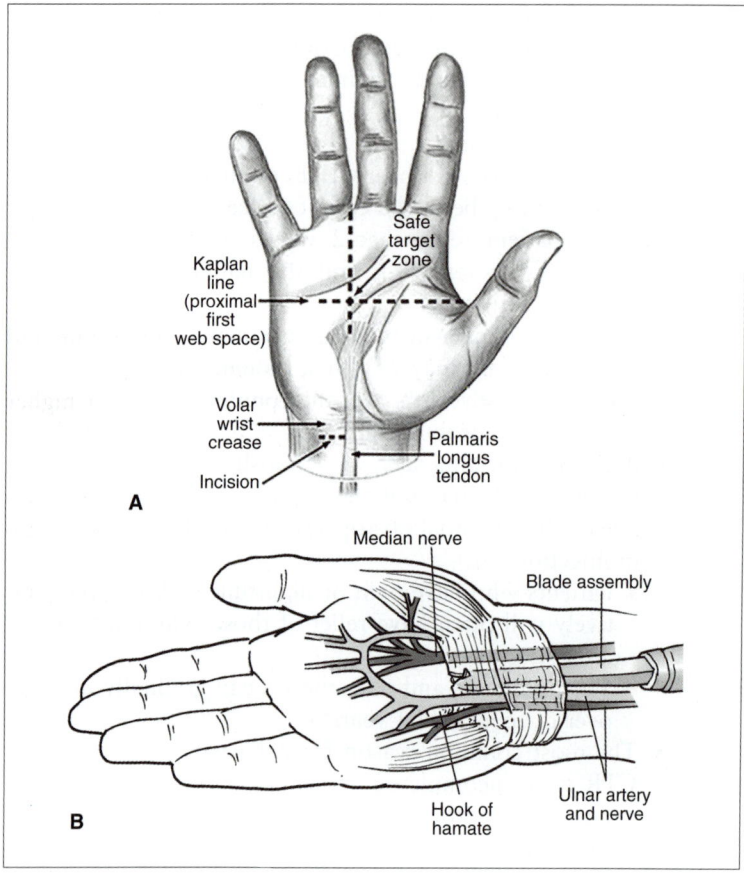

Figure 5 **A**, Illustration shows the incision for endoscopic carpal tunnel release. **B**, Illustration demonstrating how the endoscopic carpal tunnel release device is inserted into the carpal canal and the ligament is directly visualized. (Panel A reproduced with permission from Berger RA, Weiss AC: *Hand Surgery*. Lippincott Williams & Wilkins, 2004, Figure 47.6. Panel B reproduced from Diao E: Carpal tunnel release, in Colvin EC, Flatow E, eds: *Atlas of Essential Orthopaedic Procedures*, ed 2. American Academy of Orthopaedic Surgeons, 2020, p 315, Figure 7.)

- The blade is elevated just proximal to the sentinel fat and then withdrawn slowly, cutting the ligament from distally to proximally, completely releasing the transverse carpal ligament.

- Outcomes
  - Nighttime splinting has been reported to result in 75% relief at 18 months.
  - 53% to 80% of patients have initial symptom relief after corticosteroid injection; however, only 20% to 31% remained symptom free at 12 months.[5,6]
  - Long-term outcomes after open and endoscopic CTR are reported to be good or excellent in 75% to 90% of patients, with recurrence reported in 4% to 57% of cases.
    - Endoscopic CTR is associated with earlier return to work and earlier recovery of grip and pinch strength compared with open CTR but no difference at 6 months.
    - Endoscopic CTR has also been reported to have a higher risk nerve injury (usually transient) and lower risk of scar tenderness.
    - Some studies suggest a higher incidence of recurrence with techniques other than open CTR (but the numbers to support this are small).
    - The most common cause of persistent symptoms after CTR is incomplete release.

Top 10 Knowledge Drops for Your Rotation

1. CTS is the most common compression neuropathy.
2. CTS is characterized by numbness and tingling in the thumb, index and long fingers, and radial aspect of the ring finger.
3. Symptoms are often worse at night.
4. Patients may also have weakness in the hand, especially with thumb abduction and opposition.
5. The only motor branch affected in CTS is the recurrent motor branch that innervates thenar muscles, including the APB.
6. The contents of the carpal canal include the median nerve and nine tendons—FDS to the index finger through little finger, FDP to the index finger through little finger, and flexor pollicis longus.
7. If the patient has significant weakness/atrophy of the APB or EMG changes consistent with denervation, most surgeons recommend CTR rather than pursuing continued nonsurgical treatment.

8. The most significant risk of surgical release of the carpal tunnel is median nerve injury.
9. The primary advantage of endoscopic CTR is a slightly sooner return to work (approximately 2 weeks) compared with open release. At 1 year, both groups are similar.
10. The disadvantage of endoscopic CTR is a very small increase in the incidence of median nerve injury compared with open release.

TRIGGER FINGER

Epidemiology

- Entrapment tendinopathy at the hand
- Patients typically experience pain at the distal palm and locking or catching of the finger (triggering) as they flex and extend the affected digit.
- Although trigger finger is common, it is still not clear exactly what causes it.[7]
  - May be a genetic predisposition[8]

Pertinent Anatomy/Pathoanatomy

- The flexor tendon enters the flexor tendon sheath at the A1 pulley, which is just volar to the metacarpophalangeal (MCP) joint.
- It is thought that the flexor tendon developed a nodule within its substance, and that this nodule would contact the entrance of the flexor tendon sheath, leading to catching and locking as the finger flexes and extends.
  - After more careful examinations of the tendon and the A1 pulley, however, surgeons recognized that the pathology behind trigger finger is related to thickening of the A1 pulley not the tendon. This thickening is a fibrocartilaginous metaplasia that occurs within the A1 pulley itself.
- In some instances, the A1 pulley can become quite thick, greater than 5 mm (normal less than 1 mm thick).
- It is the stiffness of the A1 pulley caused by the fibrocartilaginous metaplasia that leads to the triggering of the finger.

Pertinent History/Physical Examination Findings

- Two medical conditions, diabetes and hypothyroidism, commonly worsen or potentially cause trigger finger.
  - Diabetes is the most common medical condition that exacerbates trigger finger.
- Patients often describe stiffness and a feeling of swelling in the finger.
- Sometimes the triggering is faint, leading to mild symptoms.
  - As the triggering worsens, the finger can even get stuck or locked in position (typically flexed down into the palm).
- Although some patients may not have much discomfort with the triggering, others have considerable pain localized to the A1 pulley in the palm, especially as they unlock the finger.
  - The pain tends to radiate up and down the flexor tendon sheath and the course of the flexor tendon itself.
  - Patients will often localize the symptoms to the proximal interphalangeal (PIP) joint because it is the PIP joint that ends up being locked in flexion. However, the pathology is localized to the A1 pulley at the distal aspect of the palm.
- On physical examination, patients will experience point tenderness at the A1 pulley, which is just distal to the distal palmar crease.
  - If the examiner holds mild pressure over the A1 pulley while the patient flexes and extends the finger, the examiner can often feel the triggering.
  - In certain circumstances the finger will lock during the examination, further highlighting the diagnosis.
    - If the finger does lock on physical examination, one way to painlessly unlock the finger is to hold the MCP joint flexed and slowly extend the PIP joint to release the trigger.
  - Another aspect of the physical examination to focus on is the range of motion of the PIP joint itself.
- Patients often have a mild flexion contracture of the PIP joint of 10° to 20°. It is important to document this flexion contracture as it has been shown to be associated with stiffness after trigger finger release surgery.[9]

Nonsurgical Measures

- Immobilization: Wearing a splint or guard to prevent PIP flexion and limit MCP flexion as well can be helpful to allow the inflammation around the tendon sheath that is contributing to the painful triggering to subside.
- Cortisone injection: The goal of the cortisone injection is similar, to decrease inflammation at the flexor tendon sheath.
  - Although the cortisone injection is typically given at the level of the A1 pulley (**Figure 6**), it can also be effective if given at a more distal location within the flexor tendon sheath.
  - These injections can be painful for patients because even though a small dose of steroid and lidocaine are injected into the sheath itself, there is little room in the sheath to accommodate this additional fluid.
  - A cortisone injection will routinely improve the symptoms at the A1 pulley and sometimes can even resolve the trigger finger entirely.
    - If the cortisone does wear off, it does so within 3 to 6 months after the injection.

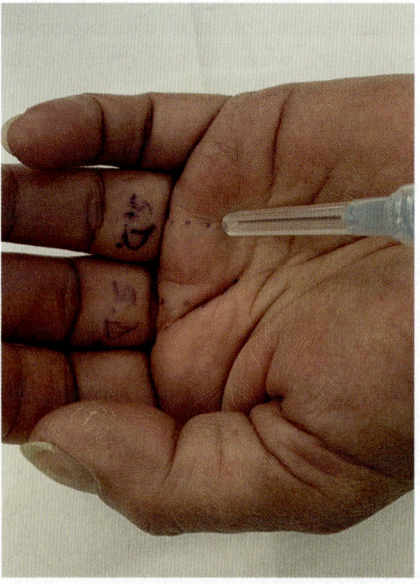

Figure 6 Clinical photograph demonstrating the injection site for cortisone for treatment of trigger finger.

Surgical Intervention

- Trigger finger can affect any digit in the hand from the thumb to the little finger. It can even affect multiple digits either individually at different times or at the same time. It is certainly possible to release multiple trigger fingers in the same surgical setting.
- A1 pulley release
  - Straightforward way to resolve the problem. Fortunately, releasing the A1 pulley itself does not significantly affect finger function over the long term.
    - Typically, trigger finger release can be performed under local anesthesia given in the subcutaneous tissues over the A1 pulley.
  - A longitudinal or transverse incision can be used, depending on surgeon's preference.
    - The neurovascular bundles to the radial and ulnar aspects of the digit are protected with blunt retractors.
    - The A1 pulley itself is exposed and then incised longitudinally to liberate the underlying FDS and FDP (**Figure** 7).
      - It is important to release the annular fibers just proximal to the A1 pulley as these can sometimes also contribute to the triggering.

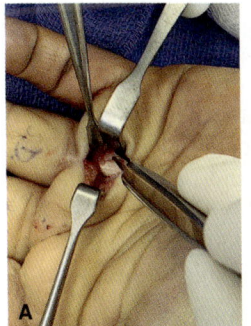 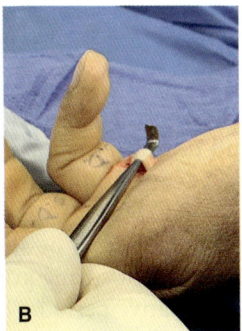 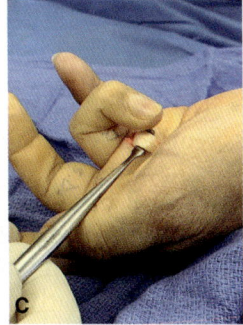

Figure 7 Surgical photographs showing A1 pulley release in a patient with trigger finger. **A**, The released A1 pulley. The thickened A1 pulley is held by a forceps. **B**, The flexor digitorum superficialis is withdrawn from the incision to demonstrate isolated proximal interphalangeal flexion. **C**, The flexor digitorum profundus is withdrawn to demonstrate composite flexion of the distal interphalangeal and proximal interphalangeal joints.

- It is also important to avoid inadvertent injury to the A2 pulley; the A2 pulley is needed to prevent bow-stringing of the flexor tendon when the finger is actively flexed.
- The standard surgical approach is a small, 1.5-cm incision over the area of the A1 pulley; however, there are other percutaneous approaches, including one that involves using a needle to release the A1 pulley.
  - Typically an 18- or 19-gauge needle is used.
    - The bevel of the needle is oriented longitudinally in line with the A1 pulley itself.
    - The needle is then used to longitudinally release the A1 pulley in a percutaneous fashion.
  - It is safest to do this on the two central digits, the long and ring fingers. At the index finger and at the little finger the neurovascular bundles are crossing obliquely near the A1 pulley and could be at potential risk with this type of percutaneous procedure.
    - At the thumb, the neurovascular bundles are also in close proximity to the center of the A1 pulley and are at risk of injury.
- Postoperative orders: After surgery, patients may begin moving their finger right away, taking care to protect the incision, so that it can heal without incident.

Outcomes

- The results of trigger finger surgery are uniformly very good with return of function and decreased palmar pain. Patients are typically very relieved to have the annoying and painful triggering resolved.
  - The palmar incision does tend to be sore for approximately 6 weeks, which can affect tight/strong gripping and heavy pushing in the early postoperative period.
- Stiffness is the most common problem after surgery.
  - Many patients benefit from the assistance of the hand therapist to regain their flexibility.
  - Stiffness can be a challenge because of postoperative scarring around the flexor tendon limiting flexor tendon excursion. Swelling of the finger can also limit the flexibility of the distal

interphalangeal (DIP) and PIP joints. Also, if the patient does have a mild flexion contracture of the PIP joint, the ligament stiffness at the PIP joint can significantly challenge regaining full flexibility.
  - Patients who have more than one trigger finger released at a time may experience more stiffness than patients with only a single digit being released.
- Another complication of trigger finger stems from incomplete release of the A1 pulley. The tendon will continue to catch and trigger in the area of an incomplete release.
  - One advantage of doing the procedure under a local anesthetic is that the patient can participate in identifying this potential complication by simply actively making a fist and flexing the finger and extending it in the operating room after the A1 pulley is released.
  - There are rare occasions where the finger continues to trigger despite complete and thorough release of the A1 pulley. In these circumstances, excising one of the slips of the FDS tendon can decrease the bulk within the flexor tendon sheath and resolve the residual triggering.

Top 10 Knowledge Drops for Your Rotation

1. The pathology of trigger finger is thickening of the A1 pulley of the flexor tendon sheath associated with fibrocartilaginous metaplasia, not from a nodule on the flexor tendons.
2. Both the FDS and the FDP tendons are within the A1 pulley at the level of the palm.
3. Patients complain of painful locking, sticking, and clicking (triggering) of their finger or thumb while they are attempting to flex and extend the finger.
4. Tenderness and palpable triggering at the A1 pulley of the affected digit are common physical examination findings.
5. For the fingers, the A1 pulley is located at the distal aspect of the palm between the distal palmar crease and the proximal digital crease.
6. There is a significant association between diabetes and the development of trigger finger.

7. Nonsurgical treatment consists of splinting and cortisone injections.
8. Surgical release of the A1 pulley is perhaps the most definitive treatment option for trigger finger.
9. A common challenge postoperatively is finger stiffness—especially if there is a mild PIP joint flexion contracture present preoperatively.
10. Recurrent trigger finger after surgical release is uncommon and is most often due to incomplete release of the A1 pulley.

FLEXOR TENDON INJURIES

Epidemiology

- The flexor tendons at the hand include both the FDS and the FDP for the fingers and the flexor pollicis longus for the thumb.
  - The flexor tendon extends from the musculotendinous junction at the mid to distal forearm out to the finger. The FDS inserts at the middle phalanx along its midsection volarly and primarily flexes the PIP. The FDP inserts at the mid to proximal aspect of the distal phalanx and flexes the DIP and PIP joints.
  - Both these tendons also help with MCP joint flexion.
- Laceration is the most frequent injury to the flexor tendon.
  - Flexor tendons can also be injured by fracture or avulsion from their insertion. This is common for the FDP and is called a jersey finger, as this injury can occur in sports when a finger gets caught on the collar of a jersey. The distal phalanx is forcibly extended, leading to rupture of the tendon from its insertion to the bone or an avulsion fracture of the tendon insertion.

Pertinent Anatomy/Pathoanatomy

- Flexor tendon injuries and lacerations have been classified anatomically by different zones of injury.
- Zone 1 injuries involve the distal aspect of the finger and include only the FDP, as the proximal edge of zone 1 is defined by the distal aspect of the insertion of the FDS.

- Zone 2 lacerations are within the flexor tendon sheath from the distal edge of the FDS insertion to the proximal edge of the A1 pulley.
- Zone 3 is from the proximal edge of the A1 pulley to the distal aspect of the carpal tunnel.
- Zone 4 is within the carpal tunnel, and zone 5 is a flexor tendon laceration proximal to the carpal tunnel in the distal forearm.

Surgical Intervention

- Flexor tendon surgery is problematic for a number of reasons.
  - The biggest concern is the battle against scar tissue adhesions that form between the tendon and the sheath or neighboring soft tissues after a flexor tendon repair.
  - Adhesions can affect the tendon at any zone of injury, but certainly zone 2, where both tendons are within the flexor tendon sheath, stands out as the most problematic.
- Zone 1 flexor tendon injuries involve the FDP tendon and its attachment to the distal phalanx.
  - These tendon injuries can occur either with an avulsion fracture off the volar surface of the distal phalanx or as a laceration or rupture of the tendon from the distal phalanx itself without a bone fragment.
  - The bone fragment can be repaired surgically with internal fixation if it is large enough.
  - If it is quite small, the bone fragment can be excised and the flexor tendon can be repaired directly to the bone using either suture anchors or by making small drill holes in the distal phalanx and tying the sutures over the dorsal aspect of the fingernail.
- Zone 2 flexor tendon lacerations were initially described, a century ago, as injuries sustained in "no man's land" because repairs in zone 2 had very poor functional outcomes.
  - Advances in flexor tendon surgery have adapted to the biggest confounding problems in zone 2: gapping of the tendon repair and scar tissue adhesions. If the flexor tendon scars during the course of healing, it will not move the finger.
    - If the repair is strong enough to allow the sutured tendon to move and glide before it heals with bridging collagen, adhesion formation can be avoided. Unfortunately, stitches

used in tendon repair are small in caliber compared with the strength of the flexor tendon and the load that the flexor tendon experiences when the finger is actively flexed.
- Originally, flexor tendon repairs were protected with a passive range of motion protocol, in which the fingers were flexed down into the palm passively. With passive motion, the flexor tendons would be gliding but they would not be loaded, thus maintaining the integrity of the suture repair.
- More recently, it has been demonstrated that a repair managed with an active range of motion protocol postoperatively compared with the passive range of motion protocol had superior functional outcomes.[10]
  - A better understanding that active motion is critical in yielding an optimal result in zone 2 flexor tendon repairs has pushed the hand surgery field to maximize repair strength to tolerate the tendon load of active motion.
  - When a strong repair can be achieved, the tendon can tolerate early active motion and patients tend to do much better. Fewer scar tissue adhesions develop and the swelling improves more rapidly.
- Techniques that strengthen a flexor tendon repair:
  - Strong caliber suture. This is generally obvious, but a large suture takes up significant space and becomes bulky, leading to impingement of the repairs site in the flexor tendon sheath. Any impingement of the repair site in the flexor tendon sheath will very rapidly lead to scar tissue adhesions. Some companies have developed a finer caliber, but stronger version of nonabsorbable suture for tendon repairs and these newer sutures were quickly adopted.
  - More suture strands crossing the repair site. If the stitch crosses the repair site four times, it is stronger than a stitch that crosses the repair site two times. A six-strand repair is even stronger. However, a six-strand repair can lead to increased bulk at the repair site, which can then lead to flexor tendon adhesions. Research has also found that a locking suture repair is stronger than a nonlocking suture repair. Regarding the technique of suture placement, a suture that enters the tendon has greater strength if it captures at least 7 to 8 mm of tendon. A small capture bite of tendon,

for example 3 to 4 mm, tends to pull out of the tendon more easily.
- Performing an epitendinous repair with a fine suture through the epitendinous layer of the flexor tendon. The larger suture is usually within the core of the flexor tendon and is called a core suture repair, whereas the finer suture circumferentially runs around the repair through the superficial, epitendinous layer of the tendon. Although the finer suture is not as strong, this type of epitendinous repair does increase the overall tendon repair strength and it leads to a smoother repair site, which will minimize catching, triggering, and adhesions about the tendon.
- Over the past decade, hand surgeons have become interested in pursuing surgeries under local anesthesia alone, without sedation.[11] This anesthesia option allows the surgeon to understand in real time exactly how their flexor tendon repair is performing. For example, after a zone 2 flexor tendon repair using a four-strand locking core suture and a running epitendinous stitch, the surgeon can ask an awake patient to flex the finger and make a fist. While the patient is attempting to flex the finger, the surgeon can identify any gapping at the repair site or any potential hang-ups in the flexor tendon sheath that the flexor tendon repair may be catching on (**Figure 8**), such as a prominent suture knots that could catch on the flexor tendon sheath. This problem could be remedied before leaving the operating room, leading to a much better functional outcome for that patient.
- Zone 3 flexor tendon repairs are not within the confines of the flexor tendon sheath and can be made a bit more bulky, allowing a surgeon to use a thicker stitch to obtain a stronger repair.
  - There are still many anatomic structures running throughout the palm that a bulky tendon repair could become hung up on or adhere to.
  - Thus, hand surgeons tend to use the same techniques for flexor tendon repair in zone 3 as they use in zone 2.
- Zone 4 injuries at the level of the carpal tunnel are very uncommon as the bone structure that shapes the carpal tunnel also protects the tendons from laceration.

Chapter 7: My Hand Hurts

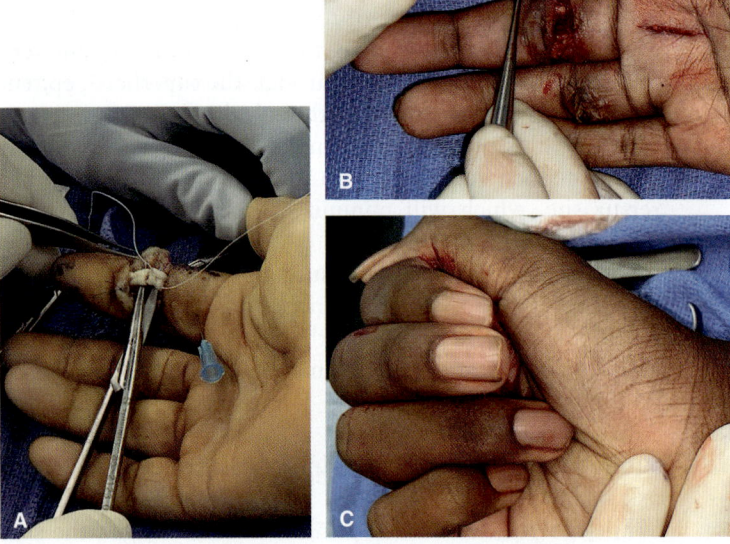

Figure 8 Surgical photographs showing stages of flexor tendon repair. **A**, Laceration of the flexor digitorum profundus being repaired with suture, taking care to reapproximate the tendon edges as precisely as possible in an effort to avoid bunching of the tendon so that the tendon can glide smoothly in the flexor tendon sheath. **B**, The flexor tendon repair site is shown. The incisions in the palm are made to retrieve the proximally retracted tendon during the initial dissection. **C**, The patient is able to maintain an active fist in the operating room after repair of the flexor digitorum profundus to the index and long fingers.

- Zone 5 injuries happen at the distal forearm.
  - There is plenty of space here at the distal forearm for a stronger repair and a thicker suture.
  - These tendon repairs tend to do better because there is no flexor tendon sheath or fibro-osseous tunnel for the tendons to traverse.

Chapter 7: My Hand Hurts

Top 10 Knowledge Drops for Your Rotation

1. Flexor tendon lacerations are characterized by the anatomic zone of injury.
2. Zone 2, between the distal edge of the FDS insertion at the middle phalanx to the proximal edge of the A1 pulley, was formerly known as "no man's land" because flexor tendon repairs in this specific zone are fraught with challenges.
3. Zone 1 injuries include the common jersey finger flexor tendon ruptures at the insertion of the FDP to the distal phalanx.
4. Flexor tendon core suture repairs are made more durable by using stronger caliber suture: for example, a 3-0 suture is stronger than a 4-0 suture, but may add more bulk to the repair.
5. Strength of the repair is also improved by having more strands of core suture; most surgeons recommend at least a four-strand core suture repair.
6. Sutures that lock to the tendon itself improve capture strength of the suture to the tendon.
7. Ensuring a 7- to 8-mm distance between the repaired end of the tendon and exit of the suture grasp into the tendon also contributes to improved repair strength.
8. Augmenting the repair with a fine running epitendinous stitch has also been found to improve pullout strength and helps resist against rupture.
9. The most common problems after a flexor tendon repair include tendon adhesions and finger stiffness with capsular contractures of the DIP, PIP, and MCP joints.
10. Although surgical treatment with the patient wide awake under local anesthesia and no tourniquet provides the surgeon with the best opportunity to assess flexor tendon repair integrity as the patient is asked to flex and extend the finger postrepair, the future of flexor tendon surgery will most likely incorporate a biologic augmentation to repairs that enhances healing and prevents the formation of adhesions in the flexor tendon sheath.

THUMB CARPOMETACARPAL ARTHRITIS

Epidemiology

- Thumb carpometacarpal (CMC) joint arthritis is characterized by pain, stiffness, and weakness at the base of the thumb.
  - It is the second most common site of degenerative disease in the hand, after arthritis of the DIP joint.
- Thumb CMC arthritis affects women more frequently than men (6:1 ratio), often in later decades of life.
  - It affects up to 25% of women older than 50 years, up to 36% of postmenopausal women, and 1 in 5 will require medical intervention to alleviate symptoms.[12]
  - The female/male difference decreases with age, with the incidence in women and men at age 75 years being 40% and 25%, respectively.[13]
- Risk factors include being female, increasing age, previous trauma, and inflammatory arthropathy. Lifetime prevalence approaches 10%.

Pertinent Anatomy/Pathoanatomy

- The thumb CMC joint is the articulation between the trapezium and first metacarpal. It is a saddle-shaped joint that allows multiple planes of motion. The concavity of each articular surface is shallow so the skeleton provides little intrinsic stability.
- The ligaments (volar anterior oblique ligament and dorsoradial ligament) are critically important for resisting the natural tendency to subluxate with pinch and grasp maneuvers.
- Studies have shown that degeneration of the anterior oblique ligament is the precursor of basal joint degenerative disease.[14]

Pertinent History/Physical Examination Findings

- Patients with thumb CMC arthritis typically present with complaints of pain at the base of the thumb, increased with loading and pinch, such as opening a jar, turning a key, or wringing out a rag.
- Examination findings:
  - Tenderness over the thumb CMC joint

Chapter 7: My Hand Hurts

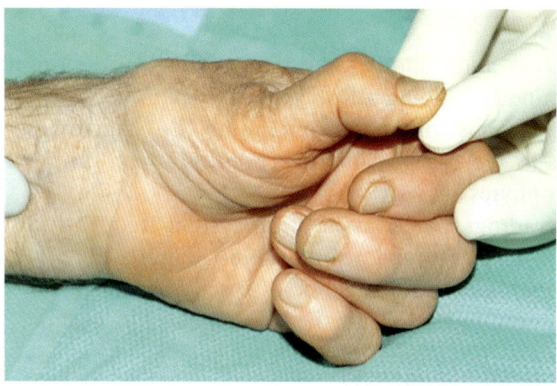

Figure 9 Photograph shows the shoulder sign and metacarpophalangeal hyperextension. (Reproduced with permission from Maschke SD, Graham TJ, Evans PJ: *Master Techniques in Orthopaedic Surgery: The Hand*, ed 3. Wolters Kluwer, 2016, Figure 26A.3.)

- Prominence over the thumb CMC joint and possible shoulder sign (**Figure 9**) consistent with subluxation of the metacarpal on the trapezium
- Positive grind test—pain or crepitus with axial loading of the metacarpal and circumduction while stabilizing surrounding joints, reflecting cartilage wear at the CMC joint (80% to 93% specificity)
- Progressive zigzag or adduction deformity with metacarpal abduction, MCP hyperextension, and first web space contracture
- The thumb MCP joint should be assessed for hyperextension, as hyperextension greater than 30° often requires intervention if the patient is going to have surgery for thumb CMC arthritis.
- Differential diagnosis includes other causes of radial-sided wrist pain:
  - de Quervain tenosynovitis, characterized by tenderness over the first dorsal compartment and pain with Finkelstein maneuver
  - Scaphotrapeziotrapezoid (STT) arthritis often will be associated with pain with radial deviation of the wrist and can be identified on radiograph as well
  - Ganglion cyst, trigger thumb, ulnar collateral ligament tear, and arthritis at the thumb MCP or radiocarpal joints

Relevant Imaging

- AP, lateral, and oblique radiographic views of the thumb should be obtained including a Robert view (true AP).
  - Radiographs will often show thumb CMC narrowing and sclerosis as well as possible subchondral cysts, subluxation, and osteophytes.
  - The radiographic classification system frequently used is the Eaton-Littler classification (**Table 1; Figure 10**).
  - Radiographs should also be assessed for arthritis in surrounding joints, most notably the STT and/or MCP joints.

Nonsurgical Measures

- Initial treatment typically includes rest, activity modification, splint immobilization with a hand-based thumb spica splint (**Figure 11**), plus/minus oral anti-inflammatory medication, if not contraindicated.
- Therapy for CMC-stabilizing exercises and modalities can be helpful as well.
- If patients have persistent or recurrent symptoms, intra-articular corticosteroid injection may be effective.

Surgical Intervention

- If symptoms persist or recur despite nonsurgical measures, surgical intervention is considered.

TABLE 1 The Four Stages of the Eaton-Littler Classification

Stage	Description
I	Subtle carpometacarpal joint-space widening
II	Slight carpometacarpal joint-space narrowing, sclerosis, and cystic changes with osteophytes or loose bodies <2 mm
III	Advanced carpometacarpal joint-space narrowing, sclerosis, and cystic changes with osteophytes or loose bodies >2 mm
IV[a]	Arthritic changes in the carpometacarpal joint as in stage III with scaphotrapezial arthritis

[a]Stage IV as modified by Eaton EG, Glickel SZ: Trapeziometacarpal osteoarthritis: Staging as a rationale for treatment. *Hand Clin* 1987;3:455-471.

Reproduced with permission from Kennedy CD, Manske MC, Huang JI: Classifications in brief: The Eaton-Littler classification of thumb carpometacarpal joint arthrosis. *Clin Orthop Relat Res* 2016;474(12):2729-2733.

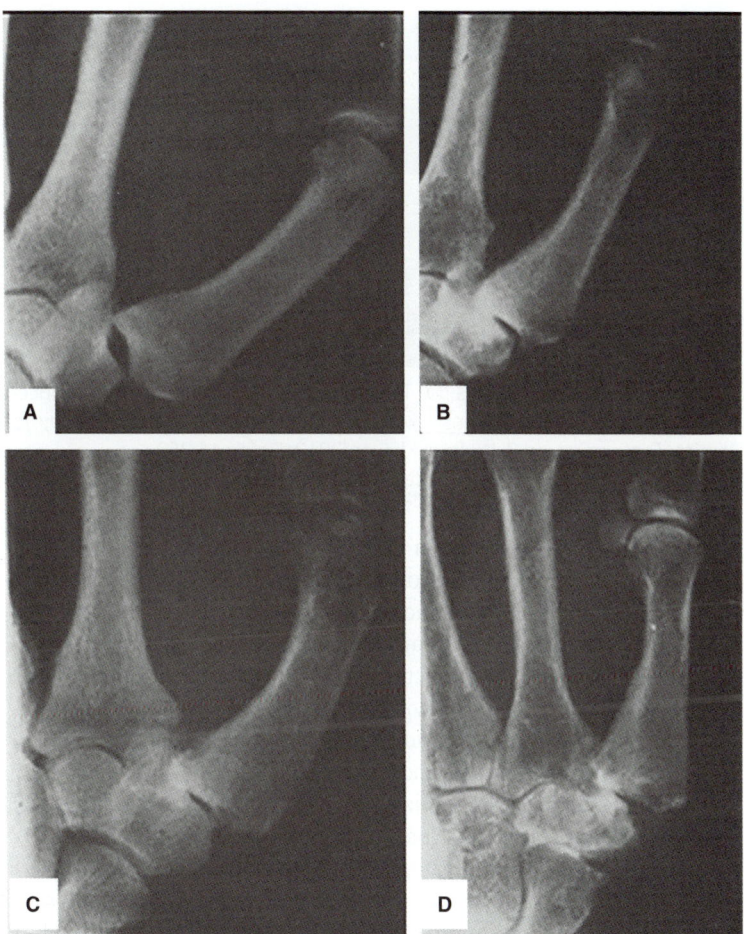

Figure 10 Radiographs show stages I (**A**), II (**B**), III (**C**), and IV (**D**) carpometacarpal arthrosis of the Eaton-Littler classification system, and as described by Eaton et al are shown. (Reproduced with permission from Eaton EG, Lane LB, Littler JW, Keyser JJ: Ligament reconstruction for the painful thumb carpometacarpal joint: A long-term assessment. *J Hand Surg Am* 1984;9:692-699. Copyright © American Society for Surgery of the Hand.)

- The thumb CMC is the most common site in the hand for which surgery is sought.
- The most frequently performed surgical intervention is trapeziectomy with or without tendon suspensionplasty.

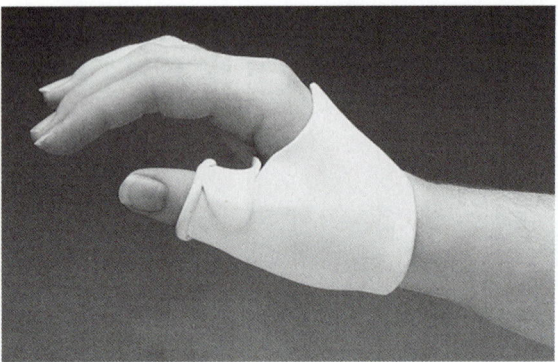

Figure 11 Photograph shows the ThumbKeeper splint (AliMed). (Reproduced with permission from Radomski MV, Trombly CA: *Occupational Therapy for Physical Dysfunction*, ed 7. Wolters Kluwer, 2013, Figure 15.25.)

- Ligament reconstruction and tendon interposition uses the flexor carpi radialis tendon for suspension (**Figure 12**).
  - Alternative methods include using a slip of the abductor pollicis longus and/or using the extensor carpi radialis longus.
  - Alternatively, trapeziectomy can be performed with a suture suspension device or without suspension at all.[15]
- The most important component of surgical intervention is excision of the trapezium.
  - It is critical to recognize potential involvement of the STT joint and to address that at the time of surgery.
  - Similarly, it is important to recognize the presence of MCP hyperextension and to consider addressing that at the time of surgery—with capsulodesis if no MCP arthrosis, MCP arthrodesis in the setting of MCP arthrosis.
- In those age 50 years or younger who perform manual labor, CMC arthrodesis is considered (20° radial abduction and 40° palmar abduction).
- Arthrodesis is contraindicated in pantrapezial arthritis (so limited to patients with stage II and III osteoarthritis).
- In patients considered young (age 50 years or younger) for trapeziectomy, treatment with denervation may be an effective option.

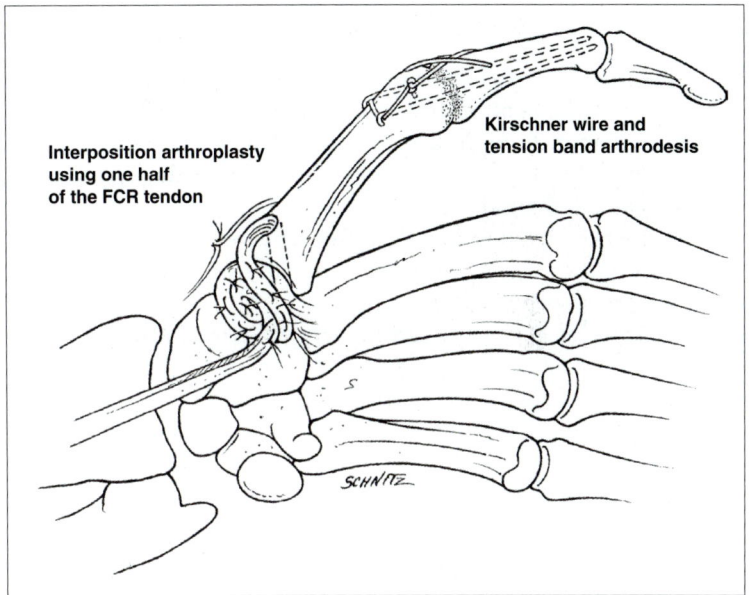

Figure 12 Schematic illustration shows ligament reconstruction and tendon interposition. FCR = flexor carpi radialis. (Reproduced with permission from Strickland JW, Graham TJ: *Master Techniques in Orthopaedic Surgery: The Hand*, ed 7. Wolters Kluwer, 2005, Figure 33.6.)

- Outcomes
  - Ligament reconstruction and tendon interposition has been shown to result in 90% to 95% patient satisfaction and pain relief as well as improved strength and grip.[16] Similar results have been reported with abductor pollicis longus suspensionplasty.[17]
  - Gray and Meals[15] reported comparable results with simple trapeziectomy with hematoma distraction (without ligament reconstruction).
  - Trapeziometacarpal arthrodesis has been reported to have a nonunion rate of 8% to 21%.[18,19]

Top 10 Knowledge Drops for Your Rotation

1. Thumb CMC osteoarthritis is the most common site for surgical management of arthritis in the hand and affects women more than men (6:1 ratio).
2. Examination of patients with CMC osteoarthritis reveals a positive axial grind test.
3. Radiographs should include a Robert view.
4. Eaton-Littler classification is frequently used; check STT on imaging as well.
5. Nonsurgical treatment can be very effective, specifically rest, activity modification, immobilization with a hand-based thumb spica splint, and cortisone injection.
6. In the surgical treatment for CMC osteoarthritis, trapeziectomy is the critical step that decreases pain and improves patient satisfaction.
7. Many surgeons prefer to suspend the thumb metacarpal base after trapeziectomy, often with ligament reconstruction using a local tendon such as the flexor carpi radialis or abductor pollicis longus.
8. Common problems after CMC arthroplasty or trapeziectomy include continued pain at the base of the thumb and radial sensory nerve irritation.
9. Possible mechanical issues after surgical treatment include settling of the thumb metacarpal base onto the distal pole of the scaphoid (loss of suspension) and intermetacarpal convergence between the base of the thumb metacarpal and the base of the index metacarpal.
10. Thumb-MCP hyperextension can cause failure of trapeziectomy procedures by inducing a Z-deformity of the thumb. MCP joint hyperextension is best addressed at the index procedure if greater than 30°.

References

1. Wessel LE, Fufa DT, Boyer MI, Calfee RP: Epidemiology of carpal tunnel syndrome in patients with single versus multiple trigger digits. *J Hand Surg* 2013;38(1):49-55.

2. Brüske J, Bednarski M, Grzelec H, Zyluk A: The usefulness of the Phalen test and the Hoffmann-Tinel sign in the diagnosis of carpal tunnel syndrome. *Acta Orthop Belg* 2002;68(2):141-145.
3. American Academy of Orthopaedic Surgeons: Management of Carpal Tunnel Syndrome Evidence-Based Clinical Practice Guideline. 2016. Available at: https://www.aaos.org/globalassets/quality-and-practice-resources/carpal-tunnel/cts_cpg_4-25-19.pdf. Accessed September 24, 2022.
4. Graham B: The value added by electrodiagnostic testing in the diagnosis of carpal tunnel syndrome. *J Bone Joint Surg Am* 2008;90(12):2587-2593.
5. Blazar PE, Emerson Floyd W, Han CH, Rozental TD, Earp BE: Prognostic indicators for recurrent symptoms after a single corticosteroid injection for carpal tunnel syndrome. *J Bone Joint Surg Am* 2015;97(19):1563-1570.
6. Ostergaard PJ, Meyer MA, Earp BE: Non-operative treatment of carpal tunnel syndrome. *Curr Rev Musculoskelet Med* 2020;13(2):141-147.
7. Makkouk AH, Oetgen ME, Swigart CR, Dodds SD: Trigger finger: etiology, evaluation, and treatment. *Curr Rev Musculoskelet Med* 2008;1(2):92-96.
8. Sood RF, Westenberg RF, Winograd JM, Eberlin KR, Chen NC: Genetic risk of trigger finger: Results of a genomewide association study. *Plast Reconstr Surg* 2020;146(2):165e-176e.
9. Baek JH, Chung DW, Lee JH: Factors causing prolonged postoperative symptoms despite absence of complications after A1 pulley release for trigger finger. *J Hand Surg Am* 2019;44(4):338.e1-338.e6.
10. Trumble TE, Vedder NB, Seiler JG III, Hanel DP, Diao E, Pettrone S: Zone-II flexor tendon repair: A randomized prospective trial of active place-and-hold therapy compared with passive motion therapy. *J Bone Joint Surg Am* 2010;92(6):1381-1389.
11. Lalonde D, Martin A: Epinephrine in local anesthesia in finger and hand surgery: The case for wide-awake anesthesia. *J Am Acad Orthop Surg* 2013;21(8):443-447.
12. Heyworth BE, Lee JH, Kim PD, Lipton CB, Strauch RJ, Rosenwasser MP: Hylan versus corticosteroid versus placebo for treatment of basal joint arthritis: A prospective, randomized, double-blinded clinical trial. *J Hand Surg Am* 2008;33(1):40-48.
13. Sodha S, Ring D, Zurakowski D, Jupiter JB: Prevalence of osteoarthrosis of the trapeziometacarpal joint. *J Bone Joint Surg Am* 2005;87(12):2614-2618.
14. Ladd AL, Weiss AP, Crisco JJ, et al: The thumb carpometacarpal joint: Anatomy, hormones, and biomechanics. *Instr Course Lect* 2013;62:165-179.

15. Gray KV, Meals RA: Hematoma and distraction arthroplasty for thumb basal joint osteoarthritis: Minimum 6.5-year follow-up evaluation. *J Hand Surg Am* 2007;32(1):23-29.
16. Tomaino MM: Ligament reconstruction tendon interposition arthroplasty for basal joint arthritis. Rationale, current technique, and clinical outcome. *Hand Clin* 2001;17(2):207-221.
17. Soejima O, Hanamura T, Kikuta T, Iida H, Naito M: Suspensionplasty with the abductor pollicis longus tendon for osteoarthritis in the carpometacarpal joint of the thumb. *J Hand Surg Am* 2006;31(3):425-428.
18. Hartigan BJ, Stern PJ, Kiefhaber TR: Thumb carpometacarpal osteoarthritis: Arthrodesis compared with ligament reconstruction and tendon interposition. *J Bone Joint Surg Am* 2001;83(10):1470-1478.
19. Taylor EJ, Desari K, D'Arcy JC, Bonnici AV: A comparison of fusion, trapeziectomy and silastic replacement for the treatment of osteoarthritis of the trapeziometacarpal joint. *J Hand Surg Br* 2005;30(1):45-49.

8

My Hip Hurts

Aaron Gipsman, MD • Eric Strauss, MD, FAAOS
Matthew A. Varacallo, MD

Introduction

Hip pain can be related to injury, overuse, arthritis, and other chronic conditions. Four categories of hip disorders are considered. Femoroacetabular impingement (FAI) is a common cause of hip pain in adolescents and adults; it is characterized by abnormal contact between the proximal femur and acetabulum. The iliopsoas functions as the strongest flexor of the hip joint. Injury to the iliopsoas can result in disabling hip and groin pain, particularly in athletic populations. Pathologic conditions of the iliopsoas include strain, tendinitis, tear, bursitis, and internal snapping

---

Dr. Strauss or an immediate family member is a member of a speakers' bureau or has made paid presentations on behalf of Arthrex, Inc., Organogenesis, Smith & Nephew, and Vericel; serves as a paid consultant to or is an employee of Arthrex, Inc., Fidia, Flexion Therapeutics, Joint Restoration Foundation, Organogenesis, Smith & Nephew, Subchondral Solutions, and Vericel; has stock or stock options held in Better PT; has received research or institutional support from Cartiheal, Fidia, and Organogenesis; and serves as a board member, owner, officer, or committee member of American Academy of Orthopaedic Surgeons, American Orthopaedic Association, and Arthroscopy Association of North America. Dr. Varacallo or an immediate family member serves as a paid consultant to or is an employee of Arthrex, Inc. Neither Dr. Gipsman nor any immediate family member has received anything of value from or has stock or stock options held in a commercial company or institution related directly or indirectly to the subject of this chapter.

hip syndrome. Hamstring injury severity can range from partial-thickness or full-thickness avulsions and retracted ruptures to chronic degenerative pathologies. Greater trochanteric pain syndrome encompasses a range of pathologies from trochanteric bursitis and lateral hip pain and snapping hip to full-thickness gluteus medius/minimus tears and tendinopathy, of which tendinopathy is the focus of this chapter. Injuries to the hip abductor complex in many ways mimic and run parallel to the pathophysiologic cascade and natural history of rotator cuff tears in the shoulder, and thus, these structures are often referred to as the rotator cuff tears of the hip.

FEMOROACETABULAR IMPINGEMENT

Epidemiology
- Most patients are younger than 40 years.
- Etiology is unknown but FAI is thought to be due to a combination of genetic and mechanical factors.
  - Activities involving repetitive hip movements at the extremes of motion, particularly hip flexion, increase the mechanical stresses on the proximal femur and acetabulum and predispose these areas to the development of a reactive bony lesion. This effect is especially pronounced in adolescents, in whom the growth pattern of the proximal femoral physis can be altered
  - Athletics associated with risk for FAI include ice hockey, soccer, dance, and football.
  - Up to 60% of active adolescents and young adults have radiographic signs of impingement, with many remaining asymptomatic.
- Males and females are at similar risk of the development of FAI but are predisposed to different patterns of impingement.
  - Pincer lesions are more common among females, which is likely related to sex-related differences in acetabular morphology.

Chapter 8: My Hip Hurts

- Males, in contrast, are more likely to have cam lesions, which is thought to be activity related.
- A unique subgroup of FAI is related to sequelae from pediatric hip conditions
  - Slipped capital femoral epiphysis classically is associated with the development of a cam lesion, whereas Legg-Calvé-Perthes disease can lead to complex deformity of the proximal femur and adaptive changes to the acetabular morphology.[1]
  - Despite the differences in etiology, these patients are treated similarly to those with more classic presentations of FAI.

Pertinent Anatomy/Pathoanatomy

- FAI occurs as a result of abnormal contact between the anterior femoral head–neck junction and anterosuperior acetabular rim with hip flexion and internal rotation. Over time, the increased contact pressure at the acetabular rim leads to injury to the cartilage and labrum.
- Cam and pincer lesions are the characteristic deformities of FAI (**Figure 1**).
  - Cam deformity is characterized by the loss of the normal spherical contour of the proximal femur at the junction of the femoral head and neck.
  - Pincer deformity occurs when the acetabular rim covers too much of the femoral head. Less commonly, a prominent anterior inferior iliac spine can also act like a pincer.
  - Approximately half of patients with FAI have mixed-type impingement with both a cam and pincer lesion, with most of the remaining patients having an isolated cam deformity.[1]
- Atraumatic hip instability is associated with FAI. Anterior bony impingement between the proximal femur and acetabulum can lever the femur posteriorly. This can worsen as the stabilizing effects of the anterior capsule and labrum attenuate, particularly among female patients with ligamentous laxity.
  - Although frank hip dislocation is uncommon, patients may experience recurrent subluxation events leading to functional limitations of hip motion and eventual posterior chondrolabral injury.

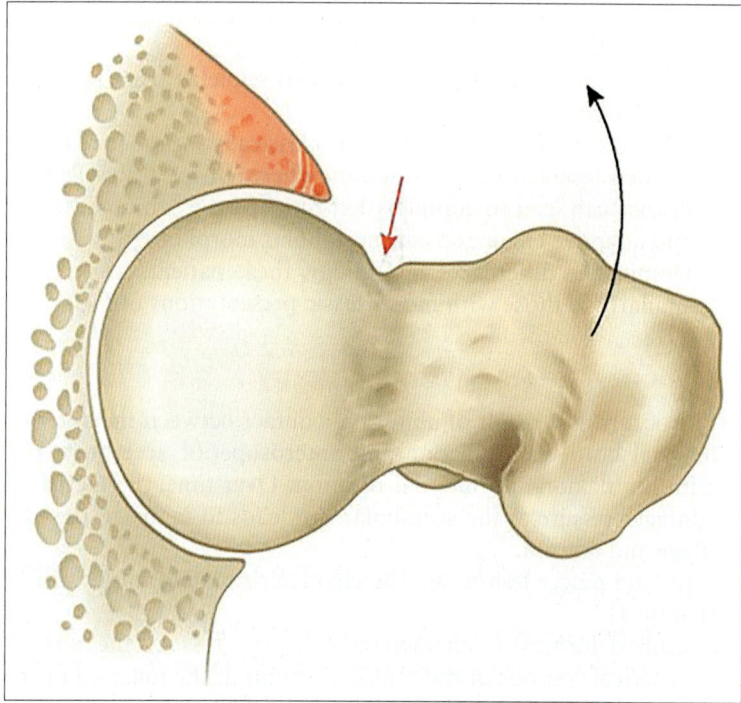

Figure 1 Illustration shows that pincer impingement (red arrow) results from abnormal acetabular morphology, whereas cam impingement (black arrow) is caused by loss of the spherical contour of the proximal femur. (Reproduced with permission from Miller MD: *Operative Techniques in Sports Medicine Surgery*. Wolters Kluwer, 2022, Figure 50.1.)

Pertinent History/Physical Examination Findings

- Patients with FAI report a gradual onset of hip and/or groin pain, typically without an inciting event.
  - Pain is worse with hip flexion, including sporting activities and sitting for prolonged periods. Mechanical symptoms, such as clicking or locking, can be indicative of a labral tear, subtle instability, or associated snapping hip syndrome.
- Examination is significant for painful and limited hip flexion and internal rotation.
  - Gait is often normal but can be antalgic in severe cases, characterized by a shortened stance phase on the affected side.

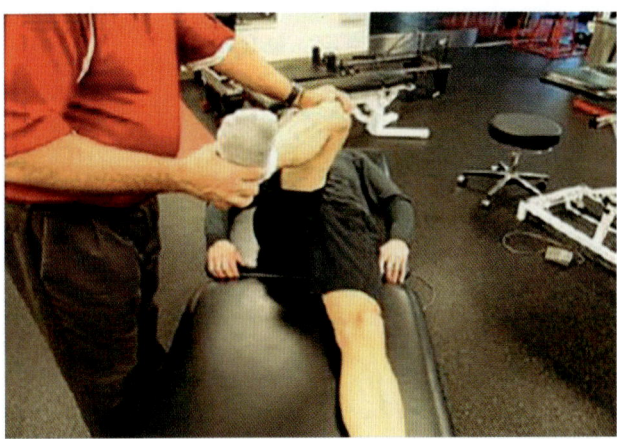

Figure 2 Photograph showing the flexion/adduction/internal rotation (or FADIR) impingement test. (Reproduced with permission from Johnson D: *Operative Arthroscopy,* ed 4. Wolters Kluwer, 2013, Figure 45.7.)

- Impingement tests have a high sensitivity with moderate specificity for FAI.[2]
  - Flexion/adduction/internal rotation (FADIR) test (**Figure 2**): Examiner passively flexes the patient's hip and knee to 90°, then adducts and internally rotates the hip. Pain and reproduction of the patient's symptoms is suggestive of anterior hip impingement.
  - Flexion, abduction, and external rotation, known as FABER or Patrick test (**Figure 3**): Patient's affected leg is placed in a figure-of-4 position, with the hip flexed, abducted, and externally rotated. The examiner stabilizes the pelvis with one hand, while applying an external rotation force to the affected limb. Hip and groin pain are suggestive of FAI, whereas buttock and low back pain are more reflective of sacroiliac or lumbar pathology.
- In patients with suspected instability, an assessment of global ligamentous laxity is obtained using the Beighton criteria.
  - The dial test can also be used to specifically evaluate for hip capsular laxity. With the patient lying supine and the knee extended, the examiner holds the limb into terminal internal rotation, then releases the force. Positive result: foot subsequently falls into more than 45° of external rotation beyond neutral

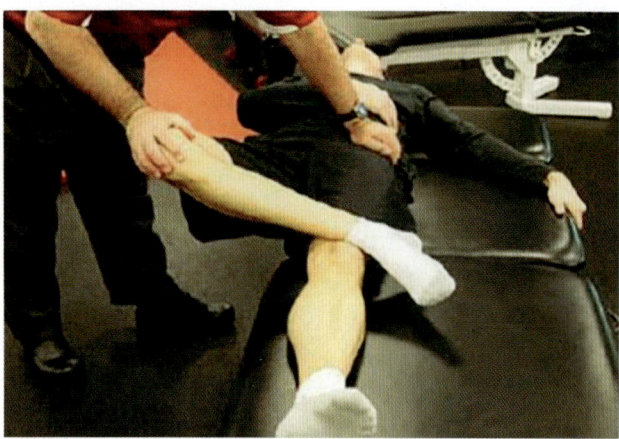

Figure 3 Photograph showing the flexion, abduction, and external fixation test, also known as FABER or Patrick test. (Reproduced with permission from Johnson D: *Operative Arthroscopy,* ed 4. Wolters Kluwer, 2013, Figure 45.9.)

Relevant Imaging

- Radiographic examination for FAI begins with an AP view of the pelvis and a frog-lateral view of the affected hip.
  - The Dunn and false-profile views are frequently used to obtain additional information about the bony morphology of the hip.
    - To obtain the Dunn view, the patient is positioned supine with the hip in neutral rotation, 45° or 90° of flexion, and 20° of abduction.
    - The false-profile view is obtained with the patient standing and facing away from the imaging plate at an angle of 65°.
  - The AP view should be carefully evaluated for joint space narrowing and subchondral sclerosis, indicative of early osteoarthritis.
  - The contour of the proximal femur should be evaluated on the frog-lateral and Dunn views, with loss of sphericity resembling a pistol grip being characteristic for a cam lesion.
    - Signs of acetabular retroversion, classically associated with pincer deformity, include the crossover sign, posterior wall sign, and the ischial spine sign.

- The alpha angle is calculated using the frog-lateral or Dunn views.
  - A best-fit circle that is centered on the femoral head is used to determine the point on the anterolateral femoral neck where a loss of sphericity occurs.
  - The alpha angle is calculated between this point and a line parallel to the longitudinal axis of the femoral neck, with a value greater than 55° reflective of cam deformity.
- Multiple parameters are used to evaluate for pincer impingement.
  - On the AP view, the lateral center-edge angle is calculated between a vertical line centered over the femoral head and the lateral edge of the acetabulum.
  - Similarly, the anterior center-edge angle can be calculated on the false profile view. A center-edge angle greater than 40° is suggestive of overcoverage and pincer impingement.
  - The Tönnis angle can also be used to evaluate for femoral head coverage on the AP view. It is determined using a horizontal line connecting the acetabular teardrops and a line tangential to the weight-bearing portion of the acetabulum, with an angle less than −10° being reflective of overcoverage.
- MRI is frequently obtained to further evaluate the patient's three-dimensional bony anatomy and identify associated soft-tissue pathology involving the labrum, cartilage, and hip musculature.
  - Bone marrow edema and cystic changes are frequently visualized on the anterosuperior aspect of the femoral neck. Chondrolabral detachment and degenerative tearing of the labrum with associated bony edema of the acetabular rim are commonly identified within its anterior and superolateral portions.[3]
  - Arthroscopic studies have found that the acetabular labrum is abnormal in greater than 90% of hips with FAI.[1]

Nonsurgical Measures

- Always begin with nonsurgical measures, including activity modification, physical therapy, and NSAIDs.
  - Patients are instructed to avoid sitting for extended periods as well as squatting and other activities involving positions of high hip flexion.

- Physical therapy focuses on strengthening of the hip flexors, hamstrings, abductors, and core musculature. Patients who do not improve with these initial treatments should receive an image-guided intra-articular corticosteroid injection.
- Symptomatic relief can be expected as quickly as 6 weeks in responsive patients.
  - However, the success of nonsurgical treatment is mixed and appears to vary according to patient age.[4]
  - Up to 85% of adolescents experience a positive response to nonsurgical treatment and can return to sports, whereas closer to 50% of adults can expect to return to normal physical activity with nonsurgical treatment alone.[5]
  - Treatment response is not associated with the presence of labral tears or the magnitude of bony deformity.[5]
  - For patients who do not obtain any symptomatic relief from an injection, an alternative diagnosis of FAI should be considered.

Surgical Intervention

- Surgery is indicated for patients with FAI in whom a trial of 3 to 6 months of nonsurgical treatment has failed, including a corticosteroid injection.[5]
  - The elements of surgery to correct FAI include femoroplasty to restore the normal spherical contour of the femoral head–neck junction, acetabuloplasty to remove the pincer lesion, and labral repair to redistribute contact pressures and restore the stabilizing suction seal.
- Hip arthroscopy is performed with the patient in the supine position (**Figure 4**).
  - The hip is distracted using a perineal post and traction boots.
    - Fluoroscopic guidance is used to localize the anterolateral portal, immediately anterior to the tip of the greater trochanter.
    - The 70° arthroscope is inserted into the joint to visualize the articular surface of the femoral head and acetabulum, also known as the central compartment.
    - An anterior working portal is then made under direct visualization of the arthroscope, slightly distal to the level of the anterolateral portal and lateral to the anterior superior iliac spine to avoid injury to the lateral femoral cutaneous nerve.

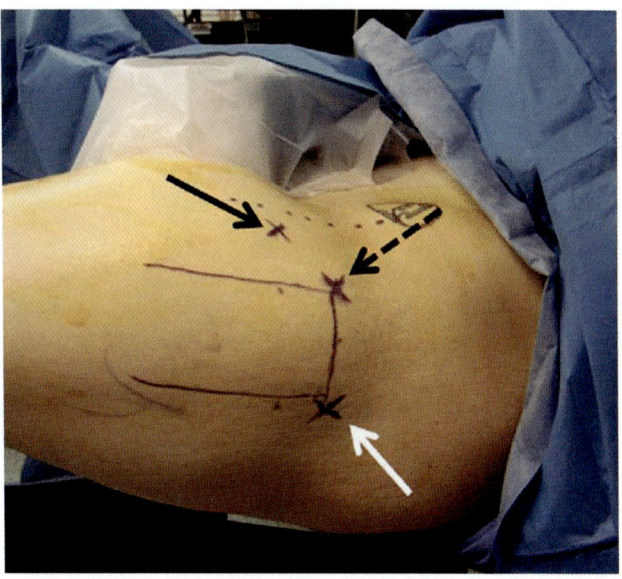

Figure 4 Photograph showing typical portals used for hip arthroscopy, which include the anterolateral (dashed arrow) and anterior (solid arrow) portals. The posterolateral portal (white arrow) is commonly used for posterior labral repair and reconstruction. (Reproduced with permission from Miller MD: *Operative Techniques in Sports Medicine Surgery*. Wolters Kluwer, 2022, Figure 50.4.)

- A capsulotomy is made between the two portals to facilitate access to the joint.
- A diagnostic arthroscopy is done in the central compartment to evaluate the cartilage and labrum.
  - Detachment of the labrum at the chondrolabral junction is typically identified between the 10-o'clock and 2-o'clock positions on the acetabular rim.
- A radiofrequency ablation device is used to débride soft tissue from the anterolateral acetabular rim, with care taken to avoid iatrogenic damage to the labral tissue.
- A motorized burr is used to resect a pincer lesion if it is present, and fluoroscopy is used to confirm adequate resection.
  - In cases without a pincer, the burr is used to remove sclerotic cortical bone at the level of the planned labral repair.

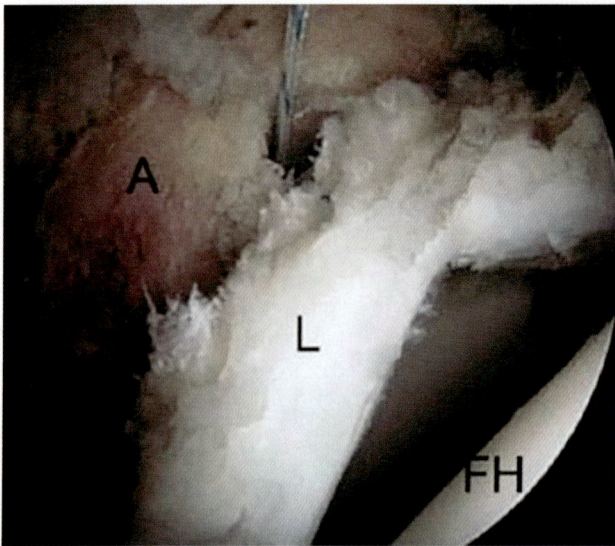

Figure 5 Arthroscopic labral repair. The arthroscope is looking down at the acetabular rim (A) and femoral head (FH). Suture repair of the labrum (L) has been performed. The articular cartilage of the acetabulum is seen in the depth of the image to the left of the femoral head. (Reproduced with permission from Johnson D: *Operative Arthroscopy*, ed 4. Wolters Kluwer, 2013, Figure 48.11G.)

- The labrum is repaired (**Figure 5**) using suture anchors, with knot-tying and knotless techniques providing similar clinical results.
  - The entry angle of the anchor should be away from the joint to minimize the risk of iatrogenic cartilage damage.
- Repair of posterior labral tears often requires a posterolateral portal that is placed posterior the tip of the greater trochanter.
- Management of chondral lesions of the acetabulum and femoral head remains controversial, with isolated débridement and microfracture most commonly used.
- With work in the central compartment complete, traction is released and the hip is flexed to 45°.

- The 70° arthroscope is directed into the extra-articular, intracapsular portion of the hip known as the peripheral compartment.
- A radiofrequency ablation device is used to elevate adherent capsule off the femoral neck and femoral head-neck junction.
- A motorized burr is then used to resect the cam lesion.
    - The hip is internally and externally rotated to access the lateral and medial edges of the lesion.
- Adequate resection with restoration of the normal spherical contour of the proximal femur is confirmed with fluoroscopy.
    - Under direct visualization of the arthroscope, the hip is brought into high flexion and internal rotation to confirm that there is no residual impingement.
- Closure of the hip capsule can then be performed with a suture passer, although the efficacy of capsular repair remains unclear.
- Postoperative rehabilitation includes toe-touch or foot-flat weight bearing on the surgical extremity with an assistive device for the first 4 weeks postoperatively.
    - Hip flexion range of motion exercises can begin immediately, with supervised physical therapy beginning by the second week.
    - Many surgeons use a hinged hip brace in the early postoperative period to prevent positions of extreme hip extension, rotation, and abduction that can place excessive tension on the labral repair.
    - By 4 weeks postoperatively, patients can be advanced to weight bearing as tolerated. Hip and core strengthening exercises are introduced and progressively increased by week 8.
    - Running and sport-specific exercises can begin between 3 to 6 months postoperatively, with return to sport expected by 1 year.
- Although hip arthroscopy is a safe and effective treatment for FAI, there is a steep surgeon learning curve that is associated with patient outcomes and the development of complications.
    - Iatrogenic chondral injury is the most common complication and occurs secondary to difficulty accessing the central compartment joint and/or improper surgical technique.

- Neurapraxia of the pudendal nerve can result from prolonged traction time or improper positioning, whereas errant placement of the anterior portal results in transient or permanent injury of the lateral femoral cutaneous nerve. Less common complications include infection, venous thromboembolism, and broken instrumentation within the hip joint.
- Postoperative hip instability is rare but can occur from extensive capsulotomy and acetabular resection in the setting of capsular laxity.
- Following hip arthroscopy, most patients can reliably expect significant reduction in pain and improved function of the hip.
  - Return to sport is high among athletes, with rates approaching 90%.[6]
  - Poorer outcomes have been reported among older patients with early osteoarthritis, particularly those with less than 2 mm of joint space remaining.
  - Longer duration of symptoms, lower patient activity level, higher alpha angles, and limited preoperative range of motion all have been associated with worse outcomes.
  - Reoperation rates by 4 years postoperatively are approximately 6%, with most patients requiring total hip arthroplasty secondary to osteoarthritis.[6]

Top 10 Knowledge Drops for Your Rotation

1. Individuals at the highest risk of the development of FAI are athletes performing hip movements at the extremes of motion, including ice hockey, soccer, dance, and football.
2. Females are more likely to have pincer impingement, whereas males are more likely to have cam lesions.
3. Slipped capital femoral epiphysis is associated with the later development of a cam lesion.
4. Patients with FAI have pain with active hip flexion and sitting for prolonged periods.
5. Radiographic examination for FAI includes an AP view of the pelvis and frog lateral, Dunn, and false-profile views of the affected hip.

6. The alpha angle is used to identify loss of sphericity of the proximal femur reflective of cam deformity, whereas the lateral center-edge and Tönnis angles are used to identify acetabular overcoverage indicative of pincer deformity.
7. Chondrolabral detachment and degenerative tearing of the labrum are commonly identified at the anterior and superolateral portions of the acetabular rim between the 10-o'clock and 2-o'clock positions.
8. Surgical correction of FAI includes femoroplasty to restore the normal spherical contour of the femoral head–neck junction, acetabuloplasty to remove the pincer lesion, and labral repair to redistribute contact pressures and restore the stabilizing suction seal.
9. The most common complications of hip arthroscopy for FAI include iatrogenic chondral injury, traction injury to the pudendal nerve, and damage to the lateral femoral cutaneous nerve from anterior portal placement.
10. Patients with less than 2 mm of remaining joint space have poorer outcomes following hip arthroscopy for FAI.

ILIOPSOAS DISORDERS

Epidemiology

- The iliopsoas is involved in 40% of patients with acute groin injuries, frequently in conjunction with an injury to the adductor musculature.[7]
  - In the chronic setting, iliopsoas conditions are present in 10% of patients presenting with hip or groin pain.
  - Female patients are more likely than males to have iliopsoas pathology, which is thought to be associated with increased hip motion secondary to underlying ligamentous laxity.
  - Activities that involve repetitive hip flexion and/or stretching to the extremes of motion, including dancing, soccer, hockey, gymnastics, and track and field, can predispose certain athletes to iliopsoas conditions.

Pertinent Anatomy/Pathoanatomy

- The iliopsoas is a composite musculotendinous structure consisting of the psoas major muscle and the iliacus muscle, which have unique origins in the lower abdomen and pelvis before combining into a single tendon distally.
  - The psoas major muscle originates from the vertebral bodies, intervertebral disks, and transverse processes of T12 through L5, and is directly innervated by the L1, L2, and L3 branches of the lumbar plexus.
  - The iliacus muscle arises from the upper two-thirds of the iliac fossa on the inner aspect of the pelvis and the lateral aspect of the sacrum and is innervated by the femoral nerve.
  - Deep to the inguinal ligament, the musculotendinous portion of the iliacus and psoas major muscles converge to form the iliopsoas tendon.
    - Proximal to the hip joint, the tendon sits within a bony groove between the anterior inferior iliac spine laterally and the iliopectineal eminence medially.
    - The tendon then courses directly superficial to the hip capsule and labrum before it inserts on the lesser trochanter of the femur. The iliopsoas tendon is therefore an extracapsular, extra-articular structure.
- A large synovial bursa exists between the iliopsoas tendon and the anterior hip capsule, which helps to reduce friction between these structures with hip motion.
  - The bursa is thin and nearly collapsed under normal conditions. In patients with iliopsoas bursitis, however, the bursa becomes inflamed and swells with fluid.
  - The close anatomic relationship between the iliopsoas tendon, hip capsule, labrum, and iliopsoas bursa frequently results in concomitant pathology between these structures.
- Snapping hip syndrome, also known as coxa saltans, is typically caused by the abnormal movement of a tendon over a bony prominence with hip motion.
  - Internal snapping occurs when the iliopsoas tendon rubs against the iliopectineal eminence, whereas external snapping happens when the iliotibial band (ITB) moves over the greater trochanter.

- Intra-articular snapping is less common but occurs when a loose body within the hip joint itself interferes with the smooth movement of the femoral head within the acetabulum.
- Acute injury of the iliopsoas will lead to a strain of the iliacus muscles or the iliacus and psoas muscles, with isolated psoas strains being uncommon.[7]
  - In the chronic setting, iliopsoas tendinitis is related to overuse and can be associated with partial tearing of the tendon.
  - An acute tendon tear of the iliopsoas tendon is rare in adults. In children and adolescents, however, an avulsion fracture of the lesser trochanter can occur because of the greater strength of the iliopsoas muscle and tendon relative to that of the developing bony apophysis.

Pertinent History/Physical Examination Findings

- Patients with iliopsoas strains, tendinitis, tears, and bursitis frequently complain of hip and/or groin pain.
  - The pain can radiate into the lower abdomen, lower back, and the upper thigh. Pain is provoked with activities that involve hip flexion and extension.
  - An injury or inciting event is frequently reported, often involving forceful hip flexion.
  - The dominant leg is more commonly involved than the nondominant leg, particularly in kicking and running athletes.
  - Recurrent injury is common, and up to 50% of patients can have a prior injury to the hip or groin.[7]
- Patients with internal snapping hip syndrome will report an audible and/or palpable snapping sensation in the inner aspect of the hip that is associated with pain.
  - Symptoms are provoked by activity, particularly those involving hip flexion.
  - Up to 40% of active individuals can have hip snapping, but most do not have symptoms.
- Physical examination should include a complete evaluation of the hip.
  - Tenderness to palpation can be present over anteromedial aspect of the hip and upper thigh.
  - Range of motion is typically normal.

- Strength testing often elicits pain with resisted hip flexion in the seated position.
- Evaluation of the snapping hip should attempt to identify the anatomic location of the pathology.
  - Many patients can voluntarily reproduce the snapping with certain movements, which is accompanied by an audible popping or clicking noise.
  - Internal snapping can be provoked by the examiner by passively moving the hip from a position of flexion, abduction, and external rotation to one of extension and internal rotation. In contrast, external snapping of the ITB over the greater trochanter occurs as the hip is flexed in neutral rotation.
- In the evaluation of the patient with hip and groin pain, it is important to differentiate iliopsoas pathology from other conditions.
  - Adductor injuries will present with pain over the medial thigh that is worsened with resisted hip adduction.
  - Sports hernia, also known as athletic pubalgia, is an overuse syndrome of the abdominal and adductor muscles that can be provoked by examination maneuvers that increase intra-abdominal pressure, such as sit-ups and Valsalva.
  - Patients with FAI and labral tears have decreased and painful motion of the hip, particularly in flexion and internal rotation.
  - In skeletally immature patients with hip or knee pain, a slipped capital femoral epiphysis should always be ruled out with diagnostic imaging.
- Iliopsoas pathology is frequently seen in conjunction with other conditions.
  - Acute strains to the iliopsoas can also involve the hip adductors, abductors, hamstrings, and/or secondary hip flexors including the rectus femoris and sartorius.
  - In the chronic setting, labral tears can occur secondary to impingement of the labrum and capsule by a pathologic iliopsoas tendon. Alternatively, inflammation of the iliopsoas bursa and tendon can occur as a result of underlying FAI and labral tearing.

Relevant Imaging

- Evaluation of a patient with suspected iliopsoas pathology should begin with standard anterior-posterior and frog-lateral hip radiographs.
  - Fracture should always be ruled out in the acutely injured patient.
  - In the chronic setting, cam and pincer lesions are reflective of underlying FAI, whereas joint space narrowing, osteophyte formation, subchondral sclerosis, and/or bony cysts are cardinal signs of hip osteoarthritis.
- The need for advanced imaging is dictated by multiple factors related to the patient and the suspected pathology.
  - MRI can identify iliopsoas strains, tendinitis, and bursitis. Furthermore, it can evaluate for intra-articular pathology involving the cartilage and labrum.
  - In certain situations, dynamic ultrasound examination is used to evaluate for a snapping iliopsoas tendon as the hip is brought through a range of motion.[8]

Nonsurgical Measures

- Treatment for any iliopsoas condition begins with nonsurgical measures.
  - Injured athletes should engage in a period of activity modification, including reduced training frequency and intensity.
  - Severe cases may require a complete cessation of sporting activity.
  - A supervised physical therapy program is frequently implemented, with a focus on hip stretching and gentle strengthening exercises of the hip flexors, hamstrings, and core musculature.
  - NSAIDs can be used on a standing basis early in the disease presentation and weaned as symptoms resolve.
- For patients who do not respond to first-line measures, an ultrasound-guided corticosteroid injection to the iliopsoas tendon and bursa can serve to reduce inflammation and improve symptoms.
  - In cases with unclear or multiple hip pathology, an injection has the added diagnostic benefit of confirming that the iliopsoas is the cause of the patient's symptoms. For patients who

do not obtain any relief from the injection, an alternative diagnosis should be considered.
- Patients with acute strains of the iliopsoas can be expected to return to athletic activities in as soon as 2 weeks postinjury.
  - Injections are very effective for snapping hip syndrome, with almost 90% of patients having sustained pain relief at four months postinjection.
  - Treatment efficacy for tendinitis and bursitis is thought to be lower, but data are currently limited.

Surgical Intervention

- Surgery is considered for patients who have persistent hip pain and limitation in function despite 3 to 6 months of nonsurgical treatment, including an injection.
  - Irrespective of the patient's underlying iliopsoas pathology, the same surgical treatment is used to lengthen the tendon and move it away from the underlying bursa, capsule, labrum, and bone.
  - Arthroscopic techniques are used to perform iliopsoas release and have similar efficacy to open surgery with reduced risk of complications.
    - Hip arthroscopy has the added benefit of evaluating and treating concomitant intra-articular pathology including FAI, loose bodies, and labral tears.
- Hip arthroscopy is performed with the patient in a supine position.
  - The hip joint is distracted with a perineal post and traction boots on the patient's foot.
  - Using fluoroscopy, an anterolateral portal is made, and the 70° arthroscope is inserted into the hip joint.
  - A diagnostic arthroscopy of the central compartment of the hip is performed and concomitant intra-articular pathology is identified.
  - An anteromedial working portal is then made under direct visualization with the assistance of the arthroscope.
  - A radiofrequency ablation wand or elongated surgical blade is used through the anteromedial portal to perform a capsulotomy between the two portals to facilitate access to the hip joint.

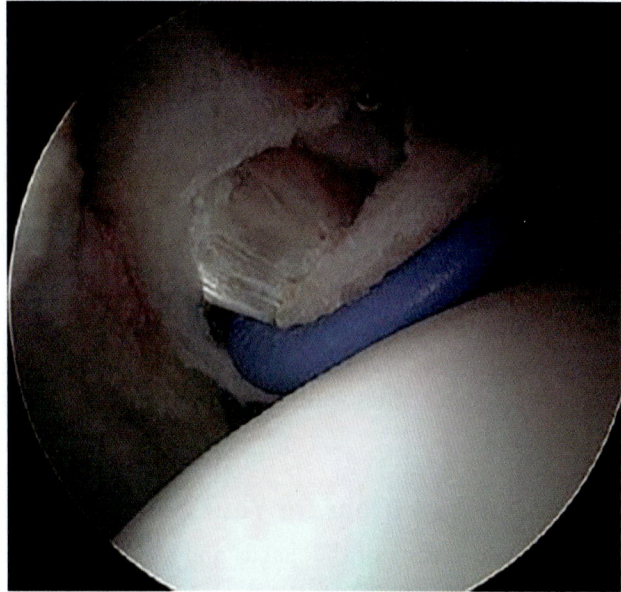

Figure 6 Arthroscopic image showing a capsulotomy being performed to expose the iliopsoas tendon. The blue electrocautery device will be used to release the tendon. (Reproduced with permission from Johnson D: *Operative Arthroscopy,* ed 4. Wolters Kluwer, 2013, Figure 49.1.)

- To expose the iliopsoas tendon, the capsulotomy is then extended anteriorly to the 3-o'clock position on the acetabulum (**Figure 6**).
- The iliopsoas tendon is visualized superficial to the capsule and labrum. The iliopsoas tendon is released using radiofrequency ablation or an elongated surgical blade until its muscular fibers are visualized.[9]
- Once the tendon is released, concomitant pathology can be addressed, such as labral repair, loose body removal, and/or resection of bony cam and pincer abnormalities from FAI.
- Postoperative rehabilitation begins with the patient being partial weight bearing with an assistive device.
  - Range of motion exercises can begin immediately, including hip flexion.

- Progression to full weight bearing and initiation of hip strengthening exercises typically occurs by 4 weeks postoperatively.
- Return to full activity without restrictions can be expected within 1 year of surgery, although many patients are able to return sooner.
- Patients can expect significant functional improvement and pain relief in their hip following surgery.
  - Patients with snapping hip syndrome should have complete resolution of the snapping symptoms.
  - Hip flexion weakness is the most common complication of surgery, although most patients eventually regain their strength.[10]
  - Symptom recurrence is uncommon but can occur, as the iliopsoas tendon regenerates within 2 years of surgical release.

Top 10 Knowledge Drops for Your Rotation

1. The iliopsoas consists of the iliacus and psoas major muscles and is the strongest hip flexor.
2. The iliopsoas tendon is an extracapsular and extra-articular structure that inserts on the lesser trochanter of the femur.
3. Internal snapping hip syndrome occurs when the iliopsoas tendon contacts the iliopectineal eminence of the pelvis.
4. Patient with internal snapping hip syndrome will report pain, popping, or clicking of the hip that is worse with hip flexion.
5. Labral tears and FAI are commonly seen in conjunction with iliopsoas pathology.
6. Dynamic ultrasound examination of the hip can be used to evaluate for a snapping iliopsoas tendon.
7. Nonsurgical treatments for iliopsoas disorders include activity modification, physical therapy, NSAIDs, and an ultrasound-guided corticosteroid injection.
8. Arthroscopic iliopsoas release is indicated for patients in whom 3 to 6 months of nonsurgical treatment failed.
9. The iliopsoas tendon is identified during hip arthroscopy by performing a capsulotomy between the 2-'clock and 3-o'clock positions on the acetabulum.
10. Hip flexion weakness is the most common complication of iliopsoas release.

HAMSTRING INJURIES

Epidemiology

- When diagnosed and managed appropriately, proximal hamstring injuries demonstrate a 95% return to sport and at least an 80% return to preinjury level of play.[11]
  - However, poor outcomes have been associated with extended recovery time and long-term disability in the setting of misdiagnosed and unmanaged injuries in addition to significant reinjury rates.
- Injuries to the proximal hamstring complex account for 12% to 26% of sporting activity–related injuries.[12,13]
  - Given the wide range of injury grades, hamstring injuries constitute varying degrees of overall dysfunction depending on the extent of involvement.[14]
- Occurring most commonly by actions of repetitive and rapid acceleration movements, injuries to the complex occur most commonly via eccentric ipsilateral hip and trunk hyperflexion and knee extension mechanisms;[13] proximal hamstring injuries remain the most common type of injury in professional athletes in general.
  - Sports with the highest incidence rates include American football, track and field, soccer, rugby, waterskiing, and surfing.
  - Skeletal maturity considerations for proximal hamstring injuries include the myotendinous junction being the most commonly injured region in adults, with the pediatric equivalent being ischial tuberosity avulsions.
- Risk factors for proximal hamstring injuries include reduced flexibility, trunk/core dysfunction and poor trunk control, muscle weakness/fatigue, and poor lumbar posture.
  - The most predictive factor for a hamstring injury is a previous hamstring injury.[15]
  - Previous hamstring injury increases the risk of reinjury twofold to sixfold.[16]

Pertinent Anatomy/Pathoanatomy

- The proximal hamstring muscle complex makes up the posterior fascial compartment of the thigh.
  - The origins consist of the long head of the posterior-medial attachment of the biceps femoris long head, the semitendinosus muscle, and the lateral crescent-shaped attachment of the semimembranosus muscle.
  - The tendons originate in the aforementioned order from the inferomedial to superolateral aspect of the ischial tuberosity.
  - The long head of the biceps femoris and semitendinosus origins together make up the conjoined tendon.
- The insertion points in the same respective order include the lateral condyle of the proximal tibia and fibular head just lateral to the styloid process (biceps femoris), the proximal medial tibial shaft (semitendinosus), and the posterior proximal medial tibial condyle (semimembranosus).
- The innervation of all the hamstring muscles except the short head of the biceps femoris is from the tibial branch of the sciatic nerve (L5, S1, S2 nerve roots).
  - The short head of the biceps femoris is innervated by the common peroneal nerve branch of the sciatic nerve (L5, S1, S2 nerve roots).
  - The sciatic nerve courses 1 cm lateral to the biceps femoris as it lies between the hamstring group and the adductor magnus.
  - The arterial supply to the entire muscle group is via the perforating branches of the profunda femoris artery, inferior gluteal artery, and the superior muscular branches of the popliteal artery.
- The pathophysiology of acute hamstring injuries entails combined explosive moments of ipsilateral hip flexion and knee extension moments, as often seen in sprinting and hurdling activity.
  - The myotendinous junction experiences the highest concentration of eccentric loading and is the most frequently injured region.[16]
- Chronic hamstring injuries and proximal hamstring tendinopathy occur progressively over time in the setting of increasing tendinopathy as the result of repetitive low forces yielding localized proximal hamstring attritional environments.[12]
  - An ensuing vicious cycle continues yielding pathologic and weakened scar tissue, which further lowers the threshold for recurrent injury.

- Ischial tuberosity avulsion injuries occur by way of the ischial apophysis, a secondary ossification center that in skeletally immature patients is the weakest element of the muscle-tendon-bone attachment continuum.[17]
  - Younger athletes are most affected, with 95% of the injuries occurring between 13 and 17 years of age.[17]

Pertinent History/Physical Examination Findings

- A comprehensive history of physical examination begins with eliciting the mechanism of injury and time of onset. The aforementioned factors will vary depending on the severity and chronicity of the injury.
  - Patients presenting with acute (partial-thickness and full-thickness) ruptures or avulsions will often recall a specific inciting event. The event is typically accompanied by a sharp stabbing pain and/or an audible pop at the onset of the injury.[15]
  - Patients presenting with chronic, degenerative tendinopathies will often be unable to identify a specific event, but rather report progressive dysfunction and increasing pain from the buttock area extending to the posterior knee with associated weakness and/or cramping with activity.[13,18]
    - Proximal hamstring tendinopathy should be considered in the differential of other overuse-type injuries affecting runners, hurdlers, and jumpers.
    - In addition, clinical suspicion should be heightened when evaluating chronic pathologies in dancers or gymnasts who perform slow-stretching exercises combined with extremes of hip flexion and knee extension.[13]
- Observation is a critical portion of the examination. Specifically, analyzing the patient for antalgic gait patterns, including the stiff-legged gait in which the patient attempts to avoid knee and hip flexion.
  - The patient should be positioned prone on the examination table and documenting for potential ecchymosis as this finding is an indication for injury to the complex.[16]
  - The ischial tuberosity should be palpated to elicit any focal areas of tenderness and/or defects. In the case of retracted ruptures, a palpable defect is present and allows the examiner to focus on the approximate degree of tendon retraction. The examiner should flex the patient's knee in the prone position

and ask the patient to resist forced extension at the knee and the defect (or pain) will be exacerbated. Comparison with the contralateral, uninjured leg can give the examiner an idea of the degree and extent of injury.[16]
- In the setting of proximal hamstring tendinopathy, additional physical examination maneuvers have varying degrees of sensitivity and specificity.
  - Modified bent-knee stretch test (sensitivity: 89%, specificity 91%): The patient is supine with both legs extended. The examiner simultaneously flexes the hip and knee followed by rapid extension of the knee. A positive test is recorded in the setting of reproducing pain in the posterior aspect of the thigh.
  - Original bent-knee stretch test (sensitivity: 84%, specificity 87%): The patient is supine with both legs extended. The hip and knee of the symptomatic extremity are maximally flexed followed by slow, passive extension of the knee. A positive test is recorded in the setting of reproducing pain in the posterior aspect of the thigh.
  - Puranen-Orava test (sensitivity: 76%, specificity 82%): The patient is standing. The hip is flexed to 90° and the knee is then actively extended while supported by a chair or table. A positive test is recorded in the setting of reproducing pain in the posterior aspect of the thigh.

Relevant Imaging

- Radiographic workup in the setting of acute and chronic injuries include an AP pelvis and lateral hip view to rule out avulsion injuries.
  - Although radiographic imaging is not mandatory, these radiographs should be pursued when clinical suspicion is present for an ischial tuberosity avulsion.[18]
- Advanced imaging is also not always warranted but should be strongly considered in cases of a suspected palpable defect and/or in the setting of failure to improve with initial nonsurgical treatment.
  - The modality of choice is MRI, although ultrasonography can also be considered.[15] However, MRI is often preferred given

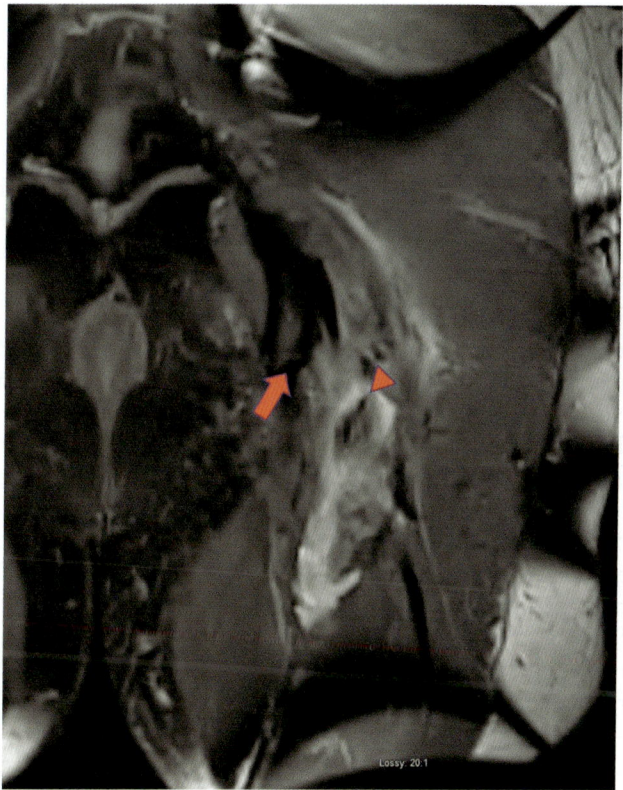

Figure 7 Coronal T2-weighted MRI of the left hip noting approximately 3 cm of retraction of the conjoined biceps femoris/semitendinosus tendon (arrowhead) origin off the posteromedial aspect of the ischial tuberosity (arrow) with associated posttraumatic hematoma in the proximal posterior thigh.

the ability to more accurately differentiate scar tissue from an acute injury.[18]
- High signal intensity can be seen on T2-weighted magnetic resonance images reflecting edema within or around the muscle in acute hamstring injuries[18] (**Figure 7**).
- However, many clinically positive diagnoses of all types of hamstring injuries fail to show any abnormality on MRI.

Nonsurgical Measures

- Nonsurgical treatment is indicated for acute hamstring strains, partial injuries, single-tendon ruptures, two-tendon ruptures with minimal retraction, and injuries in sedentary patients with significant medical comorbidities.
  - Ischial tuberosity avulsions with minimal displacement (ie, <1 cm) can also be managed nonsurgically by avoiding hip flexion and knee extension early with gradual motion progression.
- No consensus exists in the literature regarding an exact algorithm for nonsurgical management.
- The standard rest, ice, compression, and elevation (or RICE) sequence is used to minimize bleeding, swelling, and pain at the site of injury.
  - The initial 48 hours is critical to the healing phase as early immobilization and protected weight bearing may help to protect the injured tissue.[13]
  - NSAIDs are often used but remain controversial regarding their ability to reduce times to return to sport in appropriately managed nonsurgical injuries.[15,18]
  - Physical therapy in the form of graduated phases of rehabilitation and eccentric strengthening exercises should be used to reduce the risk of injury recurrence.[15,18]
- A 2011 randomized controlled clinical study demonstrated findings that shock wave therapy (SWT) is safe, effective, and superior to traditional (ie, NSAIDs and physical therapy alone) protocols alone in treatment professional athletes with proximal hamstring tendinopathy.[19]
  - Although this study yielded prospective level I evidence in favor of SWT for proximal hamstring tendinopathy, a 2017 systematic review of the overall effectiveness of SWT in common lower limb conditions cautioned the external validity and relatively small sample size of the study, and ultimately future studies are needed to elucidate the potential efficacy for SWT as an efficacious nonsurgical treatment modality.[19]
- Platelet-rich plasma has been studied in the setting of acute injuries and chronic proximal hamstring tendinopathy, yielding controversial results with respect to its clinical efficacy.[15]
  - There remains a paucity of high-quality evidence promoting its use in even high-level athletes.[13,18]

- Future recommendations for nonsurgical treatment options may include adding losartan (an angiotensin II receptor blocker) and growth factor injections such as insulinlike growth factor-1 (IGF-1), although clinical evidence supporting their use is limited at this time.[15]

Surgical Intervention

- Indications for primary surgical repair include full-thickness ruptures of all three tendons, a ruptured conjoint tendon with retraction exceeding 2.0 to 2.5 cm, or an ischial tuberosity avulsion with displacement exceeding 1.0 to 1.5 cm.
    - Chronic injuries with persistent pain and dysfunction that remain refractory to nonsurgical modalities for at least 6 months are considered for surgical management.[12]
    - Another key physical examination finding that may warrant surgical consideration earlier in the course of treatment is the presence of sciatic nerve involvement.[15]
- Primary repair (open): Surgical management of multitendon retracted ruptures involves restoration of the native tension and function via reattachment of the tendon to its osseous origin using suture anchors.[13]
    - The patient is placed prone on the surgical table and the hip is flexed at the break of the bed to facilitate exposure.
    - A transverse or vertical incision can be used, based on surgeon preference.
    - The former incision is placed in the ipsilateral gluteal crease and has the option to be extended in a T-like configuration if necessary.
    - Dissection to the underlying subcutaneous tissue leads to the gluteal fascia, which is often intact.
    - A longitudinal incision is made, and the injured hamstring tendons are encountered often in the presence of a hematoma, which is evacuated at the same time.
        - The sciatic nerve is located lateral to the tendons and in the setting of chronic pathologies may be scarred into the retracted tendons.

- Dissection and neurolysis is performed only in the chronic/scarred setting or when the patient presents with consistent debilitating symptoms preoperatively.[16]
  - Care must be taken to protect the laterally coursing sciatic nerve, which is on average 1.2 cm lateral to the most lateral aspect of the ischial tuberosity.
  - This should be noted with careful retractor placement especially before anchor placement.
- The proximal tendon edges should be débrided (not too aggressively) to maximize good tissue to invite a biologically friendly tendon-bone healing environment.
- A periosteal dissector or curet is used to clear off the ischial tuberosity before anchor placement.
- A variety of different suture anchor configurations have been described and depend on the number of tendons and total footprint compromised.
  - An X configuration is often used for anchor placement and sutures can be tied in a simple mattress configuration working from distal to proximal (**Figure 8**).
  - The knee is gently flexed during knot tying.
- This is followed by irrigation and a layered closure.
- Primary repair (endoscopic).
  - Various portals have been described but typically a three-portal technique is often used with a direct posterior portal and posterolateral portal (both in the gluteal fold), in addition to a proximal posterolateral portal (anchor placement portal).
  - A spinal needle is used under fluoroscopic guidance to localize the ischial tuberosity.
  - A 1-cm incision is used in line with the gluteal fold and a cannula is introduced.
  - The arthroscope is introduced through the posterolateral portal.
  - The subsequent portals are made under direct and fluoroscopic visualization.
  - The shaver is introduced into the hamstring bursa from the direct posterior portal.
  - The subgluteal bursectomy is performed and care is taken during the entire time to identify and visualize the sciatic nerve.

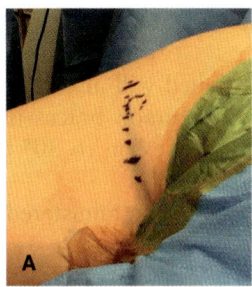
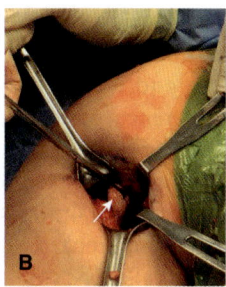
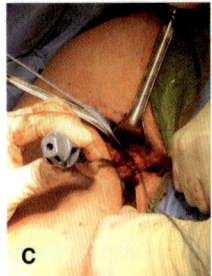
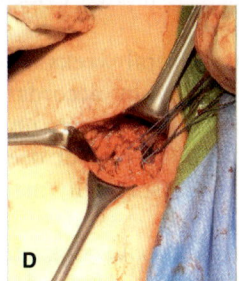
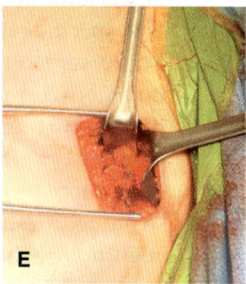

Figure 8 Intraoperative image sequence of proximal hamstring repair. A transverse incision is planned in the gluteal crease (**A**) with the patient prepped and draped in the prone position. Dissection down through the gluteal fascia leads to identification and exposure of the retracted proximal hamstring avulsion (**B**, arrow). The ischial tuberosity is prepped by debriding the bone at the native footprint and sequential anchors (**C**) are inserted. In this scenario the "X" configuration is used (**D**), and mattress configuration is used for the repair while tying down in distal to proximal fashion, yielding the final repair with all sutures tied and the native tendon reattached to the bone under physiologic tension (**E**).

- The osseous origin is débrided and anchors are placed in the same spacing fashion as in the open procedure.
- Mattress stitches are then passed through the tendon arthroscopically and the tendon is tensioned and repaired down to its anatomic osseous footprint under direct visualization.
- The portal sites are then closed in standard fashion.
- Postoperative weight-bearing status will vary depending on surgeon preference, although most protocols involve a period of

non–weight bearing or toe-touch weight bearing with crutches for ambulation.
- Brace use and type of brace applied will also depend on surgeon preference with the most common braces used include either a hip brace set to limit hip flexion to 30° to 40° or a hinged knee brace flexed to 40° to 50°.
- Postoperative oral antibiotics may be administered depending on surgeon preference.
- Postoperative deep vein thrombosis prophylaxis is recommended although there is limited evidence suggesting a consensus specific regimen.
  - Many surgeons use several weeks of aspirin for deep vein thrombosis prophylaxis in accordance with progressive weight-bearing status and return to normal mobility. A 2019 case series noted a 6.9% rate of deep vein thrombosis in both surgically and nonsurgically managed proximal hamstring injuries.
- Although both acute and chronic complete repairs improve following surgical repair, limited evidence does support that repair in the acute (within 2 months) setting demonstrates superior outcomes (patient satisfaction and pain scores) compared with chronic (>2 months) complete tears undergoing surgical repair.[20]
- Complications following surgical repair including posterior thigh numbness, postoperative hematoma, delayed wound healing (may be an issue given the location of the incision in the buttock region), sciatic nerve neurapraxia, and continued pain, especially with sitting, and/or persistent weakness when compared with the contralateral uninjured limb.
  - The most predictive risk factor for recurrent injury is a previous hamstring injury.[13]
- Acute proximal hamstring injuries with multitendon retracted ruptures and refractory proximal hamstring tendinopathies favor surgical management compared with nonsurgical treatment regimens.
  - Refractory conditions consists of patients continuing to demonstrate debilitating symptoms after 6 months of nonsurgical management in cohorts of patients with proximal hamstring tendinopathy.
  - A 2018 meta-analysis reported superior outcomes in favor of proximal hamstring avulsion repair compared with nonsurgical

treatment. The authors noted superior outcome scores favoring surgical repair in the elements of patient satisfaction rates (90.81% versus 52.94%), hamstring strength (85.01% versus 63.95%), and better Lower Extremity Functional Scale and single-legged hop test scores.[20]

Top 10 Knowledge Drops for Your Rotation

1. The proximal hamstring complex consists of the origins of the long head of the biceps femoris and semitendinosus muscles (together the conjoined tendon) as well as the lateral crescent-shaped semimembranosus attachment.
2. Proximal hamstring injury spectrum ranges from partial-thickness to full-thickness tears and multitendon retracted ruptures.
3. Acute hamstring injury history-taking pearls include an inciting event, explosive ipsilateral hip flexion/knee extension moment, stabbing pain, and audible or palpable pop.
4. Chronic hamstring tendinopathy history-taking pearls include a gradual onset of dysfunction, pain with sitting, posterior thigh to knee pain, and cramping with activity.
5. Goals of primary physical therapy rehabilitation programs are focused on optimizing function and return to sport in addition to reducing the risk of recurrent injury.
6. Partial-thickness and proximal hamstring tendinopathy often improve with nonsurgical treatment alone.
7. When nonsurgical management for appropriate pathologies has failed to improve function in 6 months, surgical intervention may be required to improve function/outcomes.
8. Limited evidence suggests improved patient satisfaction and pain scores comparing acute versus chronic repairs for complete proximal hamstring ruptures.
9. Although primary open repair remains the gold standard for treatment, emerging evidence demonstrates comparable outcomes when performed by a surgeon experienced in the technique.
10. Misdiagnosis and mismanagement of proximal hamstring ruptures yield poor outcomes.

GLUTEAL INJURIES

Epidemiology

- Given the broad clinical definitions, descriptions, and classifications used throughout the literature, the true prevalence of gluteus medius/minimus tears (GMTs) and hip abductor lesions/tendinopathy cannot be accurately estimated at this time.[21,22]
  - There is ambiguity, at least in part, because GMTs is often encompassed under the umbrella term of greater trochanteric pain syndrome (GTPS).
    - GTPS has a reported incidence rate of 1.8 per 1,000 person-years and a peak prevalence in females between the ages of 30 and 60 years.[23]
    - GMT as a distinct subset pathology is increasingly recognized as a relatively common condition in the middle-aged population and both partial and complete tears can be found in up to 20% to 25% of patients older than 50 years.[24]
- GMTs generally occur in one of four groups of patient subgroups.
  - Group 1 consists of those presenting with chronic localized lateral hip pain and MRI evidence of at least partial tears/tendinopathy without previous hip surgery.
  - Group 2 encompasses those with incidental tears at the time of hip surgery[24] (or incidentally found on MRI while working up other pathologies).
  - Group 3 includes those patients presenting on the GMT spectrum following hip reconstruction and arthroplasty procedures.
  - Group 4 occurs much less commonly via acute traumatic avulsions.

Pertinent Anatomy/Pathoanatomy

- The hip abductor complex consists of the gluteus medius, gluteus minimus, and the tensor fascia latae (TFL).
  - The gluteus minimus is deep to gluteus medius in all planes and originates along the ilium (middle gluteal line) and inserts on the anterior aspect of the greater trochanter.
  - The gluteus medius originates along the ilium and inserts via two separate insertion points (lateral and posterosuperior facets) along the greater trochanter. It is described as having at least two parts—an anterolateral portion and a longer and thicker, fan-shaped posterior portion.

- The anterolateral portion inserts on a separate lateral facet and the posterior portion inserts via the posterosuperior facet.
- The TFL originates along the iliac crest and courses distally by way of tendinous fibers joining the middle longitudinal layer of the fascia lata and eventually transitioning to the ITB, which inserts distally at the Gerdy tubercle.
- All three muscles are innervated by the superior gluteal nerve (L4, L5, S1 nerve roots), and arterial supply is from the superior gluteal artery.
- The pathophysiology of acute injuries is much rarer than chronic progressive tendinopathy and partial-thickness to full-thickness tear conversions over time.
  - Acute injuries can compromise part of the hip abductor complex, which results in larger tears that become more symptomatic as pain and weakness ensues.
  - Much more commonly, the hip abductor complex undergoes the same degenerative pathway that affects other tendons (eg, the rotator cuff) throughout the body in the form of collagen degeneration, fibroblastic and vascular proliferation, and dystrophic calcification.
    - The pathologic cascade has not been as popularly studied in the literature but has been confirmed and is documented in biopsy studies in patients undergoing hip abductor complex repair.
    - Moreover, mechanical stresses on the tendons, combined with pathologic tension and compression from adjacent anatomic structures (ie, the ITB/TFL), produce shear and frictional forces that may lead to tendinopathy.[25]

Pertinent History/Physical Examination Findings

- Acute injuries have been reported to occur with overly aggressive activities of daily living or sporting activity (eg, golfing), and full-thickness ruptures rarely occur outside of major trauma given the extensile and robust nature of the hip abductor complex.
  - Rather, multiple inciting events within a few days may lead the patient to assume a simple muscle strain, and clinical care is typically not sought until gait and compromised weight bearing occurs.

- Patient-reported symptoms pointing to chronic progressive gluteal tendinopathies include pain at night (especially when laying on the affected side), difficulty with any activities of daily living involving hip abductor motor function (ie, walking and stair climbing, recreational sports), and localized pain to the lateral aspect of the proximal thigh.
  - Patients report progressively decreasing quality of life measures that have been documented to be similar to or even worse than symptoms from end-stage hip osteoarthritis.
- Physical examination findings are fairly reproducible in this setting and include focal tenderness to palpation over the greater trochanter in addition to weakness in hip abduction and/or hip flexion muscles.
  - The patient is positioned on the contralateral side with the hip in 0° of extension and 20° of internal rotation to neutralize the abductor function of the TFL.[26] Range of motion of the hip should be documented and in isolated cases of tendinopathy should not be compromised.[21]
  - The patient is asked to ambulate, and the examiner may notice a slight or moderate limp plus or minus a Trendelenburg sign, which is positive when the patient stands on the contralateral (uninjured limb) with some support, and the symptomatic side/pelvis is noted to drop secondary to hip abductor muscle insufficiency.[21] Trendelenburg gait ensues in cases of severe hip abductor complex weakness.[26]

Relevant Imaging

- Radiographic imaging is obtained to evaluate for arthritic changes or osseous injuries about the hip and can also elucidate evidence of calcific tendinopathy (**Figure 9**) in the surrounding periarticular soft-tissue structures.
- MRI remains the best available option in diagnosing GMTs or other sources of GTPS (eg, trochanteric bursitis) and demonstrates approximately 95% specificity and 73% sensitivity level[23] (**Figure 10**).
  - The prevalence of asymptomatic GMTs is low.
  - Key diagnostic workup elements include the appropriate threshold for obtaining an MRI of the hip in patients who present with concern for an acute full-thickness avulsion or in

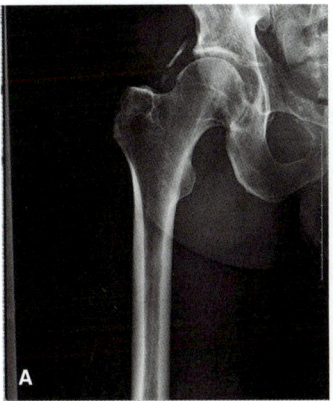
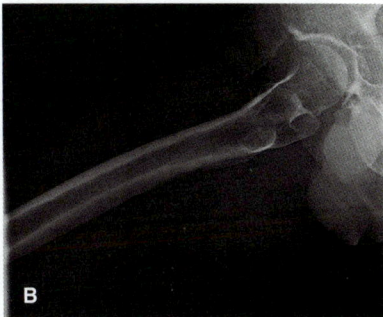

Figure 9 Right hip radiographic series demonstrating AP (**A**) and lateral (**B**) evidence of gluteal calcific tendinopathy in a patient with chronic, localized, progressive lateral hip pain.

the setting of chronic progressive tendinopathy and GMT that is refractory to initial nonsurgical treatment modalities.

Nonsurgical Measures

- Nonsurgical treatment is first line except in the setting of acute avulsions with significant weakness, Trendelenburg gait, and/or an inability to ambulate altogether, in which case early repair is advocated on MRI confirmation of the diagnosis.
- Nonsurgical measures include NSAIDs, rest/activity modification, ice, and physical therapy.
  - These modalities are successful when applied appropriately.[23]
  - Activity modification should advocate for avoiding repetitive hip abduction activities and especially avoiding sleeping on the affected side.
- Additional nonsurgical options include corticosteroid injections and extracorporeal shock wave therapy (ESWT).

Surgical Intervention

- Primary open repair
  - The patient is placed in the lateral decubitus position with the injured hip prominent.

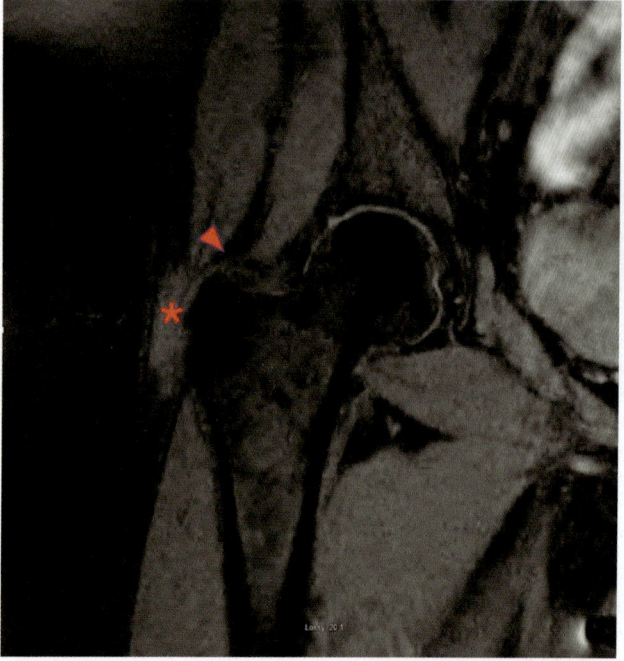

Figure 10 Right hip T2-weighted MRI sequence revealing trochanteric bursitis (asterisk) in the setting of a normal gluteal/hip abductor insertion complex (arrowhead).

- All bony prominences are well padded and an axillary roll is placed approximately at the level of the nipple.[27]
- The incision is made centered over the greater trochanter and dissection is through the subcutaneous tissue down to the level of the fascia lata.
- Longitudinal incision is commenced through the fascia, and the underlying trochanteric bursa is removed.
- The tear is identified, the tendinous edges are prepared, and the osseous footprint is débrided to stimulate an ideal biologically friendly tendon-bone healing interface.
- Suture anchors are placed at the footprint and mattress configuration stitches are passed into the torn abductor complex and the tendon is tensioned and repaired down either with knot-tying or in a knotless configuration (**Figure 11**).

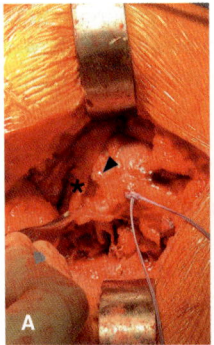 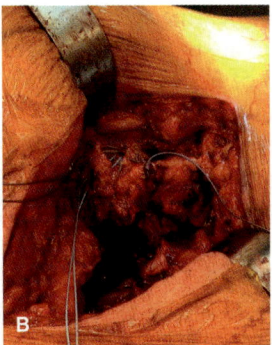 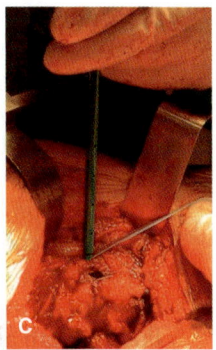

Figure 11 Intraoperative images demonstrating a full-thickness gluteus medius tear (**A**) with full-thickness retraction (asterisk) off the native footprint on the greater trochanter (arrowhead). The open technique is used to repair with knotless suture anchors in double-row fashion (**B** and **C**).

- Single-row and double-row repair techniques have been described, and a layered closure is performed after the site is irrigated.[21]
- Primary endoscopic repair: A combination of portals is used (often four).[28]
  - The same patient positioning is used for the endoscopic procedure.
  - A proximal direct lateral portal and distal direct lateral portal are made along the long axis of the femur, approximately 6 cm proximally and distally from the center point of the greater trochanter, and an anterolateral portal and posterolateral portal are made along a cross-sectional line approximately parallel with the vastus ridge through the gluteal footprint.[24]
  - Saline is injected first to insufflate the deep peritrochanteric space.
  - After the portals are established under direct visualization, a greater trochanteric bursectomy is performed and the gluteus medius and minimus tendons are identified and the injury pattern is assessed.
    - Rotation of the extremity is used to facilitate the examination of the tear footprint area.
  - After the tendinous edges are débrided and the osseous footprint burred to improve tendon-bone healing, suture anchors are placed and the tendon is tensioned and repaired back down to bone using single-row, double-row, or transosseous repair techniques.[28,29]
  - The portal sites are closed, and soft dressing is applied.

- Postoperative weight-bearing status and graduated progression is dictated by the surgeon-specific protocol but typically involves a 6- to 8-week period of non–weight-bearing or toe-touch weight-bearing restrictions with crutch use.[29]
  - Immediate full weight-bearing protocols with assistive devices have also been described.[28]
  - An abduction brace may be applied[29] but is not uniformly used across surgeon protocols.
  - In the setting of no brace use postoperatively, patients are educated on maintaining a level pelvis during gait.[28]
  - Full strength and activity is to be expected by approximately 3 to 4 months postoperatively.[29]
  - Postoperative oral antibiotics may also be prescribed, and venous thromboembolic event prophylaxis is surgeon dependent as studies are currently lacking.
    - Surgeons may prescribe aspirin for multiple weeks with consideration of the patient's gradual progression and return of full mobility.
- Results following open and endoscopic repair demonstrate a very low complication rate, and available studies note very low/negligible retear rates.
  - The most common pitfalls noted to be persistent pain, continued weakness, and failure to normalize gait/function postoperatively.
  - In the setting of advanced tendinopathy, massive tears, and revision surgery, human dermal allograft and other augmentation implants/scaffolds are considered as well.[27]
- Open and endoscopic repairs are both used and demonstrate encouraging results.
  - Kirby et al recently reported 2-year results following endoscopic repair of gluteus medius tendon tear repairs using knotless suture anchors and 90% of patients reported improved modified Harris hip scores and nonarthritic hip scores with 90% of patients noting continued improvement.[30]
  - Similar results have been reported in terms of outcomes following endoscopic repair of partial-thickness abductor tendon tear repairs and full-thickness gluteus medius and minimus endoscopic repairs at 2-year follow-up.[28,29]

Top 10 Knowledge Drops for Your Rotation

1. The hip abductor complex consists of the gluteus medius and gluteus minimus tendons in addition to the tensor fascia latae.
2. GTPS is an umbrella term encompassing trochanteric bursitis, gluteus medius/minimus partial-thickness or full-thickness tears (GMTs), and external snapping hip conditions.
3. GMTs are considered a separate subset of GTPS and most commonly affect patients older than 50 years.
4. GMTs can be found incidentally (at the time of hip surgery or following MRI during diagnostic-related workup for other conditions) or present acutely versus chronically in the setting of traumatic injury or localized pain with progressive dysfunction, respectively.
5. Acute injuries can rarely occur by way of overly aggressive activities of daily living or sporting activity (eg, golfing) and major, high-energy trauma.
6. Chronic injuries present much more commonly in the setting of increasing lateral hip pain, weakness, gait impairment, and pain at night.
7. Physical examination pearls include observation for ecchymosis, gait analysis (antalgic, Trendelenburg, or normal), and reproducible lateral hip pain plus or minus hip abductor weakness.
8. MRI is the preferred diagnostic modality and is considered in the acute setting with abrupt onset of weakness/inability to ambulate and in the event of chronic refractory episodes following nonsurgical treatment periods.
9. Nonsurgical modalities are first-line treatment (except in acute traumatic avulsions with gait dysfunction) and include physical therapy, activity modification, NSAIDs, cortisone injection, and possibly extracorporeal shockwave therapy.
10. Outcomes of open and endoscopic repairs of GMTs are encouraging with more long-term studies being needed; current studies yield promising results at 2-year follow-up in limited case series.

References

1. Clohisy JC, Baca G, Beaulé PE, et al: Descriptive epidemiology of femoroacetabular impingement: A North American cohort of patients undergoing surgery. *Am J Sports Med* 2013;41(6):1348-1356.
2. Pacheco-Carrillo A, Medina-Porqueres I: Physical examination tests for the diagnosis of femoroacetabular impingement. A systematic review. *Phys Ther Sport* 2016;21:87-93.
3. Geeslin AG, Geeslin MG, Chahla J, Mannava S, Frangiamore S, Philippon MJ: Comprehensive clinical evaluation of femoroacetabular impingement: Part 3, magnetic resonance imaging. *Arthrosc Tech* 2017;6(5):e2011-e2018.
4. Dwyer T, Whelan D, Shah PS, Ajrawat P, Hoit G, Chahal J: Operative versus nonoperative treatment of femoroacetabular impingement syndrome: A meta-analysis of short-term outcomes. *Arthroscopy* 2020;36(1):263-273.
5. Pennock AT, Bomar JD, Johnson KP, Randich K, Upasani VV: Nonoperative management of femoroacetabular impingement: A prospective study. *Am J Sports Med* 2018;46(14):3415-3422.
6. Minkara AA, Westermann RW, Rosneck J, Lynch TS: Systematic review and meta-analysis of outcomes after hip arthroscopy in femoroacetabular impingement. *Am J Sports Med* 2019;47(2):488-500.
7. Serner A, Tol JL, Jomaah N, et al: Diagnosis of acute groin injuries: A prospective study of 110 athletes. *Am J Sports Med* 2015;43(8):1857-1864.
8. Piechota M, Maczuch J, Skupiński J, Kukawska-Sysio K, Wawrzynek W: Internal snapping hip syndrome in dynamic ultrasonography. *J Ultrason* 2016;16(66):296-303.
9. Anderson CN: Iliopsoas: Pathology, diagnosis, and treatment. *Clin Sports Med* 2016;35(3):419-433.
10. Gouveia K, Shah A, Kay J, et al: Iliopsoas tenotomy during hip arthroscopy: A systematic review of postoperative outcomes. *Am J Sports Med* 2020;49(3):817-829.
11. Shambaugh BC, Olsen JR, Lacerte E, Kellum E, Miller SL: A comparison of nonoperative and operative treatment of complete proximal hamstring ruptures. *Orthop J Sports Med* 2017;5(11):2325967117738551.
12. Kayani B, Ayuob A, Begum F, Khan N, Haddad FS: Surgical management of chronic incomplete proximal hamstring avulsion injuries. *Am J Sports Med* 2020;48(5):1160-1167.
13. Chang JS, Kayani B, Plastow R, Singh S, Magan A, Haddad FS: Management of hamstring injuries: Current concepts review. *Bone Joint J* 2020;102-B(10):1281-1288.

14. Arner JW, Freiman H, Mauro CS, Bradley JP: Functional results and outcomes after repair of partial proximal hamstring avulsions at midterm follow-up. *Am J Sports Med* 2019;47(14):3436-3443.
15. Heer ST, Callander JW, Kraeutler MJ, Mei-Dan O, Mulcahey MK: Hamstring injuries: Risk factors, treatment, and rehabilitation. *J Bone Joint Surg Am* 2019;101(9):843-853.
16. Ahmad CS, Redler LH, Ciccotti MG, Maffulli N, Longo UG, Bradley J: Evaluation and management of hamstring injuries. *Am J Sports Med* 2013;41(12):2933-2947.
17. Eberbach H, Hohloch L, Feucht MJ, Konstantinidis L, Sudkamp NP, Zwingmann J: Operative versus conservative treatment of apophyseal avulsion fractures of the pelvis in the adolescents: A systematical review with meta-analysis of clinical outcome and return to sports. *BMC Musculoskelet Disord* 2017;18(1):162.
18. Chu SK, Rho ME: hamstring injuries in the athlete: Diagnosis, treatment, and return to play. *Curr Sports Med Rep* 2016;15(3):184-190.
19. Korakakis V, Whiteley R, Tzavara A, Malliaropoulos N: The effectiveness of extracorporeal shockwave therapy in common lower limb conditions: A systematic review including quantification of patient-rated pain reduction. *Br J Sports Med* 2018;52(6):387-407.
20. Bodendorfer BM, Curley AJ, Kotler JA, et al: Outcomes after operative and nonoperative treatment of proximal hamstring avulsions: A systematic review and meta-analysis. *Am J Sports Med* 2018;46(11): 2798-2808.
21. Kenanidis E, Kyriakopoulos G, Kaila R, Christofilopoulos P: Lesions of the abductors in the hip. *EFORT Open Rev* 2020;5(8):464-476.
22. Redmond JM, Chen AW, Domb BG: Greater trochanteric pain syndrome. *J Am Acad Orthop Surg* 2016;24(4):231-240.
23. Pierce TP, Issa K, Kurowicki J, Festa A, McInerney VK, Scillia AJ: Abductor tendon tears of the hip. *JBJS Rev* 2018;6(3):e6.
24. Zhu MF, Musson DS, Cornish J, Young SW, Munro JT: Hip abductor tendon tears: Where are we now? *Hip Int* 2020;30(5):500-512.
25. Grimaldi A, Mellor R, Hodges P, Bennell K, Wajswelner H, Vicenzino B: Gluteal tendinopathy: A review of mechanisms, assessment and management. *Sports Med* 2015;45(8):1107-1119.
26. Rosinsky PJ, Diulus SC, Walsh JP, et al: Development of a predictive algorithm for symptomatic hip abductor tears in patients undergoing primary hip arthroscopy. *Am J Sports Med* 2021;49(2):497-504.
27. Pascual-Garrido C, Schwabe MT, Chahla J, Haneda M: Surgical treatment of gluteus medius tears augmented with allograft human dermis. *Arthrosc Tech* 2019;8(11):e1379-e1387.

28. Nazal MR, Abraham PF, Conaway WK, et al: Endoscopic repair of full-thickness gluteus medius and minimus tears-prospective study with a minimum 2-year follow-up. *Arthroscopy* 2020;36(8):2160-2169.
29. Hartigan DE, Perets I, Ho SW, Walsh JP, Yuen LC, Domb BG: Endoscopic repair of partial-thickness undersurface tears of the abductor tendon: Clinical outcomes with minimum 2-year follow-up. *Arthroscopy* 2018;34(4):1193-1199.
30. Kirby D, Fried JW, Bloom DA, Buchalter D, Youm T: Clinical outcomes after endoscopic repair of gluteus medius tendon tear using a knotless technique with a 2-year minimum follow-up. *Arthroscopy* 2020;36(11):2849-2855.

9

My Knee Hurts

Joseph D. Lamplot, MD
Robert H. Brophy, MD, FAAOS

Introduction

Knee pain is one of the most common complaints among patients in orthopaedic clinics. Pain may result from acute trauma or from chronic degeneration of structures including the articular cartilage or meniscus. Pathologies that are frequently encountered include patellofemoral pain, meniscal tears, and ligament injuries. A thorough history and physical examination is essential in determining the etiology of the patient's symptoms and guiding treatment. Treatment options vary depending on the pathology as well as patient-specific factors and range from nonsurgical management including activity modification, bracing, and injections to surgical management, which can include débridement, repair, reconstruction, or replacement.

PATELLOFEMORAL PAIN

Patellofemoral pain (PFP), a term that encompasses a variety of pathologies involving the patellofemoral joint, is the most common chief complaint associated with the knee and typically presents as anterior knee pain. PFP is not a diagnosis in itself, because it may

---

Dr. Lamplot or an immediate family member serves as a paid consultant to or is an employee of DePuy, a Johnson & Johnson Company and has received research or institutional support from Arthrex, Inc. Dr. Brophy or an immediate family member serves as a board member, owner, officer, or committee member of the American Academy of Orthopaedic Surgeons, the American Orthopaedic Association, and the American Orthopaedic Society for Sports Medicine.

result from a variety of etiologies. Atraumatic etiologies for PFP include lateral patellar compression syndrome, chondral softening (chondromalacia patella), and patellofemoral arthritis. Traumatic etiologies include patellar instability (subluxation or dislocation), fracture, patellar or quadriceps tendinitis, and cartilage injuries of the patella or trochlea. A thorough history and physical examination is essential to determine the underlying etiology of PFP. Although an initial course of nonsurgical management is warranted in most cases of PFP, determining the cause of the patient's symptoms is essential to formulate an appropriate treatment plan. Advanced imaging studies, typically MRI, can be helpful in making a diagnosis.

Epidemiology

- PFP is the most common knee problem of patients presenting to orthopaedic clinics.
- Lateral patellar compression syndrome occurs secondary to muscular imbalance (ie, vastus medialis oblique [VMO] weakness) and causes patellar maltracking and/or tilt.
  - Most common etiology of PFP, most often affecting adolescent females
- Patellofemoral arthritis is another common cause of anterior knee pain, most commonly affecting older patients.
- Chondromalacia patella (softening of the articular cartilage of the patella) occurs in younger patients and may progress to patellofemoral arthritis.
- Acute chondral injuries are most common in young patients in the setting of patellar dislocations.
  - Commonly affect the medial facet of the patella and lateral aspect of the trochlea
- Chronic chondral lesions most frequently occur secondary to overload and are typically found in female patients age 30 to 50 years.

Pertinent Anatomy/Pathoanatomy

- Relevant bony anatomy: tibial tubercle, femoral trochlea, and patella
- Patella: Composed of smaller medial facet, larger lateral facet, and odd (distal) facet; only medial and lateral facets covered in articular cartilage

- Trochlear groove: Located at the anterior aspect of the distal femur; functions as bony constraint underlying patellofemoral stability
  - A shallow trochlear groove seen in the setting of trochlear dysplasia and associated with patellar instability
- Medial patellofemoral ligament (MPFL): Provides static stability to the patella
  - Originates posterior and proximal to the medial epicondyle at Schottle point (**Figure 1**)
  - Functions as the primary constraint to lateral patellar translation from 0° to 20° of knee flexion
- Medial and lateral retinacula: Provide static stability to the patellofemoral joint
- Dynamic stability to the patellofemoral joint conferred primarily by the VMO, which is a medial restraint to lateral translation
  - Other relevant structures: Patellar tendon and distal quadriceps tendon
- Blood supply: From the geniculate arteries

Pertinent History/Physical Examination Findings

- History: Thorough history including any injury or trauma related to the onset of anterior knee pain
  - History of instability (dislocation or subluxation)
  - Radicular or hip symptoms: Rule out the lumbar spine or hip as an etiology
  - Effusion or swelling: May suggest intra-articular pathology such as a chondral injury
  - Crepitus and mechanical symptoms: May suggest chondral pathology or arthritis
  - Exacerbating activities such as squatting, ascending, descending stairs
  - Any previous treatments and surgeries
    - If previous physical therapy: Exercises and modalities, frequency and duration of therapy, and patient's compliance
- Physical examination
  - Standing alignment and gait
    - Valgus alignment: Higher risk of patellar instability and lateral facet overload
    - A double leg and single leg squat: may demonstrate dynamic valgus collapse, suggesting VMO and/or gluteal insufficiency

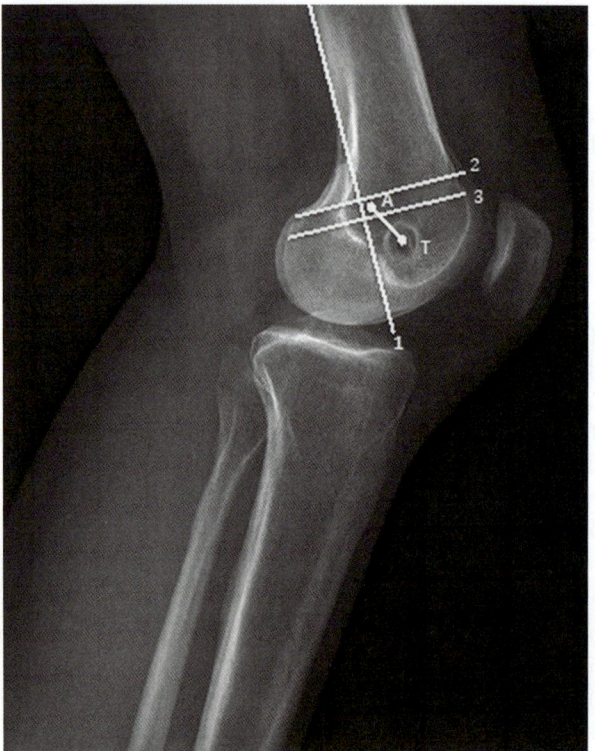

Figure 1 Lateral radiograph used to assess medial patellofemoral ligament femoral tunnel accuracy relative to Schottle point in a patient with a malpositioned femoral tunnel. Line 1 represents the posterior border of the cortex of the femur. Line 2 represents the superior border of the medial femoral condyle perpendicular to line 1. Line 3 represents the superior border of the notch parallel to line 2. Schottle point (A) is centered 1.3 mm anterior to line 1 and midway between lines 2 and 3. The center of the femoral tunnel (T). Distance from A to T in millimeters can be used to determine tunnel accuracy relative to Schottle point. (Reproduced with permission from Parikh SN: *Patellar Instability: Management Principles and Operative Techniques*, ed 1. Wolters Kluwer, 2019, Figure 38.1.)

- The patient should be asked to identify the location of maximal pain, which is particularly helpful in patients with anterior knee pain
    - Focal pain at the proximal pole near the quadriceps tendon insertion or distal pole at the patellar tendon origin may suggest overuse or tendinopathy.

- Seated examination
  - Active knee extension and flexion with the examiner's hand over the patella
    - Patellar tracking and crepitus
    - J sign or lateral maltracking of the patella as the knee moves into extension out of the bony restraints of the trochlea
  - Resisted quadriceps strength testing: Compare with contralateral side
- Supine examination
  - Hip range of motion: Identify any pain with range of motion
  - Femoral anteversion
    - Craig test (prone or supine): Palpate patient's greater trochanter and passively internally rotate hip until its most prominent aspect is at its most lateral position
  - Passive straight leg raise to assess for radicular symptoms
    - Ask patient to contract the bilateral quadriceps; then compare the muscle bulk
  - Active straight leg raise to identify presence of a lag in extensor mechanism
  - Palpate the proximal, distal, medial, and lateral aspects of the patella
  - Place posteriorly directed pressure on the patella and ask the patient to contract the quadriceps, assessing for pain (patellar compression test)
  - Assess patellar tilt and the correctability of tilt
    - With the knee in full extension, place index finger and thumb around patella and determine if there is lateral tilt. If so, assess whether this can be corrected to neutral tilt within the trochlear groove.
  - Apply lateral-directed force to the medial border of the patella to assess the amount of lateral patellar translation and for patellar apprehension
    - Normal motion: less than two quadrants of patellar translation
  - If patellar instability is present, palpate medial border of the patella and medial epicondyle, assessing for tenderness and injury to the MPFL.

- Palpate iliotibial band insertion on Gerdy tubercle and its course along the lateral femur; iliotibial band syndrome can cause anterolateral knee pain.
- Determine Beighton score to assess for generalized ligamentous laxity.
- Palpate medial and lateral infrapatellar tendon spaces: focal pain can indicate symptomatic fat pad impingement.
- Synovial bands, or plica, may be located anteromedial, anterolateral, superomedial, or superolateral, and can cause symptomatic mechanical symptoms during knee motion; these areas can sometimes be palpated or may lie deep to muscle.

Relevant Imaging

- Radiographs
  - Standardized knee radiographs: weight-bearing AP, PA Rosenberg (45°), lateral, and Merchant (or sunrise) axial radiographs
    - Axial view to assess depth of the trochlea, lateral subluxation, and tilt
    - Lateral view to evaluate trochlear morphology using criteria established by Dejour[1]
      - Also to assess for patella alta or patella baja; most often calculated using the Caton-Deschamps ratio (**Figure 2**)
    - Axial and lateral views to assess for patellofemoral joint space narrowing
- Advanced imaging: Consider whether thorough history, physical examination, standardized radiographs fail to confirm a diagnosis.
  - MRI sensitive to the presence of pathology that may be incidental and either noncontributory or minimally contributory to the patient's symptoms
    - May be obtained in the setting of patellar dislocations to assess for intra-articular loose chondral or osteochondral fragments, to assess the chondral surfaces of the patella and trochlea, and to assess other intra-articular structures, including the condyles and menisci

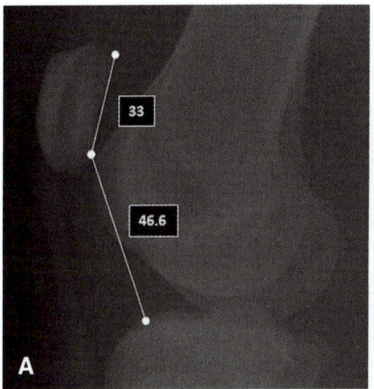 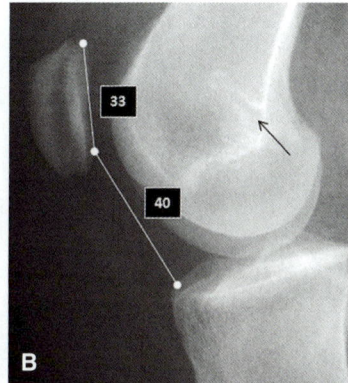

Figure 2 Patellar height measured on lateral radiograph. **A**, The preoperative Caton-Deschamps index measured 46.6/33 = 1.41. **B**, After isolated medial patellofemoral ligament (MPFL) reconstruction, the patellar height decreased to 40/33 = 1.21. The MPFL femoral tunnel is marked (black arrow). (Courtesy of Shital N. Parikh, MD, FACS.)

- Presence of an effusion often suggests an intra-articular injury; MRI should be considered in this setting because plain radiographs cannot reliably establish a diagnosis
  - Effusion with associated anterior knee pain may occur secondary to chondral injury, osteochondral injury, a loose body, or arthritis; MRI can confirm diagnosis and guide treatment.
- MRI can be used to calculate patellar indices, including the Caton-Deschamps ratio.
  - Also can be used to calculate the tibial tubercle–trochlear groove (TT-TG) distance, a measure of tibial tubercle lateralization that is associated with recurrent patellar instability[2]
    - TT-TG distance has been shown to be underestimated when measured on MRI compared with CT
- CT may be considered to assess femoral anteversion (hip to knee CT), because excessive femoral anteversion can contribute to patellar instability.
  - Can be used in a similar manner as MRI to determine the TT-TG distance (**Figure 3**)

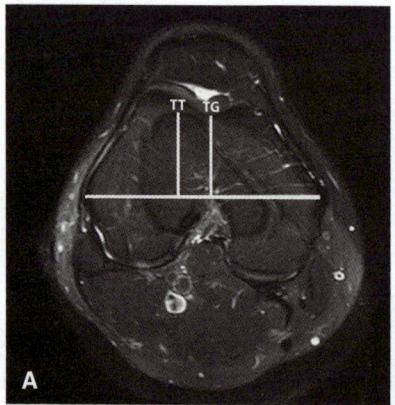

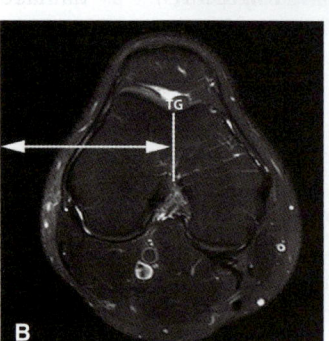
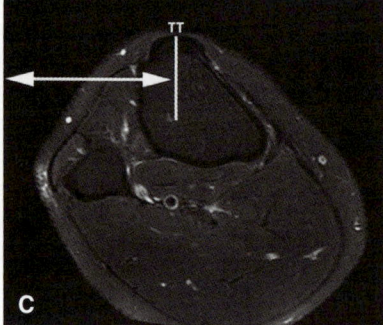

Figure 3 Measurement of tibial tubercle–trochlear groove (TT-TG) distance on MRI. **A**, Superimposed axial images of the tibia and femur showing TT-TG distance. **B** and **C**, Alternative method of determining TT-TG distance by measuring from the edge of the image (or other common landmark) and subtracting. Simple geometry may be used to correct for rotation of the limb but usually is unnecessary. (Reproduced with permission from Chew FS: *Musculoskeletal Imaging: The Essentials*. Wolters Kluwer, 2018, Figure 21.19.)

Nonsurgical Measures

- Initial treatment for most causes of anterior knee pain and should be tailored to the specific diagnosis
- NSAIDs may help with pain relief, but the most common causes of PFP are not inflammatory.

- Physical therapy with a focus on VMO, hip, and core strengthening as well as improving squat mechanics
  - A home program should be performed daily.
- A patellar cutout brace helpful in the setting of patellar maltracking
  - Compression sleeves without a patellar cutout may exacerbate symptoms; generally avoid in this setting.
- Patellar taping: to improve patellar tilt or subluxation

Surgical Intervention

- Indications depend on specific cause
- Patients with loose chondral or osteochondral fragments, which may occur in the setting of a patellar dislocation: knee arthroscopy generally indicated, as the loose fragment(s) may damage healthy surrounding articular cartilage surfaces.
  - If osteochondral fragment is sufficiently large with enough attached bone to potentially heal, fixation may be attempted with a headless compression screw.
- Skeletally immature patients: Fixation of chondral-only fragments[3] or removal of fragments
  - Cartilage restoration procedure depends on age and activity level of patient and location of the lesion(s).
- In the absence of a loose body, surgical intervention for PFP should occur only after a prolonged course of appropriate physical therapy with patient compliance.

MPFL Reconstruction

- Indications
  - Commonly performed in the setting of recurrent patellar instability with an incompetent (stretched or torn) MPFL
  - First-time patellar dislocation: If no loose bodies, patients can be treated nonsurgically, with a progressive return to activities over 6 to 12 weeks.
    - Increasing data suggest MPFL reconstruction can be considered in patients with first-time patellar dislocation with multiple risk factors for recurrence—skeletally immaturity, trochlear dysplasia, patella alta.[4]
  - Recurrent patellar instability: Associated with patellar apprehension, tenderness to palpation along the course of the MPFL

(including on either the medial epicondyle or medial patellar facet), and increased lateral patellar translation
- Effusion, particularly in the setting of a chondral or osteochondral injury
- J sign on active knee extension
  - When actively extending the knee from a flexed position, the patella will move laterally as it exits the trochlear groove
- Increased lateral patellar tilt: Examiner should determine whether correctible to neutral.
  - If lateral retinaculum is tight and tilt cannot be corrected, arthroscopic lateral retinacular release may be performed; rarely indicated in isolation
- Axial radiographs may demonstrate a bony MPFL avulsion off the medial facet of the patella or the medial epicondyle; rarely represent intra-articular loose bodies
- MRI may demonstrate midsubstance tear of the MPFL (most common) or a tear off its femoral or patellar insertion.
- Chronic patellar instability: Tear may not be identified, but previously injured scar tissue may appear wavy or redundant.
  - Chondral surfaces should be evaluated preoperatively.
    - Most common locations of chondral injuries: Medial patella facet and lateral aspect of trochlea
- Authors' preferred technique
  - With patient under anesthesia, amount of patellar translation and end point assessed and compared with contralateral side
    - If patella not fully correctible to neutral, a lateral release may be considered
  - Incision: Along the medial border of the patella from the proximal pole to approximately the midpoint of the patella
  - Dissection is carried down through layer 1 (sartorial fascia) and layer 2, which contains the native MPFL, exposing the joint capsule.
  - Blunt dissection is performed between layers 2 and 3 from the medial border of the patella toward the medial epicondyle for later graft passage
  - The capsule can be carefully incised to demonstrate the patellar articular cartilage.

- Two suture anchors are inserted as close to the cartilage as possible without violating, with the first near the proximal pole of the patella and the second just proximal to the midpoint.
  - Care must be taken to avoid penetrating the articular cartilage but also not to direct too far anteriorly so as to violate the anterior cortex of the patella.
- Because there have been no differences shown in outcomes following allograft or autograft tissue, either a semitendinosus allograft or autograft can be used.
  - The center of the graft is marked and placed midway between the two suture anchors.
  - The sutures from each of the anchors are then tied over the graft, thereby securing the graft to the patella.
- A small incision is made over the medial epicondyle.
- Dissection is carried down to the medial epicondyle, taking care to protect the saphenous neurovascular bundle.
- The saddle between the adductor tubercle and medial epicondyle is palpated and radiographically represented as Schottle point.
- A guide pin is placed at this location under fluoroscopic guidance, directed proximally and anteriorly.
  - The graft can be shuttled through to the medial incision using the previously established interval.
  - Isometry can be tested using the guide pin and passing sutures placed into the graft.
  - Once isometry is confirmed, the guide pin can be overdrilled in preparation for an interference screw.
  - The guide pin is then pulled through along with the passing sutures placed into the graft.
- The knee is placed at approximately 30° of flexion.
  - The patella should be held reduced in the trochlea and sufficient tension held on the sutures to keep it centered within the trochlea but not overtensioned.
- The interference screw is then inserted.
- Postoperative care
  - Weight bearing as tolerated with a hinged knee brace locked in full extension
    - Brace unlocked at postoperative week 6
  - Physical therapy begins within the first 2 to 4 weeks.
  - Return to sport: No sooner than 5 to 6 months after surgery

Tibial Tubercle Osteotomy

- Indications
  - Performed for chondral surface overload or in setting of recurrent patellar instability with an increased TT-TG distance
  - In setting of recurrent patellar instability, MPFL reconstruction frequently performed concomitantly with tibial tubercle osteotomy
- Approaches and techniques
  - The most common tibial tubercle osteotomy: Anteromedialization originally described by Fulkerson[5] replaces:
    - Elmslie-Trillat, or purely medializing, tibial tubercle osteotomy: Historically used to medialize the tibial tubercle in the setting of tubercle lateralization and recurrent patellar instability
    - Maquet, or purely anteriorizing osteotomy: Historically used to anteriorize the tibial tubercle in the setting of patellar overload to decrease forces across the patellofemoral joint and offload areas of chondrosis
  - Shallow anteromedialization: Osteotomy made at an angle closer to the coronal plane than the sagittal plane; performed to medialize the tibial tubercle to a greater extent than it is anteriorized
    - Most commonly used in the setting of recurrent patellar instability with an increased TT-TG distance
  - Steep anteromedialization: Osteotomy made at an angle closer to the sagittal plane than the coronal plane; performed to anteriorize the tibial tubercle to a greater extent than it is medialized
    - Most commonly used in the setting of patellar chondrosis affecting the distal and lateral aspect of the patella
  - Equipment: Commercially available cutting guide or free-hand using Kirschner wires, osteotomes
  - Keep the proximal extent of the osteotomy at least 1 cm distal to the knee joint to prevent violating the articular cartilage.
  - Protect the patellar tendon at all times.
  - Unless distalization of the tubercle is planned, as in the setting of patella alta, the distalmost aspect of the osteotomized

tibial tubercle shingle may be left intact to minimize the risk of nonunion.
- Drill holes for the screws should be made in the anterior aspect of the tubercle before performing the osteotomy cut.
- Once osteotomy is performed, the tubercle can be moved anteromedially by the templated distance.
- A Kirschner wire may be placed away from the planned location of screws to maintain the planned reduction
  - 4.5-mm cortical screws may then be placed in lag fashion (**Figure 4**).
  - A washer may be used on the proximal screw because of poor metaphyseal bone quality in that location.
- Postoperative care
  - Toe-touch weight bearing for the first 6 weeks postoperatively
  - Immediate passive range of motion from 0° to 90°
  - Straight leg raises and quadriceps sets to prevent quadriceps inhibition
  - Active and active-assisted knee extension not permitted until 6 weeks after surgery
  - Return to sport: No earlier than approximately 6 months postoperatively following a criteria-based return to sport battery of testing

Cartilage Restoration

- Indications
  - Considered in the setting of high-grade (grade 3 or 4) symptomatic chondral lesions
  - Common presenting signs and symptoms: Recurrent effusions, mechanical symptoms such as catching, pain when the patellofemoral joint is loaded, such as with deep squatting or stair climbing
  - Débridement alone, or chondroplasty, may be considered in older patients (at least age 50 years) without patellofemoral osteoarthritis, in whom the results of cartilage restoration surgery are less predictable and as a staged procedure if autologous cell-based surgery, such as

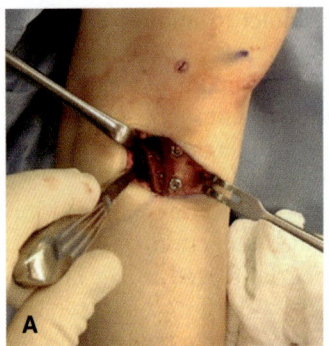
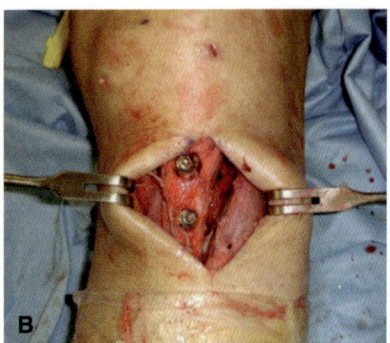
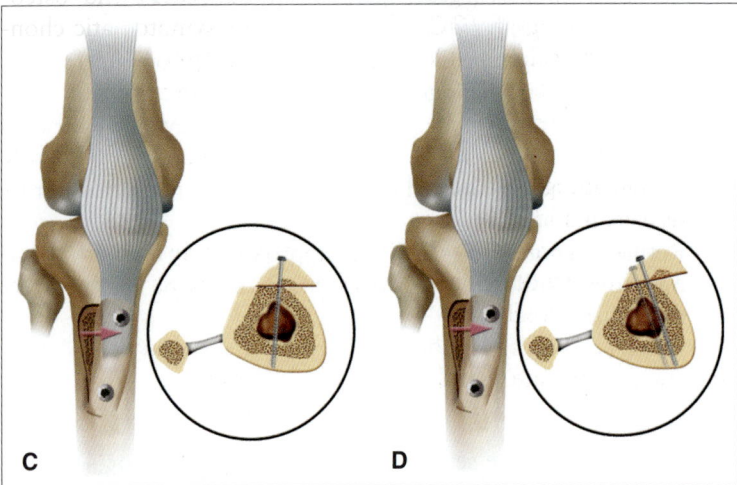

Figure 4 **A** and **B**, Demonstration of a final pictorial representation of the tibial tubercle osteotomy procedure. The broad cancellous base allows for optimal healing. **C** and **D**, A schema demonstrating a medialization cut and an oblique cut (anteromedialization), highlighting the amount of correction that can be gained. (Reproduced with permission from Cordasco F, Green D: *Pediatric and Adolescent Knee Surgery*. Wolters Kluwer, 2015, Figure 19.8.)

matrix-induced autologous chondrocyte implantation (MACI) is planned.
- MACI requires a biopsy and for the harvested cells to be expanded ex vivo before implantation.
- Chondroplasty alone may provide sufficient relief of symptoms in these patients, and the second-stage procedure is not necessary.

- Single-stage cell-based treatments also exist, most commonly in the form of particulated juvenile chondrocytes.
  - These are commercially available but often require a special order and must be used within a certain time period before expiration.
- Cell-based cartilage restoration techniques can be used only when there are no cystic changes or intralesional osteophytes within the subchondral bone.
  - Subchondral marrow edema alone without the aforementioned degenerative changes is not a contraindication for cell-based strategies.
- Osteochondral autograft transplantation (OAT) and osteochondral allograft (OCA) are options for symptomatic chondral or osteochondral lesions of the patellofemoral joint.[7]
  - OAT: For lesions less than 1.5 to 2 cm^2, depending on the size of the patient's knee
  - OCA: For larger lesions but may take longer to incorporate than autograft tissue
- Approaches and techniques
  - Typically performed via a small medial parapatellar arthrotomy; allows eversion of the patella and access to the entire patella and trochlea
    - Violate as little of the extensor mechanism as necessary to evert the patella and access the pathology.
    - Excise the retropatellar fat pad to help facilitate patellar eversion.
  - Cell-based technique (MACI or juvenile particulated chondrocytes)[6]
    - Débride lesion to a stable rim of healthy cartilage.
    - Use no. 15 blade and curets (ringed or conventional), taking care to remove the calcified cartilage layer but avoid violating the subchondral bone.
    - The lesion can then be sized before implanting the cell suspension.
    - A thin layer of fibrin glue is typically placed at the base of the lesion before inserting the cells, and then above the cells to seal them in.
    - No irrigation is used after the cells are placed within the lesion.

- Osteochondral autograft transplantation
  - Autograft plugs up to 1 cm² harvested from the intercondylar notch or from the periphery of the trochlea, most commonly the superolateral aspect of the trochlea
  - The recipient site is prepared in a similar fashion as the donor plugs are harvested.
    - The injured cartilage and subchondral bone are removed with a core harvester, typically to a depth of 1 cm.
    - When performing OAT on the patella, a guide pin and reamer are recommended rather than a manual harvester, because the subchondral bone is often harder than femoral and trochlear subchondral bone.
  - The depth of the recipient site is confirmed, and the donor plugs are carefully impacted, typically using a delivery tube, to fill the lesion.
    - It is important that the plugs are flush with the surrounding healthy articular cartilage and not proud, as this will predispose to shearing of the donor plugs and graft failure.
- Osteochondral allograft
  - Although allograft plugs are most commonly taken from a donor femoral condyle, a bulk trochlea or patella may also be used but can be difficult to procure.
    - Authors' preference: Use circular allograft plugs, which can be sized up to 18 mm² each and overlap each other
  - Measure chondral lesion, or recipient site, to determine how many and what size plugs are needed to reconstruct the defect.
  - A guide pin is then placed through a sizer, and the recipient site prepared for implantation of a donor plug.
    - Reaming is typically performed no deeper than 8 mm
  - The dimensions of the recipient site are measured, and a donor plug of those same dimensions is harvested from the OCA.
  - The plug is then impacted to fill the recipient site, and the process repeated if additional plugs are needed (**Figure 5**).
  - Although a press fit is typically used, chondral darts or headless compression screws may be considered as supplemental fixation.

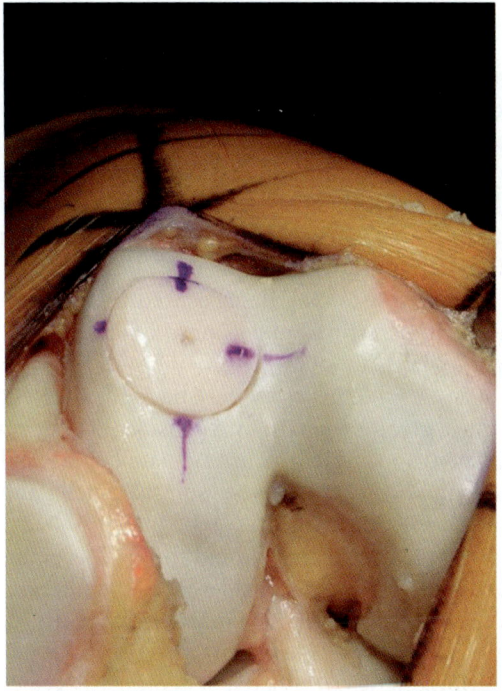

Figure 5 Photograph shows osteochondral allograft transplantation for cartilage lesions in the trochlea. (Reproduced with permission from Rubash HE: *The Adult Knee*, ed 2. Wolters Kluwer, 2020, Figure 20.3.)

- Postoperative care
  - Rehabilitation protocols vary.
  - Typically, the knee remains locked in full extension when ambulating with the assistance of crutches for at least the first 6 weeks postoperatively.
  - If early weight bearing allowed, should be with a brace locked in full extension to prevent graft shearing
  - Early motion and quadriceps contractions, including straight leg raises and quad sets, encouraged immediately
  - Return to sport: Typically no sooner than 5 to 6 months after surgery when the athlete passes a criteria-based return to sport battery of testing

Top 10 Knowledge Drops for Your Rotation

1. The most common cause of PFP is patellar maltracking resulting from a muscular imbalance, which includes a weak VMO and hip abductors.
2. A hip examination and gait assessment should be performed for all patients with knee pain, because femoral anteversion and internal tibial torsion can contribute to patellar instability as well as chondral overload.
3. The TT-TG distance may be measured using CT or MRI. The distance is underestimated by approximately 10% on MRI as compared with CT.
4. The Caton-Deschamps ratio may be used to assess for patella alta. Values greater than 1.3 are considered abnormal.
5. Factors predisposing to recurrent patellar instability include skeletal immaturity, trochlear dysplasia, patella alta, and lateralization of the tibial tubercle.
6. Lateral retinacular release should rarely, if ever, be performed in isolation and may be considered in conjunction with other procedures if the patella cannot be manually corrected to neutral.
7. An anteriorizing tibial tubercle osteotomy is typically used to decrease patellofemoral contact forces, whereas a medializing tibial tubercle osteotomy is used to treat recurrent patellar instability with increased TT-TG distance.
8. During MPFL reconstruction, the femoral insertion of the MPFL graft is at an isometric point located between the medial epicondyle and adductor tubercle. Radiographically, this is represented by Schottle point, which is just proximal to Blumensaat line and anterior to the posterior femoral cortical extension line.
9. Cell-based cartilage restoration treatments (eg, MACI, juvenile particulated chondrocyte implantation) should not be performed if there are degenerative changes of the subchondral bone.
10. When performing OAT or OCA, the implanted plugs must not sit proud relative to the surrounding articular cartilage, as this may result in shearing and graft failure.

MENISCUS TEARS

Meniscus tears are among the most common pathologies encountered by orthopaedic surgeons. Meniscus tears can be acute/traumatic, most often occurring from a twisting or pivoting injury, or degenerative, although the distinction is not always clear. They can occur in isolation or combined with a knee ligament injury, most frequently an anterior cruciate ligament (ACL) tear. Acute meniscus tears in young athletes, with or without a concomitant ACL injury, more commonly affect the lateral meniscus, whereas degenerative tears most commonly affect the posterior horn of the medial meniscus, although there is considerable overlap. The menisci play a number of important roles in the knee, including decreasing the contact forces between the tibia and femur. Therefore, the menisci should be preserved whenever possible. Because the meniscus has a limited blood supply, primarily in the periphery, not all tears are considered repairable.

Epidemiology

- Highly prevalent and occurring with an increasing frequency: increased participation in sports and fitness, greater availability of MRI[8]
  - Overall prevalence: 12% to 14%, with an increased incidence among those with ACL injury (22% to 86%)[9]
  - 10% to 20% of orthopaedic surgeries in the United States involve the meniscus
- Most common in males: 2.5:1 to 4:1
- Acute tears most common in patients ages 11 to 30 years
  - Degenerative tears most common in patients age 40 to 60 years
- Meniscus tears are commonly found in the setting of knee osteoarthritis, with more than 75% of patients with symptomatic osteoarthritis found to have a meniscus tear.[10]

Pertinent Anatomy/Pathoanatomy

- The menisci are crescent-shaped wedges of fibrocartilage located on the peripheral aspect of the tibial articular surface.
  - Red zone: Thick, peripheral vascular border that is attached to the joint capsule, with more stable capsular

attachments to the medial meniscus compared with the lateral meniscus
  - White zone: Innermost border where it tapers to a thin free edge
- The fibers that comprise the meniscus run primarily longitudinally from between the anterior and posterior root attachments.
- Healing potential depends on the vascularity, which guides surgical decision making (**Figure 6**).
  - The posterior horn has better vascularity than the body and anterior horn.
  - Peripheral 3 mm of the meniscus: well vascularized
  - Central portion: variable vascularization
  - Inner margin: avascular
- Medial meniscus: semicircular shape and broader posteriorly, covering approximately 64% of the articular surface
  - Firm attachments to the deep medial collateral ligament (MCL) and joint capsule
- Lateral meniscus: more circular shape than the medial meniscus, covering approximately 84% of the articular surface
  - The lateral meniscus posterior horn has femoral attachments via the meniscofemoral ligaments (anterior: Humphrey; posterior: Wrisberg).
  - Most patients (93%) have either an anterior or posterior meniscofemoral ligament, and 50% have both.
  - The lateral meniscus has no attachments to the fibular collateral ligament (FCL) and is attached only loosely to the joint capsule.
- The anterior horns of the menisci are connected by the intermeniscal ligament, but its function remains poorly defined.
- Important function in force transmission: axial forces through the tibiofemoral joint are converted into tensile hoop stresses
  - The meniscus increases the overall contact area and joint congruity while decreasing peak contact stresses across the tibiofemoral joint.
  - During impact loading, the meniscus acts as a shock absorber, as an intact meniscus reduces impulse loading by 20%.[11]
- The medial meniscus serves as a secondary stabilizer to anterior translation of the tibia relative to the femur, and in an ACL-deficient knee, serves as the primarily stabilizer.
- Role in joint proprioception

Chapter 9: My Knee Hurts

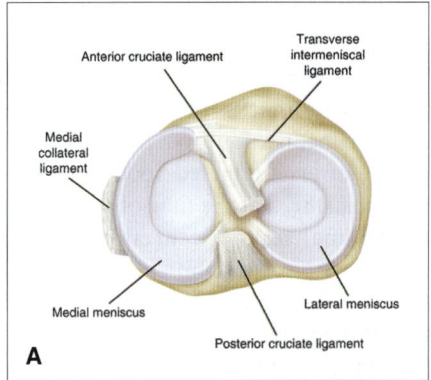

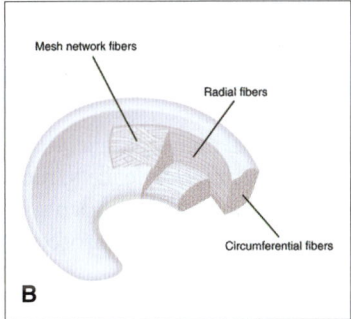
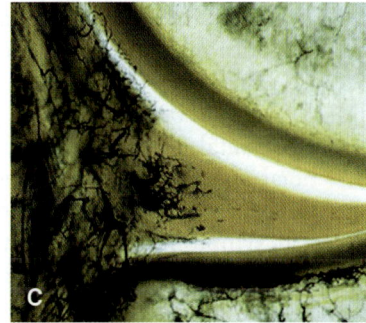

Figure 6 Meniscal anatomy. **A**, Illustration shows the axial anatomy of the menisci. The lateral meniscus is more circular in shape than the medial meniscus and has a close approximation to the insertion of the anterior cruciate ligament on the tibia. **B**, Microstructure of a meniscus. The meniscus consists of circumferential, radial, and oblique fibers. **C**, Micrograph demonstrating the vascularity of the periphery of the meniscus. Only the peripheral one-fourth to one-third of the meniscus is vascularized. (Reprinted from McCarty EC, McAllister DR, Leonard JP: Anatomy and biomechanics of the knee, in Lieberman JR, ed: *AAOS Comprehensive Orthopaedic Review*, ed 3. American Academy of Orthopaedic Surgeons, 2020, p 1247, Figure 5. Adapted with permission from Arnoczky SP, Warren RF: Microvasculature of the human meniscus. *Am J Sports Med* 1982;10:90-95.)

- The meniscus should be preserved as much as possible, and repair should be considered if the tear is located within a vascularized zone of the meniscus.
  - Subtotal medial meniscectomy has been shown to increase contact stresses across the medial compartment by 100%, whereas

subtotal lateral meniscectomy increases contact stresses by 200% to 300%.
- These marked increases in joint stresses contribute to the accelerated osteoarthritis that is observed in the setting of prior meniscectomy or meniscal injury.
- Classification: No universally agreed-upon system, but the morphology of the tear as visualized at the time of surgery may be described
  - Vertical longitudinal tears: Occur along the long axis of the meniscus in line with the circumferential fibers
    - Symptomatic tears in a vascular portion of the meniscus may be amendable to repair.
    - Radial tears occur along the axis perpendicular to the circumferential fibers, are often full thickness, and can propagate in size over time if left untreated.
      - Although the peripheral portion of these tears may be amenable to repair, the inner margin is avascular and should be débrided.
  - Horizontal cleavage tears occur in the axial plane, parallel to the tibial plateau, and result in superior and inferior leaflets, most frequently within the posterior horn of the medial meniscus.
    - If symptomatic, most commonly treated with arthroscopic partial meniscectomy of the smaller leaflet
  - Bucket-handle tears: Vertical or oblique tears with extension toward the anterior and posterior horns and displacement of the torn tissue toward or into the intercondylar notch
    - In the acute setting, if involving a vascular portion of the meniscus with good tissue quality, an attempt at repair is often warranted.
  - Complex tears: Two or more tear configurations
    - Often seen in setting of degenerative tears and most often treated with arthroscopic partial meniscectomy when symptomatic
  - Discoid menisci: Larger than normal menisci, extending further into the joint to a variable extent with complete discoid menisci filling the entire compartment of the knee
    - Rare variant most commonly encountered in pediatric patients and most frequently involve the lateral meniscus
    - Often asymptomatic, but pediatric patients may report snapping, popping, or the inability to fully extend the knee without a history of trauma

- If symptomatic: Arthroscopic partial meniscectomy, which may require saucerization back to the margins of a normal meniscus with or without repair (depending on stability of the meniscus)

Pertinent History/Physical Examination Findings

History
- Ask patient about specific inciting injury or trauma that led to the onset of the presenting signs and symptoms
  - Acute, traumatic meniscus tears most commonly occur with a twisting injury followed by swelling within the first 24 to 48 hours.
- The patient may report mechanical symptoms, such as catching, locking, popping, crepitus, or the inability to achieve full extension or flexion.
  - Mechanical symptoms, or a truly locked knee in which the knee is unable to be fully extended, typically indicate a large, displaced tear, such as bucket-handle tear or a large flap (parrot beak) tear.
- Symptoms may worsen with activities that require rotating or twisting of the knee.
  - Tears of the posterior horn or body may cause worsening of symptoms with deep squatting or bending, whereas tears of the anterior horn may exacerbate symptoms with terminal extension.
- Degenerative meniscal tears often occur without a specific trauma or inciting event.
  - Patients with degenerative tears often experience an exacerbation in symptoms after a fall or twisting event, which may suggest an acute-on-chronic event, or propagation of a degenerative tear.
- Patients often localize pain to the joint line location of the tear (medial or lateral).

Physical Examination
- Begin with a standing assessment of alignment and gait.
  - Quadriceps: Compare with contralateral side for atrophy, which can occur in the setting of a knee effusion and quadriceps inhibition
  - The knee: Assess for an effusion
  - Patellofemoral joint and knee ligaments: Rule out as concomitant injuries

- Because no single test for meniscal tear has an optimal level of sensitivity, specificity, and diagnostic accuracy, multiple provocative maneuvers can help establish a diagnosis.
  - Medial and lateral joint lines, including the posterior horns: Palpate and assess for tenderness.
  - Hyperflexion and hyperextension (bounce home) testing: Performed with patient supine to help assess for posterior horn and anterior horn pathology, respectively
  - The McMurray test: Performed by concomitantly flexing and internally rotating (lateral meniscus) and flexing and externally rotating (medial meniscus)
    - Positive result: Palpable or audible pop or click results, or the patient reports pain
  - The Thessaly test is performed with the patient standing on one leg with the knee flexed to 20°, and the patient is asked to rotate their knee and torso.
    - The examiner must ensure that the patient is twisting both their knee and torso and not their torso alone.
    - Positive result: Joint line tenderness or mechanical symptoms
  - Patients may also complain of pain with deep knee flexion while weight bearing during a squat or duck-walking.

Relevant Imaging

- Radiographs
  - Standardized knee radiographs: weight-bearing AP, posteroanterior Rosenberg (45°), lateral, and Merchant (or sunrise) axial radiographs
  - Radiographs are necessary to assess for concomitant osteoarthritis.
    - Calcification of the meniscus (chondrocalcinosis) can be found in the setting of crystalline arthroplasty (calcium pyrophosphate deposition).
  - If a patient is found to be in clinical varus or valgus, standing full-length hip to ankle alignment radiographs may be obtained to assess the patient's mechanical axis.
    - Compartment overload from malalignment may predispose the patient to meniscal pathology.
  - If patients have advanced joint degeneration on radiographs, particularly in the symptomatic compartment, MRI is unnecessary.

- Magnetic resonance imaging
  - MRI is the most sensitive diagnostic test for meniscal tear, however:
    - Has relatively high false-positive rate, particularly within the posterior horn of the medial meniscus
    - Has relatively high false-negative rate for posterior root tears and for radial tears
  - For young patients with suspected acute traumatic tears and no degenerative changes on radiographs, MRI should be considered to assess the integrity of the menisci.
  - MRI may also be considered in patients without an acute inciting event without advanced degenerative changes on radiographs in whom a course of nonsurgical treatment has failed.
  - MRI also allows for a complete assessment of the chondral surfaces and ligaments.
  - A magnetic resonance arthrogram may be considered to assess for recurrent tear among patients who have undergone prior meniscal repair or meniscectomy.
  - To be considered a tear on MRI, linear high signal must extend to either the superior or inferior surface of the meniscus.
    - The presence of a parameniscal cyst on MRI is highly correlated with the presence of a meniscal tear.
    - The presence of a "double PCL (posterior cruciate ligament)" sign or "double anterior horn" sign is diagnostic for a bucket-handle medial meniscus tear.
    - The posterior root attachments should be scrutinized, especially on coronal and sagittal images, as interruption of the root attachments can be indicated by high signal in that location (ghost sign).
- Patients with metal implants who are unable to undergo MRI can be assessed with a CT arthrogram.

Nonsurgical Measures

- Most meniscal tears can be managed initially with nonsurgical care, including physical therapy and/or anti-inflammatory agents, before surgical intervention is indicated.
  - Most notably degenerative tears without a traumatic inciting event and acute tears in patients with radiographic degenerative changes without frank mechanical symptoms

- Initial management
  - Rest and avoidance of activities that exacerbate symptoms, including twisting, pivoting, deep squatting, and running
  - Frequent ice application and elevation, especially if an effusion is present
  - Oral NSAIDs
- Supervised or at-home physical therapy: quadriceps isometrics, range of motion in pain-free arcs, gluteal and core strengthening, endurance
- A corticosteroid injection may be considered in patients with degenerative meniscal tears in the setting of degenerative changes, particularly if an effusion is present.
  - The use of corticosteroids is typically avoided in younger patients without degenerative changes.

Surgical Intervention

- Surgical intervention may be considered in patients with persistent symptoms attributable to the meniscal tear in whom nonsurgical treatment has failed.
- Important mechanical symptoms, particularly locking of the knee from a displaced meniscal fragment, are an indication for early surgical intervention.
  - The most common procedure is a partial meniscectomy with débridement/resection of the torn portion of the meniscus, and less often repair of the tear, with the treatment decision based on the location of the tear, tear type, and patient characteristics.
- Young patients with acute, traumatic meniscus tears that may be amenable to repair, patients with locking of the knee, or patients with concomitant ACL tear or other intra-articular pathology indicating more urgent surgical intervention may forego a prolonged course of nonsurgical management before surgery.
- Longitudinal tears that are often amenable to repair predominate in patients younger than 30 years, whereas complex tears that are rarely amenable to repair are most common in patients older than 40 years.
- Surgery is contraindicated in patients with severe knee osteoarthritis.

Arthroscopic Partial Meniscectomy

- Indications
  - Arthroscopic partial meniscectomy may be performed for symptomatic tears that are not amenable to repair: Tears involving the inner margin (avascular white-white zone), including parrot peak flaps, most horizontal cleavage tears, and complex tear types
  - Even if repair is attempted in the setting of a radial tear, the inner margin is unlikely to heal and may be débrided.
  - Patients with degenerative changes within the affected compartment or with poor quality meniscal tissue typically will not have a repairable tear and therefore typically undergo arthroscopic partial meniscectomy.
  - When partial meniscectomy is performed, the surgeon should take care to remove only the unstable portion of meniscus, leaving as much remaining meniscus intact as possible to minimize the risk of future joint degeneration.
- Technique
  - Supine positioning
    - Surgical leg: Positioned in a leg holder, or a post can be used to place a valgus force on the knee for visualization of the medial compartment
    - Contralateral leg: Flat on bed or placed in a well-leg holder if the bed will be flexed
  - After administration of anesthesia (general, spinal, and/or regional nerve blockade), the patient is positioned, prepped, and draped in standard fashion.
  - An anterolateral portal is established with a no. 11 blade.
  - Diagnostic arthroscopy of patellofemoral joint, medial and lateral gutters, and medial and lateral compartments
    - Displaced meniscal fragments may be found in the medial or lateral gutters.
    - To enter the medial compartment, a valgus force is placed on the knee, and to enter the lateral compartment, the leg is placed in the figure-of-4 position.
    - Depending on the location of the meniscus tear, an anteromedial portal may be made under spinal needle guidance

with the knee in the figure-of-4 position (lateral tear) or with a valgus force on the knee (medial tear).
    - The portal is made such that the tear will be accessible with arthroscopic instruments.
  - Use a probe to palpate the meniscus along its entire length from the posterior root to the anterior root and along the tibial and femoral surfaces of the meniscus, assessing for stability, reparability, and the presence of any displaced fragment.
  - Attempt to pull the posterior horn into the compartment to test the meniscocapsular attachments.
    - Assess quality of the tissue.
- If tear is not reparable: use meniscal biters and motorized shavers to remove injured, unstable tissue
  - Torn posterior horn tissue is usually best accessed with the shaver through the ipsilateral portal as the affected compartment, whereas anterior horn tissue is commonly accessed with the shaver placed through the contralateral portal.
    - Switch portals if trouble is encountered accessing the injured tissue to be débrided.
  - Degenerative tissue and complex tears often may be successfully débrided and removed with an arthroscopic shaver alone (**Figure 7**).
  - If débridement is unsuccessful using a shaver alone, arthroscopic meniscal biters may be used: straight, upbiting, left-angle and right-angle, and back biting
    - If using meniscal biters, take care to remove only injured, unstable tissue and not violate healthy, intact meniscus.
  - A shaver can be used to smooth out the edges following débridement with a meniscal biter
- Following débridement, the remaining meniscal tissue should be probed to confirm adequate débridement and a stable rim.
- Care must be taken to protect the femoral and tibial articular cartilage throughout the procedure.
- Postoperative care
  - Focus on regaining a full, symmetric range of motion and early independence with activities of daily living.

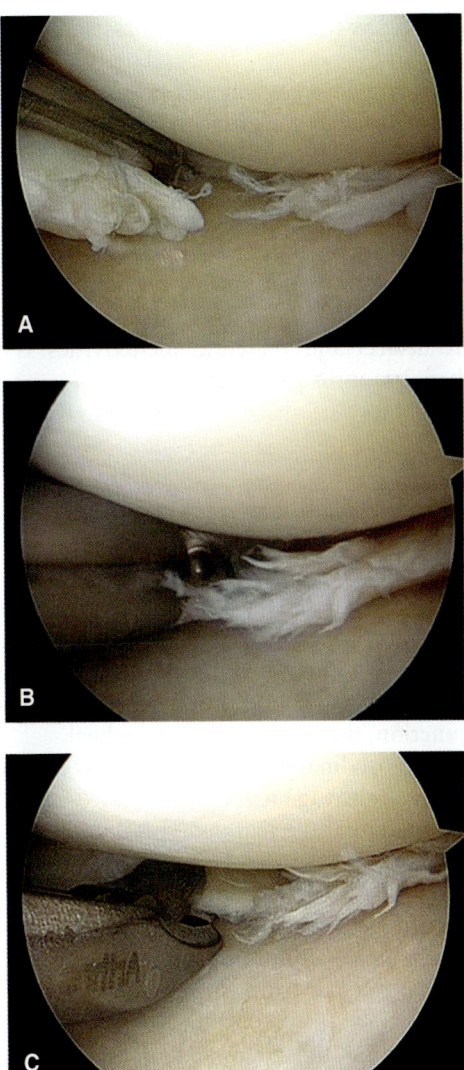

Figure 7 Arthroscopic images of the meniscus. **A**, Complex tear of the medial meniscus probed for stability. **B**, Arthroscopic shaver used to débride shredded tissue. **C**, Basket punch used to débride larger segments of the torn meniscus after the shaver removes more shredded tissue.

- Weight bearing as tolerated with the assistance of crutches or a walker
  - Wean assistive device when gait normalizes
- Ice and knee elevation for effusion control
- Immediate quadriceps activation, including straight leg raise and quad sets
- Stationary bike riding may begin within 1 month postoperatively.
- Gradual ramp up including cardiovascular endurance training (biking, swimming, elliptical) beginning approximately 1 month after surgery
- Return to sports and recreational activities is typically no sooner than 2 months postoperatively.

Meniscus Repair

- Indications
  - Considered for certain tear types that involve a vascularized portion of the meniscus
  - Most commonly performed in young patients following an acute injury, whether an isolated meniscus tear or in the setting of concomitant ACL tear
  - Repaired tears are most likely to heal if the tear occurs in the peripheral red-red zone, and the closer the tear is to the microcapsule junction, the more likely it is to heal.
    - Vertical, longitudinal tears are more likely to heal than radial or horizontal cleavage tears
  - Repair of bucket-handle tears is typically attempted in young patients when the tear involves the peripheral 50% of the meniscus.
  - Repair of degenerative meniscal tissue or in the setting of degenerative changes should rarely be attempted, as this tissue has minimal propensity for healing.
- Technique
  - Patient positioning and diagnostic arthroscopy same manner as described for arthroscopic partial meniscectomy
  - After tear is deemed repairable, use an arthroscopic shaver, rasp, or spinal needle to carefully débride and/or abrade (but not resect) the torn edges and meniscocapsular junction to stimulate a bleeding response, thereby maximizing healing potential.

- Three main techniques for meniscal repair: all-inside, inside-out, and outside-in
- All-inside technique most common technique currently; a commercially available device is used to place a suture within meniscal tissue
    - The surgeon places the needle of the disposable device through the meniscal tissue and capsule, using a pledget made of plastic or suture on the outside of the capsule.
        - Repeat in horizontal, vertical, or oblique mattress fashion with respect to the tear with a second pass of the device through meniscus and capsule.
    - The knot is carefully tightened to reduce the tear.
        - Repeat with as many all-inside devices as necessary to achieve a stable repair.
    - Advantages: Less morbidity, as no additional incisions are necessary, and a shorter surgical time
    - Disadvantages: Larger hole placed in the meniscus by the needle and the potential for misfiring of the device, in which case the pledget can become trapped in the meniscus or capsular tissue
    - The all-inside technique may be necessary for far posterior tears that may not be accessible with an inside-out technique.
    - If more than three all-inside devices are going to be used, consideration should be given to an inside-out or hybrid (all-inside and inside out) repair technique
    - Newer all-inside instruments also allow for side-to-side repair of meniscal tissue and may be considered for certain tear configurations, such as radial tears
- Inside-out meniscal repair has long been considered the gold standard of meniscal repair, but recent studies have suggested that clinical outcomes following inside-out and all-inside repairs using current implants are equivalent.[12]
    - Also used during meniscus allograft transplantation
    - Inside-out repair requires a separate incision, dissection, and retractor placement to catch needles that are passed through arthroscopic portals through the meniscus and capsule.

- Zone-specific cannulas now allow for access to almost the entire meniscus with an inside-out approach, but it remains difficult to access the anterior horn and central aspect of the posterior horn.
- The anatomic approach for an inside-out lateral meniscus repair is through a small incision made at the posterolateral joint line, with dissection carried out between the iliotibial band and the biceps femoris superficially, and deep to the lateral head of the gastrocnemius and the joint capsule.
  - Care should be taken to remain posterior to the FCL to protect it and anterior to the biceps femoris to protect the common peroneal nerve (CPN).
- On the medial side, superficial dissection is carried through the sartorial fascia, taking care to protect the saphenous neurovascular bundle.
  - Dissection is carried out posterior to the MCL and anterior to the semitendinosus muscle.
  - The semimembranosus muscle will be encountered and may be retracted posterosuperiorly
- The interval between the medial head of the gastrocnemius muscle and posterior joint capsule is identified.
  - A retractor or spoon may be placed in the deep interval to allow an assistant to safely catch the sutures as the surgeon passes them through the meniscus.
- The sutures are retrieved and tied over the capsule, thereby fixing the meniscus to the capsule.
- The inside-out approach may allow for more sutures to be placed through the meniscus, as the needle is smaller than commercially available all-inside devices.
  - Vertical longitudinal tears are often repaired in a vertical mattress fashion, with a balanced repair performed on the superior and inferior surfaces of the meniscus.
  - Radial tears may be fixed with a combination of vertical and horizonal mattress sutures.
- An inside-out technique is most commonly used for repairable anterior horn tears.
  - Includes bucket handle tears that extend into the anterior horn, or in the setting of meniscus allograft transplantation

- This technique uses spinal needles that are placed from outside the skin through the anterior horn tissue on either side of the meniscal tear.
  - Suture is then shuttled across the tear, and a small incision is made between the needles down to the level of the capsule to retrieve the sutures and tie them over the capsule in a similar fashion as the inside-out repair.

Meniscus Root Repair

- Indications
  - Meniscal root tears, which most frequently occur within the posterior roots, may be repaired in patients with minimal to no degenerative changes and without morbid obesity.
  - A torn meniscal root renders the meniscus nonfunctioning, and as such, an attempt at repair should be considered in an effort to minimize the risk of accelerated joint degeneration.[13]
- Technique
  - The authors typically use a transosseous pullout technique in which a commercially available guide is placed at the native meniscus root insertion.
    - A guide pin is inserted in this location and a short tunnel reamed in the tibia.
    - An arthroscopic suture-passing device is used to place two locked-loop sutures into the meniscal root tissue.
    - The tissue is then shuttled down the tunnel, and the sutures are tied over a cortical button or loaded into a suture anchor.
  - Isolated meniscal repairs: Authors recommend performing marrow stimulation of the intercondylar notch
    - Typically performed using a microfracture awl within the notch in an effort to deliver marrow elements and maximize the likelihood of healing
- Postoperative care
  - Protocols vary based on the type and location of meniscus repair and surgeon preference.
    - Vertical longitudinal tears: Immediate weight bearing may be permitted for many; some recommend locking the knee in extension for ambulation

- Large, bucket-handle repairs: 3 to 4 weeks of protected weight bearing
- Radial and root repairs: Weight bearing may be protected for up to 6 weeks after surgery
- Regardless of the tear pattern, quadriceps exercises including quad sets and straight leg raises commence immediately.
- Range of motion from 0° to 90° is allowed for the first 6 weeks after surgery, progressing to full range of motion for most tear types after that.
  - For radial and root tears, range of motion past 120° may not be allowed until 3 to 4 months after surgery.
- Return to sport following meniscus repair is typically no sooner than 5 months after surgery following a criteria-based return-to-play protocol.

Top 10 Knowledge Drops for Your Rotation

1. Degenerative meniscus tears without a locked knee warrant an initial course of nonsurgical management.
2. The peripheral 25% to 33% of the meniscus is vascularized. Tears involving this portion of the meniscus may be amenable to repair.
3. Medial meniscus tears are more common than lateral tears, except in acute ACL tears.
4. Degenerative meniscus tears are most common in patients older than 40 years, most commonly occur in the posterior horn of the medial meniscus, and are often complex.
5. Signal within the meniscus on MRI must extend all the way to either the femoral or tibial articular surface of the meniscus to be considered a tear.
6. The presence of a parameniscal cyst is indicative of a meniscal tear. Cysts are more common medially but more symptomatic laterally.
7. Meniscus tear is the most common indication for knee surgery.
8. Inside-out meniscal repair requires a small open incision. During the medial approach, the MCL and saphenous neurovascular bundle must be protected. During the lateral approach, the lateral collateral ligament and CPN must be protected.

9. Radial meniscus tears that extend near the capsule have significant biomechanical consequences on meniscal function. Repair of the peripheral portion of these tears and inner margin débridement should be considered to restore meniscal function.
10. Meniscus root tears render the meniscus biomechanically nonfunctional and should be repaired in most patients without advanced degeneration of the knee, although older age and elevated body mass index may be a relative contraindication.

CRUCIATE AND COLLATERAL LIGAMENT INJURIES

Knee ligament injuries are frequently encountered in athletic populations and in the setting of high-energy traumas such as motor vehicle accidents. The anterior and posterior cruciate ligaments function as the primary restraints to anterior and posterior translation of the tibia relative to the femur, respectively. Injuries may occur to each of these ligaments by either a contact (direct blow) or noncontact mechanism. The ACL is the most commonly injured knee ligament, most commonly resulting from a noncontact pivoting mechanism in athletes. The PCL is typically injured following a direct blow to the anterior aspect of the proximal tibia. MCL injuries most commonly occur following a direct blow to the lateral knee that results in a valgus force across the joint. The posterolateral corner (PLC) of the knee is composed of the FCL, popliteus tendon, and popliteofibular ligament (PFL). PLC injuries most frequently result from a direct blow to the medial aspect of the knee but may also occur from a combination of knee hyperextension, varus, and external tibial rotation. Isolated PLC injuries are also uncommon and typically occur in the setting of cruciate ligament injury (PCL more than ACL). Treatment options for knee ligament injuries vary according to the specific ligament injured, degree of injury, and patient-specific factors.

Epidemiology

- ACL injuries are occurring with an increasing frequency due in part to increased youth participation in athletics and a more active adult population, with more than 120,000 occurring annually in the United States.
  - ACL injuries account for up to 50% of knee injuries in young athletes and 60% of sport-related knee surgeries.[14]
  - Young female athletes are at a higher risk of ACL injury, as female high school athletes have been shown to have a twofold to threefold increased risk of ACL injury compared with males in the same sports.
    - Soccer and basketball are among the sports that place female athletes at the highest risk, with injury rates of 0.9% to 1.1% per season.[15]
  - Football and lacrosse place male athletes at the highest risk, with injury rates of 0.4% to 0.8% per season.
  - The overall likelihood of a multisport high school athlete sustaining an ACL tear over a 4-year career has been estimated at 5% to 10%.
- PCL injuries constitute 5% to 10% of knee ligament injuries, and isolated injuries are less common than with other concomitant ligament injuries.
  - One study reported a 2% to 3% incidence of chronic PCL insufficiency in collegiate American football players.[16]
- PLC injuries constitute a similar proportion of knee ligament injuries than PCL injuries and rarely occur in isolation, more often occurring with concomitant cruciate ligament injury.
- MCL injuries are more common than PCL and PLC injuries, making up approximately 40% of all knee ligament injuries and 10% of all athletic knee injuries.
  - Commonly occur in skiing and in contact sports including American football, rugby, hockey, and soccer
  - Commonly occur in isolation, although they also occur in combination with concomitant cruciate ligament injury

Pertinent Anatomy/Pathoanatomy

- ACL originates just lateral to the medial tibial spine, inserting onto the posteromedial wall of the lateral femoral condyle within the intercondylar notch
  - There are no fibers that attach anterior to the lateral intercondylar ridge, which is also referred to as resident's ridge and runs from proximal to distal within the lateral wall of the intercondylar notch.
  - Made of two bundles, the anteromedial and posterolateral bundles, named with respect to their tibial insertion sites (**Figure 8**)
  - Primary function: Provide rotational stability to the tibiofemoral joint while resisting anterior tibial translation
- PCL originates on the PCL facet of the posterior tibia between the posterior meniscal roots approximately 1 cm distal to the articular cartilage of the posterior tibial plateau, inserting onto the medial wall of the intercondylar notch[16]
  - Consists of a posteromedial bundle and anterolateral bundles (**Figure 9**)
  - Primary function: Act as a restraint to posterior translation of the tibia relative to the femur, with more restraint provided at increasing degrees of knee flexion
  - Three major structures of PLC: FCL, popliteus tendon, and PFL
    - FCL originates slightly proximal (1.4 mm) and posterior (3.1 mm) to the lateral femoral epicondyle and inserts onto the lateral aspect of the fibular head
    - The popliteus muscle originates on the proximal portion of the posterior tibia, and its tendon courses intra-articularly through the posterolateral aspect of the knee joint through the popliteal hiatus, inserting onto the lateral aspect of the femur.
    - The popliteus tendon courses deep to the FCL and inserts anterior and distal to the femoral insertion of the FCL, with an average of 18.5 mm between the midpoints of insertion[17] (**Figure 10**).
    - The FCL functions as the knee's primary restraint to varus stress, whereas the popliteus functions with the PCL to

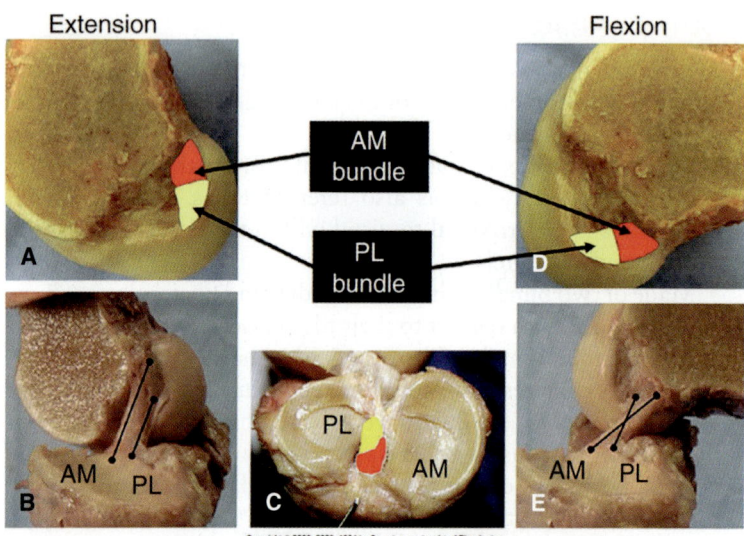

Figure 8 Photographs show the anterior cruciate ligament (ACL) anatomy. **A**, With the knee in extension, the anteromedial (AM) and posterolateral (PL) femoral insertions of the ACL are oriented vertically about the posterior aspect of the medial femoral condyle. **B**, The AM and PL bundles are parallel to each other, with the PL bundle taut. **C**, The AM and PL bundles are named according to their tibial sites of insertion. Note the close approximation to the anterior and posterior horns of the lateral meniscus. **D**, With the knee flexed, the insertions of the AM and PL bundles are oriented horizontally. **E**, The bundles cross each other, with the AM bundle taut. (Reproduced with permission from Honkamp NJ, Shen W, Okeke N, Ferretti M, Fu FH: Anterior cruciate ligament injuries, in DeLee JC, Drez D Jr, Miller MD, eds: *Orthopaedic Sports Medicine*. WB Saunders, 2010, vol 2, p 1646.)

control external tibial rotation, varus, and posterior tibial translation.
- Together with the popliteus, the PFL functions to resist external rotation of the tibia relative to the femur in knee flexion
- The MCL is composed of deep and superficial components
  - Superficial MCL (sMCL): Located in layer II of the medial knee (deep to sartorial fascia)
    - Originates posterior (4.8 mm) and proximal (3.2 mm) to the medial epicondyle of the femur and inserts on the medial

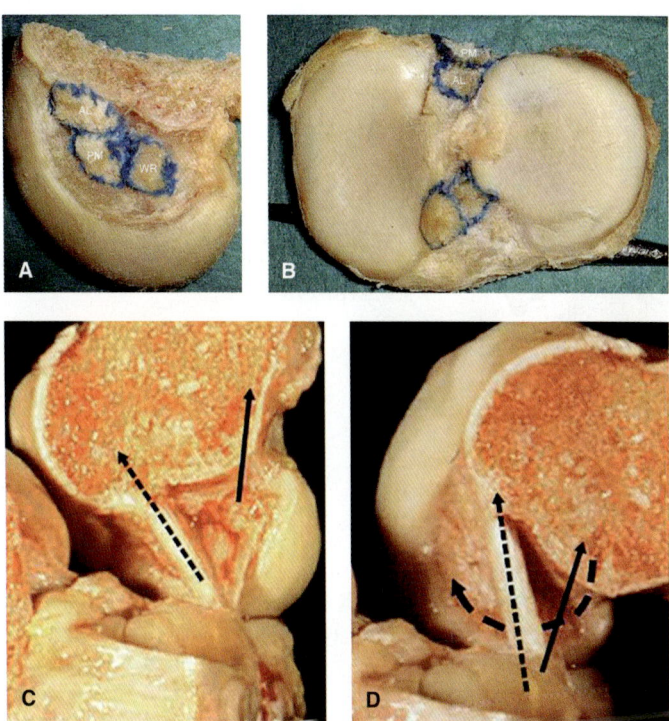

Figure 9 Photographs show posterior cruciate ligament (PCL) anatomy. **A**, Sagittal cross-section of the lateral femoral condyle showing the origins of the anterolateral (AL) and posteromedial (PM) bundles of the PCL and the ligament of Wrisberg (WR). **B**, Axial view of the tibial plateau showing the insertion sites of the AL and PM bundles of the PCL. As with the anterior cruciate ligament, the bundles of the PCL are named according to their tibial insertions. **C**, With the knee in extension, the AL bundle is loose (dashed arrow), whereas the PM bundle is taut (solid arrow). **D**, Flexion of the knee increases the tightness of the AL bundle (dashed arrow), also loosening of the PM bundle (solid arrow) as it passes between the AL bundle and the medial femoral condyle (curved dashed arrow). (Panels A and B reproduced with permission from Takahashi M, Matsubara T, Doi M, Suzuki D, Nagano A: Anatomic study of the femoral and tibial insertions of the anterolateral and posteromedial bundles of the human posterior cruciate ligament. *Knee Surg Sports Traumatol Arthrosc* 2006;14[11]:1055-1059. Panels C and D reproduced with permission from Amis AA, Gupte CM, Bull AMJ, Edwards A: Anatomy of the posterior cruciate ligament and the meniscofemoral ligaments. *Knee Surg Sports Traumatol Arthrosc* 2006;14:257-263.)

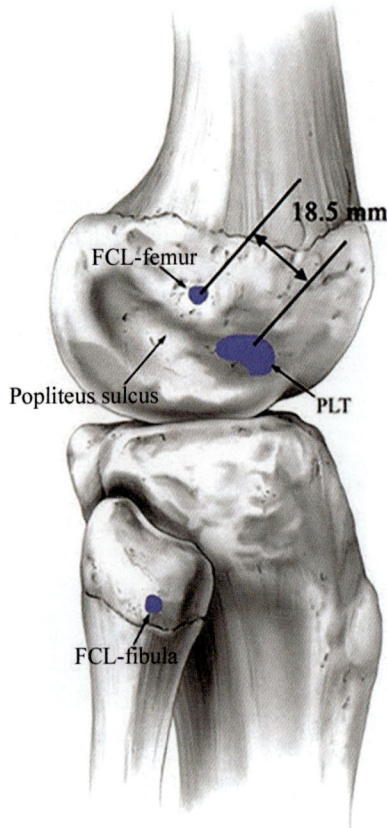

Figure 10 Illustration of a right knee showing the fibular collateral ligament (FCL) attachment sites on the femur and fibula, as well as the popliteus tendon (PLT) attachment site in the popliteus sulcus on the femur. The average distance between the femoral attachment sites is also noted. (Reproduced with permission from LaPrade RF, Ly TV, Wentorf FA, et al: The posterolateral attachments of the knee: A qualitative and quantitative morphologic analysis of the fibular collateral ligament, popliteus tendon, popliteofibular ligament, and lateral gastrocnemius tendon. *Am J Sports Med* 2003;31[6]:854-860.)

aspect of the proximal tibial an average of 61.2 mm distal to the joint line[18]
- The tibial attachment is deep and posterior to the pes anserine tendons, and caution should be taken to avoid injury to the sMCL when harvesting these tendons.
- Deep MCL: Located in layer III of the medial knee (along with the joint capsule); composed of meniscofemoral and meniscotibial fibers
- The sMCL functions as the primary stabilizer to valgus stress at all angles of knee flexion, whereas the deep MCL is a secondary stabilizer.

Pertinent History/Physical Examination Findings

History
- Detailed history including injury mechanism, symptoms at the time of injury, current symptoms, and previous history of knee injury or surgery
- ACL injuries often create an audible or palpable pop in the knee and result in immediate knee swelling and difficulty bearing weight, but patients may be unable to recall exactly how the injury occurred.
  - An acute knee effusion typically indicates the presence of intra-articular pathology, and although common in the setting of ACL injury, may also occur with other pathologies including meniscal tear, patella dislocation, osteochondral injury, fracture, or PCL injury.
- PCL injury should be suspected in the setting of a high-velocity motor vehicle accident with dashboard injury (direct blow to proximal tibial in a flexed knee position) but can also occur following a load (ie, tackle) to a hyperflexed knee and plantarflexed foot or with a hyperextension injury mechanism.
  - Can occur from a variety of mechanisms: direct blow to the knee resulting in a varus or external rotatory moment, noncontact or contact hyperextension injury, knee dislocation
  - In the setting of PLC injury, associated neurovascular injuries are not uncommon and most frequently involve the CPN, so a peripheral vascular examination and assessment of motor strength and sensation must be performed.
- MCL injuries occur from a valgus stress to the knee, and a contact mechanism is more common than a noncontact mechanism.
  - Although injury more commonly occurs at the sMCL femoral insertion, distal MCL tears have inferior healing rates and residual laxity.
  - A complete distal rupture can result in a Stener lesion in which the torn ligament retracts superficial to the pes anserine tendons and is unable to heal to bone, thereby resulting in persistent valgus instability.

Physical Examination
- Begin with a standing assessment of alignment and gait (if able).
  - Varus thrust may suggest chronic PLC injury

- Supine examination: begin with the unaffected knee, assessing range of motion and a ligamentous examination
- Examination of the injured knee
  - Inspection, noting the presence of swelling as well as any abrasions or bruising, which may indicate direct trauma
  - The patient should be asked to fire the quadriceps muscles bilaterally and muscle bulk and tone assessed.
  - Active and passive range of motion should be measured and is often restricted in the setting of acute injury with effusion.
  - Assess for tenderness to palpation along the joint lines and the course of the MCL and FCL.
    - Focal joint-line tenderness may suggest meniscal or chondral injury.
  - Additional meniscal testing may be performed as tolerated.
- Ligamentous testing: Typically performed last, because may cause discomfort to the patient
  - Lachman test for anterior tibiofemoral laxity: Most commonly used maneuver to assess ACL integrity
    - Graded 1 to 3 based on the amount of anterior translation of the tibia relative to the femur in comparison to the normal contralateral knee, with less than 5 mm considered grade 1, 5 to 10 mm grade 2, and greater than 10 mm grade 3
    - The end point may also be defined as A (present) or B (not present).
  - The patient's knee can be flexed to 90° and both anterior drawer (ACL) and posterior drawer (PCL) testing performed.
    - Posterior drawer testing may be similarly graded from 1 to 3
      - In a grade 1 injury, the tibial plateau remains anterior to the femoral condyles.
      - In a grade 2 injury, the plateau is flush with the femoral condyles.
      - In a grade 3 injury, the plateau moves posterior to the condyles.
  - To assess the integrity of the FCL, varus stress testing should be performed at 0° and 30° and graded in comparison with the intact contralateral knee.
    - The injury is graded from 0 to 3, with up to 5 mm of lateral joint opening defined as grade 1, 6 to 10 mm grade 2, and greater than 10 mm without end point grade 3.

- Instability to varus stress at both 0° and 30° suggests a combined ligament FCL and cruciate ligament injury, whereas instability at 30° alone suggests an isolated FCL injury.
- The dial test may be performed to assess the integrity of the popliteus and PFL.
  - This test may be performed prone or supine, and the bilateral feet are externally rotated with the knees flexed to 30° and 90°.
  - A 10° increase in external rotation on the injured knee relative to the uninjured knee suggests a PLC injury (popliteus and/or PFL).
  - Asymmetry at 30° alone suggests an isolated PLC injury, whereas asymmetry at both 30° and 90° suggests a combined PLC and cruciate ligament injury.
- A posterolateral drawer test may also be performed to assess the integrity of the PLC.
- The integrity of MCL is assessed with valgus stress testing at 0° and 30°
  - Similar to FCL injury, a grade 1 injury demonstrates less than 5 mm of medial joint opening, grade 2 is 6 to 10 mm, and grade 3 greater than 10 mm
  - Instability to valgus stress testing at both 0° and 30° suggests a combined MCL and cruciate ligament injury, whereas instability at 30° alone suggests an isolated MCL injury.
- Thorough neurovascular examination, including peripheral pulses, sensation in all lower extremity nerve distributions, and graded motor strength
  - CPN injuries are common in the setting of knee dislocations and PLC injuries and must be evaluated.
  - In the setting of a known or suspected knee dislocation, ankle-brachial indices should be obtained to rule out vascular injury, even if peripheral pulses are present and symmetric.
  - Knee dislocations may occur in patients with obesity with low-energy mechanisms, and a high suspicion for neurovascular injury must be maintained in these patients when presenting with knee ligament injury.

Relevant Imaging

- Radiographs
  - Standardized knee radiographs, including weight-bearing AP, PA Rosenberg (45°), lateral, and Merchant (or sunrise) axial radiographs should be obtained.
    - An avulsion fracture of the proximal lateral tibia (Segond fracture) represents an avulsion of the anterolateral ligament and is highly associated with an ACL rupture.
    - A tibial spine fracture represents injury to the ACL tibial insertion.
    - A sulcus terminalis fracture in the lateral femoral condyle is specific but not sensitive for an ACL tear
    - In the setting of PCL injury, a fragment of bone may be avulsed along with the injured ligament and its tibial insertion, and this may be visualized on lateral radiograph.
  - Stress radiographs may be obtained and compared with the contralateral side to assess for PCL injuries (kneeling), MCL injuries (supine valgus stress), and lateral collateral ligament injuries (supine varus stress) (**Figure 11**).
- Advanced imaging
  - MRI: Diagnostic imaging modality of choice to confirm a diagnosis of ligament injury
    - In the setting of ACL rupture, fluid-sensitive sequences may demonstrate a bone bruise involving the middle third of the lateral femoral condyle at the sulcus terminalis and the posterior aspect of the lateral tibial plateau.
    - When assessing for PLC injury, scrutinize MRI for injury to the FCL, popliteus tendon, PFL, and biceps femoris tendon
    - In the setting of MCL injury, the location of injury (proximal, midsubstance, distal) should be determined
      - Distal injuries have inferior healing capacity compared with other locations, and the injured ligament can displace superficial to the pes tendons (Stener), warranting repair or reconstruction.
  - Low-grade (1 or 2) isolated MCL injuries may not warrant immediate MRI.

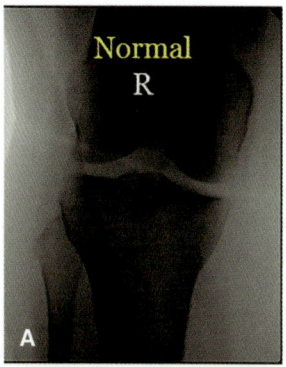
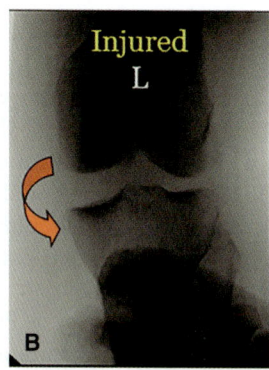
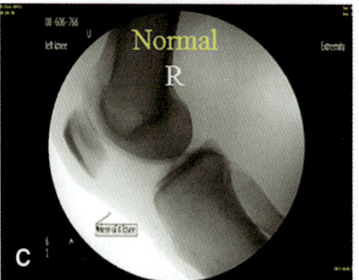
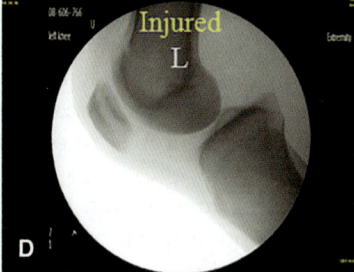

Figure 11 Stress images of a multiple ligament–injured knee. **A** and **B**, AP radiographic valgus stress views of uninjured right and injured (arrow) left knees, respectively. **C** and **D**, Lateral fluoroscopic posterior stress views of the same right and left knees, respectively.

Nonsurgical Measures

- An attempted course of nonsurgical treatment including physical therapy, a home exercise program, and activity modification may be considered in patients with ACL tears who are not involved in cutting/pivoting sports or heavy manual labor.
- Nonsurgical management should be attempted for most PCL injuries and should focus on quadriceps strengthening while avoiding hamstring activation.
  - For isolated grade I and II PLC injuries, a course of nonsurgical management including bracing followed by functional rehabilitation may be attempted.
- Most MCL injuries can be managed nonsurgically with bracing and functional rehabilitation.

Surgical Intervention

- Indications
  - If a patient with ACL injury continues to have episodes of knee instability after nonsurgical treatment, such as buckling or giving way with activities of daily living or vocational activities, ACL reconstruction should be considered.
  - ACL reconstruction should be considered as the first treatment option for most active patients who want to resume cutting and pivoting sports.
  - Surgical indications for PCL injury include displaced bony avulsion fractures, combined ligamentous injuries, and grade III injuries in athletes.
  - Surgical indications for MCL injury include distal avulsions in which the torn tissue is displaced superficial to the pes anserine tendons (Stener lesion) and persistent valgus instability despite initial nonsurgical treatment, most commonly in the setting of concomitant ACL reconstruction.
- Techniques
  - ACL reconstruction
    - Surgical repair has a limited role in the management of ACL injury, and the decision to reconstruct the ACL should consider the patient's age, activity level, and goals.
    - Various graft choices for ACL reconstruction, including multiple autograft and allograft options
      - Caution should be taken when considering the use of allograft tissue in young athletes, as higher failure rates have been reported in this setting.[19]
      - The most commonly used autografts include bone-patellar tendon-bone, hamstring (semitendinosus alone or with gracilis), and quadriceps tendon
    - The authors' preferred technique for a bone-patellar tendon-bone autograft ACL reconstruction:
      - Incision from the inferior pole of the patella to the medial aspect of the tibial tubercle
      - The central third of the patellar tendon (9 to 11 mm wide) is incised from the inferior pole of the patella distally to the tibial tubercle.
      - A sagittal saw is used to harvest first a rectangular tibial bone plug measuring 20 to 25 mm in length and the same

width as the harvested tendon, then a triangular patellar bone plug 18 to 22 mm in length and the same width as the harvested tendon.
- The graft is brought to the back table, and a rongeur and Metzenbaum scissors are used to trim the bone plugs, usually to a diameter of 9 or 10 mm.
  - Excess bone is retained for later patellar harvest site bone grafting during closure.
  - A small drill is used to make holes in the bone plugs and shuttling sutures passed through the holes.
- Standard diagnostic arthroscopy is then performed.
- A motorized shaver is used to débride the torn ACL tissue.
- A combination of motorized shaver and electrocautery is used to expose the posterior wall of the lateral aspect of the intercondylar notch.
- A tibial tunnel drill guide is inserted via the anteromedial portal and placed at placed at the native ACL tibial footprint.
  - The posterior aspect of the anterior horn of the lateral meniscus as well as the anterior aspect of the PCL may be used as a reference point for tibial tunnel guide pin placement.
- A guide pin is inserted through the tibial drill guide at this location and overreamed using a reamer matching the tibial bone plug diameter.
- A femoral tunnel drill guide is inserted through the anteromedial portal and placed at the 10:30 (right knee)/1:30 (left knee) clock position on the lateral wall of the intercondylar notch, ensuring an adequate rim of bone posteriorly to prevent posterior wall blowout.
- A beath pin is inserted through the femoral drill guide at this location and similarly overreamed using a reamer matching the femoral bone plug diameter to a depth equal to the femoral bone plug length.
- Bone debris is removed using a motorized shaver.
- A shuttling suture is pulled through the femoral tunnel using a beath pin, and the looped end of the suture is then retrieved from the tibial tunnel.

- Using this shuttling suture, the ACL graft is shuttled through the tibial tunnel and knee joint such that the femoral bone plug is pulled into the femoral tunnel.
- An interference screw is then placed within the femoral tunnel, although suspensory fixation (cortical button) may be used per surgeon preference.
- The surgeon then pulls traction on the distal sutures (passed through distal bone plug) while taking the knee through a full range of motion to remove creep from the graft (cycling).
- With the knee at or near full extension and a posterior drawer applied to the tibia, an interference screw is inserted into the tibial tunnel.
- The surgeon performs a Lachman test to ensure that there is no persistent laxity following tibial fixation.
- Immediate postoperative weight bearing as tolerated or partial weight bearing for 1 to 6 weeks per surgeon preference
  - Rehabilitation commences immediately with quadriceps strengthening and a focus on regaining terminal extension early in the postoperative phase.
  - Return to sport is based on a criteria-based program including recovery of quadriceps strength compared with the contralateral side (limb-symmetry indices) and elimination of high-risk movement patterns such as dynamic knee valgus.
    - Athletes are typically not allowed to return to cutting or pivoting sports for at least 6 months, although recent data suggest 8 to 12 months may be optimal to reduce risk for reinjury.
- PCL reconstruction
  - Graft choices include hamstring autograft and multiple allograft options.
    - Current evidence suggests similar outcomes whether autograft or allograft tissue is used.[20]
  - Techniques: Transtibial single-bundle or double-bundle reconstruction, tibial inlay technique
  - Immediate postoperative weight bearing as tolerated or partial weight bearing for less than 6 weeks per surgeon preference
    - Bracing according to surgeon preference

- Rehabilitation commences immediately with quadriceps strengthening, avoiding active knee flexion and resisted hamstring exercises for at least 6 weeks after surgery.
- Prone passive knee flexion is allowed, starting immediately.
- Athletes typically are not allowed to return to cutting and pivoting sports until at least 6 months after surgery.
- PLC reconstruction
  - Examination under anesthesia is performed, including varus stress testing at 0° and 30° and a dial test at 0° and 30°.
  - For isolated varus instability without posterolateral rotatory instability, only one femoral tunnel may be necessary at the native FCL femoral insertion.
    - However, if there is injury to the popliteus or PFL resulting in posterolateral rotatory instability, two femoral tunnels may be necessary.
  - The authors prefer the Larson technique, and the following description includes two femoral tunnels:[21]
    - The anterior tibialis allograft is typically used.
      - The graft is opened and thawed on the back table and its diameter measured using a graft sizer.
      - One end of the graft is whipstitched using heavy nonabsorbable suture.
    - An incision is made from approximately 2 cm proximal to the lateral epicondyle to a location halfway between Gerdy tubercle and the anterior aspect of the fibular head.
      - The incision is carried down to the iliotibial band and fascia overlying the biceps femoris.
    - The CPN is palpated posterior to the biceps femoris, carefully dissected free, and protected posteriorly for the remainder of the case.
    - A neurolysis may be performed as necessary to release adhesions and scarring, which is common in the subacute or chronic setting.
    - The fibular head is palpated, and a combination of electrocautery and a periosteal elevator may be used to develop planes anterior and posterior to the fibular head in preparation for fibular tunnel drilling.
    - A guide pin is placed through the fibular head in a slightly anterolateral to posteromedial direction.

- Taking care to protect the CPN and prevent fibular head blowout, the guide pin is inserted and overreamed with a reamer matching the size of the graft diameter.
- The guide pin is removed and a shuttling suture placed to maintain the fibular tunnel. Next, the lateral epicondyle is palpated, and an incision is made through the iliotibial band directly overlying the lateral epicondyle.
- Dissection is carried down to the native FCL femoral insertion, which is located just posterior and proximal to the lateral epicondyle.
- A beath pin is then inserted at the native FCL femoral insertion and directed in a proximal and anterior position to avoid the trochlea and other tunnels for concomitant ligament reconstruction (ACL, PCL).
- The tunnel is then overreamed using a reamer matching the size of the graft diameter.
- A second parallel beath pin is then placed 18.5 mm proximal and anterior to the femoral FCL guide pin and overreamed in similar fashion.
- Shuttling sutures are then pulled through each of the femoral tunnels for later graft passage.
- The graft is then shuttled through the fibular tunnel.
- A large Kelly clamp is used to develop a plane from the femoral tunnels beneath the iliotibial band to the fibula to shuttle the graft proximally.
- The anterior limb of the graft (reconstructing the PFL) should pass deep to the posterior limb of the graft (reconstructing the FCL).
- The posterior limb is shuttled into the FCL tunnel.
- An interference screw is placed within the lateral collateral ligament tunnel.
- Next, with the knee in approximately 30° of flexion, the anterior limb is held up to the aperture of the anterior femoral tunnel and measured.
- 25 to 30 mm of graft is pulled into the tunnel, and any excess graft removed before pulling into the tunnel.
- A whipstitch is then placed into this limb in a similar fashion as the FCL limb.
- The graft is then shuttled into the PFL tunnel.

- With the knee in approximately 30° of flexion and a valgus stress placed, the PFL limb is fixed with an interference screw in similar fashion as the FCL limb.
- Weight bearing is restricted for the first 2 weeks postoperatively or longer per surgeon preference.
  - Rehabilitation commences immediately with quadriceps strengthening as well as seated and supine active and passive knee flexion and extension.
  - Because PLC reconstructions are rarely performed in isolation, rehabilitation guidelines for other ligaments reconstructed should be adhered to.

Top 10 Knowledge Drops for Your Rotation

1. The ACL is composed of an anteromedial and posterolateral bundle, whereas the PCL is composed of an anterolateral and posteromedial bundle.
2. The Lachman and pivot shift tests are used to assess the integrity of the ACL. The Lachman test assesses for excessive anterior translation of the tibia, whereas the pivot shift test assesses for anterolateral rotatory instability.
3. Most MCL injuries are successfully managed nonsurgically. Injuries at the tibial insertion, particularly when the ligament is displaced superficial to the pes anserine tendons (Stener lesion), have a lower propensity for healing and may warrant surgical treatment.
4. PCL injuries typically occur with a posteriorly directed force onto the tibia of a flexed knee, such as a dashboard injury during a motor vehicle accident.
5. CPN injuries may occur in the setting of posterolateral PLC injuries. Neurovascular injuries are common in the setting of knee dislocations and should be suspected in the setting of low-energy knee ligament injuries in patients with obesity.
6. The lateral intercondylar ridge, or resident's ridge, is located within the lateral wall of the intercondylar notch. There are no native ACL fibers that attach anterior to this ridge.

7. The most common reason for failure of ACL reconstruction is tunnel malpositioning. The femoral tunnel is often placed excessively high in the notch (vertical tunnel) and/or excessively anterior.
8. Following ACL reconstruction, the surgeon and physical therapist should emphasize the importance of early recovery of terminal extension and quadriceps strengthening.
9. Failure rates following ACL reconstruction using allograft in young, athletic populations are three to four times higher than ACL reconstructions using autograft.
10. When performing a PLC reconstruction, the CPN is located posterior to the biceps femoris and must be identified and protected throughout the case.

References

1. Kazley JM, Banerjee S: Classifications in brief: The Dejour classification of trochlear dysplasia. *Clin Orthop Relat Res* 2019;477(10):2380-2386.
2. Shu L, Ni Q, Yang X, Chen B, Wang H, Chen L: Comparative study of the tibial tubercle-trochlear groove distance measured in two ways and tibial tubercle-posterior cruciate ligament distance in patients with patellofemoral instability. *J Orthop Surg Res* 2020;15(1):209.
3. Fabricant PD, Yen YM, Kramer DE, et al: Fixation of traumatic chondral-only fragments of the knee in pediatric and adolescent athletes: A retrospective multicenter report. *Orthop J Sports Med* 2018;6(2):2325967117753140.
4. Martin RK, Leland DP, Krych AJ, Dahm DL: Treatment of first-time patellar dislocations and evaluation of risk factors for recurrent patellar instability. *Sports Med Arthrosc Rev* 2019;27(4):130-135.
5. Ferrari MB, Sanchez G, Kennedy NI, Sanchez A, Schantz K, Provencher MT: Osteotomy of the tibial tubercle for anteromedialization. *Arthrosc Tech* 2017;6(4):e1341-e1346.
6. Brophy RH, Wojahn RD, Lamplot JD: Cartilage restoration techniques for the patellofemoral joint. *J Am Acad Orthop Surg* 2017;25(5):321-329.
7. Hinckel BB, Pratte EL, Baumann CA, et al: Patellofemoral cartilage restoration: A systematic review and meta-analysis of clinical outcomes. *Am J Sports Med* 2020;48(7):1756-1772.
8. Chambers HG, Chambers RC: The natural history of meniscus tears. *J Pediatr Orthop* 2019;39(6, suppl 1):S53-S55.

9. Fox AJ, Wanivenhaus F, Burge AJ, Warren RF, Rodeo SA: The human meniscus: A review of anatomy, function, injury, and advances in treatment. *Clin Anat* 2015;28(2):269-287.
10. Jarraya M, Roemer FW, Englund M, et al: Meniscus morphology: Does tear type matter? A narrative review with focus on relevance for osteoarthritis research. *Semin Arthritis Rheum* 2017;46(5):552-561.
11. Rodeo SA, Monibi F, Dehghani B, Maher S: Biological and mechanical predictors of meniscus function: Basic science to clinical translation. *J Orthop Res* 2020;38(5):937-945.
12. Fillingham YA, Riboh JC, Erickson BJ, Bach BR Jr, Yanke AB: Inside-out versus all-inside repair of isolated meniscal tears: An updated systematic review. *Am J Sports Med* 2017;45(1):234-242.
13. Cinque ME, Chahla J, Moatshe G, Faucett SC, Krych AJ, LaPrade RF: Meniscal root tears: A silent epidemic. *Br J Sports Med* 2018;52(13):872-876.
14. Kaeding CC, Léger-St-Jean B, Magnussen RA: Epidemiology and diagnosis of anterior cruciate ligament injuries. *Clin Sports Med* 2017;36(1):1-8.
15. Gornitzky AL, Lott A, Yellin JL, Fabricant PD, Lawrence JT, Ganley TJ: Sport-specific yearly risk and incidence of anterior cruciate ligament tears in high school athletes: A systematic review and meta-analysis. *Am J Sports Med* 2016;44(10):2716-2723.
16. Bedi A, Musahl V, Cowan JB: Management of posterior cruciate ligament injuries: An evidence-based review. *J Am Acad Orthop Surg* 2016;24(5):277-289.
17. Serra Cruz R, Mitchell JJ, Dean CS, Chahla J, Moatshe G, LaPrade RF: Anatomic posterolateral corner reconstruction. *Arthrosc Tech* 2016;5(3):e563-e572.
18. Serra Cruz R, Olivetto J, Dean CS, Chahla J, LaPrade RF: Superficial medial collateral ligament of the knee: Anatomic augmentation with semitendinosus and gracilis tendon autografts. *Arthrosc Tech* 2016;5(2):e347-e352.
19. Kaeding CC, Pedroza AD, Reinke EK, et al: Change in anterior cruciate ligament graft choice and outcomes over time. *Arthroscopy* 2017;33(11):2007-2014.
20. Chahla J, von Bormann R, Engebretsen L, LaPrade RF: Anatomic posterior cruciate ligament reconstruction: State of the art. *Joint Disorders Orthop Sports Med* 2016;1(5):292-302.
21. Treme GP, Salas C, Ortiz G, et al: A biomechanical comparison of the Arciero and laprade reconstruction for posterolateral corner knee injuries. *Orthop J Sports Med* 2019;7(4):2325967119838251.

10. I Need a Joint Replacement

Melvyn A. Harrington, Jr, MD, FAAOS, FAOA
Javad Parvizi, MD, FRCS, FAAOS • Matthew Blue, MD
Graham Goh, MD • Brian I. Nwannunu, MD

INTRODUCTION

Osteoarthritis is one of the leading causes of pain and disability. It is caused by the degeneration of articular cartilage. The hip and knee are two of the most commonly affected joints. Hip and knee arthritis can commonly be managed nonsurgically to alleviate pain and improve patient function. However, when nonsurgical measures are unsuccessful, total hip or knee arthroplasty can be considered. Total joint arthroplasty is one of the most commonly performed elective surgical procedures in the United States, with an annual volume projected to exceed two million procedures over the next decade. The outcomes of total joint arthroplasty are excellent overall, with most patients experiencing decreased pain and improved function for many years.

Dr. Harrington or an immediate family member serves as a paid consultant to or is an employee of Zimmer; has received research or institutional support from Smith & Nephew; and serves as a board member, owner, officer, or committee member of American Orthopaedic Association, Arthritis Foundation, and J. Robert Gladden Society. Dr. Parvizi or an immediate family member has received royalties from Corentec; serves as a paid consultant to or is an employee of Corentec, Ethicon, Fidia Pharm, Heraeus, Jointstem, KCI/3M (Acelity), MicroGenDx, Peptilogics, Tenor, and Zimmer Biomet; and has stock or stock options held in Acumed, LLC, Alphaeon, Ceribell, Corentec, Hip Innovation Technology, Intellijoint, Joint Purification Systems, MDValuate, MicroGenDx, Molecular Surface Technologies, Nanooxygenic, Parvizi Surgical Innovations and Subsidiaries, PRN-Veterinary, PRN-Veterinary, and Sonata. None of the following authors or any immediate family member has received anything of value from or has stock or stock options held in a commercial company or institution related directly or indirectly to the subject of this chapter: Dr. Blue, Dr. Goh, and Dr. Nwannunu.

Epidemiology

- Osteoarthritis: a degenerative disease of synovial joints that causes a progressive loss of articular cartilage
  - Primarily affects older individuals and has a significant economic and social burden
- Incidence
  - Hip osteoarthritis: approximately 100 per 100,000 individuals per year[1]
  - Knee osteoarthritis: 200 per 100,000 individuals per year[1]
  - Both hip and knee osteoarthritis are expected to increase in conjunction with the increase in the elderly population and the incidence of obesity.[2]
- Difficult to place value on the social burden
  - Many patients report decreased enjoyment of activities or altogether missing key life events because of the discomfort imparted by arthritis of the hip and knee.
  - It has been estimated that osteoarthritis causes an economic burden of approximately 3% of the gross domestic product as a result of the work hours missed by patients with hip and knee pain caused by osteoarthritis.[3]

Pertinent Anatomy/Pathoanatomy, Pathophysiology, and Risk Factors

- Both the knee and hip are classic examples of synovial joints, which allow movement and distribute the weight of the body.
  - Joint ends are capped with articular cartilage.
  - Five types of cartilage throughout the human body:
    - Fibroelastic cartilage, as seen in the meniscus of the knee
    - Fibrocartilage, often seen at tendon or ligament insertions
    - Elastic cartilage, found in the auricle of the external ear among other places
    - Physeal cartilage, found in the growth plates of bones
    - Hyaline or articular cartilage—focus of this chapter
  - Each cartilage type serves a different structural function and has slightly different composition to help facilitate the individual function.
- Hyaline (articular) cartilage is composed of chondrocytes (cells) and extracellular matrix.

- Embryologically, chondrocytes are derived from chondroblasts, which come from the mesenchymal stem cell lineage.
  - This is a complex, multistep process that involves several transcription factors that dictate stem cell differentiation, migration, and ultimate formation of hyaline cartilage.
  - Key transcription factor involved in this process is SOX-9.
- When fully developed, the chondrocytes are responsible for the production of collagen, proteoglycans, and various enzymes.
  - They are also the metabolically active component of hyaline cartilage.
- Chondrocytes respond to both mechanical stimuli (changes in mechanical load or hydrostatic pressure) and chemical stimuli (cytokines and growth factor response).
- The noncellular aspect of hyaline cartilage is the extracellular matrix.
  - When listed in order of decreasing percentage of cartilage weight, this matrix is composed of water, collagen, proteoglycans, and small amounts of noncollagenous proteins.
  - Water makes up anywhere from 65% to 80% of the mass of cartilage depending on the layer of cartilage being sampled.
    - The total water content of cartilage decreases with normal aging.
    - However, with the pathologic process of osteoarthritis there is an increase in water content of cartilage.
    - This increase leads to increased permeability, decreased strength, and decreased Young modulus of elasticity.
  - Collagen accounts for approximately 10% to 20% of total cartilage mass.
    - Hyaline cartilage is composed of 90% to 95% type II collagen.
      - The small remaining portion is varying amounts of type V, VI, IX, and XI collagen.
    - The function of collagen is to provide the tensile strength and overall structural framework of the extracellular matrix.

- Proteoglycans are the last major contributor to extracellular matrix composition.
  - They make up 10% to 15% of cartilage weight and provide the hydrophilic behavior and compressive strength of cartilage.
  - As their name suggests, proteoglycans are composed of a core protein heavily glycosylated with chondroitin and keratan sulfate glycosaminoglycan subunits.
  - Aggrecan is the most abundant proteoglycan in hyaline cartilage and is responsible for the hydrophilic behavior of the extracellular matrix.
- Normal articular cartilage is composed of three distinct layers or zones—with distinct chemical composition, collagen orientation, and chondrocyte morphology—before the tidemark (**Figure 1**).
  - Outermost zone (layer in contact with synovial fluid): the superficial (tangential) zone
    - Characterized by flat chondrocytes and type II collagen fibers that run parallel to the surface of the joint
    - Has highest concentration of collagen and lowest concentration of proteoglycans of all the layers
  - Next layer: intermediate zone
    - Thickest zone of the hyaline cartilage
    - The collagen fibers are arranged in an oblique and often random orientation.
  - Final zone: deep (basal) layer
    - Has round chondrocytes that are arranged in columns
    - Has the highest concentration of proteoglycans and lowest concentration of collagen
    - The collagen fibers of the deep layers are arranged perpendicular to the joint surface.
- Articular cartilage composition changes with normal aging, and these changes differ from the changes seen in osteoarthritis.
  - Although an increasingly common pathology in older adults, osteoarthritis is a distinct pathology different from the normal aging process.

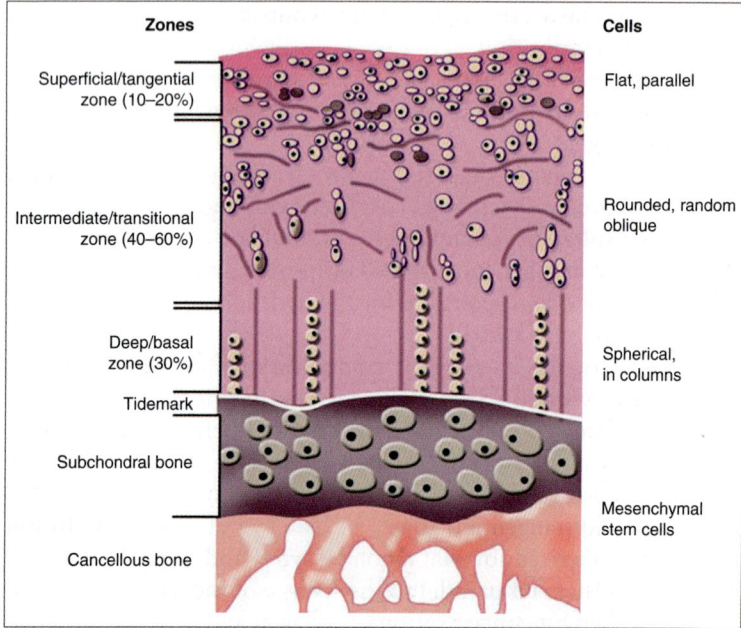

Figure 1 Illustration shows articular cartilage zones demonstrating the morphology and orientation of the cells in each layer. (Reproduced with permission from Clohisy J, Beaule P, Della Valle C, Callaghan JJ, Rosenberg AG, Rubash HE, eds: *The Adult Hip*. Wolters Kluwer, 2014, Figure 4-1.)

- Both normal aging and osteoarthritis show a decrease in the number of chondrocytes present in the articular cartilage.
  - The chondrocytes that remain tend to be larger and in the setting of late osteoarthritis cluster together.
  - The water content of the articular cartilage differs between the two processes.
    - Normal aging: cartilage tends to dry out, with an overall decreased water content, which, along with an increase in glycation of proteins, leads to a higher Young modulus (stiffer, less elastic)

- Osteoarthritis: cartilage changes lead to a softening of the cartilage, which leads to an increased water content, resulting in a decreased Young modulus
- Differences are also seen in the collagen present in the cartilage.
    - Normal aging: collagen becomes increasingly cross-linked, which leads to increased brittleness
    - Osteoarthritis: increased collagenase activity, resulting in disorganized collagen fibrils and subsequently, less brittle cartilage
- Important chemical distinctions can also be made in the composition of proteoglycans and their respective glycosaminoglycan subunits.
    - In both normal aging and osteoarthritis, there tends to be a decrease in proteoglycan size; the difference lies in the ratio of the glycosaminoglycan subunits.
        - Normal aging: increased keratan sulfate to chondroitin sulfate ratio
        - Osteoarthritis: increased ratio of chondroitin sulfate to keratan sulfate
- A pathologic process, osteoarthritis produces inflammation and degradation not seen with normal aging.
    - Increase in inflammatory cytokines (interleukins 1 and 6, tumor necrosis factor alpha) results in synovial inflammation, leading to a vicious cycle of joint destruction.
        - The inflammatory cytokines result in an increase in matrix metalloproteases such as stromelysin, which function to break down the extracellular matrix.
        - This increased damage results in further release of inflammatory cytokines and the cycle continues to propagate.
    - This cycle of joint destruction can be seen on a gross level as well.
        - Early stages of osteoarthritis: mild inflammatory changes to the synovium
        - Middle phase: synovium becomes hypervascular because of its prolonged inflamed state

- As the friable cartilage becomes damaged, it leads to changes in the bone, with the subchondral bone attempting to remodel and forming sclerotic edges.
- Eventually, osteophytes form from the pathologic activation of endochondral bone formation using the Indian hedgehog signaling pathway, and ultimately bone cysts develop.
- Risk factors for developing osteoarthritis?
  - Complex and not entirely well understood concept
    - Few known modifiable risks factors for its development
    - Pathogenesis is multifactorial and linked to both systemic and local factors
  - Risk increases as patients age and with patient body habitus
  - Possible differences in patient's risk based on sex, ethnicity, race (hormonal factors), nutrition, and even specific genes[2]
    - Systemic factors are often nonmodifiable, but it is important to have a good understanding of these factors to properly counsel patients.
  - Local factors, specific to a given joint
    - Anatomic abnormalities and malalignment
    - Occupation, history of injury, or even sports participation can alter the risk of the development of arthritis.
    - Local factors are often more modifiable, but it can be difficult to tease out the influence of local effects from the more systemic risks.

Pertinent History/Physical Examination Findings

- Symptoms: pain in the joint, stiffness, functional limitations, and often mechanical symptoms such as instability, locking, and catching.
- Inspection: Look at body habitus, limb alignment, and check for the presence of an effusion.
- Evaluate patient's gait; patients with arthritis often have a shortened stride length and with knee arthritis an increased adductor moment (antalgic limp).
- Check range of motion; range of motion often decreases as arthritis progresses.

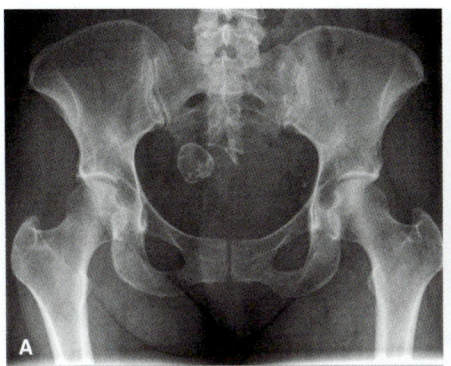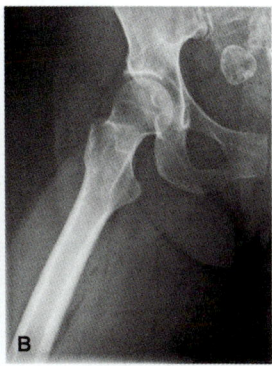

Figure 2 **A**, AP radiograph of the pelvis. **B**, Lateral radiographic view of the right hip.

- Evaluate the patient holistically, keeping in mind comorbidities because they can ultimately affect treatment options and outcomes.

Relevant Imaging

- Radiography: main imaging modality
  - Hip: AP view of the pelvis and lateral view of the affected hip (**Figure 2**)
    - Some physicians will recommend a false profile view or cross-table lateral view.
    - The lumbar spine also should be evaluated because this can affect symptoms and treatment.
  - Knee: AP, lateral, and patellofemoral view weight-bearing views (**Figure 3**)
  - Radiographic findings of osteoarthritis: joint-space narrowing, osteophyte formation, subchondral sclerosis, and cysts
- Advanced imaging such as MRI is rarely beneficial and should not be routinely ordered in the setting of osteoarthritis.

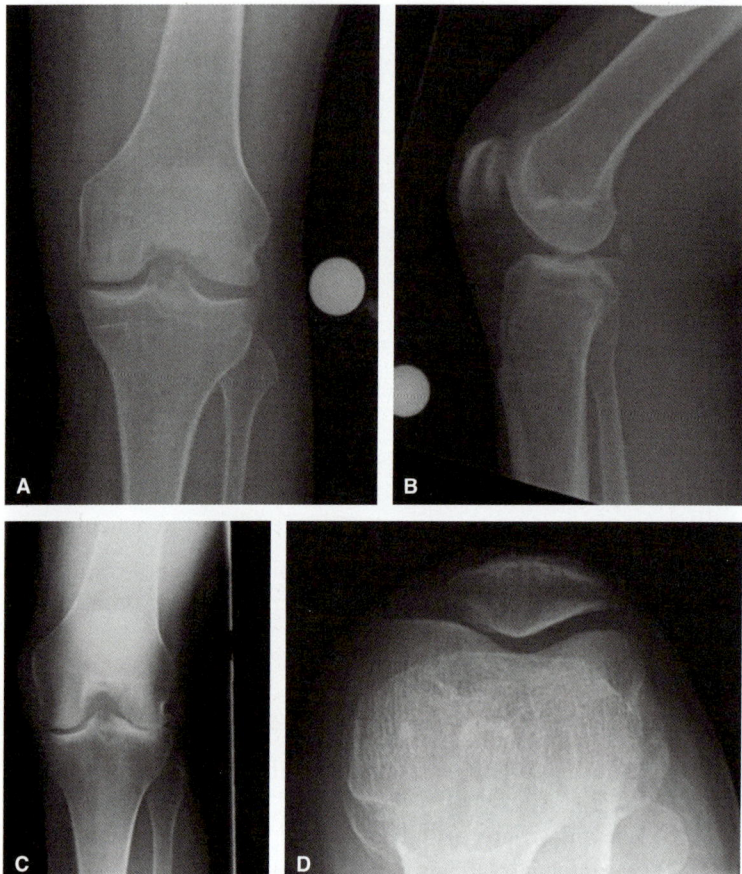

Figure 3 Radiographs of the left knee. **A**, AP view. **B**, Lateral view. **C**, Rosenberg view. **D**, Sunrise view. (Reproduced with permission from Miller MD, Dempsey IJ, eds: *Making the Diagnosis in Orthopaedics: A Video-Enhanced Guide to Identifying Musculoskeletal Disorders*. Wolters Kluwer, 2019, Figure 1-5.)

Top 10 Knowledge Drops for Your Rotation

1. Osteoarthritis is defined as a degenerative disease of synovial joints that causes a progressive loss of articular cartilage.
2. Hip and knee osteoarthritis is a major cause of disability in the United States.
3. Articular cartilage is found in synovial joints and is one of the five main types of cartilage.
4. Chondrocytes are derived from chondroblasts and are the main cell in articular cartilage.
5. SOX-9 is the main transcription factor involved in chondrocyte differentiation.
6. Osteoarthritis results in increased water content of the cartilage.
7. Type II collagen is the main type of collagen found in articular cartilage.
8. Aggrecan is the most abundant proteoglycan in articular cartilage.
9. The main patient complaint of osteoarthritis is pain.
10. The main imaging modality for diagnosis of arthritis is radiographs; advanced imaging is rarely needed.

TOTAL KNEE ARTHROPLASTY

Total knee arthroplasty (TKA) is a valuable intervention for patients who have severe daily pain along with radiographic evidence of arthritis or degenerative joint disease (DJD) of the knee. The natural history of DJD is typically progression of disease, leading to increasing pain and disability. Over time, symptoms usually become more severe, frequent, and debilitating.

Pertinent History/Physical Examination Findings

- Key findings in patient history: pain that is better with rest and worse with increased activities, stiffness, swelling, subjective instability or giving away of the knee, and history of prior knee injury or surgery

- Key findings on physical examination: progressive varus or valgus deformities, an antalgic gait, limp, muscle atrophy, effusion, joint line or patellofemoral tenderness to palpation, painful and limited range of motion, and crepitus
- Certain activities classically affected in patients with DJD of the knee: pain with walking and weight bearing; difficulty descending steps, standing from the seated position, and getting in and out of a car
- Radiographs: decreased joint space, osteophytes, subchondral sclerosis, and bone cysts

Nonsurgical Measures

- Health and behavior modifications: physical therapy, weight loss, and knee braces
- Pharmacotherapy: acetaminophen and topical and oral NSAIDs are strongly recommended, whereas glucosamine and/or chondroitin sulfate have a limited recommendation
- Intra-articular injections: corticosteroids are recommended. Hyaluronic acid injections are not recommended.

Surgical Intervention

- Knee replacement surgery is typically reserved for those patients in whom several methods of nonsurgical treatment have failed.
- Surgical management for DJD of the knee can be further subdivided into nonarthroplasty and arthroplasty options.
  - Nonarthroplasty options: osteotomy, arthroscopy, and synovectomy
  - Arthroplasty options: unicompartmental knee arthroplasty, TKA
    - Unicompartmental knee arthroplasty
      - Indications as delineated by Kozin et al[4] and Kozin and Scott:[5] isolated medial compartmental DJD (no lateral compartment arthritis, only mild patellofemoral arthritis on Merchant view); no lateral joint line tenderness; intact anterior cruciate ligament (in wear pattern on lateral radiograph of the knee, posterior tibial bone loss indicates disrupted anterior cruciate ligament because the tibia has shifted anteriorly without the anterior cruciate ligament restraint, exposing the posterior tibia to contact stresses from the distal femoral condyles); noninflammatory arthritis; weight

less than 82 kg; correctable varus deformity (less than 5° deformity); patient age older than 60 years; flexion contracture less than 5°; range of motion greater than 90°
- These criteria served as the foundation for patient selection for years, yet recent studies and surgeons have questioned those previously established thresholds and have expanded indications to include no age limit, higher body mass index, and acceptance of greater angular deformity measurements (increasing the flexion contracture to less than 15°, and less than 10° varus or 5° valgus deformity)[6]
- Technique of TKA
  - Incision
    - Classically, anterior longitudinal midline incision made from approximately three to four fingerbreadths above the superior pole of the patella proximally to the inferior medial aspect of the tibial tuberosity distally
    - General principles to consider for TKA incisions: prior scars should be taken into consideration to preserve vascularity, preexisting anterior longitudinal scars should be incorporated when possible, and when parallel anterior longitudinal scars are present, the one most lateral should be used if possible
      - If it is not possible to use a prior incision, a wide skin bridge of at least 8 cm should be allowed between the new incision and previous scar.
      - Horizontal scars can be crossed at right angles, and short oblique scars may be ignored.
  - Arthrotomy approaches
    - After the skin incision has been made, full-thickness skin flaps are created and then an arthrotomy can be performed.
    - Most common arthrotomy approaches: medial parapatellar, subvastus (Southern), and midvastus
      - Medial parapatellar approach: quadriceps tendon is cut longitudinally from proximal to distal along its medial border, leaving a cuff of tendon 5 to 10 mm wide, then the arthrotomy is carried further distally, skirting along the medial border of the patella and patellar tendon

- Subvastus approach: blunt dissection is carried from the medial intermuscular septum; a transverse incision is made at the midpatella through the medial retinaculum inferior to the vastus medialis and is stopped once the patellar tendon is reached, and then a second incision is made along the medial border of the patellar tendon to the tibial tubercle
- Midvastus approach (**Figure 4**): blunt finger dissection is begun at the superomedial pole of the patella in the midsubstance and through the full thickness of the vastus medialis muscle, and is extended parallel to its fibers, to a maximum of 4 cm proximal medial to this starting

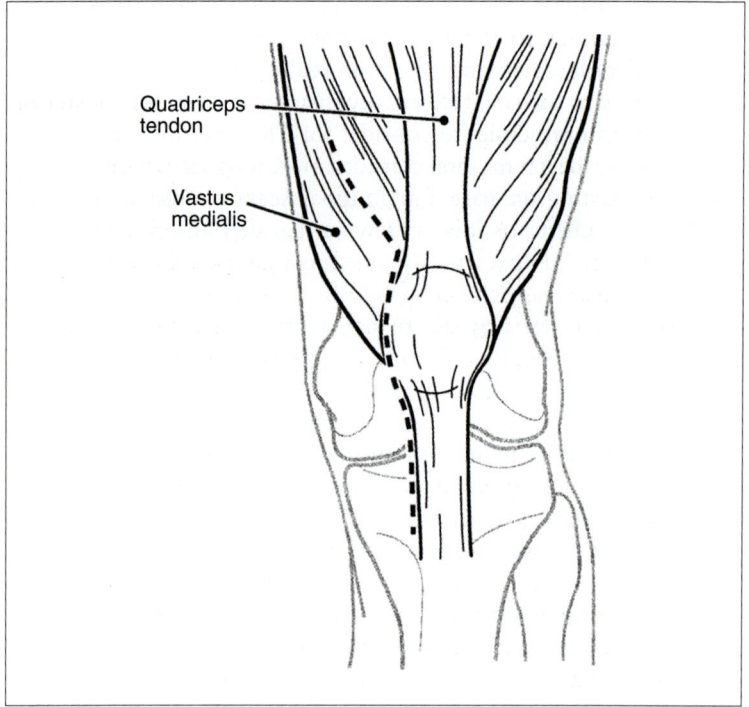

Figure 4 Illustration shows the midvastus approach to the knee. (Reprinted from Engh GA, Holt BP, Parks NL: A midvastus muscle splitting approach for total knee arthroplasty. *J Arthroplasty* 1997;12[3]:322-331. Copyright 1997, with permission from Elsevier.)

Chapter 10: I Need a Joint Replacement

point, then the incision is taken similar to the previous approaches distally along the medial border of the patellar tendon to the tibial tubercle
- The decision regarding which approach to use is determined by surgeon preference, as the most current data indicate that the results following TKA using any of these approaches are similar.[7]
- Bone preparation
  - Either the femur or the tibia can be prepared first for a TKA
  - Standard bone cuts for any TKA:
    - Distal femoral condylar resection
    - Anterior and posterior condylar resections
    - Anterior and posterior chamfer resections from the distal femur
    - Transverse proximal tibial resection
    - Retropatellar cut in patellar resurfacing
    - Intercondylar box cut—performed only for posterior-stabilized designs
  - The order of the bone cuts and decision of whether to use a cruciate-retaining TKA or posterior-stabilized (cruciate-substituting) TKA is determined by surgeon preference.
  - Classically, bone cuts are made to align the implanted knee prosthesis perpendicular to the mechanical axis of the lower extremity, thereby distributing weight-bearing forces evenly between medial and lateral compartments (**Figure 5**).
    - Some surgeons have begun advocating for making bone cuts relative to the kinematic axis of the knee, a technique that seeks to restore the native tibia varus and femoral valgus as opposed to referencing the mechanical axis of the lower extremity.[8]
- Femoral component rotation
  - Making accurate cuts is essential to obtaining proper size and rotation of the final femoral component, and achieving appropriate femoral rotation is critical for patellar tracking.
  - There are four basic techniques to setting femoral rotation.
    - Three use femoral anatomic landmarks and are known as measured resection techniques for achieving appropriate femoral rotation.

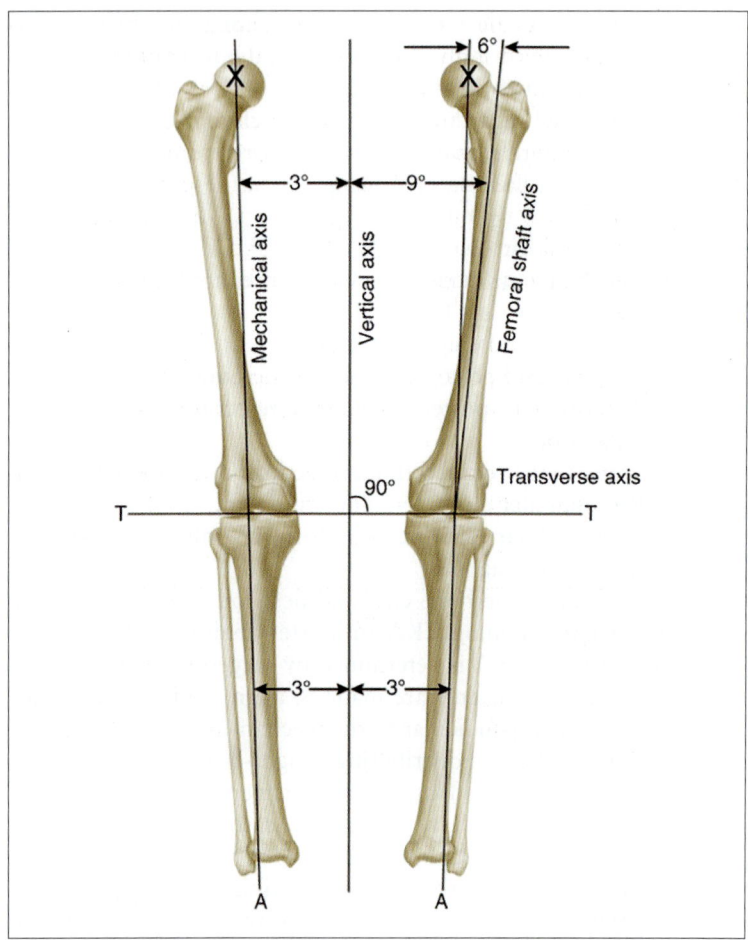

Figure 5 Illustrations demonstrate mechanical and anatomic axes of the lower extremities. A = anatomic, T = transverse (Reprinted from McCarty EC, McAllister DR, Leonard JP: Anatomy and biomechanics of the knee, in Lieberman JR, ed: *AAOS Comprehensive Orthopaedic Review*, ed 3. American Academy of Orthopaedic Surgeons, 2019, p 1250.)

- Perpendicular to the Whiteside line (the trans-sulcus line, which is a line drawn from the top of the intercondylar notch to the deepest part of the femoral trochlea)[9]
- Parallel to the transepicondylar axis
- Aligning the cutting block in 3° of external rotation relative to the posterior condylar axis (**Figure 6**)
  - The fourth technique—gap balancing—is independent of femoral anatomic landmarks, instead using the flat proximal tibial resection and ligament balance to set femoral rotation.
  - Most surgeons use a combination of all four techniques and multiple reference points to help reduce any error in setting the rotation of the femoral component.
- Tibial rotation
  - At least three ways have been described to orient the rotational alignment of the tibial component.

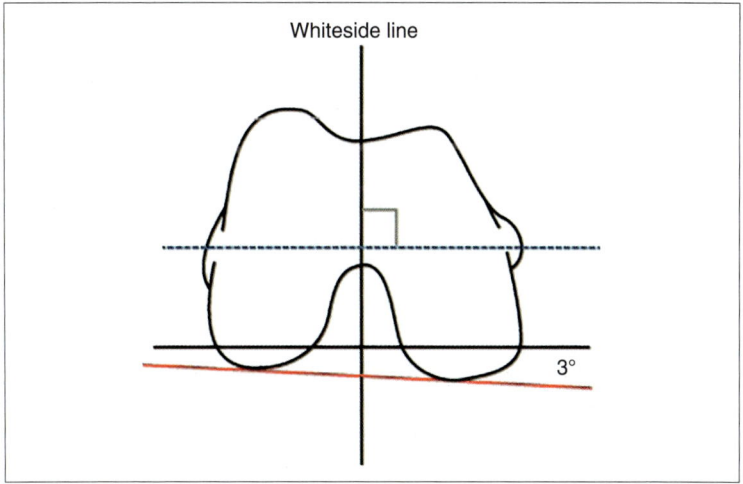

Figure 6 Drawing shows references for rotational alignment on the distal femur demonstrating the epicondylar axis, the posterior condylar axis, and Whiteside line. (Reproduced with permission from Zikria B, ed: *The Johns Hopkins High-Yield Review for Orthopaedic Surgery*. Wolters Kluwer, 2019, Figure 2-7.)

- The first method is to use an asymmetric or anatomic tibial tray that mimics the cut surface of the tibia and apply the tray anatomically.
- The second method is to align the tibial rotation based on the tibial tubercle; the most commonly used landmark is the junction between the medial and central thirds of the tubercle.
- The third method is known as floating the tibia component during the trial range of motion, which allows the fixed femoral component articulation to set the rotation of the tibial component to achieve proper patellar tracking.
- No matter which method is chosen, it is important to avoid internal rotation of the tibial component, because this can result in significant patellar tracking problems.
- Patellar resurfacing
  - Often, but not always performed during TKA
  - Patellar preparation can be done at any point in the procedure.
    - Preparation immediately following the initial approach can facilitate exposure for the rest of the procedure.
    - The patella cut can be performed using a patellar cutting jig, mill, or freehand technique with an oscillating saw.
  - Regardless of technique, the goal is to make a flat cut and place the patellar button superiorly and medially to help achieve optimum patellar tracking within the femoral trochlea.
    - A caliper is used to assess the patellar thickness before the cut and after the patella is resurfaced.
    - Care must be taken to avoid overstuffing the patellofemoral compartment, as this can adversely affect flexion and tracking.
    - A minimum of 12 mm of patellar bone stock must remain after patellar resection, because less than 12 mm of bone stock is associated with a higher risk of postoperative patella fracture and osteonecrosis.
- Balancing the knee
  - After component positioning is achieved, trial component insertion and reduction are performed.
  - At this time, final balancing of the knee is assessed and any necessary adjustments are performed to ensure flexion and extension gap symmetry.

- The flexion gap is the space created by the tibial cut surface and the posterior femur.
 - The extension space is created by the tibia and distal femur.
 - The collateral ligaments form the sides of these rectangular spaces.
- The goal of balancing the knee is to achieve equal flexion and extension gaps with symmetric tension on the collateral ligaments.
- **Table 1** provides a general guide to aid in correcting gap asymmetries during the trial phase.
- Fixation strategies
  - TKA components can be fixed with either bone cement or press-fit technique.
  - Cementation is currently the primary mode of TKA fixation in the United States, but press-fit designs are gaining popularity.
  - When cement technique is used, polymethyl methacrylate is used for fixation of the components.
    - Before cementation, it is important to prepare the cut bony surfaces by using pulsatile lavage to thoroughly irrigate the bone, remove all debris, and then subsequently dry the bone completely with suction and dry gauze.
    - It is important to remove all excess cement particles from the joint to avoid third-body wear.
  - Although cemented fixation of TKA components remains the gold standard, increasing demand among young and active patients, coupled with an increasing life expectancy, has spurred growing interest in the use of press-fit options.[10]

TABLE 1 Techniques to Balance the Flexion and Extension Gaps in Total Knee Arthroplasty

		Extension Gap	
		Tight	**Loose**
Flexion Gap	Tight	Use thinner tibial insert Resect additional tibia	Augment distal femur Anteriorize femoral component Downsize femoral component (anterior referencing system only)
	Loose	Release posterior soft tissues Resect additional distal femur Augment posterior only	Use thicker tibial insert

- Midterm to long-term studies have demonstrated no significant differences in the clinical outcomes between the cemented and cementless groups.
- One such study concluded that over a minimum 8-year postoperative period the mean ranges of knee movement and radiologic results were similar in both groups, no osteolysis was identified in either group, and the rate of survival of the femoral and tibial components was 100% in both groups at final follow-up.[11]
- Constraint in implant design
  - One of the keys to long-term success in TKA is knee joint stability.
    - Soft-tissue balancing in the coronal plane is performed by releasing the contracted ligament on the concave side of the deformity.
    - The extent of the releases will be based on the degree of deformity.
  - Cruciate-retaining or cruciate-substituting (posterior-stabilized) implants (**Figure 7**)

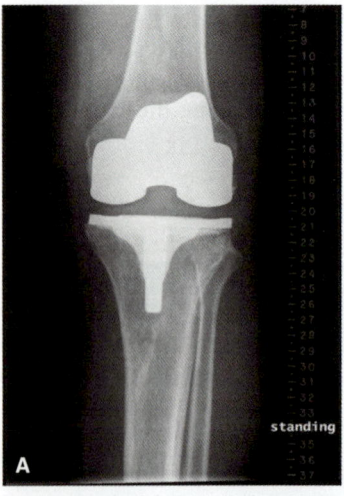 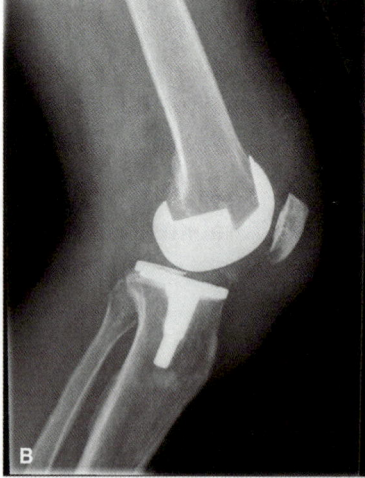

Figure 7 **A**, AP and lateral (**B**) radiographs demonstrating a cemented posterior-stabilized total knee arthroplasty.

- After the coronal plane stability has been established, standard implants, including cruciate-retaining or posterior-stabilized knee implants, may be used.
- A posterior-stabilized implant provides stability in the sagittal plane and prevents posterior translation of the tibia relative to the femur, but it does not provide an increase in coronal plane stability.
- Constrained implants
  - It can be difficult to obtain adequate coronal plane soft-tissue balancing in severely deformed knees.
    - When ligament balancing is not possible and there is persistent varus or valgus laxity, more constraint is required.
    - In this setting, a constrained prosthesis design should be used to prevent medial or lateral instability and recurrent deformity.
  - Constrained designs have tibial posts that are higher and wider in comparison with standard posterior-stabilized designs.
    - Useful for coronal plane instability where a collateral ligament is still present although lax
- Hinge implants
  - In the setting of a severely damaged knee where there is an incompetent or absent ligament, or hyperextension, a constrained design will not provide adequate stabilization of the joint, and a hinge design must be used.
  - The hinge design allows for the restoration of knee joint stability that the other less constrained designs cannot provide in the severely damaged knee, particularly when there has been massive bone loss and absent ligament support.
  - Gradations in constraint improve stability and are useful in certain settings, but it is also important to keep in mind that increasing constraint leads to increased loads to the implant fixation interfaces, which can carry a risk for earlier failure rates.
  - The least amount of constraint necessary should therefore be used. Still, joint stability is one of the key goals to long-term success of TKA.[12]

- Postoperative management
  - Rehabilitation protocols vary but typically include early mobilization and initiation of weight-bearing activities, early range of motion, appropriate pain management, and weaning off assistive devices as tolerated.
  - Current analgesic strategies use a multimodal approach to pain management.
  - Antibiotics are typically administered for one or two doses postoperatively.
  - Patients should also be placed on a venous thromboembolism prophylaxis protocol, although the exact regimen used varies by surgeon.
  - Patients are typically discharged, either to home or to an inpatient rehabilitation facility.
  - Surgeries can also be performed on an outpatient basis in appropriately selected patients.
  - Once strength, mobility, and balance are regained, patients can resume low-impact sport activities such as cycling, swimming, walking, hiking, golf, or bowling.
  - Higher impact activities such as basketball, soccer, and football are generally discouraged.
- Outcomes
  - Survivorship of TKA is related to appropriate alignment and balance.
    - In patients with correct positioning of the tibial and femoral components both axially and rotationally, there was considerable improvement in functional outcome and excellent long-term clinical survivorship.[13]
    - Recently reported survival rates were noted to be above 85% at up to 23 years of follow-up, with favorable gains for pain and functionality.[14]
  - Most patients have high overall satisfaction rates with good to excellent results.
  - Lower satisfaction rates: younger patients (younger than 50 years), morbidly obese patients (body mass index greater than 40 kg/m^2), patients with prior reconstructive surgery, and patients receiving workers' compensation
    - These patients deserve special consideration and should undergo counseling before surgical intervention.

Chapter 10: I Need a Joint Replacement

Top 10 Knowledge Drops for Your Rotation

1. Surgical management for DJD of the knee can be subdivided into arthroplasty and nonarthroplasty options. The nonarthroplasty surgical options, which are primarily for the knee, include osteotomy, arthroscopy, and synovectomy. The arthroplasty options include unicompartmental knee arthroplasty or TKA.
2. There are general principles to consider for TKA incisions and these include the following: prior scars should be taken into consideration to preserve vascularity, preexisting anterior longitudinal scars should be incorporated when possible, and when parallel anterior longitudinal scars are present, the one most lateral should be used if possible.
3. The most common arthrotomy approaches include the medial parapatellar, subvastus (Southern), and midvastus approaches. The most current data indicate that the results following TKA using any of these approaches are similar.
4. There are six standard bone cuts for any TKA: (1) distal femoral condylar resection, (2) anterior and posterior condylar resections, (3) anterior and posterior chamfer resections from the distal femur, (4) transverse proximal tibial resection, (5) retropatellar cut in patellar resurfacing, and (6) the intercondylar box cut, which is performed only for posterior-stabilized designs.
5. Classically, bone cuts are made to align the implanted knee prosthesis perpendicular to the mechanical axis of the lower extremity; more recently, some surgeons have advocated for making bone cuts relative to the kinematic axis of the knee.
6. There are four basic techniques to setting femoral rotation, three of which use femoral anatomic landmarks: (1) perpendicular to the Whiteside line, (2) parallel to the transepicondylar axis, or (3) aligning the cutting block in 3° of external rotation relative to the posterior condylar axis. The fourth technique is known as the gap balancing technique and is independent of femoral anatomic landmarks.
7. Three methods have been described to orient the rotational alignment of the tibial component: (1) use of an asymmetric tray that mimics the cut surface of the tibia and apply the tray anatomically, (2) alignment of the tibial rotation based on

the tibial tubercle; most commonly the junction between the medial and central thirds of the tubercle, and (3) the method known as floating the tibial component during the trial range of motion.
8. During knee balancing, the flexion gap is the space created by the tibial cut surface and the posterior femur. The extension space is created by the tibia and distal femur. The collateral ligaments form the sides of these rectangular spaces.
9. TKA components can either be fixed with bone cement or press-fit technique. Cementation is the primary mode of TKA fixation currently in the United States, but press-fit designs are gaining popularity.
10. Gradations in constraint improve stability and are useful in certain settings, but it is also important to keep in mind that increasing constraint leads to increased loads to the implant fixation interfaces, which can carry a risk for earlier failure rates.

TOTAL HIP ARTHROPLASTY

- Indications
  - The primary indication for total hip arthroplasty (THA) is the same as for knee arthroplasty—functionally limiting pain.
    - This pain is generally described by patients as an achy pain located in the groin and is often aggravated by activity and improved with rest.
    - At the time of surgical intervention, the pain is often advanced to the point that oral medications no longer provide relief.
    - Patients often express difficulty with ambulation, particularly going upstairs and often with activities such as putting on shoes and socks.
  - Imaging typically shows decreased joint space and osteophyte formation.
  - On examination, clinicians will see painful range of motion of the hip and gait changes as previously described.
- Templating
  - Templating is the use of preoperative imaging combined with various computer programming to predict the size and position of implants before surgery.

- This allows the surgeon to ensure availability of implants, predict and account for possible areas of difficulty in the surgery, and more accurately reproduce hip biomechanics and leg length.
- AP pelvis radiograph is used when creating a template.
  - It is important to ensure this radiograph is centered over the pubis and the femur is correctly positioned in approximately 10° to 15° of internal rotation.
- Establish the patient's leg length discrepancy by using a horizontal line to connect the ischial tuberosities of the pelvis.
  - When drawing this line, make sure to take the line out past the lateral cortex of the femur on each side.
  - Mark the most proximal aspect of the lesser trochanter and measure the distance between this point and the horizontal line.
  - When completed bilaterally, these values should be equal in a patient without a leg length discrepancy.
  - Any difference is the leg length discrepancy (**Figure 8**).
- The computer software will often measure the diameter of the femoral head/acetabulum and give a predicted acetabular

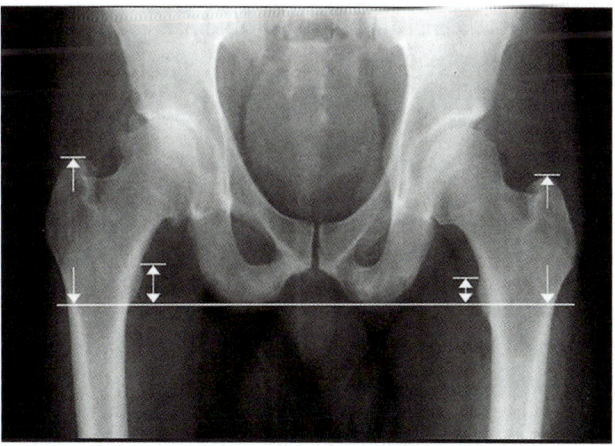

Figure 8 Leg length discrepancies can be determined on an AP radiograph of the pelvis by measuring the distance between a fixed reference line on the pelvis and references on the femur. In this case a line is drawn along the ischium on each side, and measured relative to the greater or lesser trochanters as shown by the arrows.

component size based on the specific implant the surgeon selects for the procedure.
- After this size is determined, the cup is placed into approximately 40° to 45° of abduction with the medial border of the cup at the ilioischial line and the inferior border of the cup level with the inferior aspect of the teardrop.
- Likewise, the computer software will provide femoral component sizes based on the specific implant selected.
  - The surgeon selects the stem size, head size, and neck-shaft angle that appropriately fits the patient and restores appropriate offset (distance between the center of rotation of the femoral head and a line bisecting the long axis of the femur) and leg length.
- Technique
  - Approaches
    - When performing a THA, one of the first decisions to be addressed is the surgical approach.
      - There are several approach variations, and to the young surgeon or medical student they can easily become complicated and confusing.
      - These approaches can be grouped according to location of the skin incision, whether anterior, lateral, or posterior.
  - Anterior approach
    - The patient is positioned supine, and an intraoperative radiograph, brought in from the contralateral side, is often used.
    - Skin incision is made approximately 2 cm distal and 3 cm lateral to the anterior superior iliac spine.
      - This incision is general 8 to 10 cm long and angles slightly lateral over the tensor fascia lata muscle.
    - This approach uses the superficial interval between the tensor fascia lata (superior gluteal nerve) and the sartorius (femoral nerve).
      - The deep plane is between the rectus femoris (femoral nerve) and gluteus medius (superior gluteal nerve).
      - When performing superficial dissection, care must be taken to avoid injury to the lateral femoral cutaneous nerve.
      - Care must be taken to identify and ligate the ascending branch of the lateral femoral circumflex artery.

- As deep dissection proceeds, the plane between the rectus femoris and the gluteus medius will be identified first.
  - The rectus is detached from both of its origins, which will allow retraction of the rectus femoris and iliopsoas medially.
  - The gluteus medius will be retracted laterally to expose the hip capsule.
- The leg is placed into an adducted and externally rotated position to put the capsule on stretch and perform a capsulotomy.
  - This exposes the hip joint, allowing femur and acetabular preparation as described next.
- Lateral approach
  - Can include both the direct lateral and anterior lateral and the variations of these approaches
    - Patient is generally prepped in the lateral position.
  - Intraoperative fluoroscopy generally is not used, although some providers do obtain intraoperative radiographs.
  - The starting point is usually 5 cm proximal to the greater trochanter and the incision is carried distal for approximately 8 cm.
    - There is no true muscular or nervous plane.
  - The superficial dissection is made through the fascia lata
    - The split fascia lata is then retracted anteriorly to expose the tendon of the gluteus medius.
    - The gluteus medius fibers that attach to the fascia lata are then detached using sharp dissection.
    - Care should be taken when splitting the fascia lata not to progress more than 3 to 5 cm above the greater trochanter because of the risk of the superior gluteal nerve.
  - An anterior flap is raised by taking the anterior aspect of the vastus lateralis, gluteus minimus, and gluteus medius off the bone to expose the underlying capsule, which can be opened to allow for preparation of the femur and acetabulum.
- Posterior approach
  - One of the most common approaches
  - Patient positioned laterally with the hip undergoing surgery facing up
  - Intraoperative radiographs occasionally used but fluoroscopy is rare

- The starting position for the incision is lateral to the posterior superior iliac spine and runs distal over the greater trochanter.
  - Again, there is no internervous plane
- The dissection is carried through subcutaneous fat to the fascia lata. After incising the fascia lata, the gluteus maximus is split.
  - This gives access to the short external rotators, which are detached off the femur.
- After tagging and retracting the short external rotators, the capsule is identified and incised, giving access to the femur and acetabulum.
- Bone preparation
  - The bone preparation for a THA involves both acetabular preparation and femur preparation.
  - Generally, the femoral neck cut is made first, which allows access to the acetabulum.
    - This cut is made approximately 1 cm above the lesser trochanter at an angle equal to the anatomic angle of the neck.
    - Care should be taken to ensure the anterior cortex cut is equal or distal to the posterior cortex as this helps avoid retroversion of the femoral component.
  - After removal of the femoral head, the head can be sized, and the acetabulum can be prepped.
  - The labrum and other soft tissues are removed.
  - Then the acetabulum can be reamed.
    - Generally, the initial reaming is done with a reamer that is smaller than the templated acetabular size.
    - The first reaming is directed more medial.
    - Medialization is done until there is good cancellous bone medially, taking care to not penetrate the medial wall unless controlled penetration is needed for proper cup coverage.
    - After obtaining proper medialization, the acetabulum is reamed circumferentially to obtain a centralized reaming of the acetabulum.
    - The reaming is considered complete when there is good circumferential bite of the reamer and a hemispherical acetabulum, usually 4 to 5 mm larger than the diameter of the head measured.

- The goal for cup positioning is between 20° and 30° of anteversion and 35° to 45° of abduction.
- At this point, the trial or final component can be placed, and attention is turned to the femur.
  - Different systems vary in terms of exact methods but in general the femoral canal is opened with a box osteotome, and a canal reamer is used to start the first broaches.
- After this, the canal is sequentially reamed or broached up to the templated size.
  - Care should be taken to clear the intramedullary bone from the lateral aspect of the femur to avoid varus stem placement.
- After the correct stem is identified, the trial femoral components are placed, the hip is reduced, and leg length and stability are assessed.
  - The general goal is to place the femur in a position that matches the normal femoral anteversion of 10° to 15° and to maintain limb length that is equal to the contralateral side.
- Cementing in THA
  - The type of fixation used to secure THA hardware can be divided into two main categories, cemented and cementless fixation.
    - The current trends in orthopaedic surgery have progressed toward cementless fixation.
      - This technique can be further subdivided into ingrowth or ongrowth based on the design of the implant; the main concept of fixation remains the same.
    - With cementless fixation, the stability of the implant relies on the development of a biologic interface between the bone and the implant (**Figure 9**).
    - Cemented fixation uses polymethyl methacrylate as a grout to form an interlocking bond between the implant and the bone.
      - This technique is used less commonly in modern arthroplasty, but it is still used for severe osteoporosis, bone that has been irradiated, and femur anatomy that has an enlarged metaphyseal region that lacks a solid isthmus and therefore would make supporting a cementless design difficult.

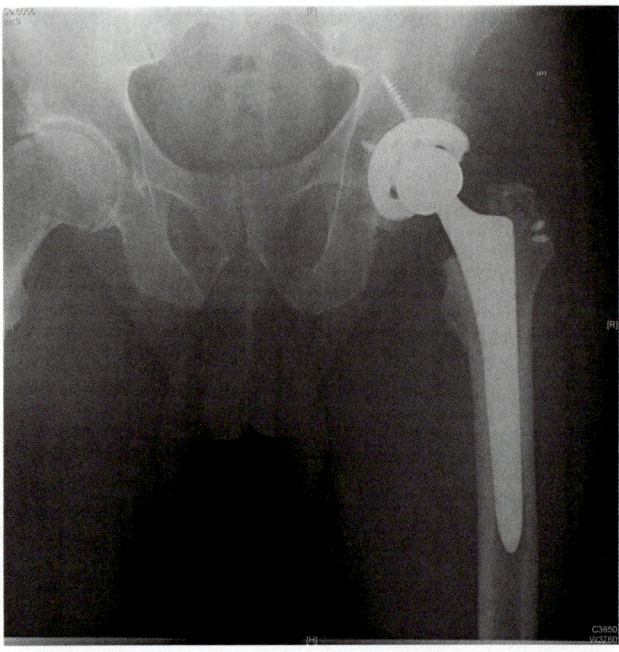

Figure 9 AP radiograph of the pelvis demonstrating a noncemented left total hip arthroplasty.

- When cement is used, certain techniques can optimize the cement-prosthesis interface and improve fixation strength.
  - Vacuum mixing is used to reduce cement porosity, which results in a reduced number of stress points in the cement and improves fixation.
  - The femoral canal is prepped with pulsatile lavage and thoroughly dried.
  - A cement restrictor is placed 2 cm beyond the tip of the stem.
  - The cement is injected into the canal in a retrograde manner, and then the column is pressurized.
  - The canal is completely filled with cement to allow for an even 2-mm mantle of cement around the entire prosthesis.
  - When placing the stem, care must be taken to ensure the stem is centered within the canal and not in varus or valgus (this can increase the stress on the cement interface).

Chapter 10: I Need a Joint Replacement

- Regarding the acetabulum, there are rare instances when an acetabular cup is cemented into position.
- Generally, however, a biologically fixed (press-fit) acetabulum is used, even in the setting of a cemented femoral component; known as a hybrid construct.
- Cemented acetabular components have been shown to fail at a higher rate than press-fit components.
- Postoperative management
  - Rehabilitation protocol varies by surgeon.
  - Patients are typically allowed to bear weight as tolerated and early ambulation is encouraged.
  - For patients who undergo a posterior approach for THA, posterior hip precautions are generally used following surgery, including avoiding excessive flexion and internal rotation of the hip.
  - Patients receive a dose of preoperative antibiotics before incision and at least one (sometimes more) following surgery.
  - Patients should also be started on a venous thromboembolism prophylaxis protocol, although the exact regimen used varies by surgeon.
  - Most modern literature suggests a multimodal strategy for pain control with minimization of opioids.

Top 10 Knowledge Drops for Your Rotation

1. Pain that limits function is the main indication for surgery.
2. Preoperative templating allows the surgeon to ensure availability of implants, predict and account for possible areas of difficulty in the surgery, and more accurately reproduce hip biomechanics and leg length.
3. Anterior, lateral, and posterior approaches to the hip are available. They all have benefits and drawbacks; long-term results are similar, and it is surgeon preference.
4. The anterior approach uses the superficial interval between the tensor fascia lata (superior gluteal nerve) and the sartorius (femoral nerve).
5. Care must be taken to avoid injury to the lateral femoral cutaneous nerve with the anterior approach.

6. With the lateral approach, care must be taken when splitting the fascia lata not to progress more than 3 to 5 cm above the greater trochanter because of risk of injury to the superior gluteal nerve.
7. The femoral neck cut is made approximately 1 cm above the lesser trochanter at an angle equal to the anatomic angle of the neck.
8. The goal for cup positioning is between 20° to 30° of anteversion and 35° to 45° of abduction.
9. The general goal for femoral placement is to place the femur in a position that matches the normal femoral anteversion of 10° to 15° and to maintain limb length that is equal to the contralateral side.
10. Early ambulation, deep vein thrombosis prophylaxis, and 24 hours of antibiotics are recommended following surgery.

PERIPROSTHETIC JOINT INFECTIONS

Total joint arthroplasty (TJA) is one of the most commonly performed elective surgical procedures in the United States, with an annual volume projected to exceed two million procedures over the next decade. Despite the success of TJA, complications can occur. Periprosthetic joint infection (PJI) is a rare but devastating complication that has been suggested to be the main cause of failure in modern TJA.[15] Because of increasing life expectancies as well as the lifelong risk of bacterial seeding on the implant, the absolute number of PJIs will invariably increase. Recently, several evidence-based guidelines were introduced to standardize the approach to a patient with a suspected PJI, including the AAOS Clinical Practice Guideline on Diagnosis of Periprosthetic Joint Infection[16] as well as the Proceedings of the 2018 International Consensus Meeting (ICM) on Periprosthetic Joint Infection.[17]

Epidemiology

- PJI affects approximately 0.5% to 2% of patients undergoing TKA and 0.5% to 1% of patients undergoing THA.

- Data from six international arthroplasty registries found the average hip and knee infection burden to be 0.97% and 1.03%, respectively.[18]
  - The higher rate of PJI following TKA has been attributed to the greater mobility and poorer soft-tissue coverage of the knee joint.
- The incidence of PJI is highest in the first 2 years postoperatively.
  - Using the Medicare 5% national sample administrative data set comprising 69,000 patients undergoing elective TKA who were followed longitudinally from 1997 to 2006, the rate of PJI was 1.5% within the first 2 years compared with 0.5% at 2 to 10 years after joint replacement.[19]
- This disastrous complication significantly increases the mortality risk and diminishes the quality of life of orthopaedic patients.
- Hospitalization costs can be as much as 52% to 76% higher than in uninfected patients.
  - The combined annual hospital costs related to PJI of the hip and knee is estimated to reach $1.85 billion by 2030, posing a substantial economic burden to the health care system.
- Multiple risk factors for PJI have been proposed, with current evidence supporting some factors more than others (**Table 2**).
  - Patient factors that increase the risk of PJI overlap greatly with those that predispose to postoperative infections.
    - Most common risk factors: obesity, diabetes mellitus, tobacco use, malnutrition, rheumatoid arthritis, immunocompromised status secondary to malignancy or immunosuppressive drugs, factors that may compromise the integrity of dermal barrier may allow direct inoculation of bacteria into the surgical site, such as active skin ulceration, chronic venous insufficiency, psoriasis, intravenous drug use, and other causes of poor wound healing
  - Any patient with an active infection in the perioperative period will have an increased risk of PJI because of the risk of transient bacteremia and hematogenous seeding of the prosthesis.
    - Such patients should be strongly advised against proceeding with elective TJA.
    - In contrast, there is still a paucity of evidence on the implications of asymptomatic bacteremia and poor dentition.

TABLE 2 Patient-Specific Risk Factors for Periprosthetic Joint Infection

Moderate evidence
Obesity
Limited evidence
Diabetes, especially uncontrolled diabetes Tobacco use Immunocompromised status (other than HIV), including transplant, malignancy Inflammatory arthritis Prior prosthetic joint infection Peripheral vascular disease Cardiac disease (arrhythmia, coronary artery disease, congestive heart failure, other) Renal disease Liver disease (hepatitis, cirrhosis, other) Mental health disorders (including depression) Malnutrition Preoperative anemia Alcohol use
Based on expert opinion only
Active infection Anticoagulation status, active thromboprophylaxis Autoimmune disease HIV status Institutionalized patients Prior bariatric surgery

Adapted with permission from the American Academy of Orthopaedic Surgeons Evidence-Based Clinical Practice Guideline for Diagnosis and Prevention of Periprosthetic Joint Infections. https://www.aaos.org/globalassets/quality-and-practice-resources/pji/pji-clinical-practice-guideline-final-9-18-19-.pdf. Accessed March 11, 2019.

- Surgery-related risk factors include the location of arthroplasty, whether primary or revision arthroplasty is performed, duration of surgery, perioperative hyperglycemia, need for nonautologous blood transfusion, and postoperative complications such as hematoma or wound dehiscence.
- To assess a patient's individualized probability of the development of PJI, a simple and validated risk calculator was recently developed by the 2018 ICM.[20]

Pertinent Microbiology

- Establishing a microbiologic diagnosis in PJI allows surgeons to formulate a surgical plan and optimize antimicrobial therapy, thereby maximizing the chance of treatment success.

- Microbial identification also provides valuable prognostic information for patients and guides perioperative counseling.
  - The virulence of the microorganism and its sensitivities to intravenous as well as oral antimicrobial agents for long-term suppression are several factors affecting the overall treatment plan.
- The most frequent pathogens implicated in PJI are gram-positive cocci.
- The timing of infection is the most important clue on the identity of the causative microorganism.
  - Early-onset (less than 3 months after surgery): *Staphylococcus aureus*, gram-negative bacilli, anaerobes, or polymicrobes
  - Delayed-onset (3 to 12 months after surgery): coagulase-negative staphylococci, *Cutibacterium* spp or enterococci
  - Late-onset (more than 12 months after surgery): *S aureus*, gram-negative bacilli, or beta-hemolytic streptococci. However, cultures are often negative.
- Other factors affecting the microbiology of PJI include a history of concomitant or preceding infection, known colonization with *S aureus* or other resistant organisms, and patient comorbidities.
  - Fungal (most frequently *Candida* spp) or mycobacterial infections may be encountered in immunocompromised patients.
- The most important virulence factor is the formation of biofilm on the implant surface, during which the bacteria adhere, multiply, encase themselves in glycocalyx and coalesce, forming a protective barrier that decreases the diffusion of antimicrobial agents and confers resistance to antimicrobial mechanisms.
  - The biofilm likely accounts for the delayed development of PJI weeks to months after arthroplasty, as well as the difficulties in pathogen isolation especially in cases of indolent, late-onset PJI.
  - As the metabolic rate of organisms within a biofilm declines substantially, antibiotic suppression may produce an initial clinical response in some cases, but this is often followed by delayed relapse within days to months in the absence of implant removal.

Pertinent History/Physical Examination Findings

- Early onset: acquired during implantation or contiguous spread through wound dehiscence

- Cardinal signs of acute inflammation are frequently present, including pain, erythema, warmth, swelling at incision site, wound drainage or dehiscence, joint effusion, and fever.
  - Frequently associated with hematoma formation
- Delayed onset: acquired during implantation
  - Indolent course presenting as joint pain
  - Sinus tract with drainage may be present.
  - Fever is infrequent (less than 50%) and physical examination is usually normal.
  - Early loosening of the implant may be seen, making it difficult to distinguish from aseptic failure.
  - The character of pain may offer clues to the diagnosis: persistent joint pain (in PJI) versus pain with motion and weight bearing that is relieved with rest (in mechanical loosening).
- Late onset: due to hematogenous spread (eg, urinary tract infection)
  - Acute onset of systemic symptoms may be seen in a previously well-functioning joint (as described for early onset).
  - Dislocation can occur.
  - The source of infection is found in fewer than half of cases.
- Asymptomatic
  - It is well established that a varying degree of clinically relevant PJI may be detected in some cases of presumed aseptic loosening based on positive intraoperative cultures.[21]
  - Consequently, it is imperative that intraoperative cultures be taken during revision procedures regardless of the preoperative diagnosis.

Relevant Investigations

- The general approach to diagnosis of a PJI is twofold:
  - The presence or absence of a joint infection must be confirmed.
  - The infecting microorganism(s) must be isolated and its susceptibility elucidated.
- Although not useful for the diagnosis of PJI, plain radiographs should still be ordered to exclude differential diagnoses of pain and instability.
- Several diagnostic criteria have been proposed: 2011 Musculoskeletal Infection Society criteria, 2013 ICM criteria, 2013 Infectious Disease Society of America guidelines, and most recently, the 2018 ICM criteria[17] (**Figure 10**).

Major criteria (at least one of the following)	Decision
Two positive cultures of the same organism	Infected
Sinus tract with evidence of communication to the joint or visualization of the prosthesis	

		Minor Criteria	Score	Decision
Preoperative Diagnosis	Serum	Elevated CRP _or_ D-Dimer	2	≥6 Infected
		Elevated ESR	1	
	Synovial	Elevated Synovial *WBC* _or_ *LE* (++)	3	2-5 Possibly Infected*
		Positive Alpha-defensin	3	
		Elevated Synovial PMN %	2	0-1 Not Infected
		Elevated Synovial CRP	1	

	*Inconclusive preoperative score _or_ dry tap	Score	Decision
Postoperative Diagnosis	Preoperative score	-	≥6 Infected
	Positive Histology	3	4-5 Inconclusive**
	Positive Purulence	3	
	Positive Single Culture	2	≤3 Not Infected

* For patients with inconclusive minor criteria, operative criteria can also be used to fulfill definition for PJI.
** Consider further molecular diagnostics such as next-generation sequencing.

Figure 10 Evidence-based criteria for the diagnosis of periprosthetic joint infections as recommended by the 2018 International Consensus Meeting. CRP = C-reactive protein, ESR = erythrocyte sedimentation rate, LE = leukocyte esterase, PJI = periprosthetic joint infection, PMN = polymorphonuclear leukocytes. (Reprinted from Parvizi J, Tan TL, Goswami K, et al: The 2018 definition of periprosthetic hip and knee infection: Validated criteria. *J Arthroplasty* 2018;33[5]:1309-1314.e2. Copyright 2018, with permission from Elsevier.)

- Diagnosis of PJI often relies on laboratory results from peripheral blood and synovial fluid, microbiologic evaluation, histologic examination of periprosthetic tissue, intraoperative findings, and in some cases, radiographic evaluation (**Table 3**).
- To aid surgeons in the diagnosis, an algorithm was recently proposed by the 2018 ICM[22] (**Figure 11**).
- Despite the greater sensitivity of synovial fluid tests (alpha-defensin, leukocyte esterase, synovial C-reactive protein, white blood cell count, and polymorphonuclear leukocyte percentage compared with culture-based tests),[23] microbiologic identification

TABLE 3 Investigations to Aid in the Diagnosis of Periprosthetic Joint Infection

Investigations	Advantages	Disadvantages
Peripheral Blood Tests		
ESR and CRP	Cheap and accessible High sensitivity >90%	Nonspecific marker False-negative result when organism is slow growing or less virulent
D-dimer	Cheap and accessible Higher sensitivity and specificity than ESR and CRP Guides timing of reimplantation	Relatively new marker with limited evidence High variability in laboratory measurement and reporting
IL-6	Higher sensitivity and specificity than ESR and CRP	Relatively new marker with limited evidence High costs and technical skills required
Synovial Fluid Analysis		
WBC and PMN%	Cheap and accessible High sensitivity and specificity	Varies based on timing of infection (acute versus chronic) False-negative result when organism is less virulent, premature antibiotic False-positive result in corrosion reactions
Leukocyte esterase	Cheap and accessible High sensitivity and specificity Point-of-care test Not influenced by preoperative antibiotics	Blood contamination can affect colorimetric changes (but overcome with centrifugation)
Alpha-defensin	High sensitivity and specificity Point-of-care test (for lateral flow test) Not influenced by preoperative antibiotics	Expensive Lateral flow test is less sensitive (~80%) False-positive in crystal-deposition arthritis, corrosion reactions
CRP	High sensitivity and specificity Combination with other synovial biomarkers yields high accuracy	False-negative when organism is less virulent
Intraoperative		
Frozen section histopathology	Results obtained intraoperatively Not influenced by preoperative antibiotics	Only moderate sensitivity False-negative when organism is less virulent Potential for sampling error High costs and technical skills required

CRP = C-reactive protein, ESR = erythrocyte sedimentation rate, IL-6 = interleukin-6, PMN% = polymorphonuclear neutrophil percentage, WBC = white blood cell count

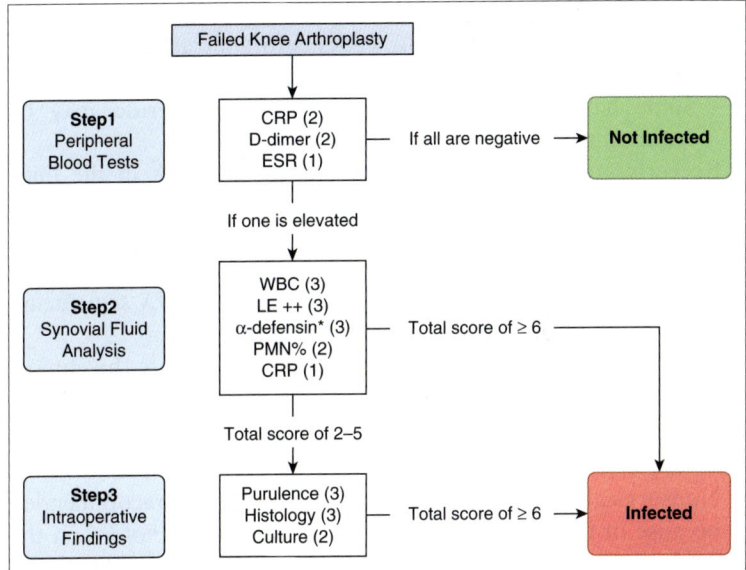

Figure 11 Diagnostic algorithm to guide the selection of laboratory tests. CRP, C-reactive protein; ESR, erythrocyte sedimentation rate; WBC, white blood cell count; LE, leukocyte esterase; PMN%, polymorphonuclear neutrophil percentage. Points are stated in parentheses. *Does not need to be performed routinely. (Data from Shohat N, Tan TL, Della Valle CJ: Development and validation of an evidence-based algorithm for diagnosing periprosthetic joint infection. *J Arthroplasty* 2019;34[11]:2730-2736.e1. Copyright 2019, with permission from Elsevier.)

still plays a major role in any diagnostic algorithm as it guides antibiotic selection and provides prognostic information.
- For patients presenting with fever or other systemic signs of infection, two sets of blood cultures should be obtained.
- Three to six intraoperative periprosthetic tissue specimens should be collected; if pus is encountered, this should be aspirated in a sterile tube and sent for culture.
• Establishing a microbiologic diagnosis remains challenging, with an estimated 7% to 39% of patients having negative cultures despite clear clinical evidence of infection, a phenomenon also known as culture-negative PJI.
  - The most important cause of this is the premature administration of antibiotics before obtaining samples from the infected joint.

- This has prompted the AAOS to recommend withholding antibiotic therapy for at least 2 weeks before intraoperative specimen collection to improve culture yield.
  - Some have proposed that an even longer period may be required to culture certain fastidious organisms.
- Recently, molecular tests to detect bacterial DNA in the joint have been developed to improve the diagnosis of PJI, particularly in the setting of negative cultures.
  - These include multiplex polymerase chain reaction and, more recently, non-Sanger-based high-throughput DNA sequencing (also known as next-generation sequencing).
  - However, further research is necessary to evaluate the clinical utility of these molecular tests.

Nonsurgical Measures

- Nonsurgical management of PJI is generally not recommended because of the persistence of infection within the biofilm on the implant surface, though it may be appropriate for patients who are poor candidates for surgery.
- Chronic oral antimicrobial suppression should be guided by cultures of aspirated joint fluid.
- Most importantly, patients should be counseled on the high risk of relapse and the importance of medication adherence.

Surgical Intervention

- Surgical intervention is required not only to manage the infection but also to confirm the diagnosis of PJI in indeterminate cases that require additional diagnostic criteria to be fulfilled based on intraoperative findings and sampling of infected periprosthetic tissue (**Figure 10**).
- Key factors influencing the surgical plan: duration of symptoms, presence of a sinus tract, available soft-tissue coverage, stability of the implant, infecting microorganism and its susceptibility to oral and/or intravenous antimicrobial agents, and the patient's willingness and ability to undergo more than one surgical intervention.
- Surgical options can be classified into three approaches: irrigation and débridement with retention of the prosthesis, or exchange of the prosthesis in one or two stages.
  - In certain cases, salvage options such as arthrodesis or amputation may be required to eradicate the infection.

- Débridement, antibiotics, irrigation, and retention or irrigation and débridement.
  - Indications: Early postoperative PJI (less than 3 months postoperatively) or acute hematogenous PJI (at least 3 months postoperatively with short duration of symptoms less than 3 weeks). In both situations, there should be the absence of a sinus tract, stable implants, good soft-tissue cover, and an identified organism that is susceptible to oral antimicrobial therapy.
  - Outcomes: wide variation in the literature (50% to 70%); some evidence suggests higher failure rates for acute hematogenous PJI or infections caused by virulent organisms
  - Technique: aggressive débridement of nonviable soft or osseous tissues, exchange of modular components (preferably), inspection of component interfaces for loosening, copious irrigation with pulsatile lavage
  - Antibiotics: intravenous antibiotics for 4 to 6 weeks, then oral antibiotic suppression for 6 months
- Two-stage exchange arthroplasty
  - Indication: late PJI that cannot be managed with débridement, antibiotics, irrigation, and retention
  - Technique: First stage involves resection of all components (including cement), aggressive débridement, and antibiotic-loaded cement spacer insertion (articulating or nonarticulating spacer). During component removal, efforts should be made to minimize bone loss.
  - Intravenous antibiotics is recommended for at least 2 weeks; switching to oral antibiotics may be feasible depending on organism susceptibility. Antibiotics should be administered for a total of 4 to 6 weeks in the interim.
  - There are currently no tests available to determine the optimal timing of reimplantation, although D-dimer has been suggested to be a useful marker. Erythrocyte sedimentation rate and C-reactive protein should not be used to guide this decision. Aspiration before second stage may be performed, which has been shown to be highly specific but with variable sensitivity. To minimize false-negative results, antibiotics should be withheld for 2 weeks after completion and before aspiration.
  - Second stage involves removal of the spacer, aggressive débridement, and reimplantation. New components should be

semiconstrained or fully constrained depending on ligamentous functioning and stability of the joint. Bone loss should be addressed. Mode of fixation may be cemented, cementless using diaphyseal-engaging stems, or hybrid.
- Repeat débridement with spacer exchange should be performed if there is suspicion of persistent infection. Culture and sensitivity results from the first stage can be used to guide antibiotic selection for the new spacer.
- Postoperative antibiotics should be continued only until intraoperative cultures confirm no growth. If cultures are positive, chronic antibiotic suppression should be considered.
- Outcomes: Success rates are 80% to 90%. Higher failure in patients with prior failed irrigation and débridement.
- One-stage exchange arthroplasty
  - Performed in 85% of specialized centers in Europe, less common in North America
  - Indications: infecting organism and sensitivity determined preoperatively
  - Contraindications: systemic sepsis, failure of two or more one-stage procedures, extensive soft-tissue involvement, infection involving neurovascular bundles, organism with high virulence, culture-negative PJI
  - Technique: similar to two-stage procedure. Radical débridement should be performed without a tourniquet so that nonbleeding (nonviable) tissues may be identified. Antibiotic-loaded cement specific for the organism susceptibility should be used.
  - Outcomes: Generally comparable with two-stage exchange arthroplasty (ie, 10% to 20%)

Top 10 Knowledge Drops for Your Rotation

1. PJI is perhaps the most devastating complication in arthroplasty.
2. The rate of PJI is highest in the first 2 years following arthroplasty. This ranges between 0.5% to 2.0% for TKA and 0.5% to 1.0% for THA.
3. The timing of infection can give clues to the mechanism of infection, identity of the infecting organism, and expected clinical manifestations. However, time definitions for PJI are not

always clear-cut, particularly in patients for whom the diagnosis is delayed.
4. PJI should be suspected in any patients with a joint replacement and signs and symptoms of inflammation (including joint pain, warmth, erythema, induration at the incision site, sinus tract or persistent wound drainage, wound dehiscence, joint effusion, or fever).
5. The diagnosis of PJI remains a challenge. Several diagnostic criteria have been proposed.
6. Major criteria considered confirmatory of PJI are the presence of a sinus tract and the same pathogen isolated on two or more intraoperative or a combination of preoperative synovial fluid aspiration cultures and intraoperative tissue cultures.
7. Peripheral blood tests and joint aspiration should be performed (unless a sinus tract is present or débridement is planned). Although synovial fluid tests have the highest accuracy, microbiologic isolation using cultures is key for prognostication and guiding treatment.
8. Surgical treatment of PJI can be categorized into three main approaches: irrigation and débridement, two-stage exchange arthroplasty, or one-stage exchange arthroplasty. Key factors influencing the surgical plan consist of the duration of symptoms, presence of a sinus tract, available soft-tissue coverage, stability of the implant, infecting microorganism and its susceptibility to oral and/or intravenous antimicrobial drugs, and patient's willingness and ability to undergo more than one surgical intervention.
9. Although seemingly advantageous, débridement and retention of the implant has highly variable success rates (50% to 70%), which should be maximized by adhering to strict indications.
10. Two-stage exchange arthroplasty remains the gold standard for treatment in North America (80% to 90% success rate). This involves component removal with spacer insertion and an interim period of intravenous antibiotics, followed by reimplantation.

PERIPROSTHETIC FRACTURES

Periprosthetic fractures (PPFs) are an increasingly common complication following TJA. By definition, these are fractures that occur above, below, or around the prosthetic stem, which can occur intraoperatively or postoperatively. PPF is one of the most common indications for revision surgery. Implant, surgeon, and patient factors all contribute to the risk of this complication. Although PPFs may present in many different configurations, it is important to understand the classification systems and principles of management, as this will determine the optimal treatment strategy for each patient.

Epidemiology

- The increasing incidence of PPF directly correlates with the growth in the annual volume of TJA, which reflects the increasing life expectancies and higher activity levels among older patients.
- Several studies have shown that patients with PPF have a similar or higher mortality rate than patients with hip fractures or native distal femur fractures.
- For TKA, femoral supracondylar PPFs are the most common, with an incidence of 0.3% to 2.5% after primary TKA, although this can reach up to 38% in revision cases.
  - In contrast, tibia PPFs are relatively less common, with an incidence of 0.4% to 1.7% in primary TKA and 0.9% in revision TKA.
  - PPFs of the patella have an incidence of 0.2% to 21%, which can increase with the use of patellar resurfacing.
- For THA, femoral PPFs have an incidence of 0.1% to 18%, whereas acetabular PPFs are rare with an incidence of 0.07% to 0.4%.
  - PPF is reported to be the third leading cause of revision THA in the first 2 years postoperatively and the second leading cause of revision in the long term.
- The most pertinent risk factor for PPF is advanced age, which predisposes to osteoporosis and recurrent falls, and is also considered a major risk factor in itself.

- Female sex, rheumatoid arthritis, and neurologic disorders are additional risk factors.
- Causes of increased osteolysis (eg, polyethylene wear, metal-on-metal reactions) and periprosthetic bone loss also increase the risk of PPF.
- Surgical factors include the use of cementless prostheses and revision procedures. Specific risk factors for TKA and THA are outlined in **Table 4**.

Pertinent Anatomy/Pathoanatomy

- To improve surgical decision making, numerous classification systems have been proposed for each bone and each joint that take not only the fracture localization but also the fracture type, implant stability, and bone quality into consideration.
  - The most common classification systems used are outlined in **Table 5**.
    - The Unified Classification System was proposed as a common classification system that can be applied to every anatomic region of the body, regardless of the precise location of the fracture.[24]

TABLE 4 Surgical Risk Factors for Periprosthetic Fractures

Fracture Location	Risk Factors
TKA femur	Implant: rotationally constrained components Technical: anterior femoral notching (controversial)
TKA tibia	Implant: Long-stemmed component Previous tibial tubercle osteotomy
TKA patella	Implant: noncemented, metal backed, central single peg Technical: asymmetric resection, overresection (minimum thickness is 13 mm), extensive lateral release (transection of superior geniculate artery), maltracking
THA femur	Implant design: noncemented Technical errors (eg, overaggressive rasping)
THA acetabulum	Implant design: noncemented, elliptical, threaded cup Technical: underreamed cup (≥2 mm), overmedialization Hip dysplasia Radiation therapy

THA = total hip arthroplasty, TKA = total knee arthroplasty

TABLE 5 Most Commonly Used Classification Systems for Periprosthetic Fractures

Fracture Location	Classification System

TKA femur	Lewis and Rorabeck
	    Type I: Nondisplaced, component stable
	    Type II: Displaced, component stable
	    Type III: Displaced, component loose or failing

TKA tibia	Felix and associates
	    Type I: Fracture of tibial plateau
	    Type II: Fracture adjacent to tibial stem
	    Type III: Fracture of tibial shaft, distal to component
	    Type IV: Fracture of tibial tubercle

TKA patella	Ortiguera and Berry
	    Type I: Intact extensor mechanism, component stable
	    Type II: Disrupted extensor mechanism, component stable or loose
	    Type III: Intact extensor mechanism, component loose
	        A: Good bone stock (patella thickness ≥10 mm)
	        B: Poor bone stock (patella thickness <10 mm or marked comminution)

THA femur	Vancouver
	    A: Trochanteric region
	        AL: Lesser trochanter
	        AG: Greater trochanter
	    B1: Around stem or just below it, component stable
	    B2: Around stem or just below it, component loose, good bone stock
	    B3: Around stem or just below it, poor bone stock
	    C: Well below stem

THA acetabulum	Paprosky
	    Type 1: Intraoperative (component insertion)
	        A: Recognized, component stable, fracture undisplaced
	        B: Recognized, component unstable, fracture displaced
	        C: Not recognized
	    Type 2: Intraoperative (component removal)
	        A: Good bone stock (≥50%)
	        B: Poor bone stock (<50%)
	    Type 3: Traumatic
	        A: Component stable
	        B: Component unstable
	    Type 4: Spontaneous
	        A: Good bone stock (≥50%)
	        B: Poor bone stock (<50%)
	    Type 5: Pelvic discontinuity
	        A: Good bone stock (≥50%)
	        B: Poor bone stock (<50%)
	        C: Associated with pelvic radiation

THA = total hip arthroplasty, TKA = total knee arthroplasty

- Although not as widely used, the Unified Classification System represents a practical tool that can be used to approach all PPFs.
- This simple mnemonic system was devised by the authors:
  - Type A, Apophyseal (to which, one or more soft-tissue structures are attached; ie, avulsion fracture)
  - Type B, Bed of the implant (B1, component stable; B2, component loose; B3, component loose and poor bone stock)
  - Type C, Clear of the implant
  - Type D, Dividing one bone that supports two joint replacement
  - Type E, Each of two bones supporting one joint replacement
  - Type F, Facing or articulating with an implant
- Anatomic considerations are specific for each type of PPF.
  - The acetabulum column theory is important when approaching any fracture of the acetabulum.
    - Anterior and posterior columns form an inverted Y
    - Anterior column: anterior ilium (gluteus medius tubercle), anterior wall and dome, iliopectineal eminence, and lateral superior pubic ramus
    - Posterior column: quadrilateral surface, posterior wall and dome, ischial tuberosity, and greater/lesser sciatic notches
    - When encountering PPFs intraoperatively, evaluating posterior column integrity and stability is crucial
  - For PPF of the distal femur, femoral notching of the anterior cortex, which can occur during the anterior femoral bone cut when saw cuts into the anterior femoral cortex, has been postulated to play a major role.
    - This finding may be seen on postoperative radiographs (**Figure 12**) and its prevalence following TKA has been estimated at 3.5% to 41%.
    - Although cadaver studies have demonstrated that femoral notching led to a 39% decrease in torsional strength and 18% decrease in bending strength of the distal femur, long-term follow-up studies have concluded that the clinical significance of this finding remains controversial.
    - Nonetheless, manipulation of the knee should be avoided in TKAs with a notch.

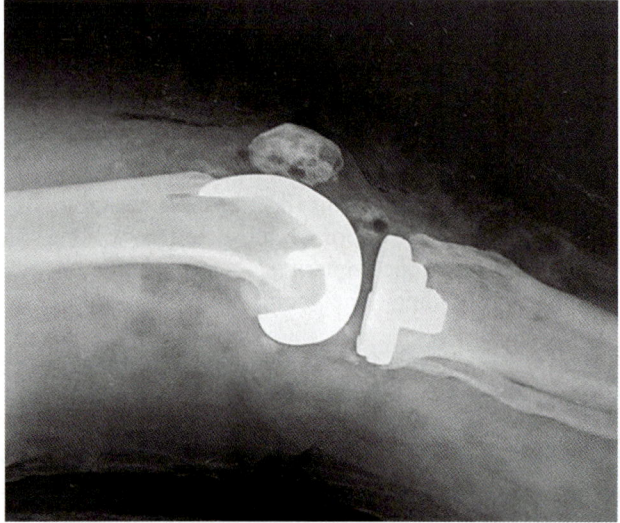

Figure 12 A lateral radiographic view of the knee demonstrates notching of the anterior femoral cortex.

Pertinent History/Physical Examination Findings

- History about the trauma (if any) and mechanism of injury
- Comorbidities and chronic medications can give clues on the underlying etiology of the fracture.
- Assess for increasing hip or knee pain on weight bearing or reduced mobility because of joint problems before the fracture, which may suggest preexisting loosening of the implant.
  - Loosening because of infection must also be excluded by determining whether there is a history of pain with rest, swelling, erythema, prolonged wound drainage, or a sinus tract.
- Lower extremity examination
  - Deformity of the affected limb and skin bruising are obvious signs supporting the diagnosis.
  - Forceful palpation and excessive motion of the limb should be avoided because this can lead to further displacement of the fracture.
  - Extensor lag may be present in patella PPFs.
  - Neurovascular status and condition of the overlying skin should be properly documented.

Relevant Investigations
- Standard AP and lateral radiographs form the basis of fracture diagnosis and classification.
  - Signs of loosening should be identified, which include fracture through the cement mantle, displacement of the component, and/or complete radiolucent lines of 2 mm or greater at the bone-cement interface around the prosthesis.
    - Previous radiographs may be used for comparison if they are available.
- Complex fracture patterns may not be easily classified on plain radiographs, often requiring a CT scan to aid in the diagnosis.
- If there is history suggestive of septic loosening, erythrocyte sedimentation rate and C-reactive protein level should be checked and a joint aspiration performed if any of the laboratory results are elevated.

Principles of Management
- Goals of treatment: achieve a painless and stable joint with restoration of alignment and maintenance of prosthesis fixation.
- Ideally, the selected treatment strategy should permit early range of motion so that the patient can return to function as soon as possible.
- Multiple treatment algorithms have been formulated based on the respective classification systems, but general principles of treatment are best summarized by the Unified Classification System:
  - Type A. Importance of the attached soft-tissue structures should be assessed; if unimportant, the fracture can be managed nonsurgically, even if displaced
  - Type B1. Management would depend on the existing surgical or nonsurgical management of the fracture type, provided that implant stability is confirmed
  - Type B2. Revision with a longer stem
  - Type B3. Complex reconstruction required
  - Type C. Implant can be ignored if the fracture is sufficiently distant from it. Principles of management follow those employed as if the implant was not present
  - The treatment of type D and E fractures is complex and beyond the scope of this chapter

- For fractures of the acetabulum after hip hemiarthroplasty, the most common example of a type F fracture, nonsurgical measures with protected weight bearing may be used.
- A delayed conversion to THA may be considered if patient is still symptomatic.
- If the initial displacement is substantial, early surgical intervention should be considered.

Treatment of Specific Fractures

- The type of fixation depends on implant stability, fracture pattern, bone quality, amount of bone stock, and need for augments.
  - Fixation should be accomplished with minimal damage to the surrounding tissue.
- TKA femoral fractures
  - In the Rorabeck classification, nondisplaced fractures with stable implants are managed nonsurgically with casting or bracing, whereas displaced fractures with stable implants are managed with internal fixation.
    - Fractures with unstable components, regardless of bone quality, are always managed with revision surgery using a long stem, with or without bone grafting.
  - Fixation can be achieved using open reduction and internal fixation (ORIF) with plating or a retrograde intramedullary nail (IMN).
    - Plating
      - Plates can be nonlocking (conventional) or locking, which can be subdivided into variable-angle or fixed-angle locking plates.
      - The most common method of fixation is ORIF with fixed-angle plating.
      - Complications related to plate fixation include nonunion (especially with the extensile approach compared with submuscular approach) and malunion (especially with minimally invasive techniques).
      - Locking plating typically requires non–weight-bearing status for several weeks.
    - Retrograde IMN
      - Best suited for distal diaphyseal fractures

- Patient must have a femoral component with an open-box design for IMN access and sufficient bone stock in the distal fragments for locking fixation.
    - Care must be taken to ensure that the nail does not impinge on the polyethylene bearing or patellar component.
    - Compared with nonlocking plating, the use of IMNs has the advantage of reduced surgical time and intraoperative blood loss, as well as lower risk of nonunion and need for revision surgery.
  - Previous studies have compared the use of retrograde IMNs and locking plates for supracondylar femoral fractures and concluded that each option has its own advantages and disadvantages, but the clinical outcomes, such as nonunion and revision rates, were similar.[25]
  - The complication rate after retrograde IMN and locking plate fixation is 15% to 20%.
    - Common complications include infection, hardware failure, nonunion, malunion, and mortality.
  - For patients with PPFs in the setting of loose implants, revision TKA with a diaphyseal engaging stem is the choice of treatment because it provides rotational stability to the implant.
    - ORIF of the fracture is performed in the same setting.
  - In elderly patients as well as patients with poor bone quality or bone stock (comminuted fractures), treatment with fracture resection and distal femoral replacement is recommended.
- TKA tibial fractures
  - Rare
  - If the fracture is nondisplaced with stable implants, nonsurgical treatment may be feasible.
  - If the implant has loosened, PPF should be managed with revision with stemmed implants, with or without bone grafting.
  - Displaced fractures with stable implants should be managed with ORIF.
  - Occasionally, a revision endoprosthesis is required if implants are unstable and bone stock is poor.
- TKA patellar fractures
  - Type I fractures are most common.
    - Patients are frequently asymptomatic and the fracture is identified on routine follow-up radiographs.

- This type of PPF may be managed with a controlled motion brace initially locked in extension, with increasing amounts of flexion permitted as time progresses.
- Type II is a disruption of the extensor mechanism and associated with a high rate of complications (50%) and recurrent operations (42%). Extensor reconstruction is necessary.
- When the component is loose (type II or III), component revision should be performed if bone stock is good (type IIIA) and patellectomy performed if bone stock is insufficient to permit resurfacing (type IIIB).
- THA femoral fractures
  - A longitudinal split in the calcar may be encountered when implanting a tapered proximally coated stem and can be managed with stem removal, cabling, and reinsertion.
  - If the implant is still unstable, a stem that bypasses the fracture and achieves diaphyseal fixation may be needed.
  - Wedge taper cementless stems are associated with proximal femoral fractures in the early postoperative period, whereas cylindrical fully porous-coated stems are associated with distal femoral fractures.
  - If the component is loose and unstable, ORIF and component revision is necessary. If the component is still well fixed, observation and protected weight bearing is required if the fracture is small and nondisplaced.
  - Alternatively, ORIF may be necessary for significantly displaced fractures.
  - Management of late fractures is guided by the Vancouver classification (**Figure 13**).
  - Main considerations include whether the stem is loose and whether loosening is caused by the fracture or occurred before the fracture.
    - Type AG: Nonsurgical management if minimal displacement, or else may need ORIF with wires, cables, or claw-plate. Limiting hip abduction may decrease the risk of displacement. In the presence of severe osteolysis, bone stock may be inadequate for fixation and fracture healing; hence ORIF is not recommended.
    - Type AF: Nonsurgical management with protected weight bearing, even if displaced

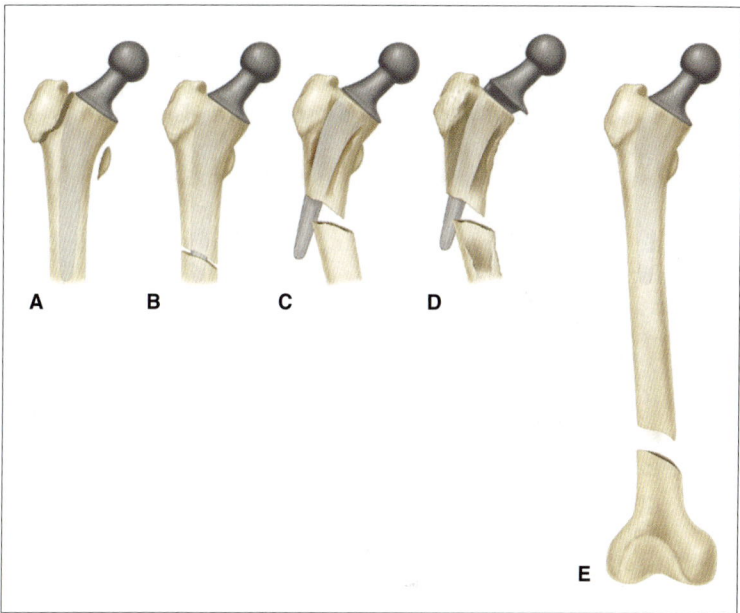

Figure 13 Illustration shows the Vancouver classification of periprosthetic hip fractures. Type A fractures (**A**) include greater and lesser trochanteric fractures. Type B fractures occur around or just below the implant and include B1 fractures with a well-fixed stem (**B**), B2 fractures around a loose stem (**C**), and B3 fractures around a loose stem with poor bone stock (**D**). Type C fractures (**E**) occur well distal to the femoral prosthesis. (Reprinted from McPherson MD, Thompson SR, eds: *Review of Orthopaedics*, ed 7. Figure 5-32. Copyright 2015, with permission from Elsevier.)

- Type B1: ORIF with locking plate, cerclage wires/cables proximally, and bicortical screws distal to stem is needed. May require strut allograft.
- Type B2: Revision THA using a diaphyseal engaging cementless revision stem (fully porous coated cylindrical or tapered fluted modular implant may be used). Fracture fragments are secured proximally around revision femoral implant using wires or cables. Recent studies suggest that good results may be achieved with ORIF in select cases.

- Type B3: Revision THA with augmentation. This can be achieved with allograft (younger patients) or using a proximal femoral replacement (older or low-demand patients).
- Type C: ORIF using standard osteosynthesis techniques
- THA acetabular fracture
  - Most commonly caused by a vertical, incomplete split of the posterior column due to underreaming (≥2 mm) in sclerotic bone; can also occur during impaction of the acetabular component
  - Intraoperative fractures that are stable should be managed nonsurgically with the addition of supplemental screws to the cup
    - If unstable, pelvic stabilization should be performed with single or double plating of the posterior column before implanting the final cup—if there is insufficient bone, bone grafting or the use of porous augments should be considered and associated with a porous cup with screws.
  - Postoperative fractures are managed based on etiology.
    - Traumatic fractures with a stable component can be managed nonsurgically.
    - Unstable fractures require revision with a porous cup with supplemental screws, or a cage with a cemented cup; plating of the columns may be added if necessary.
    - Acute pelvic discontinuity is managed in a manner similar to that of unstable fractures. In chronic pelvic discontinuity caused by severe osteolysis, revision surgery using a cage-cup reconstruction can be performed.
    - Alternatively, if bone quality is poor, a two-stage technique can be used—first, ORIF and reconstruction of bone loss are performed; second, a revision cup is implanted after fracture consolidation.
- Postoperative complications
  - PPFs are a rare but potentially disastrous complication following TKA and THA.
  - Postoperative complications of PPF are similar to those of any fractures (eg, nonunion, malunion, infection, hardware failure).
  - Prosthesis loosening is common.

Top 10 Knowledge Drops for Your Rotation

1. The increasing incidence of PPFs directly correlates with the growth in the annual volume of TJA.
2. PPFs may present in many different configurations; therefore, it is important to understand the classification systems and principles of management because this will determine the optimal treatment strategy for each patient.
3. For TKA, femoral supracondylar PPFs are the most common, with an incidence of 0.35% to 2.5%. For THA, femoral PPFs are the most common, with an incidence of 0.1% to 18%.
4. The most pertinent risk factor for PPF is advanced aged. Surgical factors include the use of cementless prostheses and revision procedures.
5. All patients should be assessed for increasing hip or knee pain while bearing weight or reduced mobility caused by joint problems before the fracture. This will suggest preexisting loosening of the implant.
6. Complex fracture patterns may not be easily classified on plain radiographs, often requiring a CT scan to aid in the diagnosis.
7. The goals of treatment should be to achieve a painless and stable joint with restoration of alignment and maintenance of prosthesis fixation.
8. The type of fixation depends on implant stability, fracture pattern, bone quality, amount of bone stock, and need for augments.
9. Distal femoral PPFs may be managed according to the Rorabeck classification.
10. Proximal femoral PPFs may be managed according to the Vancouver classification.

References

1. Cui A, Li H, Wang D, Zhong J, Chen Y, Lu H: Global, regional prevalence, incidence and risk factors of knee osteoarthritis in population-based studies. *EClinicalMedicine* 2020;29-30:100587.
2. Chaganti RK, Lane NE: Risk factors for incident osteoarthritis of the hip and knee. *Curr Rev Musculoskelet Med* 2011;4(3):99-104.

3. Felson DT, Lawrence RC, Dieppe PA, et al: Osteoarthritis new insights. Part 1: The disease and its risk factors. *Ann Intern Med* 2000;133(8):635-646.
4. Kozinn SC, Marx C, Scott RD: Unicompartmental knee arthroplasty. A 4.5-6-year follow-up study with a metal-backed tibial component. *J Arthroplasty* 1989;4 suppl:S1-S10.
5. Kozinn SC, Scott R: Unicondylar knee arthroplasty. *J Bone Joint Surg Am* 1989;71(1):145-150.
6. Berend KR, Lombardi AV Jr, Adams JB: Obesity, young age, patellofemoral disease, and anterior knee pain: Identifying the unicondylar arthroplasty patient in the United States. *Orthopedics* 2007;30(5 suppl):19-23.
7. Bonutti PM, Zywiel MG, Ulrich SD, et al: A comparison of subvastus and midvastus approaches in minimally invasive total knee arthroplasty. *J Bone Joint Surg Am* 2010;92(3):575-582.
8. Howell SM, Howell SJ, Kuznik KT, et al: Does a kinematically aligned total knee arthroplasty restore function without failure regardless of alignment category? *Clin Orthop Relat Res* 2013;471(3):1000-1007.
9. Patel AR, Talati RK, Yaffe MA, McCoy BW, Stulberg D: femoral component rotation in total knee arthroplasty: An MRI-based evaluation of our options. *J Arthroplasty* 2014;29(8):1666-1670.
10. Gwam CU, George NE, Etcheson JI, Rosas S, Plate JF, Delanois RE: Cementless versus cemented fixation intotal knee arthroplasty: Usage, costs, and complications during the inpatient period. *J Knee Surg* 2019;32(11):1081-1087.
11. Choy W, Yang D, Lee K, Lee S, Kim K, Chang S: Cemented versus cementless fixation of a tibial component in LCS mobile-bearing total knee arthroplasty performed by a single surgeon. *J Arthroplasty* 2014;29(12):2397-2401.
12. Sculco TP: The role of constraint in total knee arthroplasty. *J Arthroplasty* 2006;21(4):54-56.
13. Ganesh RR, Saravanan A, Govardhan RH, Muhammad Ismail ND, Sathish M: Long term outcome analysis of fixed bearing total knee arthroplasty. *Int J Orthop Sci* 2018;4(3):56-61.
14. Kim YH, Kim JS, Choe JW, et al: Long-term comparison of fixed bearing and mobile bearing total knee replacements in patients younger than fifty-one years of age with osteoarthritis. *J Bone Joint Surg Am* 2012;94(10):866-873.
15. Koh CK, Zeng I, Ravi S, Zhu M, Vince KG, Young SW: Periprosthetic joint infection is the main cause of failure for modern knee arthroplasty: An analysis of 11,134 knees. *Clin Orthop Relat Res* 2017;475:2194-2201.
16. American Academy of Orthopaedic Surgeons: *Clinical Practice Guideline on the Diagnosis and Prevention of Periprosthetic Joint*

Infections. AAOS Quality & Practice Resources, n.d. https://www.aaos.org/search/?q=clinical+practice+guideline+periprosthetic+joint+infection. Accessed April 17, 2023.

17. Parvizi J, Tan TL, Goswami K, et al: The 2018 definition of periprosthetic hip and knee infection: An evidence-based and validated criteria. *J Arthroplasty* 2018;33:1309-1314.e2.
18. Springer BD, Cahue S, Etkin CD, Lewallen DG, McGrory BJ: Infection burden in total hip and knee arthroplasties: An international registry-based perspective. *Arthroplasty Today* 2017;3:137-140.
19. Kurtz SM, Ong KL, Lau E, Bozic KJ, Berry D, Parvizi J: Prosthetic joint infection risk after TKA in the Medicare population. *Clin Orthop Relat Res* 2010;468:52-56.
20. Tan TL, Maltenfort MG, Chen AF, et al: Development and evaluation of a preoperative risk calculator for periprosthetic joint infection following total joint arthroplasty. *J Bone Joint Surg* 2018;100:777-785.
21. Jacobs AME, Bénard M, Meis JF, van Hellemondt G, Goosen JHM: The unsuspected prosthetic joint infection: Incidence and consequences of positive intra-operative cultures in presumed aseptic knee and hip revisions. *Bone Joint Lett J* 2017;99-B:1482-1489.
22. Shohat N, Tan TL, Della Valle CJ, et al: Development and validation of an evidence-based algorithm for diagnosing periprosthetic joint infection. *J Arthroplasty* 2019;34(11):2730-2736.e1.
23. Carli AV, Abdelbary H, Ahmadzai N, et al: Diagnostic accuracy of serum, synovial, and tissue testing for chronic periprosthetic joint infection after hip and knee replacements: A systematic review. *J Bone Joint Surg* 2019;101:635-649.
24. Duncan CP, Haddad FS: The Unified Classification System (UCS): Improving our understanding of periprosthetic fractures. *Bone Joint Lett J* 2014;96-B:713-716.
25. Shin Y-S, Kim H-J, Lee D-H: Similar outcomes of locking compression plating and retrograde intramedullary nailing for periprosthetic supracondylar femoral fractures following total knee arthroplasty: A meta-analysis. *Knee Surg Sports Traumatol Arthrosc* 2017;25:2921-2928.

11 My Foot and Ankle Hurt

Lauren E. Geaney, MD, FAAOS
Jonathan R. Kaplan, MD, FAAOS
MaCalus V. Hogan, MD, MBA, FAAOS, FAOA

Introduction

Foot and ankle pathology is very diverse, ranging from deformity to trauma to sports injuries to arthritis and everything in between. As with all musculoskeletal complaints, it is imperative to understand the anatomy in order to understand the pathology. For students, understanding pertinent history, physical examination findings, and management options will be beneficial on orthopaedic surgery rotations. It is important to provide an overview of some of the most common pathologies affecting the foot and ankle: hallux valgus, hallux rigidus, posterior tibial tendon dysfunction, Achilles tendinopathy, and ankle instability. Hallux valgus is often referred to as a bunion. It is a progressive deformity in which the

---

Dr. Geaney or an immediate family member serves as a paid consultant to or is an employee of Paragon 28, Smith & Nephew, Novastep, and Vilex LLC; has received research or institutional support from Arthrex, Inc.; and serves as a board member, owner, officer, or committee member of American Orthopaedic Foot and Ankle Society and Connecticut Orthopaedic Society. Dr. Kaplan or an immediate family member has received royalties from Novastep; serves as a paid consultant to or is an employee of Medline, Novastep, and Vilex; has stock or stock options held in GLW Medical Innovation; and serves as a board member, owner, officer, or committee member of American Orthopaedic Foot and Ankle Society. Dr. Hogan or an immediate family member is a member of a speakers' bureau or has made paid presentations on behalf of Journal for Bone and Joint Surgery - Miller Review Course and Zimmer and serves as a board member, owner, officer, or committee member of AAOS Board of Special Societies, American Orthopaedic Foot and Ankle Society, International Society of Arthroscopy, Knee Surgery, and Orthopaedic Sports Medicine, J. Robert Gladden Society, and Nth Dimensions Education Solutions, Inc.

Chapter 11: My Foot and Ankle Hurt

first metatarsal translates medially while the toe begins to drift laterally, resulting in a prominence medially, which may become painful with time. Hallux rigidus (also referred to at times as hallux limitus) is arthritis of the metatarsophalangeal joint of the great toe and can eventually result in difficulty with shoe wear, painful range of motion, and disability. Posterior tibial tendon dysfunction, or the adult acquired flatfoot deformity, is a common problem in the field of orthopaedic foot and ankle surgery. Initially thought to be due to failure of the posterior tibial tendon, it is now found to be much more complex because it not only involves deficiency of the posterior tibial tendon but also progressive failure of the supporting ligamentous structures. Achilles tendon pathology includes insertional Achilles tendinopathy and complete tendon rupture, both of which are discussed. Distinct physical examination findings and imaging help identify the specific diagnosis. Management of tendon pathology is dependent on patient's desired functional outcomes. Finally, lateral ankle instability can contribute to both long-term functional and mechanical instability in patients. Medical students should be provided with information to properly identify and offer treatment options for lateral ankle instability. Grasping the following concepts of all of these diagnoses presented here will assist with success on orthopaedic surgery rotations.

HALLUX VALGUS

Epidemiology

Incidence

- 23% of adults aged between 18 and 65 years
- 35.7% of adults older than 65 years have hallux valgus[1,2]

Demographics

- Risk factors
  - Somewhat related to tight shoe wear in females[3]
  - Increased age[2]
  - Genetics (particularly in juveniles and young adults)[4]

- Anatomy[1,3,4]
  - Longer first metatarsal
  - Round first metatarsal head
  - Lateral displacement of sesamoids
  - First ray/first tarsometatarsal instability
  - Pes planovalgus

Public Health Considerations

- Hallux valgus has been associated with the choice of shoe wear. A study evaluating monozygotic and dizygotic female twin pairs concluded that hallux valgus was associated with a constrictive toe box during the fourth decade rather than share genetic factors.[5]
- A recent systematic review similarly showed an association between high-heeled shoe wear and hallux valgus.[6]

Pertinent Anatomy/Pathoanatomy

Soft Tissue

- The anatomy around the first metatarsophalangeal (MTP) joint is complex; an understanding of this anatomy is critical for successful surgical correction. The medial and lateral sesamoids are plantar to the first metatarsal head and separated by a crista. The flexor hallucis brevis has two insertions, one on each of the sesamoids.
- There are four structures that are attached to the lateral sesamoid, including one head of the adductor hallucis, the lateral metatarsosesamoid ligament, the intermetatarsal ligament, and the lateral capsule. The only medial structures attached to the first metatarsal head are the medial collateral ligament and the medial sesamoid ligament[4] (**Figure 1**).
- As the medial capsule becomes attenuated, the first metatarsal begins to drift medially with respect to the sesamoids because there are no soft-tissue connections between the first and second metatarsals. As the first metatarsal head drifts medially, the two sesamoids with their respective heads of the flexor hallucis brevis become displaced laterally with respect to the metatarsal head and this causes a valgus moment on the proximal phalanx. Additionally, the abductor hallucis, which was a medial structure, translates plantarly, resulting in a pronation moment on the proximal phalanx. As the metatarsal head continues to displace, the extensor hallucis longus (EHL) and flexor hallucis longus (FHL)

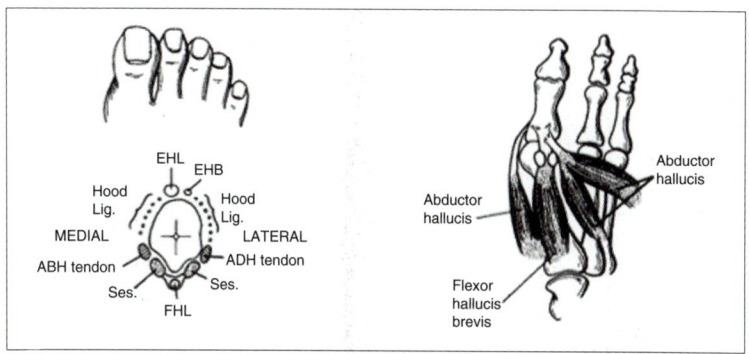

Figure 1 Drawings showing the anatomy of the normal first metatarsophalangeal joint. ABH tendon = abductor hallucis tendon, ADH tendon = adductor hallucis tendon, EHB = extensor hallucis brevis, EHL = extensor hallucis longus, FHL = flexor hallucis longus, Ses = sesamoid. (Reproduced from Coughlin MJ: Hallux valgus. *Instr Course Lect* 1997;46:357-391.)

also displace medially and also act as a valgus force on the proximal phalanx further contributing to the deformity[4] (**Figure 2**).

- The dorsomedial cutaneous nerve (a branch of the superficial peroneal nerve) is the structure that is most commonly placed at risk during surgical correction. The nerve follows a medial

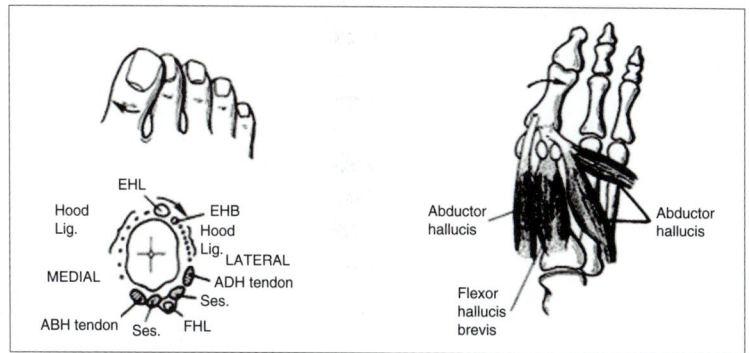

Figure 2 Drawings showing the anatomy of the first metatarsophalangeal joint with hallux valgus. ABH tendon = abductor hallucis tendon, ADH tendon = adductor hallucis tendon, EHB = extensor hallucis brevis, EHL = extensor hallucis longus, FHL = flexor hallucis longus, Ses = sesamoid. (Reproduced from Coughlin MJ: Hallux valgus. *Instr Course Lect* 1997;46:357-391.)

plantar to dorsal course and commonly has a large medial branch that crosses approximately 2 cm proximal to the first MTP joint.[7]

Bony/Articular Structures

- The first MTP joint includes not only the articulation between the first metatarsal and the proximal phalanx but also between the medial and lateral sesamoid and the metatarsal head. The first metatarsal may be rounded or chevron shaped and articulates with the concave surface of the proximal phalanx.
- The range of motion of the first MTP joint is normally 35° of plantar flexion and 75° of dorsiflexion.[8]
- With hallux valgus, it should be noted that the angle between the articular surface and the first metatarsal (the distal metatarsal articular angle [DMAA]) may be increased. This will differentiate a congruent deformity from an incongruent deformity (**Figure 3**). If the DMAA is increased, the articular surface will be facing laterally and will result in a congruent joint. Alternatively, if there

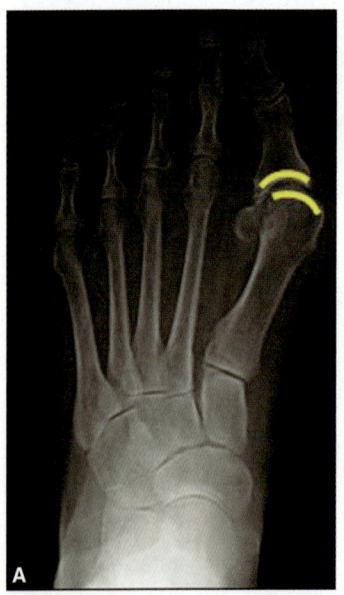
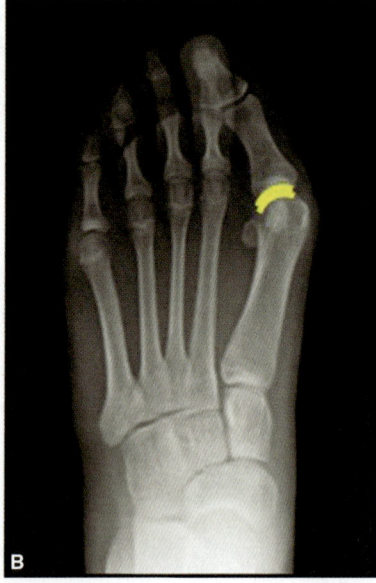

Figure 3 AP radiographs of two feet with a normal distal metatarsal articular angle (DMAA) and an incongruent joint (**A**) and with an increased DMAA and a congruent joint (**B**).

is a normal DMAA and the articular surface is perpendicular to the shaft of the metatarsal, as the proximal phalanx shifts into valgus, this will result in an incongruent joint.

Pertinent History/Physical Examination Findings

- History
  - Patients will most often present with complaints of pain over the medial eminence, particularly with shoe wear.
  - As the hallux valgus progresses, transfer metatarsalgia may develop, which may result in pain and/or calluses under the second metatarsal head.
  - Consideration for treatment should include assessment of comorbidities such as diabetes, particularly with neuropathy, history of neuromuscular disease, or inflammatory arthritis.
- Physical examination
  - Patients will have a prominent medial eminence. The great toe will then shift into valgus and pronate.
  - It is important to evaluate the foot for any calluses. In particular, calluses will often develop under the medial great toe as the toe begins to pronate. Calluses under the second metatarsal head may develop as a result of transfer metatarsalgia.
  - The first MTP motion should be evaluated next to determine any stiffness or pain.
  - Any instability of the first tarsometatarsal (TMT) joint must be evaluated and compared with the opposite side. Although this is important to evaluate, there is some controversy about how to accurately quantify first TMT joint instability.[9]
  - Palpate the medial eminence and first MTP joint as well as the medial and lateral sesamoids. The lesser MTP joints should be inspected for any tenderness or deformity.
  - Numbness of the great toe may be a result of the dorsomedial cutaneous nerve being stretched over the medial eminence (and should be noted before surgery).

Relevant Imaging

- AP, oblique, and lateral images are necessary for evaluation of hallux valgus. The diagnosis of hallux valgus is based on an increase in the hallux valgus angle (HVA) and the 1-2 intermetatarsal angle (1-2 IMA), which are calculated on the AP images.

- Sesamoid views may sometimes be helpful to help evaluate the sesamoid position as well as to determine if there is any arthritis between the sesamoid and the first metatarsal head. This may also be a tool to help determine if there is rotation of the first metatarsal head.[1]
- Radiographic angles are necessary for surgical planning.
  - The HVA is calculated by measuring the angle between the first metatarsal and the proximal phalanx.[10]
  - The 1-2 IMA is calculated as the angle between the shafts of the first and second metatarsal.
  - An HVA greater than 15° and a 1-2 IMA above 9° are considered evidence for a hallux valgus deformity[10] (**Figure 4**).
  - The DMAA is obtained to determine whether a joint is congruent or incongruent. The angle is calculated as the angle between the distal articular surface and the longitudinal surface of the first metatarsal.[1] An angle greater than 10° is considered

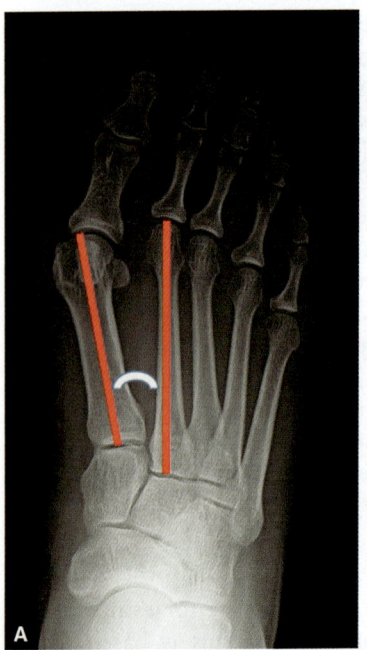
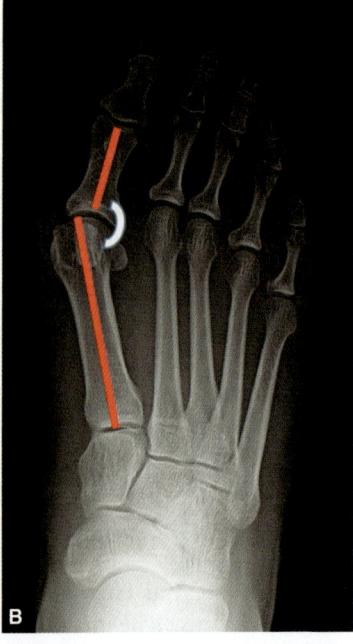

Figure 4 AP radiographs of mild hallux valgus deformity with 1-2 intermetatarsal angle of 12° (**A**) and a 27° hallux valgus angle (**B**).

abnormal and evidence of a congruent joint. An angle less than 10° is normal and suggests an incongruent deformity.
- Congruency of the joint in this hallux valgus scenario indicates that the articular surface is abnormally tilted laterally (elevated DMAA).
- Incongruency of the joint in hallux valgus indicates a soft-tissue imbalance, with contracture of lateral-sided soft-tissue structures around the great toe MTP joint (normal DMAA).

Classification of Deformity

- Mild deformity: HVA between 15° and 20° and a 1-2 IMA between 9° and 11°
- Moderate deformity: an HVA between 20° to 40° and a 1-2 IMA between 11° and 16°
- Severe deformity: an HVA greater than 40° and an IMA greater than 16°[1,10]

Nonsurgical Measures

- Nonsurgical management of hallux valgus is fairly limited considering nonsurgical management has not been shown to reduce the deformity or prevent the progression of hallux valgus.[9]
- Nonsurgical management of hallux valgus is aimed at reducing the pain related to the prominence.
  - Patients should be advised to wear wider and deeper shoes.
  - Softer material such as mesh or soft leather tends to be more flexible to accommodate the prominence.
  - If the deformity is flexible, toe spacers may help reduce the prominence.[1]
  - Orthotics may be of limited benefit.[11]

Outcomes/Current Data Include the Following Studies

- Nakagawa et al[11] recruited 65 patients older than 20 years with an HVA over 20° and a symptomatic bunion who were interested in nonsurgical management. These patients were noted to have a significant decrease in their visual analog scale score at 6 months after wearing the orthotics. However, although the effect was still

statistically significant, the effect of the orthotic diminished at the 12-month mark.
- A 2-year follow-up study[12] showed that 81% of patients continued to use the orthotics at the 24-month mark. This study confirmed no radiographic change in the HVA or IMA.

Surgical Intervention

Indications
- A painful deformity that is persistent despite attempted shoe wear modifications
- Counseling patients is critical to ensure that they have reasonable expectations specifically regarding shoe wear postoperatively.
- The indications for specific techniques are mostly related to the degree of deformity as well as whether the joint is congruent or incongruent.

Techniques—Top Three

Chevron Bunionectomy

Applied Anatomy/Approaches (Relevant Landmarks)
- A distal soft tissue (a modified McBride procedure [soft-tissue release without sesamoidectomy]) may be performed with the chevron bunionectomy and is usually performed first.
  - An incision is initially made in the first web space and dissection is carried down to the lateral sesamoid.
  - A toothed laminar spreader may be placed between the metatarsals to allow better visualization.
  - The attachments to the lateral sesamoid are then released sequentially including:
    - The head of the adductor hallucis tendon is released off the lateral sesamoid.
    - Lateral suspensory sesamoid ligament is released from proximal to distal.
    - The lateral capsule is pie-crusted.
    - The intermetatarsal ligament is released from distal to proximal.
  - Alternatively, a release of the lateral suspensory sesamoid ligament may be completed through the first MTP joint after exposure.

- The chevron osteotomy is next completed by making a medial incision over the medial eminence extending approximately halfway down the shaft of the first metatarsal.
- Dissection is completed down to the medial capsule, being sure to carefully retract the dorsomedial cutaneous nerve that runs just dorsal to the incision.
- An incision in the medial capsule is made and the capsule carefully elevated dorsally and plantarly being sure to preserve two robust cuffs of tissue to allow for a capsulorrhaphy at the end of the procedure.
- The medial eminence is next shaved off before completing the bunionectomy.
- The chevron bunionectomy is a V-shaped cut centered at the distal metatarsal head (**Figure 5**).
- After this is complete, the metatarsal head is translated laterally.
- This may be fixed with many different options but is often held in position with a single screw from dorsal to plantar being sure not to penetrate the plantar metatarsal head or the articular surface.
- After the translation is complete, the overhanging medial bone is shaved down in line with the medial foot.
- Some redundant capsule may be excised and a capsular imbrication performed.

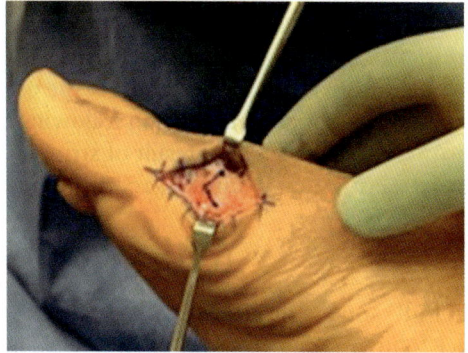

Figure 5 Photograph showing planned osteotomy for a chevron bunionectomy.

Indications for Particular Technique
- Mild deformity, usually with a 1-2 IMA less than approximately 13° and an HVA less than 20°.

Fixation Strategies
- Typically a single compression screw is used across the chevron bunionectomy.
- However, an absorbable screw may also be used[9] as well as Kirschner wire (K-wire) fixation.[13]
- More recently an intramedullary plate has been introduced as a fixation option for chevron bunionectomies.[14]

Postoperative Orders
- Patients are generally allowed to bear weight on the heel directly after surgery.
- Patients are advised to elevate the foot as often as possible to decrease swelling and possibly lower the rate of wound healing complications that can be related to excessive swelling.
- Patients are allowed to bear weight as tolerated in the postoperative shoe for 6 weeks and then transition into a regular supportive shoe.
- Some providers may recommend a toe spacer or strapping of the toe for up to 12 weeks following surgery.

Pearls and Pitfalls
- It is very important to ensure that the osteotomy is translated directly lateral to avoid shortening or lengthening the first metatarsal when translated the metatarsal head. The surgeon similarly must avoid plantar flexion or dorsiflexion at the osteotomy site.
- Osteonecrosis is a potential complication following chevron bunionectomies thought to occur as a result of stripping of the plantar and lateral periosteum;[9] unnecessary stripping of the bone should be avoided.

Outcomes
- Kaufmann et al[13] sought to determine what factors were related to recurrence following chevron bunionectomies. They found that the radiographic factors that contributed to recurrence were an

increased preoperative IMA and HVA and preoperative DMAA and sesamoid position.
- Matsumoto et al[14] published data on intramedullary fixation following chevron osteotomies. An average of 17.8° of correction of the HVA and 7.4° improvement in the IMA were found. Translation of the head of the metatarsal 6.5 mm was achieved and all patients had a successful union.
- A technique with a longer plantar limb on the chevron bunionectomy has been introduced to correct more severe deformities. Song et al[15] performed a retrospective analysis of 36 patients with moderate deformity and 36 patients with severe deformity using the extended distal chevron osteotomy technique. There was significant improvement in all radiographic angles within normal values for both the moderate and severe deformities. Eighty-two percent of patients in the moderate group and 81% of the patients in the severe group rated outcome as good to excellent.[15]
- Quality of life may also be improved for patients with hallux valgus following chevron bunionectomy. Surgery improved the Short Form-36 (SF-36) scores for general health, emotional well-being, role limitations due to personal or emotional problems, physical functioning, and bodily pain. Age and duration of symptoms were related to lower postoperative scores for emotional well-being and bodily pain.[16]

Scarf Bunionectomy

Applied Anatomy/Approaches (Relevant Landmarks)

- A modified McBride lateral soft-tissue release may be used before the scarf bunionectomy (see aforementioned description of chevron bunionectomy).
- The medial first metatarsal and first MTP joint is exposed by making a medial incision over the medial eminence extending approximately from the proximal phalanx distally to the first TMT joint proximally.
- A dissection is completed down to the medial capsule, being sure to carefully retract the dorsomedial cutaneous nerve that runs just dorsal to the incision.
- An incision in the medial capsule is made and the capsule carefully elevated dorsally and plantarly, being sure to preserve two robust cuffs of tissue to allow for a capsulorrhaphy at the end of the procedure.

- A complete dorsal release of the periosteum is important for fixation, but care must be taken to avoid overdissection dorsolaterally or plantarly and disruption of the vascular supply to the metatarsal head.
- Before making the osteotomy incision, a K-wire may be passed to guide the cut from the medial metatarsal head, approximately 5 mm proximal to the articular cartilage and at the dorsal one-third to two-third junction of the width of the metatarsal head. The K-wire is aimed toward the fourth metatarsal head and in a slight plantarward direction to avoid lengthening or shortening the metatarsal head as it is translated.
- The scarf bunionectomy is then completed with three separate cuts. The initial cut is a longitudinal cut that is sloping plantarward from distal to proximal. The proximal and distal cuts are then made at approximately 55° to 60°[1,9] (**Figure 6**).
- After ensuring that there are no periosteal connections between the shaft and the metatarsal head, the distal metatarsal is translated laterally and rotated medially. The reduction is then held with wires and two screws are generally placed to compress the osteotomy.
- The overhanging bone is then resected in line with the medial foot and smoothed down to avoid prominences. Some redundant medial capsule may be excised and a capsular imbrication performed using 0 or 2-0 absorbable sutures in a pants-over-vest fashion.

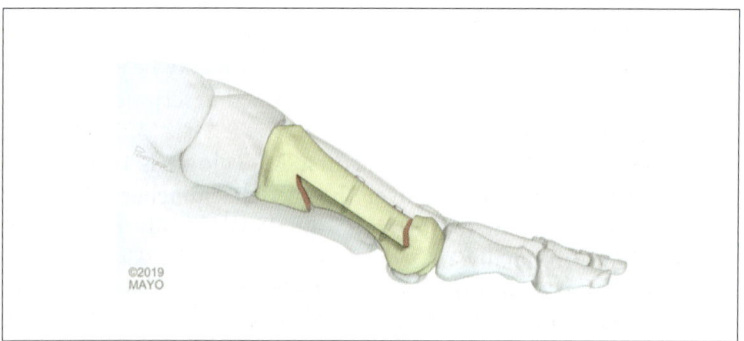

Figure 6 Illustration showing medial approach to the scarf osteotomy. (Reprinted from Shi GG, Whalen JL, Turner NS III, Kitaoka HB: Operative approach to adult hallux valgus deformity: Principles and techniques. *J Am Acad Orthop Surg* 2020;28(10):410-418.)

Indications for Particular Technique
- Moderate to severe bunion deformities

Fixation Strategies
- In general, two compression screws are placed across the osteotomy.

Postoperative Orders
- Patients are generally allowed to bear weight on the heel immediately after surgery.
- Patients are advised to elevate the foot as often as possible to decrease swelling and possibly lower the rate of wound healing complications that can be related to excessive swelling.
- Patients are allowed to bear weight as tolerated in the postoperative shoe for 6 weeks and then transition into a regular supportive shoe.
- Some providers may recommend a toe spacer or strapping of the toe for up to 12 weeks following surgery.

Pearls and Pitfalls
- It is important to avoid lengthening or shortening the first ray. To accomplish this, a K-wire may be placed under fluoroscopic guidance to ensure that the distal metatarsal is being translated directly lateral. If the metatarsal is shortened, this may result in transfer metatarsalgia where the load is placed on the second metatarsal head resulting in overload and pain. Lengthening of the metatarsal can result in stiffening of the first MTP joint. It is also important not to plantarflex or dorsiflex the metatarsal during translation.

Outcomes
- A long-term study evaluated 75 patients (88 feet) in Hong Kong with an average 92-month follow-up. Mean overall American Orthopaedic Foot and Ankle Society (AOFAS) scores improved from 29.6 to 86.83 points and the visual analog scale score improved from 6.61 to 0.66. The average HVA correction was 25.42° and average IMA correction was 8.49°. However, the 8- to 10-year recurrence rate of the HVA over 20° was 31.8% with a higher preoperative HVA more likely to result in recurrence.[17]
- Law et al[18] found that scarf bunionectomy for severe deformity had excellent patient-reported outcomes and radiographic outcomes regardless of severity of deformity at 2-year follow-up.

- A recent abstract described a retrospective study of 22 male patients (26 feet) who underwent scarf bunionectomy and in whom there was a significant improvement in both patient-reported outcomes and radiographic outcomes. There was improvement in visual analog scale score and SF-36 physical scores. IMA improved from 15.9° to 8.7° and HVA improved from 36.1° to 15.1°. These results were maintained over 7.6 years.[19]
- A midterm retrospective cohort similarly showed improvement in radiographic parameters at an average of 13 months postoperatively. Patients had improvement of IMA from 14.3° to 7.9° and improvement of HVA from 32° to 11°. Only two patients reported complications—one with a symptomatic screw and the other with a fracture at the osteotomy site.[20]
- A recent study measured postoperative foot width on radiographs following scarf bunionectomy. The change in the foot width was minimal and on average the width was reduced 2%. Those with larger deformities had a decrease in width, whereas those with smaller deformities had a paradoxical increase in foot width.[21]

Lapidus Bunionectomy

Applied Anatomy/Approaches (Relevant Landmarks)

- A modified McBride procedure may be used for lateral soft-tissue release.
- The approach to the Lapidus procedure begins with a dorsal incision over the first TMT joint. The EHL is identified, the tendon sheath is opened, and the tendon is retracted laterally (if the incision is dorsomedial, retract the tibialis anterior tendon medially).
- In incision is then made directly over the capsule to expose the first TMT joint. An elevator is placed into the joint to free the capsule and allow full exposure down to the plantar aspect of the joint.
- Using a combination of tools such as a chisels, curets, and microsagittal saws, the cartilage is removed from the joint. The joint is irrigated and evaluated until all of the cartilage has been sufficiently removed. The joint is then prepared either using a chisel in a fish-scaling manner or by using a small drill to penetrate the subchondral bone.
- The joint is reduced and compressed with a pointed reduction clamp and held in place with a K-wire. When the first metatarsal and 1-2 IMA are sufficiently reduced, joint fixation is

accomplished with either two crossing cannulated screws, a plate, or a combination of techniques.
- After the first metatarsal is corrected, the medial eminence of the first metatarsal may be shaved down. This is performed through an incision directly over the medial eminence.
- The medial capsule is split and the medial eminence shaved down with a saw. A capsular imbrication is completed following removal of the medial eminence.

Indications for Particular Technique

- The Lapidus bunionectomy a fusion of the first TMT joint and is indicated for moderate to severe bunions or for cases with hypermobility of the first ray. This can also be considered in cases where the patient has a flatfoot for first TMT joint arthritis.[1]

Fixation Strategies

- Options for fixation include crossing cannulated screws or plating. Newer techniques include intramedullary nailing.

Postoperative Orders

- Postoperatively, patients typically do not bear weight for 6 to 12 weeks.
- The patient's foot is usually immobilized initially in a splint and after suture removal the transition is made into a boot or cast based on the surgeon's preference.

Pearls and Pitfalls

- Whenever performing a fusion, nonunion or malunion is a potential complication. In particular with this technique, a dorsiflexion malunion must be avoided. The first TMT joint is approximately 30 mm deep and approached dorsally. It is imperative that the plantar aspect of the joint be meticulously prepared to avoid this complication. Additionally, a clamp placed dorsally could accentuate a dorsiflexion force, so this should be monitored as well.

Outcomes

- Studies have recently been evaluating the effect of early weight bearing on union rates for Lapidus bunionectomies.

- One recent review of 8 clinical trials with 12-month minimal follow-up concluded that there was a 3.61% rate of nonunion with early weight bearing less than 2 weeks after surgery.[22]
- Another recent study evaluated the addition of a crossing screw into the middle cuneiform with an average follow-up of 9.3 months. They reported a 96.7% union rate, a 6.8° improvement in the IMA, and 14.8° improvement in the HVA.[23]
- Barp et al[24] evaluated different constructs in their patient population in a retrospective review. A total of 147 patients were treated with an intraplate compression screw, a solid crossing screw, and a single screw with a locking plate all performed by a single surgeon. The overall nonunion rate was 6%, with 4% requiring hardware removal. There was no statistical significance between the different fixation constructs.

Top 10 Knowledge Drops for Your Rotation

1. Hallux valgus is a complex disorder that generally starts with relative laxity of the medial capsule.
2. During surgical dissection, the dorsomedial cutaneous nerve is at risk for injury.
3. Nonsurgical management generally consists of modified shoe wear and toe spacers.
4. Surgery is indicated when nonsurgical treatment and shoe wear modification have failed.
5. Physical examination focused on the first MTP joint should assess range of motion, pain, and sensation as well as the ability or inability to reduce the joint.
6. Physical examination should also include assessment of the first TMT joint, specifically for laxity.
7. Surgical treatment is generally determined by the degree of deformity.
8. A mild deformity can be managed with a distal first metatarsal osteotomy such as a chevron bunionectomy.
9. A moderate to severe deformity can be managed with a proximal first metatarsal osteotomy such as a scarf bunionectomy.
10. First TMT joint laxity or a moderate to severe deformity can be managed with a Lapidus bunionectomy.

Chapter 11: My Foot and Ankle Hurt

HALLUX RIGIDUS

Epidemiology

Incidence
- The first MTP joint is the most common location of arthritis in the foot.[25]
- 10% of adults have symptomatic hallux rigidus, although it is predicted that many more have radiographic evidence of arthritis.[25]

Demographics
- Risk factors
  - Occurs more often in females than males
  - Family history: those with a family history are more likely to have bilateral disease versus unilateral disease in those with a history of trauma.[26]
  - Flatter or chevron-shaped metatarsal head[27]
  - Patients with trauma to the great toe, either a single event or repetitive microtrauma, are at risk for the development of hallux rigidus.[25]
  - There does not seem to be any relationship to Achilles tendon tightness, foot positioning, first metatarsal elevation, or first ray hypermobility.[26]

Pertinent Anatomy/Pathoanatomy

- The plantar plate is an important part of the anatomy of the first MTP joint. The plantar plate complex includes the medial and lateral sesamoid, the two heads of the flexor digitorum brevis, the plantar plate, and other ligaments that contribute to the stability of the first MTP joint.[28]
- The EHL extends past the MTP joint and inserts distal to the interphalangeal joint. The EHL functions as a dorsiflexor of the first MTP joint.
- The FHL lies plantarly and inserts on the distal phalanx. The FHL travels between the two sesamoids plantarly and has the main function of plantarflexing the first MTP joint.
- The first MTP joint consists of the first metatarsal articulating with the proximal phalanx. The cartilage of the first metatarsal

head extends to the dorsal surface to accommodate the proximal phalanx when the joint is in dorsiflexion.
- The first metatarsal head is convex whereas the proximal phalanx is concave. On the plantar aspect of the first metatarsal head, there are two grooves separated by the cristae to articulate with the medial and lateral sesamoids.[28]
- The range of motion of the first MTP joint is normally 35° of plantar flexion and 75° of dorsiflexion.[5]
- With normal movement and gait, the first MTP joint dorsiflexes, resulting in repetitive compressive loads on the dorsal aspect of the joint. This results in wear of the dorsal cartilage and dorsal osteophytes and eventual full-thickness cartilage loss.[5]

Pertinent History/Physical Examination Findings

History

- Patients may describe a remote injury to the great toe or may have been involved in sports that could cause repetitive microtrauma to the first MTP joint, such as running.
- Patients usually complain about pain and stiffness.
- Hallux rigidus is notable for the large dorsal bony spurs that develop on the first metatarsal head. These spurs can lead to pain with shoe wear because of their prominence.
- The spurs also block dorsiflexion and cause pain when the proximal phalanx dorsiflexes into the bone spur. Because of this, activities that require great toe dorsiflexion tend to exacerbate pain. Some activities would include standing on tiptoe, certain yoga poses, squatting down with the toes flexed (as while gardening), doing push-ups, or planks or walking uphill.
- Because of the loss of motion and pain at the great toe, patients will often offload the medial foot by supinating and placing the pressure more laterally. Over time, these patients will often complain about pain over the lesser MTP joints as a result of overload.[25]

Physical Examination

- The dorsal osteophyte of the first metatarsal head results in a prominence that is notable on examination.
- Patients often have swelling and tenderness when palpating the spur.

- Range of motion of the first MTP joint is limited, particularly in dorsiflexion. In later stages, there will also be loss of plantar flexion.
- Range of motion should always be compared with the opposite side, particularly if there is no hallux rigidus contralaterally.
- A grind test should also be performed by placing axial load to the first MTP joint to determine whether there is pain in the midrange of motion.
- The sesamoids should be palpated plantarly to determine whether there is metatarsal-sesamoid arthritis.

Classification

- The most commonly referenced classification for hallux rigidus was described by Coughlin and Shurnas[26] in 2003. This classification system takes into account both radiographic findings and clinical examination findings (**Table 1**).

TABLE 1 Coughlin and Shurnas Classification System

Grade	Dorsiflexion	Radiographic Findings	Clinical Findings
0	40°-60° (20% loss of normal motion)	Normal	No pain. Only stiffness and loss of motion
1	30°-40° (20%-60% loss of normal motion)	Dorsal osteophyte. Minimal joint-space narrowing, periarticular sclerosis and flattening of the metatarsal head	Mild or occasional pain and stiffness at the extremes of motion
2	10°-30° (50%-75% loss of normal motion)	Dorsal, lateral, possible medial osteophytes with flattened appearance to the metatarsal head; less than one-fourth of the dorsal joint space is involved on the lateral radiograph; mild to moderate joint-space narrowing and sclerosis; sesamoids not involved	Moderate to severe pain and stiffness. Pain occurs just before maximum dorsiflexion and maximum plantar flexion
3	≤10° (75%-100% loss of normal motion) loss of plantar flexion as well (often ≤10°)	Same as in grade 2 but with substantial narrowing, cystic changes, more than one-fourth of the dorsal joint space is involved on the lateral radiograph, sesamoids enlarged, cystic and/or irregular	Constant pain and substantial stiffness at the extremes of range of motion but not a midrange
4	Same as in grade 3	Same as in grade 3	Same as in grade 3 but with hindrance of passive motion

Reprinted with permission from Coughlin MJ, Shurnas PS: Hallux rigidus: Grading and long-term results of operative treatment. *J Bone Joint Surg Am* 2003;85(11):2072-2088.

- Grade 0 hallux rigidus: normal radiographs and slightly diminished dorsiflexion compared with the normal side.
- Grade 1 hallux rigidus: radiographic findings with minimal joint-space narrowing and a dorsal osteophyte of the first metatarsal head. Patients will begin to note a more significant loss of dorsiflexion at this stage.
- Grade 2 hallux rigidus: Radiographs show more flattening of the metatarsal head, mild-to-moderate joint-space narrowing, and 50% to 75% loss of dorsiflexion compared with the opposite side.
- Grade 3 hallux rigidus: More substantial narrowing on radiographs and more than one-fourth of the dorsal joint space involved on lateral radiographs with or without changes to the sesamoids. Dorsiflexion is very limited and there may be some loss of plantar flexion as well.
- Grade 4 hallux rigidus: Has all the components of grade 3 hallux rigidus with the addition of pain during the mid-range of motion of the MTP joint (as opposed to grades 1 through 3. which only have pain at the extremes of motion) (**Figure 7**).

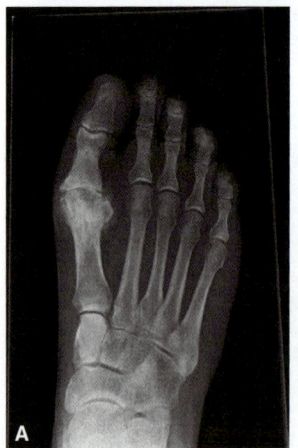
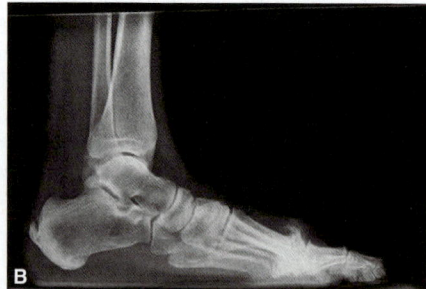

Figure 7 Stage 4 hallux rigidus. **A**, AP radiograph shows loss of joint space with some hallux valgus deformity. **B**, Lateral radiograph shows a large dorsal osteophyte and loss of joint space.

Relevant Imaging

- Radiographs are the gold standard for evaluating hallux rigidus.
- Standard views include AP, oblique, and lateral views.
    - In early stages of hallux rigidus, osteophytes begin to develop. These are most commonly on the dorsal first metatarsal head and the dorsal proximal phalanx at the articular margin on the lateral view.
    - With time, a plantar flexion contracture of the first MTP joint may develop, which can lead to elevation of the first metatarsal or metatarsus elevatus.
    - AP views will often show bone spurs on the medial and lateral proximal phalanx or first metatarsal head with squaring of the metatarsal head.
    - As arthritis progresses, there will be more noticeable joint-space narrowing. Subchondral cysts may begin to develop in the metatarsal head.
    - It is also important to note any malalignment.
- A sesamoid view may also be obtained to evaluate the articulation between the first metatarsal head and the sesamoids. Osteophytes of the sesamoids or narrowing of the joint space are seen in patients with arthritis.

Nonsurgical Measures

- Patients may be treated with oral or topical anti-inflammatory medications to help control symptoms.
- They may also find improvement with shoe wear modifications. If a patient has pain primarily over the dorsal bone spur, then appropriate shoe wear may improve pain. Softer or leather materials tend to be better tolerated because they are more flexible and can stretch to accommodate any prominences. They may also find that a deeper toe box allows for more space and less irritation of the prominence.
- Alternatively, for later stage arthritis where there is pain either in midrange or end range of motion, a device that limits dorsiflexion of the great toe is of benefit. This can be in the form of a stiffer shoe or a Morton extension device, which is a stiff shank under the medial ray to prevent motion of the first MTP joint.[8]

- Intra-articular corticosteroid injections may be of short-term benefit. Cortisone works as a strong local anti-inflammatory agent to help decrease pain in the joint.

Outcomes
- A recent review evaluated the current literature regarding the nonsurgical management of hallux rigidus. Although it was noted that most interventions showed some improvement, it was concluded that there is poor evidence to support intra-articular cortisone injections for pain relief and fair evidence against the use of intra-articular cortisone injections for long-term efficacy. There was no good evidence recommending any intervention because of the lack of high-quality studies.[29]
- Grice et al in 2017 published outcomes retrospectively looking at the efficacy of foot and ankle corticosteroid injections. In a study of 22 patients with hallux rigidus who received an injection, 91% had significant benefit from the injection. However, this benefit only extended beyond 3 months in three of these patients (14%), suggesting that this may be helpful for short-term relief.[30]

Surgical Interventions
Indications

Key Findings on History
- Patients are indicated for surgery if nonsurgical management has been attempted and was unsuccessful.

Key Findings on Examination
- On examination, patients will have pain with range of motion of the first MTP joint and pain with palpation dorsally over the first MTP joint.
- They will usually have a large prominence over the dorsal first metatarsal head at the location of the osteophyte.

Key Laboratory Findings
- Radiographs will show evidence of dorsal osteophytes of the first metatarsal head and/or the proximal phalanx on lateral images.
- AP and oblique images will often also show medial and lateral osteophytes and may show joint-space narrowing depending on the stage of the disease.

Techniques—Top Three

Cheilectomy

Applied Anatomy/Approaches (Relevant Landmarks)

- Dorsal approach
  - An incision is made dorsally over the medial ray, centered over the first MTP joint.
  - Sharp dissection is performed down to the EHL tendon.
  - The tendon sheath is then opened and the EHL tendon is released off the dorsal capsule for the full extent of the incision.
  - The EHL tendon is retracted laterally and a midline incision is made in the capsule of the first MTP joint extending the length of the incision (**Figure 8**).
- After the capsule is retracted out of the way, the dorsal spurs are identified.
- A rongeur is used to remove the osteophytes at the base of the proximal phalanx. The joint is then plantarflexed to expose the dorsal first metatarsal head osteophyte. Either a saw or a chisel may be used to remove the dorsal osteophyte.
- It is generally recommended that at least one-third of the dorsal surface of the first metatarsal head be excised.

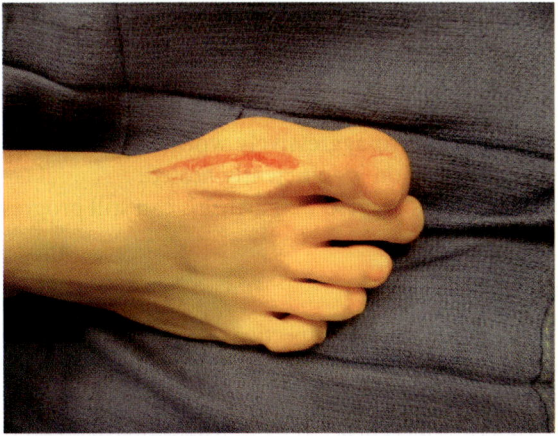

Figure 8 Photograph showing standard dorsal exposure to the first metatarsophalangeal joint.

Indications for Particular Technique
- A cheilectomy alone is indicated in Coughlin and Shurnas grade 1, 2, and 3 disease with less than 50% loss of cartilage.
- This may also be an appropriate procedure in patients with low physical demands and who are only having symptoms related to the prominence alone.

Postoperative Orders
- A soft dressing and a stiff-soled shoe are used and patients are allowed immediate weight bearing.
- Deep vein thrombosis prophylaxis is based on patient risk factors but in general is not indicated for the procedure alone.
- Stitches are removed at approximately 10 to 14 days postoperatively.
- After removal of stitches, the patient is encouraged to begin range of motion and transitioning into regular shoe wear.
- Patients may require physical therapy if the range of motion is not progressing adequately.

Pearls and Pitfalls
- Understanding and counseling patient expectations is critical before any surgery.
- Patients should know that although pain relief is fairly consistent, improvement in range of motion is less so.
- It is important to be aggressive with the dorsal cheilectomy and remove one-third of the metatarsal head to allow optimal improvement in range of motion.
- It is also important to aggressively work on mobilizing the joint as soon as the incision is sufficiently healed.
- It should be communicated that arthritis can still progress despite a cheilectomy.

Outcomes
- Sidon et al performed a retrospective review evaluating 165 patients with an average of 6.6 years of follow-up. Patients with grade 1 through 3 hallux rigidus in whom nonsurgical management failed and who underwent a cheilectomy were included in the study. Patient satisfaction surveys showed that 69% were satisfied or very satisfied with the results and most had improvement in their pain level.

Twenty-nine percent had recurrence of pain following the surgery. More than 70% had complete relief of their symptoms, whereas 13% had no relief. Five percent underwent a subsequent surgery at an average of 3.6 years following initial cheilectomy.[31]

Interposition Arthroplasty

Applied Anatomy/Approaches (Relevant Landmarks)

- The dorsal approach previously described is used similarly for an interposition arthroplasty.
- However, rather than splitting the capsule in the midline, a proximally based flap of capsule is carefully elevated off the first MTP joint.
- After the joint is exposed, the dorsal spur of the first metatarsal is removed as in a hallux cheilectomy.
- The base of the proximal phalanx is then removed with a saw to create some space to accommodate the interposition. It is important bevel the resection proximally to keep the proximal plantar phalanx intact with the plantar plate attachments to avoid a cock-up deformity.
- The dorsal capsule is then interposed in the space by resurfacing over the metatarsal head. A stitch is then passed from each corner of the dorsal capsular flap to the medial or lateral plantar plate respectively.

Indications for Particular Technique

- Interposition arthroplasty is a reasonable alternative for patients with more advanced arthritis who are not candidates for a hallux cheilectomy, but who require or desire some preserved range of motion. This may include patients who are dancers or yoga instructors, for example.

Postoperative Orders

- Postoperative protocol is identical to that of a hallux cheilectomy.

Pearls and Pitfalls

- Although interposition arthroplasty is a good option for patients who require range of motion, it should be emphasized that this may not relieve pain entirely.

- It is also unlikely that the patient will regain normal range of motion, especially if they did not have normal motion before surgery.
- Because of the plantar plate attachment to the proximal, plantar base of the proximal phalanx, it is very important that this attachment is not removed while excising the base of the phalanx. If this is removed, a cock-up deformity can develop.

Outcomes

- In 2017 Aynardi et al retrospectively reviewed 133 patients who underwent the procedure with an average follow-up of 62.2 months. They found that outcomes were rated excellent in 65.4% and good in 24.1%, with fair or poor results in 10.5%. Unfavorable outcomes included six patients with a cock-up deformity of the first MTP joint or metatarsalgia in 17.3%. The procedure was unsuccessful in five patients, three of whom were converted to fusion.[32]
- A long-term outcome study assessing capsular interposition retrospectively evaluated 64 patients with an average of 11.3 years of follow-up. There was significant improvement in visual analog scale scores, SF-12 physical and mental scores, and Foot Function Index scores. Patient satisfaction score was an average of 7.4 on a 10-point scale. Four patients (9.5%) required conversion to a fusion at an average of 6.1 years following their initial surgery.[33]

First MTP Joint Fusion

Applied Anatomy/Approaches (Relevant Landmarks)

- The dorsal incision is again used for an MTP joint fusion.
- If a plate is going to be used, it is important that the periosteum be split the length of the plate and elevated to accommodate it.
- A 360° release of the MTP joint is performed to allow the first MTP joint to be hyperplantarflexed to gain exposure to the two surfaces. Any large osteophytes may then be removed with a saw or rongeur.
- A cup-and-cone preparation of the surfaces is often used for primary joint fusion. Many implant companies have reamers specific to this procedure to allow joint preparation. A K-wire is first inserted into the center of the metatarsal head and

advanced down the center of the first metatarsal shaft. AP and lateral radiographs are then obtained to confirm appropriate position of the wire. A cone-shaped reamer appropriate to the specific size of the patient's metatarsal head is then advanced over the wire. The metatarsal head is reamed until the cartilage and subchondral bone is removed and there is bleeding bone visualized.
- In a similar manner, the wire is then advanced down the shaft of the proximal phalanx and the position is confirmed on radiographs. The corresponding sized cup-shaped reamer is then advanced and the bone is again reamed until bleeding bone is seen. The surfaces may then be further prepared by drilling with a drill or K-wire.
- The great toe is then positioned into physiologic positioning. This includes approximately 10° to 15° of dorsiflexion with respect to the floor and 5° to 15° of valgus.[34]
- The first MTP joint is held provisionally in place with one or two K-wires. A flat plate is placed against the plantar aspect of the foot to simulate weight bearing and confirm the appropriate position of fusion. AP and lateral radiographs are also obtained to confirm position of the fusion and good compression across the joint.
- If a single compression screw is to be used, it is usually passed percutaneously from distal medial to proximal lateral across the MTP joint. Following placement of this screw, a second crossing screw may be placed or a dorsal neutralization plate can be placed.
- After all hardware has been placed, final radiographs are obtained to evaluate hardware position, fusion position, and compression across the joint. The wound is irrigated and the dorsal capsule is closed over the plate followed by closure of the skin.

Indications for Particular Technique

- First MTP joint fusion is the surgery of choice for a patient with more advanced disease, specifically grades 3 or 4, with significant loss of joint space, cartilage, and motion recognized on examination but pain in the midrange of motion.
- This is also an excellent option for patients with deformity or neuromuscular disorders.[25]

- Patients with some comorbidities should be counseled before undergoing any foot and ankle surgery. In particular, patients with diabetes should have their diabetes controlled and it is generally recommended that hemoglobin A1C be less than 8 mg/L or 7.5 mg/L before undergoing surgery of the foot and ankle to lower risk of complications.[35] Smokers should be counseled on smoking cessation, most importantly before undergoing a fusion. In particular, cigarette smoking is known to increase perioperative complication rates including nonunion, delayed union, infection, delayed wound healing, and persistent pain.[36]

Fixation Strategies
- There are multiple options for fixation of the first MTP joint. The critical factors to lead to a successful fusion include good compression and strong fixation, which can be achieved through many different fixation constructs. Fixation ranges from crossing cannulated screws to dorsal plating to a combination of the two.

Postoperative Orders
- A soft dressing and a stiff-soled shoe are used, and patients are allowed immediate weight bearing. Patients may alternatively wear a short walking boot.
- Patients should be advised to elevate the limb to decrease swelling, manage pain, and allow the soft tissues to heal.
- Deep vein thrombosis prophylaxis is based on patient risk factors but in general is not indicated for the procedure alone.
- Stitches are removed at approximately 10 to 14 days postoperatively.
- The stiff-soled postoperative shoe or boot is used for up to 12 weeks postoperatively depending on the progress of fusion. Patients rarely require physical therapy after this surgery unless required for gait training.

Pearls and Pitfalls
- Position of the fusion is critical for function. Ten degrees to 15° of dorsiflexion is recommended to allow normal roll-through during gait. If the toe is too dorsiflexed, it

will result in difficulty with shoe wear and if too plantarflexed, the patient can jam the toe during roll-through, and this can lead to hyperlaxity of the interphalangeal joint to accommodate.
- Radiographs should also be checked to evaluate for any evidence of nonunion. Patients who use nicotine products and those with diabetes or vascular insufficiency may be particularly prone to nonunion and should be followed closely.
- When preparing the joint, it is important to remove all the sclerotic bone, but care should be taken to avoid removal of too much bone. If the medial ray is shortened too much, the patient could be at risk for transfer metatarsalgia (pain under the second metatarsal head).

Outcomes (Current Data)
- DeSandis et al reviewed 53 patients who underwent first MTP fusion over a 6-year period. All 53 patients progressed to a successful fusion and had improvement in performing activities of daily living along with their SF-12 scores and Foot and Ankle Outcome Score. Eighty-five percent of patients were satisfied or highly satisfied. Fifty-three percent of patients had limitations in shoe wear, specifically the height of a heel that could be worn. Patients had increased ability to participate in walking, jogging, running, and treadmill activities.[37]
- Lunati et al recently published prospective results of patients undergoing first MTP fusion to determine if age was a factor for union. In a total of 143 patients (79 patients younger than 65 years and 64 patients older than 65 years), there was no difference in outcomes despite more comorbidities in the older group. Visual analog scale and SF-36 physical and mental component summaries all increased significantly at the 6- and 12-year postoperative time point. Both cohorts had similar complication rates.[38]
- Kannan et al reviewed 409 consecutive fusions in 385 patients. One hundred seventeen patients with a plate and screw construct were compared with 94 patients with a solid screw construct. A union rate of 91.4% was reported. Of the 35 nonunions, only 10 were symptomatic. There was no difference in complications between the two constructs.[39]

Top 10 Knowledge Drops for Your Rotation

1. Patients with hallux rigidus will often complain of pain with dorsiflexion activities (performing heel raises, yoga, reaching above the head, walking uphill) and pain with shoe wear related to the dorsal prominence.
2. Patients may report a history of a single trauma or repetitive trauma such a running.
3. On physical examination, patients will have a painful dorsal prominence, pain with range of motion, loss of dorsiflexion first, then loss of plantar flexion.
4. On physical examination, the grind test can help determine whether there is cartilage loss centrally in the MTP joint.
5. A prominence related to a bunion can be distinguished by looking at the position of the great toe and whether it is straight or shifting into valgus.
6. Radiographs are critical to determine the stage of disease. Early arthritis has large dorsal bone spurs only; more advanced disease has loss of joint space.
7. Nonsurgical options for hallux rigidus include Morton extension/stiff shank insert versus stiff shoes, anti-inflammatory agents, cortisone injections.
8. Cheilectomy alone is the preferred surgical option when joint space is preserved on radiographs and pain is related to the large prominence and pain at the extremes of motion.
9. First MTP joint fusion is the gold standard for advanced arthritis with loss of cartilage and loss of motion and/or the need for deformity correction.
10. Interposition arthroplasty is a reasonable alternative for patients with later stage arthritis but who require range of motion.

POSTERIOR TIBIAL TENDON DYSFUNCTION

Epidemiology

- Most commonly presents in patients in their fifth or sixth decades
- More common in females than males
- Risk factors: obesity, diabetes, and hypertension. Occasionally a history of trauma or corticosteroid use

- Differential diagnosis: accessory navicular syndrome, tarsal coalitions, traumatic isolated spring ligament tears
- Young adult males with PTTD symptoms should be referred to rheumatology specialists to rule out inflammatory arthropathy

Pertinent Anatomy/Pathoanatomy

- Soft tissue
  - PTT
    - Deep posterior compartment of the leg
    - Origin: Posterior tibia, intraosseous membrane, and posterior fibula
    - Insertion: Primarily on medial tuberosity and medial cuneiform with secondary insertions on the middle/lateral cuneiforms, and second through fifth metatarsals
    - Innervation: Tibial nerve
    - Blood supply: Primarily posterior tibial artery with additional distal supply from anterior tibial artery
      - Hypovascular area 2.2 cm proximal to through 0.6 cm distal to medial malleolus[40]
    - Function: Inverts hindfoot; adducts and supinates forefoot. Locks transverse tarsal joint to allow toe-off
    - Antagonist: Peroneus brevis
  - Flexor digitorum longus
    - Origin: Posterior tibia
    - Insertion: Plantar second through fifth toe distal phalanx bases
    - Innervation: Tibial nerve
    - Runs superficial (plantar) to the FHL at the knot of Henry
  - Spring (calcaneonavicular) ligament
    - Origin: sustentaculum tali of the calcaneus
    - Insertion: inferior/inferomedial navicular
    - Function: Stabilize medial longitudinal arch
  - Deltoid ligament
    - Superficial layer: tibionavicular, tibiocalcaneal, and posterior tibiotalar
    - Deep layer: anterior tibiotalar and deep posterior tibiotalar
    - Function: Prevents valgus tilting of the talus and eversion of the hindfoot, and provides stability of the ankle to external rotation and pronation

Pertinent History
- Patients will typically present early with pain along the medial ankle and hindfoot. As the disease progresses, pain develops along the lateral hindfoot due to subfibular impingement or development of subtalar arthritis. Patients will initially note pain with physical activity that eventually becomes more constant as the deformity progresses. Often patients will have a long-standing history of flatfoot that has become symptomatic and begun to progressively collapse. It is important to determine whether there is a history of trauma as an initiating event because this may be a sign of an acute PTT tear or spring ligament tear.

Pertinent Physical Examination
- Assessment of alignment in standing position will often show hindfoot valgus with pronation of the foot. In some patients there will be increased forefoot abduction, which is referred to as the too many toes sign.
- Ankle alignment should be assessed for any valgus deformity. While the patient is standing, it is imperative to have the patient perform a single leg heel rise (SLHR) to determine whether the PTT is intact. The patient is then examined in a seated position. Palpate for any tenderness along the PTT, deltoid and spring ligaments, as well as along the ankle, subtalar, and transverse tarsal joints. There may also be swelling or bogginess over the PTT suggestive of thickening and tendinosis.
- Range of motion of the ankle, hindfoot, and transverse tarsal joints is important, including assessment of whether the hindfoot valgus and forefoot abduction and pronation are passively correctible or rigid in nature.
- With the hindfoot corrected to neutral, the forefoot should be checked for any residual fixed forefoot supination.
- The Silfverskiöld test should be performed to assess for any gastrocnemius or Achilles tendon contractures. This is done by examining the ankle dorsiflexion with the knee extended and again with the knee flexed to 90°. It is normal if the ankle can be dorsiflexed above neutral in both the flexed and extended positions of the knee. If the dorsiflexion is limited with the knee extended but not flexed, there is tightness in the gastrocnemius; however, if dorsiflexion is limited with the knee both extended and flexed, then there is tightness in the Achilles tendon.

Relevant Imaging

- Radiographs
  - Weight-bearing radiographs to adequately demonstrate the true extent of the deformity
  - Ankle AP/oblique/lateral radiographs
    - Presence of any valgus tilting of the talus suggestive of tearing of the deltoid ligament
  - Foot AP/oblique/lateral, and hindfoot alignment radiographic views
    - AP foot radiographs: There may be an increase in the talo–first metatarsal angle (normal 15° to 30°) and talonavicular uncoverage because of abduction across the transverse tarsal joint.
    - Lateral foot radiographs: There may be an increase in Meary angle (lateral talo–first metatarsal angle, normal −4° to +4°), decrease in calcaneal pitch (normal 18° to 20°), and decrease in medial cuneiform to floor height (normal 18 mm).
    - Hindfoot alignment view (**Figure 9**): Hindfoot valgus with the center of the calcaneus being lateral to the axis of the tibia.
  - Presence of arthritis should be noted in the subtalar joints, transverse tarsal joints, or tibiotalar joint
- Advanced imaging is often not needed on initial evaluation; perform MRI or CT in cases where nonsurgical measures have failed.
  - MRI will show tenosynovitis, tearing or thickening of the PTT along with spring ligament tearing, or the presence of any arthritis of the hindfoot joints. This allows for assessment of the deltoid ligament as well.
  - CT: assessment for hindfoot arthritis
    - Three-dimensional weight-bearing CT scans have become beneficial in evaluating the true hindfoot deformity.[41]

Classification

The most commonly accepted classification of PTTD is that originally described by Johnson and Strum with stages I, II, and III and subsequently modified by Myerson to include stage IV. Understanding the stages is important for describing the deformity but also for surgical intervention.

- Stage I, PTT tenosynovitis: No/minimal deformity. +SLHR

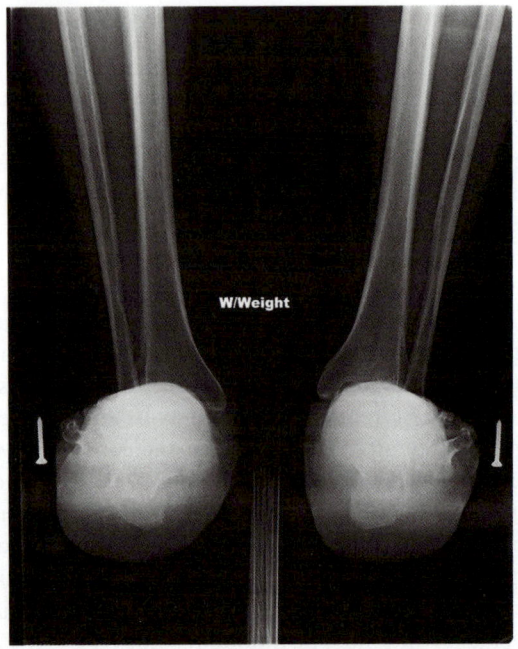

Figure 9 Radiograph showing hindfoot alignment.

- Stage II, PTT tear/dysfunction: Flexible deformity (passively correctable), −SLHR
  - IIa: No/minimal forefoot abduction (less than 30% talonavicular uncoverage)
  - IIb: Forefoot abduction (greater than 30% talonavicular uncoverage)
- Stage III, PTT tear/dysfunction, hindfoot arthritis: Rigid deformity (not passively correctable), −SLHR
- Stage IV, PTT tear/dysfunction, deltoid ligament tear/dysfunction: Ankle and hindfoot valgus, −SLHR

Nonsurgical Measures

Nonsurgical management should be considered the first line of treatment for PTTD regardless of the stage of the deformity. Depending on severity of symptoms, a period of immobilization in a boot or walking cast may be required. NSAIDs as well as physical therapy may aid in alleviating symptoms. Additionally, medial arch support of some type is often recommended to offload the PTT and the medial longitudinal arch. For stage 1 deformity, this includes custom orthotics with medial posting/medial heel lift. For stage II deformity, this includes either a University of California Berkeley Laboratory orthosis with medial posting or a custom short articulated ankle-foot orthosis. For stages III and IV deformities, an ankle-foot orthosis or Arizona brace provides more support than a custom orthotic. Short-term studies have shown good benefit with these orthotic devices in stage I and II deformities; however, long-term studies are lacking demonstrating prolonged effectiveness or prevention of progression of deformity.

Surgical Intervention

Surgical treatment is often indicated when nonsurgical treatment modalities for at least 3 months have failed. The specific surgical intervention is often based on the stage of the deformity.

- Stage I: Tenosynovectomy. Consider addition of medial displacement calcaneal osteotomy in setting of hindfoot valgus to protect PTT.
- Stage IIa: PTT débridement with flexor digitorum longus tendon transfer, medial displacement calcaneal osteotomy, +/− spring ligament repair/reconstruction, +/− gastrocnemius recession or Achilles tendon lengthening.
  - After the hindfoot has been corrected, the surgeon evaluates for the presence of residual forefoot supination. If present, a Cotton medial cuneiform opening wedge osteotomy or a first tarsometatarsal plantar flexion arthrodesis is added.
- Stage IIb: Same as IIa; however, increased abduction across talonavicular joint can be corrected through Evans lateral column lengthening (opening wedge osteotomy of the lateral calcaneus) or calcaneocuboid joint opening wedge arthrodesis.
- Stage III: Hindfoot arthrodesis, +/− gastrocnemius recession or Achilles tendon lengthening; traditionally involved triple arthrodesis (subtalar, talonavicular, and calcaneocuboid joint). Studies have shown good outcomes with double arthrodesis (subtalar and talonavicular joints).
- Stage IV: Similar treatment to stages II or III; however, additional treatment of the tibiotalar joint and incompetent deltoid ligament is required. For the flexible valgus ankle deformity, a

deltoid ligament reconstruction is performed. For a rigid valgus ankle deformity, a tibiotalocalcaneal or pantalar arthrodesis (ankle, subtalar, talonavicular, and calcaneocuboid joints) is performed.

Top 10 Knowledge Drops for Your Rotation

1. PTT anatomy: Primarily inserts on medial navicular. Hypovascular area 2 to 6 cm proximal to insertion site.
2. Knot of Henry: Flexor digitorum longus is superficial (plantar) to FHL.
3. Spring ligament: Originates from sustentaculum tali of calcaneus and inserts on inferomedial navicular.
4. Ability to perform SLHR infers intact PTT.
5. Silfverskiöld test is used to determine presence of gastrocnemius or Achilles contracture.
   a. Dorsiflexion limited only in knee extension: gastrocnemius tightness
   b. Dorsiflexion limited in knee extension and flexion: Achilles tightness
6. Meary angle = lateral talofirst metatarsal angle. Normally −4° to +4°: In PTTD there will be an increase in Meary angle.
7. Stages of PTTD
   I = PTT tenosynovitis: + SLHR
   IIa = PTT tear: −SLHR, flexible deformity without forefoot abduction
   IIb = PTT tear: −SLHR, flexible deformity with forefoot abduction
   III = PTT tear: SLHR, rigid deformity (arthritis)
   IV = PTT tear: −SLHR, deltoid ligament tear/incompetence → valgus ankle
8. Arch support should include medial posting (medial lift) to offload PTT/medial arch.
9. Surgical correction of hindfoot valgus usually includes a medial calcaneal osteotomy.
10. Surgical correction of forefoot supination includes Cotton medial cuneiform osteotomy or first tarsometatarsal plantar flexion arthrodesis.

ACHILLES TENDINOPATHY AND TENDON RUPTURE

Epidemiology

- Approximately 6% of the general population complains of Achilles tendon pain throughout their lifetime.[42]
- Insertional Achilles tendinopathy (IAT) accounts for approximately 20% of all Achilles tendon disorders.[43]
- Causes of IAT
  - Haglund deformity
  - Tendinous calcification
  - Enthesophytes (bone spurs)
- IAT risk factors
  - Overweight
  - Use of fluoroquinolones and statins
  - Chronic diseases (eg, diabetes, rheumatoid arthritis, and hypercholesterolemia)
- Achilles tendon ruptures are most common among young male patients (20 to 39 years of age).[44]
- Tendon rupture risk factors
  - Weekend warrior
  - Fluoroquinolone antibiotic class
  - Steroid injections

Pertinent Anatomy/Pathoanatomy

- This is the strongest and largest tendon in the human body.[45]
- Surrounded by a paratenon (ie, false sheath).
- The Achilles tendon is a confluence of the following muscles:
  - Medial gastrocnemius
  - Lateral gastrocnemius
  - Soleus
  - Plantaris
- Inserts into the calcaneal tuberosity.
- Blood supply of the Achilles tendon is from the posterior tibial artery.
- Blood supply of the Achilles tendon insertion is an arterial plexus, which surrounds the calcaneus and is supplied by the posterior tibial and fibular arteries.[46,47]

- There is a hypovascular zone of the Achilles tendon 2 to 6 cm proximal to its insertion site.
  - This zone is the most common site of tendon pathology.
- Mechanism of injury
  - Traumatic
    - Usually during a sporting event
  - Sudden forced plantar flexion
  - Sudden dorsiflexion in a plantarflexed foot

Pertinent History/Physical Examination Findings

- IAT history
  - Patients may have tenderness to palpation about insertion of Achilles tendon.
  - They may have heel swelling and/or redness.
  - They may mention pain with activity and stiffness at rest.
  - Patients may also mention pain while wearing shoes that enclose the heel.
- Physical examination findings[48]
  - Limited ankle dorsiflexion and plantar flexion weakness
  - Firm, tender, prominence on the posterior aspect of the heel where the Achilles tendon inserts
- Achilles tendon rupture
  - History
    - Patients are typically active but not all are.
    - They may have heel pain and report hearing a pop while running/jogging.
  - Physical examination findings
    - Patients may not be able to bear weight on the injured side.
    - Patients may have bruising and swelling around the Achilles tendon and foot.
    - Thompson test: With the patient prone, squeeze the calf of the injured side.
      - Examination is considered positive when the calf is squeezed and plantar flexion of the ipsilateral ankle is not observed.
    - Have the patient lie prone on an examination table. Then ask the patient to bend their knees to 90°. The injured side will have increased resting dorsiflexion (will be more parallel to examination table) compared with the noninjured side (**Figure 10**).

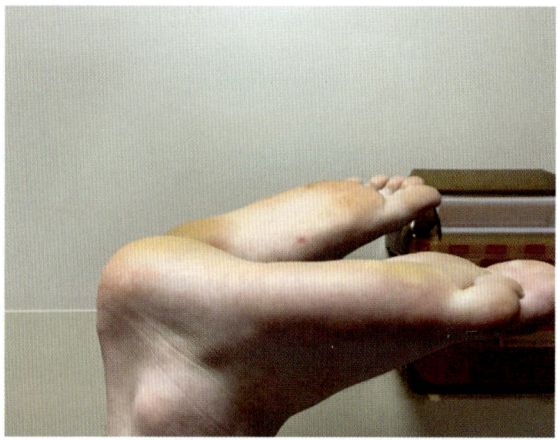

Figure 10 Photograph shows increased resting ankle dorsiflexion with the patient in the prone position and knees flexed. These findings suggest Achilles tendon rupture.

- Most patients will have a palpable gap at the rupture site.
  - Palpation gap test: With the patient prone, palpate the Achilles tendon as it inserts into the calcaneal tuberosity. Continue palpating proximally. There may be an indentation where the tendon is torn.
- There will be increased passive dorsiflexion and weakness to active ankle plantar flexion on motor examination testing.

Relevant Imaging

Insertional Achilles Tendinopathy

- Standard three-view radiographic imaging is clinically useful. Lateral view identifies calcifications within the Achilles tendon, Haglund deformities, fractures, etc (**Figure 11**).
- MRI can also identify IAT pathology (eg, globular Achilles tendon due to its chronicity) (**Figure 12**).

Achilles Tendon Rupture

- Standard three-view radiographic imaging will not identify soft-tissue pathology (tendon rupture).

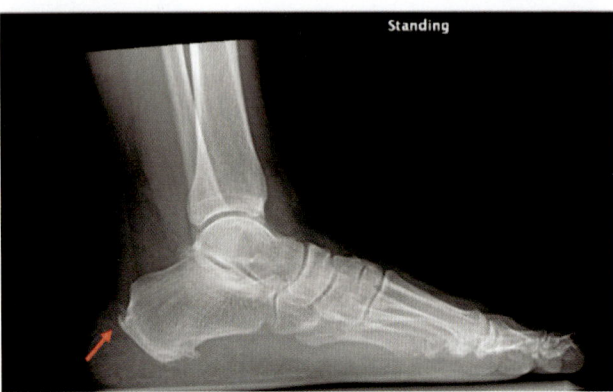

Figure 11 Radiograph shows small dorsal calcaneal (arrow) in a patient with insertional Achilles tendinopathy.

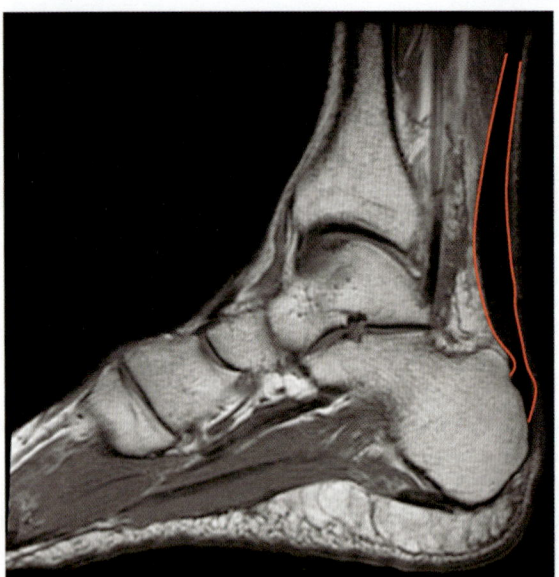

Figure 12 Sagittal T1 magnetic resonance image showing globular contour to the Achilles tendon is consistent with insertional Achilles tendinopathy. There is superimposed small interstitial tearing involving the distal Achilles tendon.

- Ultrasonography may be used as a confirmatory test in the diagnosis of partial or complete acute Achilles tendon rupture. It is reliable in evaluating the location, type, and distance between the two ruptured ends.
- MRI may also be used as a confirmatory test in the setting of equivocal physical examination findings or evaluation but is less dependable when attempting to differentiate between complete and partial tears (**Figures 13 and 14**).

Nonsurgical Measures

Insertional Achilles Tendinopathy

- Activity and shoe modification, NSAIDs (oral and/or topical), nitroglycerin patches, along with functional rehabilitation (Graston therapy).

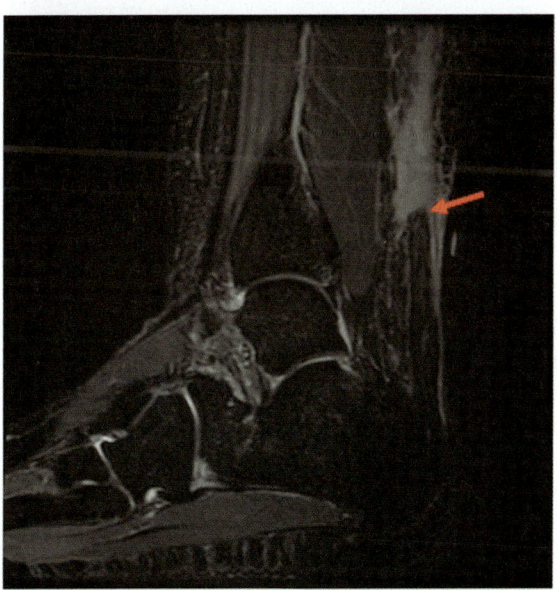

Figure 13 Sagittal T2 magnetic resonance image showing complete Achilles tendon tear (arrow) approximately 7.5 cm proximal to the calcaneal tuberosity with 2-cm gap and additional small foci of interstitial tears within the proximal and distal tendon.

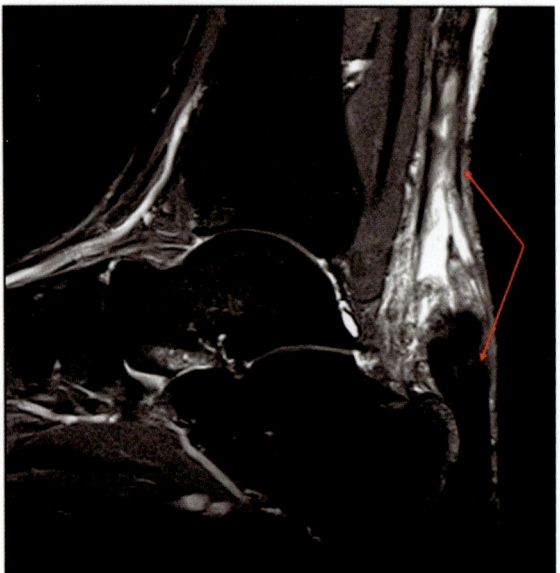

Figure 14 Sagittal T2 magnetic resonance image showing near full-thickness tear of the Achilles tendon (arrow) noted within the middle third of the tendon. Only a tiny, attenuated tendon fiber bridges the 2.6-cm gap in the tendon.

Achilles Tendon Rupture

- Cast immobilization is typically for 2 weeks or up to 8 weeks. The patient's foot will be in equinus (plantarflexed) for the first 2 to 4 weeks and neutral for the last 2 to 4 weeks. This is to prevent excessive dorsiflexion, which would stress the injury further.[49]
- Functional rehabilitation is also important for treatment.

Outcomes

- According to van der Vlist et al,[50] all active treatments for IAT have better outcomes than watching and waiting. However, there is no single treatment that is superior to the others.
- For Achilles tendon ruptures, functional rehabilitation was found to be superior to long-term cast immobilization in reducing rerupture rates and comparable to surgical repair in functional

improvement. However, nonsurgical and surgical rerupture rates are 12.6% and 3.5%, respectively.[49]
- A systematic review by Ochen et al[51] reported nonsurgical versus surgical complication rates (1.6% versus 4.9%, respectively) for management of tendon ruptures.

Surgical Intervention

Insertional Achilles Tendinopathy

- Indications
  - Persistent pain in patients in whom nonsurgical treatment has been exhausted for a period of 3 to 6 months[52]
  - Haglund deformity continuing to cause pain and discomfort after unsuccessful nonsurgical management

Achilles Tendon Rupture

- Despite the growing popularity of rehabilitation, surgical repair of the Achilles tendon is still a more reliable treatment.[49]
- Indications
  - Acute ruptures as defined by injury occurring within 6 weeks of presentation
  - Chronic rupture that functionally limits the patient
  - Failed functional rehabilitation

Surgical Techniques

Insertional Achilles Tendinopathy

- Surgical options
  - Achilles tendon débridement + FHL transfer
    - Typically used in patients older than 55 years with tendon degeneration greater than 50%
    - Midline, posterolateral, or posteromedial incision
    - FHL tendon augmentation
    - Achilles tendon reattached with two bone anchors
    - Outcomes
      - In 2015, Hunt et al reported an AOFAS score of 92 out of 100 points and an 87% satisfaction rate. There were several wound complications within the 39-patient sample size.[53]

- Haglund deformity excision
  - May be performed open or arthroscopically
  - The bony prominence and bursa are identified, and an incision is made.
  - The deformity is excised or shaved down, and the Achilles tendon is débrided and reattached to its insertion.
  - The incision is closed, and the foot is placed in a splint.
  - Outcomes
    - In 2016, Gillis and Lin reported an average AOFAS score of 87 out of 100 points for 14 patients and 16 feet. One patient experienced a wound infection that resolved with incision and drainage.[54]

Achilles Tendon Rupture

- Surgical options
  - Open end-to-end Achilles tendon repair
  - Indication: Acute ruptures (less than 6 weeks from initial injury)
    - The defect is identified, and a posteromedial approach is taken to avoid damage to the sural nerve (**Figure 15**).
    - A 3-inch incision is made, and each end is sewn with suture (**Figure 16**).

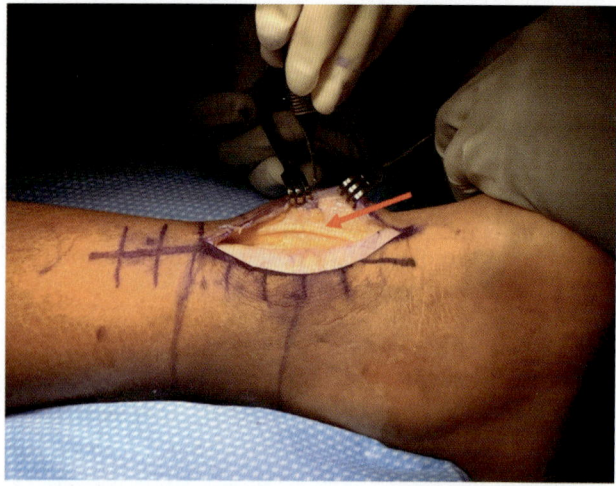

Figure 15 Intraoperative photograph of the sural nerve (arrow).

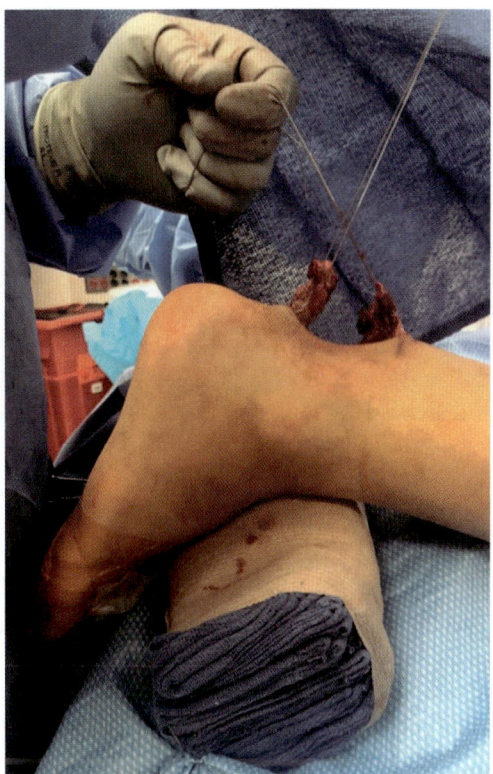

Figure 16 Surgical photograph showing the distal and proximal ends of ruptured Achilles tendon before reattachment.

- The proximal and distal ends are brought together using the suture so that the tendon is intact and under normal tension (**Figure 17**).
- The incision is closed and a splint is placed with the foot and ankle mildly plantarflexed.
- Percutaneous repair
- Indication: Ideal for patients who are concerned about the appearance of scars
  - This approach requires three small incisions over the site of the rupture.

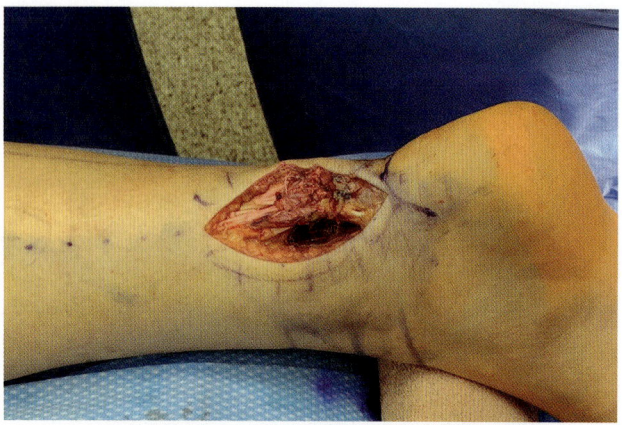

Figure 17 Intraoperative photograph of reattached Achilles tendon.

- The proximal and distal ends of the tendons are sutured, and traction is applied to both ends.
- The proximal and distal ends are sutured again, and the suture is tied before closing the incisions.
- Reconstruction with V-Y gastrocnemius advancement
- Indication: Chronic ruptures with a defect measuring less than 2 cm but may be used for defects up to 5 cm[55]
  - An incision is made posteromedial or posterolateral to the Achilles tendon rupture.
  - The shape of a V is made into the aponeurosis and the Achilles tendon is débrided.
  - The Achilles tendon is repaired using the Krakow method (special way to anchor sutures and bring both ends of the tendon together).
  - The V that was made in the aponeurosis is then pulled down to close the gap and attached to the soleus with suture.
  - The incision is then closed.
  - The patient's foot is placed in a splint for 4 to 6 weeks.
  - Note: Benefits of reconstruction include it being an economically conscious method to use because it does not require expensive implants. In addition, it allows patients to

perform single heel raises and regain strength of the tendon postoperatively.[55]
- FHL transfer +/− V-Y advancement of gastrocnemius
- Indication: Chronic ruptures with a defect larger than 2 cm (patient needs to have a functioning tibial nerve).
  - An incision is made posteromedial or posterolateral to the Achilles tendon rupture.
  - The amount of space between ruptures should be measured and the length of the turndown flap should be determined.
  - The FHL tendon should be harvested and transferred into the bone tunnels, which are made by drilling into the posterior calcaneus.
  - Screws are used to fix the FHL tendon to the bone tunnel and the incision should be closed with suture.
  - The patient's foot is placed in a splint for 4 to 6 weeks.

Outcomes
- In 2019, Lin et al[55] found that patients who underwent reconstruction with V-Y gastrocnemius advancement had a mean AOFAS score that increased from 59.25 ± 12.28 (range, 40 to 75) preoperatively to 96.55 ± 3.75 (range, 90 to 100) at final follow-up.
- Patients undergoing FHL transfer tend to experience dysfunction of the FHL and should not be used as a mainstay in treatment in younger patients.[55]

Relevant Landmarks
- The sural nerve should be identified and avoided (**Figure 15**).
- An intact plantaris tendon can be used to determine the desired length of the repair.

Fixation Strategies
- Not applicable

Postoperative Orders
- Weight-bearing status
  - No weight bearing for 3 to 4 weeks
  - Controlled ankle motion boot for 2 to 3 weeks

- After injury, patients are allowed to progress to low-impact activities during a 6-month period.
- Once they have successfully progressed with low-impact activity, patients are allowed to begin progressing to high-impact activities after 6 months has passed.

Antibiotics
- None

Venous Thromboembolism Prophylaxis
- Aspirin 325 mg once a day until patient has resumed wearing a shoe

Suggested Pain Regimen
- Ibuprofen 600 mg three times a day for 3 days, then one to two 5-mg oxycodone tablets every 4 hours as needed, acetaminophen 500 mg every 4 to 6 hours, gabapentin 300 mg twice a day for 10 days

Pearls and Pitfalls
- Potential complications
  - Sural nerve injury
  - Infection
  - Delayed wound healing/hypertrophic scars
  - Gastrocnemius and soleus muscle weakness
  - Deep vein thrombosis[49]
- What to look for clinically:
  - Patient report of lateral ankle, lateral column of the foot, and fourth and fifth toes with burning sensation
  - Warmth, erythema, lower leg pain, purulent drainage at the incision site
  - Wound dehiscence or thickened skin along the incision
  - Patient unable to or has trouble doing a single leg toe raise on the affected side or muscle atrophy present
- What to look for radiographically
  - Soft-tissue inflammation

Top 10 Knowledge Drops for Your Rotation

1. There is a hypovascular zone of the Achilles tendon 2 to 6 cm proximal to its insertion site, which is the most common area of Achilles tendon pathology.
2. Patients with IAT will have pain at the insertion of the Achilles tendon.
3. Nonsurgical treatment for IAT includes physical therapy and heel lifts.
4. Surgical treatment for IAT includes insertional Achilles tendon débridement with reattachment with or without an FHL transfer.
5. An FHL transfer is indicated if greater than 50% of the Achilles tendon is excised.
6. Patients with an acute Achilles rupture are often weekend warriors and often describe a pop or a sensation of getting kicked from behind at the time of injury.
7. Critical physical examination finding in Achilles tendon rupture includes the Thompson test: With the patient prone, squeeze the calf of the injured side. Examination is considered positive when the calf is squeezed and plantar flexion of the ipsilateral ankle is not observed.
8. Patients with an acute Achilles tendon rupture will also have loss of resting plantar flexion in the prone position when compared with the opposite side.
9. Nonsurgical treatment for an acute Achilles tendon rupture may be indicated in certain patients depending on their goals of treatment.
10. Surgical options include open repair, mini-open repair, or percutaneous repair.

LATERAL ANKLE INSTABILITY

Epidemiology

- Ankle injuries are among the most common orthopaedic injuries both in the general and athletic populations.
- Approximately 40% of sports-related injuries involve ankle sprains.

Chapter 11: My Foot and Ankle Hurt

- Clinicians dichotomize lateral ankle sprains into mechanical and functional pathologies.
  - Patients with a mechanical injury have ligamentous damage.
  - Patients with functional pathology sense their ankle as being weak or unstable.

Pertinent Anatomy/Pathoanatomy

- The lateral ankle ligamentous complex is composed of the anterior talofibular ligament (ATFL), calcaneofibular ligament (CFL), and posterior talofibular ligament.
- Of those three ligaments, the ATFL is most commonly injured first because of its decreased strength and anatomic position.
- The ATFL is often torn at its midpoint or avulsed from the talus.
- An inversion force with the ankle in plantar flexion is the most common mechanism of injury.[56]

Pertinent History/Physical Examination Findings

- History
  - Patients may report general soreness, weakness, limited range of motion, swelling, general decreased function, or tenderness of the injured ankle.[57]
  - They may also report a sensation of instability or not trusting their ankle.
  - Inquire about:
    - Timing of injury
    - Mechanism of injury
    - Ability to bear weight following the injury
    - History of previous or recurrent ankle sprains
      - If yes, does this apply to the currently injured ankle or contralateral ankle
    - Hearing an audible pop or crack
- Physical examination findings
  - Inspect the lower extremities bilaterally first for any abnormalities.
  - Ensure that the contralateral ankle is consistently used as a comparison to the injured side and pay special attention to the lateral ligamentous complex throughout the examination.

Chapter 11: My Foot and Ankle Hurt

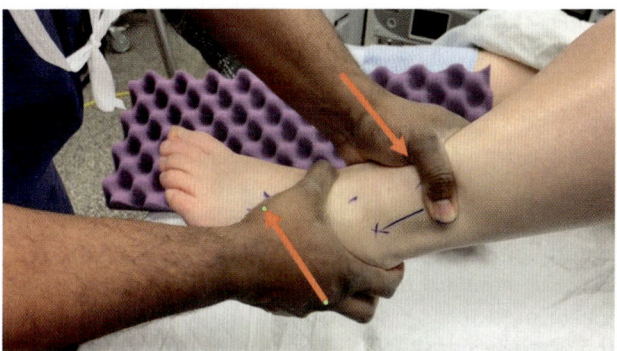

Figure 18 Photograph showing the preoperative anterior drawer test.

- Palpate the dorsalis pedis and posterior tibial pulses, elicit areas of tenderness, and determine the severity of active edema if present.
- Check passive and active range of motion.
- Test the patient's strength against resistance.
- Note any lack of sensation, numbness, or tingling.
- Perform special tests such as the anterior drawer test and talar tilt test as these can assist in diagnosing ATFL and CFL pathologies, respectively[58] (**Figures 18** and **19**).
- Be sure to use the Ottawa ankle rules during the assessment of the patient's ankle pain.

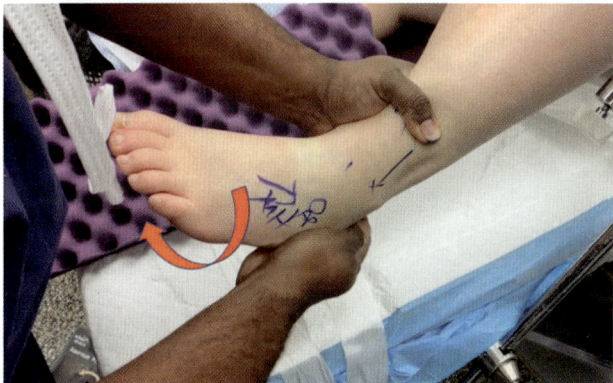

Figure 19 Photograph showing the preoperative talar tilt test.

- This set of rules is especially helpful in excluding ankle fractures in the emergent setting.[59]

Relevant Imaging

- Standard three-view radiographic imaging is used to rule out concomitant injuries (eg, fractures, deltoid and syndesmotic sprains). However, ligamentous pathology cannot be seen with radiographs.
- MRI is the standard diagnostic tool for ligamentous pathology. It is also used to assess associated pathology (eg, syndesmotic injury, osteochondral injury, os trigonum) (**Figure 20**).
- Diagnostic ultrasonography is becoming more popular within the sports medicine community to identify soft-tissue pathology.
- CT is rarely used.

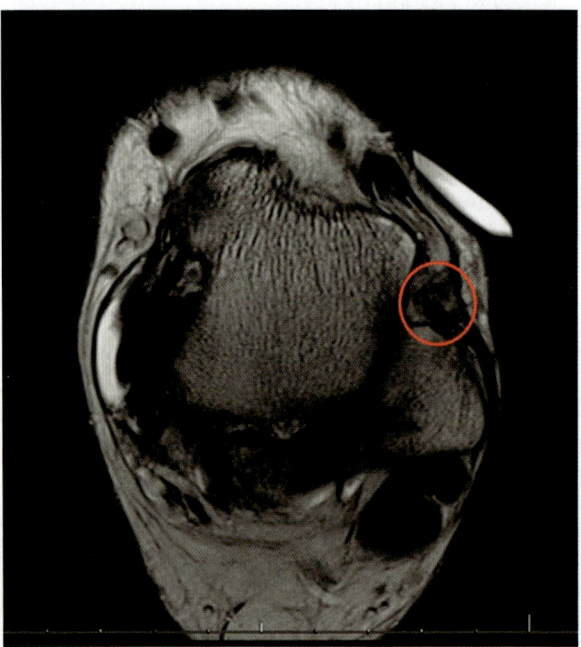

Figure 20 Axial magnetic resonance image depicting grade 3 anterior talofibular ligament sprain.

Nonsurgical Intervention

- Indications
  - Patient able to bear weight at time of injury
  - Minimal pain present
- Options
  - Rest, ice, compression, and elevation and walking boot initially
  - Functional rehabilitation, proprioceptive training, peroneal tendon strengthening, semirigid ankle bracing, and shoe modifications
  - Outcomes:
    - A recent systematic review reported good outcomes with all of these methods.[60]

Surgical Intervention

- Indications
  - Continued pain after nonsurgical measures attempted
  - Functionally unstable ankle sprains
- Surgical options[61]
  - Anatomic
    - Direct repair: open or arthroscopically
    - Reconstruction: autograft or allograft
    - Augmentation (eg, suture tape)
  - Nonanatomic
    - Checkrein tenodesis
  - Ancillary procedures
    - Consider lateral calcaneal slide osteotomy for varus hindfoot
- Pearls
  - More than 50 surgical procedures have been described for ankle instability. However, the direct repair (eg, Broström-Gould) option is the standard approach.
    - Advantages: low cost, simple, minimally invasive, and low complication rates
    - Contraindications: insufficient ligamentous tissue, previous failed stabilization procedures, high body mass index, and generalized ligamentous laxity
      - Generalized ligamentous laxity is an independent predictor of poor outcomes and a risk factor of recurrent instability.[62]

- A 26-year follow-up study reported excellent functional outcomes of 32 ankles that underwent the Broström procedure for chronic lateral ankle instability.[63] Of the 31 patients, 91% described their ankle function as good or excellent.
- Broström-Gould approach (**Figure 21**)
  - Direct repair and reinsertion of both ATFL and CFL. Both ligaments are reinforced with inferior extensor retinaculum and distal fibular periosteum.
- Arthroscopic Broström procedure
  - Reconstructs the ATFL but not the CFL
  - Peroneal tendon and superficial peroneal nerve are at risk
  - A recent meta-analysis showed improved AOFAS scores at 6 months and 1 year, improved visual analog scale scores at 6 months and 1 year, and quicker return to weight bearing with the arthroscopic approach.[64]

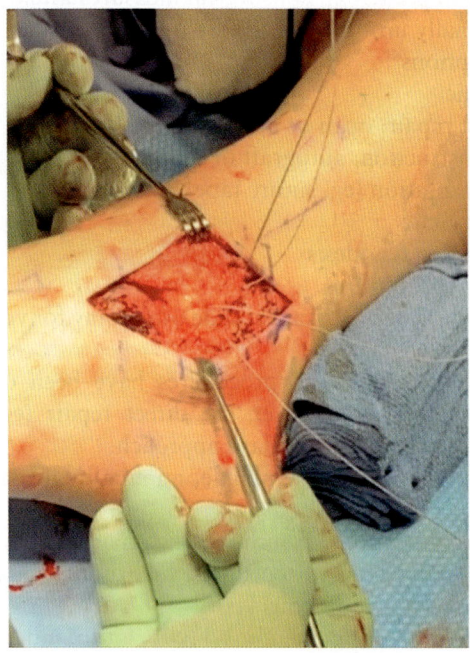

Figure 21 Intraoperative photograph of complete modified Broström procedure.

Top 10 Knowledge Drops for Your Rotation

1. An inversion force with the ankle in plantar flexion is the most common mechanism of injury.
2. The lateral ankle ligamentous complex is composed of the ATFL, CFL, and posterior talofibular ligament. Of those three ligaments, the ATFL is most commonly injured first because of its decreased strength and anatomic position.
3. While obtaining the history from the patient, be sure to ask about generalized laxity. Always ask patients if they have a history of previous ankle sprains.
4. The anterior drawer test is a key component of the physical examination in patients with lateral ankle instability.
5. The talar tilt test is also an important physical examination finding.
6. MRI is the standard diagnostic tool for ligamentous pathology. It is also used to assess associated pathology (eg, syndesmotic injury, osteochondral injury, os trigonum) (**Figure 20**).
7. Initial treatment for an ankle sprain includes functional rehabilitation, proprioceptive training, peroneal tendon strengthening, semirigid ankle bracing, and shoe modifications.
8. The modified Broström approach (ie, Broström-Gould) involves direct repair and reinsertion of both ATFL and CFL. Both ligaments are reinforced with inferior extensor retinaculum and distal fibular periosteum.
9. Generalized ligamentous laxity is an independent predictor of poor outcomes and a risk factor of recurrent instability.
10. Nonanatomic lateral ligament repair is generally reserved for failed anatomic repairs or for patients with severe laxity such as Ehlers-Danlos syndrome.

References

1. Ray JJ, Friedmann AJ, Hanselman AE, et al: Hallux valgus. *Foot Ankle Orthop* 2019;4(2):1-12.
2. Nix SE, Smith M, Vicenzino B: Prevalence of hallux valgus in the general population: A systematic review and meta-analysis. *J Foot Ankle Res* 2010;3:21.
3. Nix SE, Vicenzino BT, Colling NJ, Smith MD: Characteristics of foot structure and footwear associated with hallux valgus: A systematic review. *Osteoarthritis Cartilage* 2012;20(1):1059-1074.

4. Perera AM, Mason L, Stephens MM: Current concepts review: The pathogenesis of hallux valgus. *J Bone Joint Surg* 2011;93:1650-1661.
5. Munteanu SE, Menz HB, Wark JD, et al: Hallux valgus, by nature or nurture? A twin study. *Arthritis Care Res (Hoboken)* 2017;69(9):1420-1428.
6. Barnish MS, Barnish J: High-heeled shoes and musculoskeletal injuries: A narrative systematic review. *BMJ Open* 2016;6:e010053.
7. Solan MC, Lemon M, Bendall SP: The surgical anatomy of the dorsomedial cutaneous nerve of the hallux. *J Bone Joint Surg Br.* 2001;83B(2):250-252.
8. Kunnasegaran R, Thevendran G: Hallux Rigidus: Nonoperative treatment and orthotics. *Foot Ankle Clin N Am* 2015;20(1):401-412. .
9. Shi GG, Whalen JL, Turne NS, Kitaoka HB: Operative approach to adult hallux valgus deformity: Principles and techniques. *J Am Acad Orthop Surg* 2020;28:410-418.
10. Welck MJ, Al-Khudaira N: Imaging of hallux valgus: How to approach the deformity. *Foot Ankle Clin N Am* 2019;23:183-192.
11. Nakagawa R, Yamaguchi S, Akagi R: Clinical and radiographic outcomes of foot orthosis for hallux valgus: A prospective one-year follow-up study. *Foot Ankle Orthop* 2016;1(1):1.
12. Nakagawa R, Yamaguchi S, Kimura S, et al: Efficacy of foot orthoses as nonoperative treatment for hallux valgus: A 2-year follow-up study. *J Orthop Sci* 2019;24(3):526-531.
13. Kaufmann G, Sinz S, Giesinger JM, et al: Loss of correction after chevron osteotomy for hallux valgus as a function of preoperative deformity. *Foot Ankle Int* 2019;40(3):287-296.
14. Matsumoto R, Gross CE, Parekh SG: Short-term radiographic outcome after distal chevron osteotomy for hallux valgus using intramedullary plates with an amended algorithm for the surgical management of hallux valgus. *Foot Ankle Spec* 2018;12(1):25-33.
15. Song JH, Kang C, Hwang DS, Lee GS, Lee SB: Comparison of radiographic and clinical results after extended distal chevron osteotomy with distal soft tissue release with moderate versus severe hallux valgus. *Foot Ankle Int* 2019;40(3):297-306.
16. Koken M, Guclu B: The effect of hallux valgus surgery on quality of like. *J Am Podiatr Med Assoc* 2020;110(5):1-4.
17. Weng-lo N, Kwok-Bill C, Yuk-Nam Y: Long-term clinical outcomes of scarf osteotomy in regional hospital in Hong Kong. *J Orthop Traum Rehab* 2019;27(1):28-32.
18. Law GW, Tay KS, Lim JW, et al: Effect of severity of deformity on clinical outcomes of scarf osteotomies. *Foot Ankle Int* 2020;41(6):705-413.
19. Scott DJ, Ford SE, Alejandro SF, et al: Outcomes of modified scarf osteotomy for male hallux valgus. *Foot Ankle Orthop* 2020;5(4):10.

20. Alolayan LI, Alshehri MH, Almohawis AH, et al: Midterm outcome after correction of hallux valgus deformity using scarf osteotomy in adult population. *J Health Spec* 2017;5(2):91-94.
21. Tenenbaum SA, Herman A, Bruck N, et al: Foot width changes following hallux valgus surgery. *Foot Ankle Int* 2018;39(11):1272-1277.
22. Crowell A, Van JC, Meyr AJ: Early weightbearing after arthrodesis of the first metatarsal-medial cuneiform joint: A systematic review of the incidence of nonunion. *J Foot Ankle Surg* 2018;57(6):1204-1206.
23. Langan TM, Greschner JM, Brandao RA, et al: Maintenance of correction of the modified Lapidus procedure with a first metatarsal to intercuneiform cross-screw technique. *Foot Ankle Int* 2020;4(4):428-436.
24. Barp EA, Erickson JG, Smith HL, et al: Evaluation of fixation techniques for metatarsocuneiform arthrodesis. *J Foot Ankle Surg* 2017;56(3):468-473.
25. Anderson MR, Baumhauer JF: Current concepts review: Hallux rigidus. *Foot Ankle Int* 2018;3(2):1-11.
26. Coughlin MJ, Shurnas PS: Hallux rigidus: Demographics, etiology and radiographic assessment. *Foot Ankle Int* 2003;24(10):731-743.
27. Michelson JD, Janowksi JW, Charlson MD: Quantitative relationship of first metatarsophalangeal head morphology to hallux rigidus and hallux valgus. *Foot Ankle Surg* 2018;24:435-439.
28. Lucas DE, Hunt KJ: Hallux rigidus: Relevant anatomy and pathophysiology. *Foot Ankle Clin N Am* 2015;20(1):381-389.
29. Kon Kam King C, Loh J, Zheng Q, Mehta K: Comprehensive review of non-operative managmenet of hallux rigidus. *Cureus* 2017;9(1):e987.
30. Grice J, Marsland D, Smith G, Calder J: Efficacy of foot and ankle corticosteroid injections. *Foot Ankle Int* 2017;38(1):8-13.
31. Sidon E, Rogero R, Bell T, et al: Long-term follow-up of cheilectomy for treatment of hallux rigidus. *Foot Ankle Int* 2019;40(10):1114-1121.
32. Aynardi MC, Atwater L, Dein E, et al: Outcomes after interpositional arthroplasty of the first metatarsophalangeal joint. *Foot Ankle Int* 2019;38(5):514-518.
33. Vulcano E, Chang A, Solomon D, Myerson M: Long-term follow-up of capsular interposition arthroplasty for hallux rigidus. *Foot Ankle Int* 2018;39(1):1-5.
34. Rammelt S, Panzner I, Mittlmeier T: Metatarsophalangeal joint fusion: Why and Hows? *Foot Ankle Clin N Am* 2015;20:465-477.
35. Wukich DK, Crim BE, Frykberg RG, Rosario BL: Neuropathy and poorly controlled diabetes increase the rate of surgical site infection after foot and ankle surgery. *J Bone Joint Surg Am* 2015;96(10):832-839.
36. Bettin CC, Gower K, McCormick K, et al: Cigarette smoking increases complication rate in forefoot surgery. *Foot Ankle Int* 2015;36(5):488-493.

37. DeSandis B, Pino A, Levin DS, et al: Functional outcomes following first metatarsophalangeal arthrodesis. *Foot Ankle Int* 2016;37(7):715-721.
38. Lunati MP, Manz WJ, Maidman SD, et al: Effect of age on complication rates and outcomes following first metatarsophalangeal arthrodesis for hallux rigidus. *Foot Ankle Int* 2020;41(11):1347-1354.
39. Kannan S, Bennett A, Chong HH, et al: A multicentre Retrospective Cohort Study of first metatarsophalangeal joint arthrodesis. *J Foot Ankle Surg* 2020;60(3):436-439.
40. Manske M, McKeon K, Johnson J, McCormick J, Klein S: Arterial anatomy of the tibialis posterior tendon. *Foot Ankle Int* 2020;36(4):436-443.
41. Lintz F, Welck M, Bernasconi A, et al: 3D biometrics for hindfoot alignment using weightbearing CT. *Foot Ankle Int* 2017;38(6):684-689.
42. Kujala UM, Sarna S, Kaprio J: Cumulative incidence of Achilles tendon rupture and tendinopathy in male former elite athletes. *Clin J Sport Med* 2005;15(3):133-135.
43. Caudell GM: Insertional Achilles tendinopathy. *Clin Podiatr Med Surg* 2017;34(2):195-205.
44. Lemme NJ, Li NY, DeFroda SF, Kleiner J, Owens BD: Epidemiology of achilles tendon ruptures in the United States: athletic and nonathletic injuries from 2012 to 2016. *Orthop J Sports Med* 2018;6(11):2325967118808238.
45. O'Brien M: The anatomy of the Achilles tendon. *Foot Ankle Clin* 2005;10(2):225-238.
46. Zantop T, Tillmann B, Petersen W: Quantitative assessment of blood vessels of the human Achilles tendon: An Immunohistochemical Cadaver Study. *Arch Orthop Trauma Surg* 2003;123(9):501-504.
47. Knobloch K, Kraemer R, Lichtenberg A, et al: Achilles tendon and paratendon microcirculation in midportion and insertional tendinopathy in athletes. *Am J Sports Med* 2006;34(1):92-97.
48. Chimenti RL, Cychosz CC, Hall MM, Phisitkul P: Current concepts review update: Insertional Achilles tendinopathy. *Foot Ankle Int* 2017;38(10):1160-1169.
49. Park SH, Lee HS, Young KW, Seo SG: Treatment of acute Achilles tendon rupture. *Clin Orthop Surg* 2020;12(1):1-8.
50. van der Vlist AC, Winters M, Weir A, et al: Which treatment is most effective for patients with Achilles tendinopathy? A living systematic review with network meta-analysis of 29 randomised controlled trials. *Br J Sports Med* 2021;55(5):249-256.
51. Ochen Y, Beks RB, van Heijl M, et al: Operative treatment versus non-operative treatment of Achilles tendon ruptures: Systematic review and meta-analysis. *BMJ* 2019;364:k5120.

52. Barg A, Ludwig T: Surgical strategies for the treatment of insertional Achilles tendinopathy. *Foot Ankle Clin* 2019;24(3):533-559.
53. Hunt KJ, Cohen BE, Davis WH, Anderson RB, Jones CP: Surgical treatment of insertional Achilles tendinopathy with or without flexor Hallucis longus tendon transfer: A prospective, randomized study. *Foot Ankle Int* 2015;36(9):998-1005.
54. Gillis CT, Lin JS: Use of a central splitting approach and near complete detachment for insertional calcific Achilles tendinopathy repaired with an Achilles bridging suture. *J Foot Ankle Surg* 2016;55(2):235-239.
55. Lin YJ, Duan XJ, Yang L: V-Y tendon plasty for reconstruction of chronic Achilles tendon rupture: A medium-term and long-term follow-up. *Orthop Surg* 2019;11(1):109-116.
56. Chan KW, Ding BC, Mroczek KJ: Acute and chronic lateral ankle instability in the athlete. *Bull NYU Hosp Jt Dis* 2011;69(1):17-26.
57. Hertel J, Corbett RO: An updated model of chronic ankle instability. *J Athl Train* 2019;54(6):572-588.
58. Czajka CM, Tran E, Cai AN, DiPreta JA: Ankle sprains and instability. *Med Clin North Am* 2014;98(2):313-329.
59. Bachmann LM, Kolb E, Koller MT, Steurer J, ter Riet G: Accuracy of Ottawa ankle rules to exclude fractures of the ankle and mid-foot: Systematic review. *BMJ* 2003;326(7386):417.
60. Petersen W, Rembitzki IV, Koppenburg AG, et al: Treatment of acute ankle ligament injuries: A systematic review. *Arch Orthop Trauma Surg* 2013;133(8):1129-1141.
61. Yasui Y, Murawski CD, Wollstein A, Takao M, Kennedy JG: Operative treatment of lateral ankle instability. *JBJS Rev* 2016;4(5):e6.
62. Park KH, Lee JW, Suh JW, Shin MH, Choi WJ: Generalized ligamentous laxity is an independent predictor of poor outcomes after the modified Broström procedure for chronic lateral ankle instability. *Am J Sports Med* 2016;44(11):2975-2983.
63. Bell SJ, Mologne TS, Sitler DF, Cox JS: Twenty-six-year results after Broström procedure for chronic lateral ankle instability. *Am J Sports Med* 2006;34(6):975-978.
64. Attia A, Taha T, Mahmoud K, et al: Outcomes of open versus arthroscopic Broström surgery for chronic lateral ankle instability: A systematic review and meta-analysis of comparative studies. *Ortho J Sports Med* 2021;9(7):23259671211015207.

12. Spine—My Back Is Killing Me

S. Elizabeth Ames, MD, FAAOS
Emmanuel Menga, MD, FAAOS

Introduction

Low back and neck pain are encountered in routine clinical evaluation and in emergent settings. Evaluation requires a comprehensive understanding of common conditions that affect the spine including myofascial conditions, spinal stability, or neurologic function. Assessment must focus on face-to-face patient evaluation, including the history of the current episode and previous experiences. There are three goals—to rule out high-risk conditions, to understand contributing factors, and to create a clinical diagnosis based on history and physical examination and confirm with imaging and other modalities. The diagnosis is supported by patient-reported symptoms, knowledge of anatomy, the overall physical examination, and neurologic assessment of spinal cord health (myelopathy) and nerve root function (radiculopathy). Specific etiologies such as tumor, spinal trauma and instability, and spinal infections may require immediate treatment; others such as degenerative processes can often be managed nonsurgically before surgical intervention is considered.

Dr. Menga or an immediate family member has received royalties from Evolution Spine and serves as a paid consultant to or is an employee of Evolution Spine and Globus Medical. Neither Dr. Ames nor any immediate family member has received anything of value from or has stock or stock options held in a commercial company or institution related directly or indirectly to the subject of this chapter.

Epidemiology

- Prevalence of spine-related pain in the general population: 20% to 30%
  - No substantial studies assess the effect of race on back pain; there are variable reports on the effect of sex.
  - Pain incidence peaks at ages 20 to 60 years for Americans (which has a substantial effect on the workforce), with limited information about elderly patients.
  - In 2016, low back and neck pain accounted for the third highest US health care spending at $87.6 billion and low back pain accounted for 3% to 4% of emergency department visits.[1]
  - Up to 85% of patients presenting with axial spine pain have nonspecific etiologies, making diagnosis and treatment difficult.
- Radiculopathy is irritation of a nerve root causing symptoms in the distribution served by that nerve; usually occurs secondary to the degenerative process in the spinal column but can relate to tumor, trauma, or other conditions.
  - Lumbar radiculopathy has an estimated prevalence of 9.8 cases per 1,000 in the lumbosacral spine.
    - Prior history of axial low back pain is a well-established risk factor.
  - Cervical radiculopathy is similar and known to peak in the sixth decade in both males and females.
- Myelopathy is the leading cause of spinal cord dysfunction in adults worldwide.
  - Clinical diagnosis with cumulative symptoms that can include weakness, dysfunction of gait and balance, hand function, bowel and bladder dysfunction resulting from spinal cord compression.
  - Degenerative processes, hypertrophy, or calcification of vertebral structures can lead to narrowing of the spinal canal.
    - These changes are classically associated with aging but can be aggravated by trauma, or related to encroachment of the spinal cord by tumor, infection, or instability from trauma.
    - The spinal cord travels through the cervical and thoracic spine and then variably extends over the proximal lumbar spine and ends as the conus most commonly at the thoracolumbar junction.

Chapter 12: Spine—My Back Is Killing Me

- Most lumbar and sacral spine levels are composed of nerve roots, but upper lumbar lesions may generate symptoms more consistent with spinal cord/conus cord injury.

Pertinent Anatomy/Pathoanatomy

- The spinal column is integrated, interdependent, and dynamic.
  - The spine is a series of specific anatomic structures from the base of the skull to the tip of the coccyx.
  - The functional spinal unit—vertebral structures over two levels and the intervening disk—is important to understand from both structural and biomechanical points of view (**Figure 1**).
  - Classically this has been described as three columns: the anterior column (anterior two-thirds of the vertebral body), the middle column (posterior one-third of the vertebral body and ligaments, pedicles, and neural elements), and the posterior column (the lamina, spinous process).[2]
  - The three columns of the spine are consistent throughout the spine and relevant to evaluating spinal trauma and the bony stability of the spine.
- Each region of the spine has morphologic variations that help support posture, provide mobility, and protect the spinal cord and nerve roots.
  - The anatomy review here focuses on a basic foundation that supports the process of initial patient evaluation; it is not comprehensive.
  - There are many anatomic terms in the spine that are not used consistently in a clinical setting; clinical terms are included in parentheses where relevant.
- Vertebra structure
  - Each vertebra consists of two parts: a ventral body deep to anything palpable and a dense cortical posterior structure called the dorsal vertebral arch (posterior elements) (**Figures 1** and **2**).
    - The arch consists of the osteochondral joints (facets), lamina, two transverse processes, and spinous process.
      - It also carries the posterior ligaments and extensor musculature (not discussed in this chapter).
    - The structures of the posterior arch vary by spinal region, and some of these structures and the spinal erector muscles are palpable.

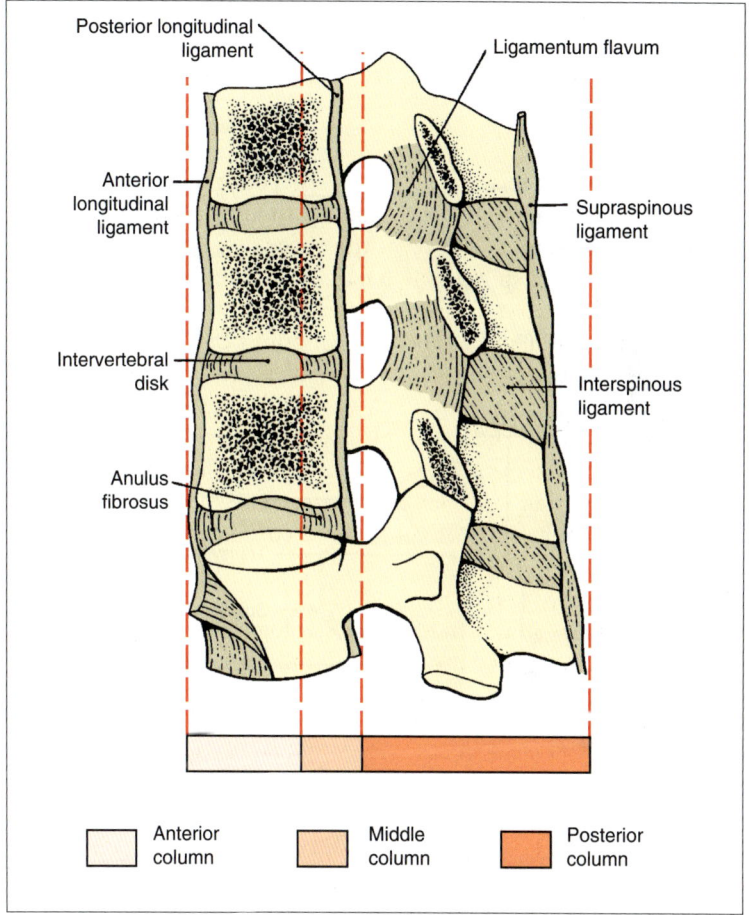

Figure 1 Illustration shows the division of the spine into three columns. The three-column concept in viewing the thoracolumbar spine is helpful in determining the stability of various injuries. Fractures involving all three columns are unstable, and those affecting one column are stable. (Modified with permission from Denis F: The three-column spine and its significance in the classification of acute thoracolumbar spinal injuries. *Spine [Phila Pa 1976]* 1983;8[8]:817-831.)

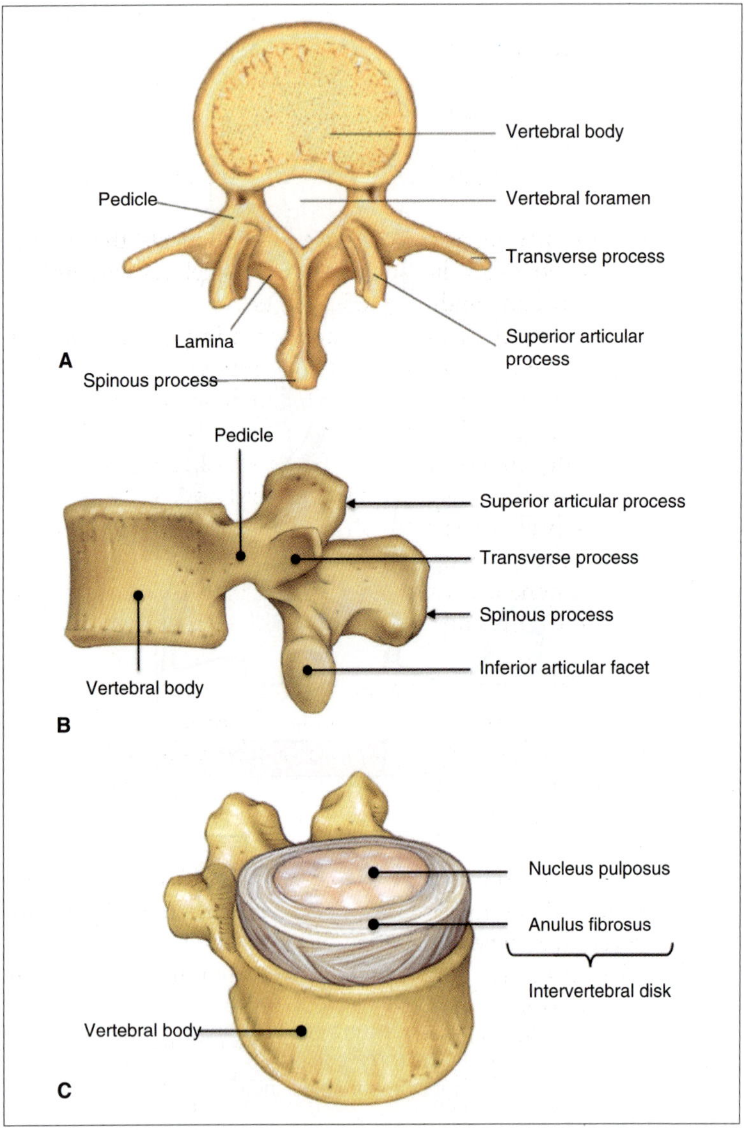

Figure 2 Illustrations showing the spine anatomy. **A**, Axial view of typical lumbar vertebra. **B**, Side view of typical lumbar vertebra. **C**, Oblique view of typical lumbar vertebra and disk. (Panel C reproduced with permission from Pope TL, Harris JH, eds: *Harris and Harris' The Radiology of Emergency Medicine*, ed 5. Wolters Kluwer, 2012.)

- The vertebral bodies are deep structures that consist of end plates, trabecular bone, and a cortical shell.
  - They are accompanied by the vascular and neurologic structures that supply the extremities.
- Anterior and middle structures
  - The anterior column is made up of vertebral bodies and disks.
    - Vertebral size increases craniocaudally, reflects the importance as a load-bearing structure, and correlates with ability to resist fracture and mechanical stress.
    - Each region demonstrates changes that imply function; for example, the lumbar and cervical bodies are slightly higher in the front, and the thoracic vertebrae have specialized processes to support the rib cage.
  - The end plates support the intervertebral disk, a fibrocartilaginous structure that connects two vertebral bodies.
    - Intervertebral disk size and shape vary from region to region, but the intrinsic structure is the same.
    - Two components: a semifluid mass called the nucleus pulposus and concentric fibrous lamellae called the anulus fibrosus.
    - The nucleus resists compression and is integrated with the chondral end plates and the anulus fibrosus.
    - The anulus fibrosus is composed of fibrous lamellar bands that are predominantly vertical in orientation; it connects the vertebral bodies and resists tension forces and torsion.
      - The connection to the vertebral bodies blends with the vertebral periosteum and the longitudinal ligaments through Sharpey fibers.
      - The disk is metabolically active but has limited vascularity.
      - The peripheral vascular plexus of the anulus fibrosus and the vessels adjacent to the cartilage of the end plate and bone/disk interface are the sources of nutrients.
  - Ligaments are found both anteriorly and posteriorly.
    - Two major ligaments accompany the vertebral bodies: anterior longitudinal ligament, posterior longitudinal ligament, and the ligamentum flavum.

- The anterior longitudinal ligament extends along the ventral surface from the skull to the sacrum.
  - The deep fibers adhere to the anterior surface of the vertebra and are only loosely attached to the anterior anulus fibrosus of the disk.
- The posterior longitudinal ligament is closely applied to the posterior anulus fibrosus and less integrated with the vertebral bodies.
- Posterior structures
  - The lamina is the roof of the spinal canal.
    - Primarily cortical and less vulnerable to trauma or disease than other areas
    - Continuous with the pars, the facets, the pedicles, and the spinous process and one of the most common anatomic structures encountered in spinal procedures
    - The central nerve canal is directly below the lamina.
  - Facet joints
    - Cervical facet joints oriented to allow significant rotation; lumbar facet joints oriented to allow flexion and extension with limits on rotation
    - Size varies but structure is the same; all have hyaline cartilage surface, supportive capsule, and nutrition typical of other joints in the body
    - True synovial joints with synovial membrane, hyaline cartilage, and a fibrous capsule
  - Pars articularis—area between the facets and lateral aspect of the lamina
    - Resists translation forces, particularly at C2 and L5; respective clinical examples are a hangman's fracture or isthmic spondylolisthesis
    - Roofs the lateral part of the spinal canal and contributes to the opening the nerve roots use to exit the spine (foramen)
  - The pedicles of the vertebra above and below are the superior and inferior boundaries of the intervertebral foramen.
    - The foramina are spaces that allow the nerves to exit.
      - The foraminal floor is disk structures and ligaments, and the roof includes the facet joints.
      - Degenerative changes and tumor, trauma, and congenital disorders all affect the size of the foramen.

- The pedicles are primarily cortical and reliably sized and oriented.
  - Pedicles connect the posterior elements with the anterior vertebral body.
  - The relationship between the pedicle and landmarks is well defined at most levels, and easily confirmed with imaging.
  - Neural elements are closely applied in all regions, and vascular elements in some. These characteristics have made pedicle instrumentation a surgical workhorse particularly in the lumbar spine.
- The 24 vertebrae of the spine are divided by region; the regions are determined by overall alignment and individual anatomic features that are most evident in the posterior column.
  - Four anatomic regions—cervical, thoracic, lumbar, and sacral
  - Three biomechanical transition zones—cervicothoracic, thoracolumbar, and lumbosacral—carry equal importance.
  - By convention the spine is defined in two planes: coronal (looked at from the front or back) and sagittal (looked at from the side).
    - A third plane—axial—defines much of the space available for the neurologic elements.
    - All three planes are important to clinical evaluation.
  - Alignment and anatomy are closely related but also affected by external forces such as gravity and motion.
- Four regions to the spinal column—cervical (C1-7), thoracic (T1-12; characterized by the presence of ribs), lumbar (L1-5), and a conjoined sacrum
  - Each is built to respond to the forces it experiences (**Figure 3**).
- In the cervical region, C3-6 are relatively uniform in shape and design (**Figure 4**).
  - Cervical vertebrae carry the least weight in the spine.
  - The neural canal is filled by the spinal cord, and the nerve roots have short, nearly horizontal transitions out of the canal.
  - The vertebral artery (**Figure 5**) travels directly through bone structure in the cervical spine, which affects risk of injury both traumatic and surgical.

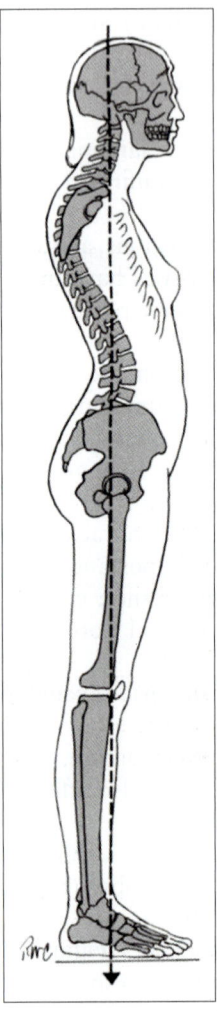

Figure 3 Illustration shows the cervical spine is lordotic, the thoracic spine is kyphotic, and the lumbar spine lordotic again. This keeps the head balanced over the feet when standing. (Reproduced with permission from MediClip image copyright © 2003 Lippincott Williams & Wilkins. All rights reserved.)

- The cervical disks are accessible through anterior dissection of the neck with safe access to structures affecting the cord and roots; posterior access is more difficult.
- The posterior bone structures are small, but instrumentation techniques are available including pedicle access at C7.

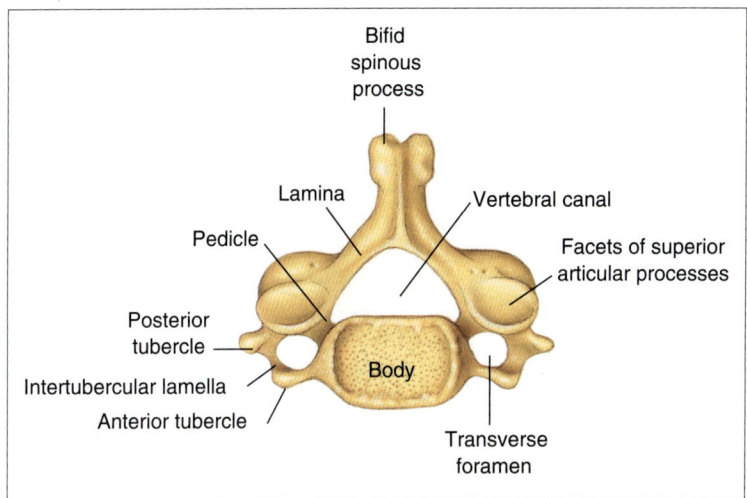

Figure 4 Illustration shows the superior view of cervical vertebra. Note the large foramen for the vertebral artery and the position of the canal for the spinal cord. (Reproduced with permission from Anatomical Chart Company © Wolters Kluwer. All rights reserved.)

- The atlantoaxial complex—occiput, C1, and C2—forms a complex articulation that allows rotation of the head.
  - C1 is a bony ring that can be thought of as similar to a standard vertebra without the body.
  - Embryologically the body of C1 has become the dens of C2, a prominence arising from the body of C2. C1 rotates around C2, supported primarily by ligaments (**Figure 6**).
    - It is critical to understand this relationship in detail when assessing patients with either high-impact and low-impact trauma.
  - The course of the vertebral artery is closely applied to the posterior ring of C1, risking injury with surgical dissection.
  - The posterior arch of C2 is substantial, and the inferior processes are typical of the rest of the cervical spine.
    - C2 is also the end vertebra of the cervical lordosis.
    - For both these reasons C2 is often included in surgical constructs.

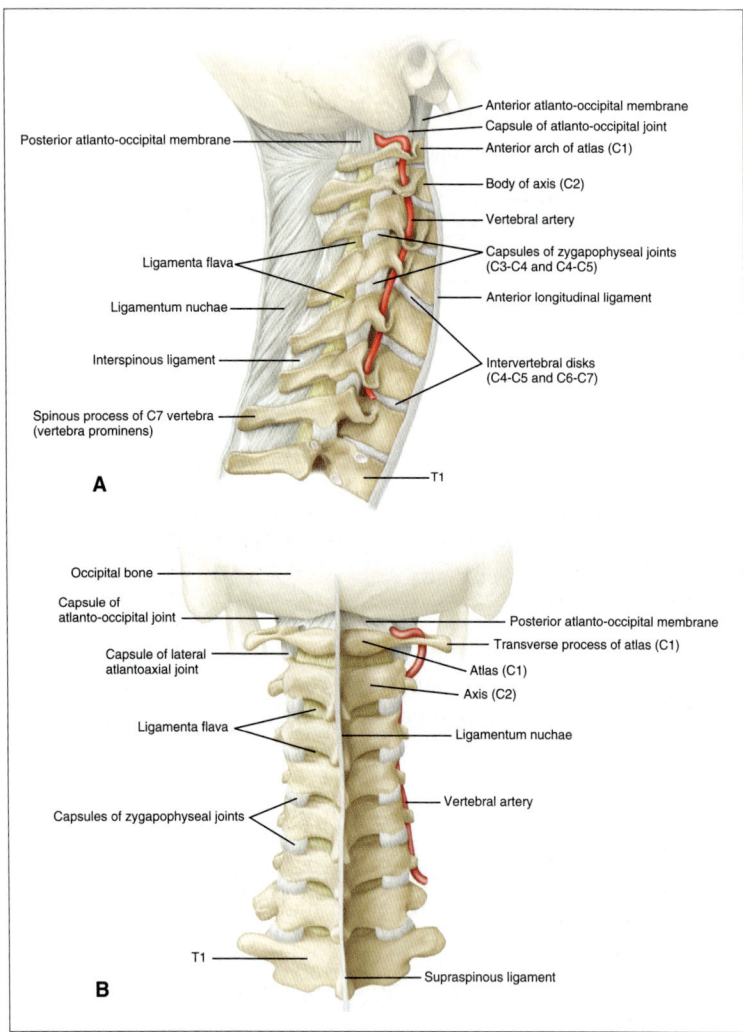

Figure 5 **A**, Illustration shows the course of the cervical vertebra in the lateral view. **B**, Illustration shows the course of the vertebral artery at C1-C2. (Reproduced with permission from Pansky B, Gest TR, eds: *Lippincott's Concise Illustrated Anatomy: Head & Neck*. Wolters Kluwer, 2014, vol 3. p 57. Figure 1.9I.)

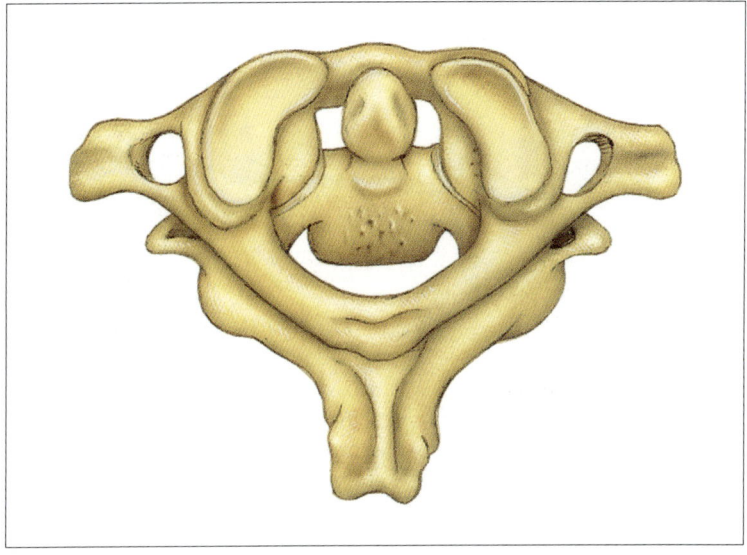

Figure 6 Superior view drawing shows the relationship between C1 and the odontoid of C2. (Reproduced with permission from Anatomical Chart Company © Wolters Kluwer. All rights reserved.)

- The cervicothoracic junction is an area of high stress and rapid transition, with stress coming from the highly mobile cervical spine meeting the stiffer, rib-bound thoracic spine.
  - The anterior anatomy of this region is important to know because airway, esophagus, great vessels, and the sternoclavicular junction are closely spaced to the spine.
  - C7 is a transitional vertebra.
    - The inferior portion of the body is relatively larger than the superior portion and the spinous process is also large and distinct.
- All 12 thoracic vertebrae connect to ribs.
  - Body size is approximately halfway between the cervical and lumbar vertebrae.
  - The posterior elements are more robust than the cervical spine, but the space available for the spinal cord is smaller (**Figure 7**).

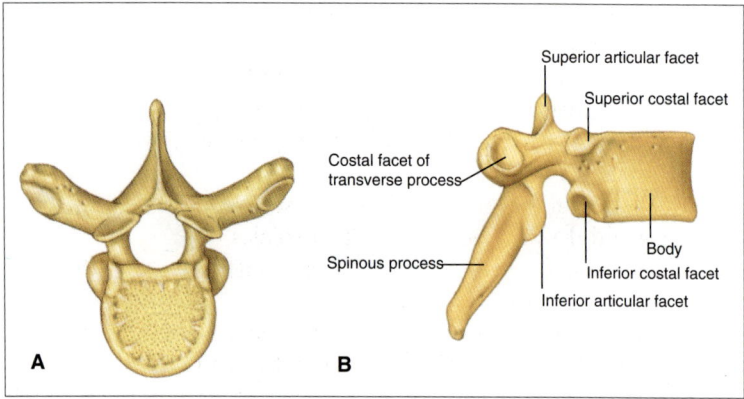

Figure 7 Illustrations showing a typical thoracic vertebra (**A**) and the seventh thoracic vertebrae (**B**). (Reproduced with permission from Anatomical Chart Company © Wolters Kluwer. All rights reserved.)

- The pedicle height increases from T1 to T12 but the width remains small.
- The spinous processes are long and triangular and hang down at 60° in adaptation to upright stature; rib articulation is a better indicator of spinal level on radiographs.
- The thoracic vertebra often exhibits growth or developmental variation with clinical effects.
- The thoracolumbar junction is the end of the lumbar spine and transitions to the less mobile thoracic spine.
  - It has the most gradual sagittal change and individual vertebra may be characterized as neutral.
  - It is at the junction point of two long lever arms (upper body and lower body) and is highly vulnerable to traumatic forces.
    - Has implications for instrumentation choices.
  - Axial rotation of the thoracic vertebral column is more extensive than in the lumbar region, and the opposite occurs for flexion.
  - The lumbar facets are oriented in the sagittal plane to provide stability during movement.
  - There are posterior element anatomic changes from T10 to L2 that are important to consider.

- L2-L5 are the workhorse levels of the spine.
  - The anterior vertebral bodies are robust to support the weight of the upper body—the width is larger than the anteroposterior diameter, for example.
  - The arch structures are short, stout, and relatively consistent in shape and angle.
  - The neural foramina are large because of the size of the bodies and the high position of the pedicles.
  - The articular processes are larger and shaped differently than other levels.
  - The superior articular facets are concave and face each other; the inferior articular facets from the level above are extensions of the laminae that direct laterally and thus lock themselves into the complex.
  - The degree of direction in both the lateral and ventral planes varies from L1 to L5 as the spine shifts from facilitating rotation in the thoracic levels to facilitating flexion and extension in the lumbar region.
- The lumbosacral junction is also anatomically distinct in bone structure.
  - The sacrum consists of five fused vertebrae (**Figure 8**) as a triangular complex that supports the spine and connects it to the pelvis.
  - The posterior aspect forms a depression that gives origin to the inferior parts of the paraspinal muscles.
  - The sacral region has been defined as three zones: the vertebral structures at S1, the remaining sacrum from the body of S2 to the tip of the coccyx, and the ilia.
  - The sacroiliac joints[3] are best described as an articular cavity that transfers loads between the spine and lower limbs.
    - Only minimal movement is allowed by well-developed ligaments and the irregular shape to the articular surfaces.
    - The sacroiliac joints permit stable yet flexible support to the upper body and connection to the basic platform provided by the pelvis.
    - The erector spinae and gluteus maximus act as interdependent control forces for the spine, pelvis, and hip joints.

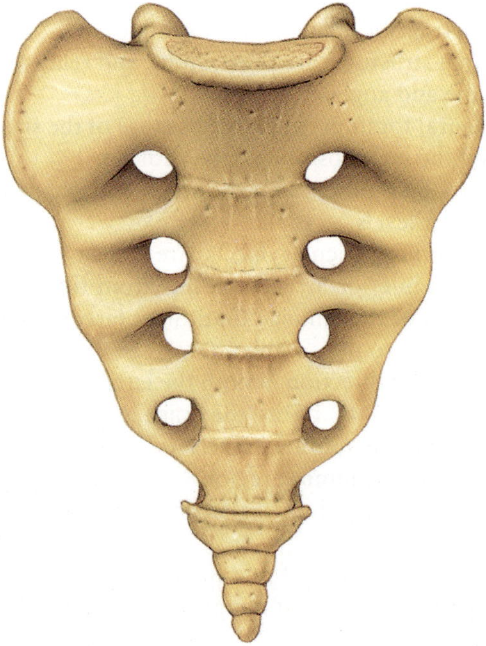

Figure 8 Illustration showing the anterior view of the sacrum. (Reproduced with permission from Anatomical Chart Company © Wolters Kluwer. All rights reserved.)

- Neural elements (**Figures 9** and **10**)
  - Two major types of neural elements within the spinal column: central (spinal cord) and radicular (nerve roots).
    - The spinal cord usually terminates in the conus at L2 or L3 because of the disparity of growth in the vertebral column compared with the spinal cord.
    - It begins at the brainstem and continues downward to the conus usually between T11 and L2.

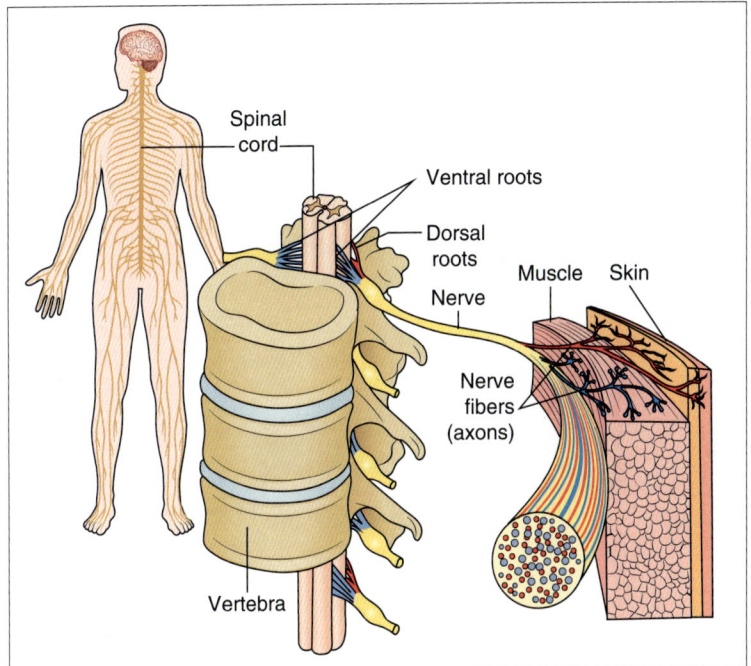

Figure 9 Schematic drawings show the relationship between vertebral bodies, spinal cord, and existing dorsal and ventral nerve roots. (Reproduced with permission from Lippincott's Professional Development Programs, 2012. © Wolters Kluwer. All rights reserved.)

- The orientation of neurologic columns and vascularity has clinical importance in patients with spine conditions and should be carefully studied.
- The conus has a distal taper continuous with the L4-S1 nerve roots in the canal and consists of S2-S5 and coccygeal nerve segments.
  - It is generally oval with an anterior sulcus and posterior promontory; the transverse diameter is 8 to 11 mm, which leaves room for the cauda equina composed of all distal nerve roots.
  - The conus gives rise to the lumbar sympathetic, sacral somatic, and sacral parasympathetic nerve supply, which are crucial for sexual function. The conus terminates as the filum terminale that stabilizes the spinal cord.

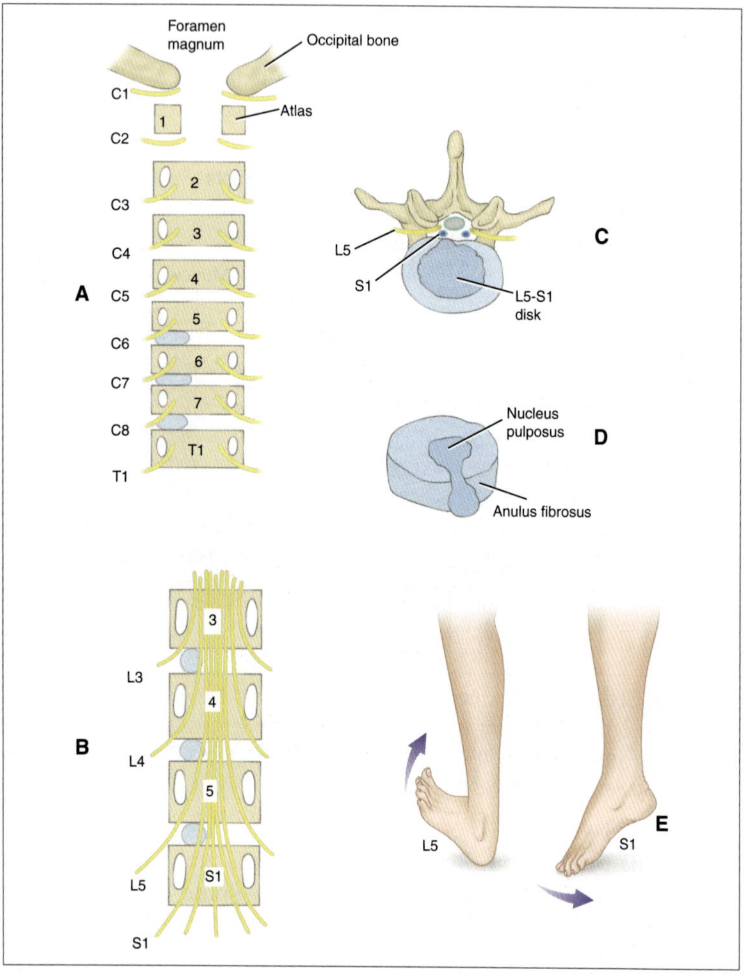

Figure 10 **A** and **B**, Illustrations show the relationship that might exist between a herniated nucleus pulposus and spinal nerve roots. Note the relationship between the root number and the vertebral body, which changes at C7-T1. **C**, Posterolateral herniation of the nucleus pulposus of the intervertebral disk with pressure on the S1 nerve root. Note that L5 root is lateral to the herniation and may not be affected. **D**, An intervertebral disk that has herniated its nucleus pulposus posteriorly. **E**, Each nerve root will have a different physical examination finding. L5 (big toe and foot extension) and S1 (ankle flexion) are shown. (Reproduced with permission from Splittgerber R, ed: *Snell's Clinical Neuroanatomy*, ed 8. Wolters Kluwer, 2018.)

- Nerve roots convey sensory information from the periphery to the spinal cord and regulate the motor activity of the limbs.
  - Composed of motor, sensory, and autonomic fibers
  - Five regional divisions—8 cervical roots, 12 thoracic, 5 lumbar, 5 sacral, and 1 coccygeal
  - Each root emerges from the spinal cord at a specific level as an anterior (ventral) and posterior (dorsal) root on each side.
    - The anterior roots carry the motor neurons and preganglionic autonomics, and the posterior roots carry the fibers that return sensory information.
    - Cervical nerves emerge from the canal above the named vertebra (ie, C3 root above C3 vertebra), but there are eight of them so C8 emerges above T1.
      - This results in all lower roots emerging from the canal below their named vertebra (ie, L4 root below L4 pedicle).
  - From C1 to L1, the spinal nerve roots have a short distance to travel to the foramen where they exit the spine.
    - Caudal to L1, the roots travel along the spinal column to exit at their level.
      - These pairs travel in the dural sac resembling a horse's tail (cauda equina).
    - The meninges cover the nerve roots as they travel and fuse with the nerve as it leaves to become its outer coating before it joins the lumbar plexus.
    - Nerve root compression alters conduction and compromises nutritional support.
      - Varying causes of inflammation coupled with varying degrees of compression contribute to the pain response and neurologic deficits seen clinically.
- Innervation of the vertebral column itself is derived from the sympathetic system and from branches of the spinal nerves.
  - Two rami—anterior and posterior—support the anterior wall muscles, prevertebral flexors such as iliopsoas, and the spinal extensors.
  - Trunk muscles must have sufficient strength to ensure stability and movement control.
  - The spinal extensors are predominantly type I muscle fibers to provide endurance.

- Posture and endurance change with factors such as decreased extensor muscle strength with age.
  - Biomechanical forces experienced by the spinal column change in response.
  - The vertebral column adapts with functional spinal unit changes that can affect the space available for the neural elements.
- Associated structures
  - Neural architecture is dominated by the lumbar plexus (**Figure 11**).
    - The lumbar plexus is formed by the ventral rami of the first through fourth lumbar spinal nerves.[4]
      - It is a network of fibers on the posterior abdominal wall, much of it within the substance of psoas major.
      - The greatest concentration of nerves is located along the transverse processes of L3 to L5 and extends over the ala of the sacrum and the sacroiliac joint.

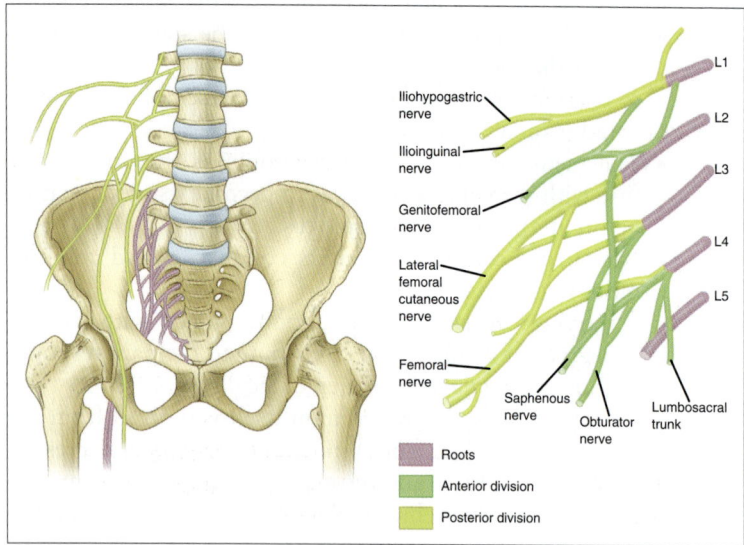

Figure 11 Illustrations show the lumbar plexus is formed by the segmental nerves T12 through L5. The lower portion of the plexus merges with the upper portion of the sacral plexus to form the lumbosacral trunk. (Reproduced with permission from Anderson MK, Parr GP, Hall SJ, eds: *Foundations of Athletic Training: Prevention, Assessment, and Management*, ed 7. Wolters Kluwer, 2021.)

- The position of the lumbar plexus makes it vulnerable to injury during minimally invasive surgical approaches.
  - The lumbar plexus produces branches that innervate the lower abdomen, genitalia, and parts of the lower limb through the iliohypogastric nerve, ilioinguinal nerve, lateral femoral cutaneous nerve, and genitofemoral nerve.
- The vascular structures relevant to the lumbar spine begin with the aorta.[5]
  - The aortic bifurcation is most commonly at L4 or L5 (**Figure 12**).
  - At each level, a segmental artery connects the aorta to the posterior blood supply.
    - This vessel can be highly variable at L5 and presents significant bleeding risk during a retroperitoneal approach.

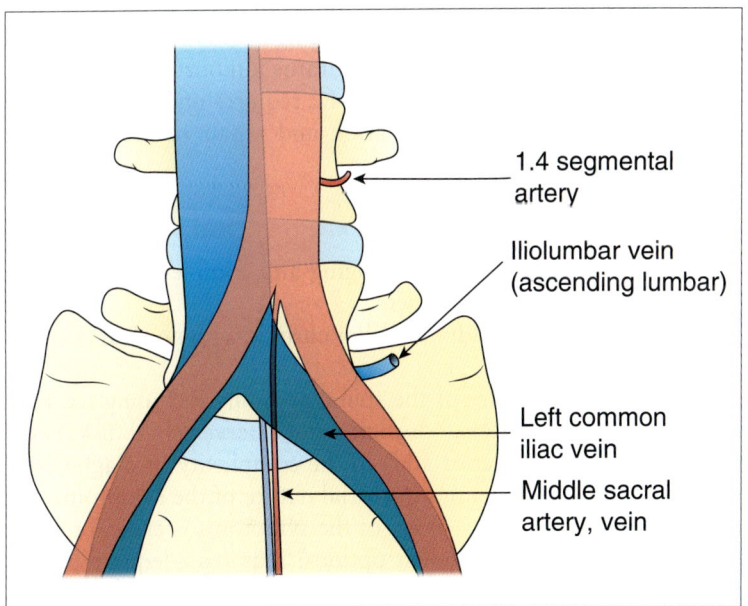

Figure 12 Illustration shows the typical vascular pattern overlying the L4-L5 and L5-S1 disk spaces. (Reproduced with permission from Zdeblick TA, Albert TJ, eds: *Master Techniques in Orthopaedic Surgery: The Spine*, ed 3. Wolters Kluwer, 2014.)

- This is also true of the iliolumbar branch at the common iliac bifurcation.
- The iliolumbar vein travels laterally 3 to 4 cm below the bifurcation and tracks medially to laterally along the body of the L5 vertebra.
- It typically courses between the lumbosacral plexus and the obturator nerve, and it drains the iliac fossa, iliacus, and psoas muscles as well as L4 and L5.
- Retroperitoneal or transthoracic approaches require understanding intrathoracic and intra-abdominal anatomy. Details are beyond the scope of this chapter, but one muscular structure is important.
  - Access to the thoracolumbar spine frequently requires diaphragmatic mobilization.
  - The diaphragm is a dome-shaped structure that attaches to the undersurface of the 11th and 12th ribs and forms crura bilaterally along the upper lumbar spine.
    - The medial and lateral arcuate ligaments of the diaphragm arc over the psoas and quadratus lumborum, respectively.
    - Complete access from T11-L2 requires undermining these ligaments and mobilization and repair of the diaphragmatic crus.

Pertinent History/Physical Examination Findings

- Neck and back pain are challenging and complex problems for patients and medical providers.
  - The pain can be insidious and/or chronic with no clear etiology of the symptoms.
  - The intricate nature of the spinal anatomy including the ligaments, muscle, fascia, bony anatomy, intervertebral disk, nerve roots, and spinal cord adds to the complexity in diagnosis of spinal pain and the multifactorial nature of the symptoms.
  - Understanding the etiology of the symptoms is critical to providing adequate treatment options; requires adequate patient history and physical examination, and correlation of the history of illness and physical examination findings with imaging as needed.
- The provider should be thorough and systematic in obtaining adequate history related to the patient's symptoms including

possible nontraumatic, traumatic, psychosocial, and idiopathic causes for symptoms.
  - The provider must understand and be able to differentiate between myofascial pain, discogenic/axial pain, radicular pain, neurogenic pain.
    - These are classified based on description of symptoms, physical examination findings, and correlation with imaging findings as needed.
    - Pain should be assessed or described as localized or focal midline or paraspinal muscle pain, radiating pain to a dermatomal or nondermatomal, or nonspecific, distribution to assess for myofascial pain, axial pain, radicular pain, or neuropathic pain.
  - The provider should inquire about symptoms of paresthesia, including numbness and or tingling, weakness, gait instability, and changes in bowel and bladder habits.
  - Identification of pain-inciting factors and activities providing pain relief may also provide some insight on the etiology of symptoms and possible treatment options or treatment expectations.
- Physical examination remains a critical tool in diagnosis and management of patients.
  - Correlation of the patient history and physical examinations findings are essential to determine the degree of physical and functional impairment associated with the patient's symptoms.
  - Adequate physical examination requires thorough understanding of myotome function, grading (**Tables 1 and 2**), and dermatomal nerve distribution (**Figure 13**).
- Adequate physical examination begins with observation and assessment of gait patterns.
  - Posture, changing position to guard against or relieve pain, muscle fullness or atrophy, and spinal or limb deformity all are critical and can provide clues to diagnosis or possible symptom etiology.
  - Gait patterns should be observed to evaluate functional status and impairment related to pain versus neuromuscular deficit.
- Range of motion of relevant spine segments, including flexion, extension, and rotation of the cervical and lumbar spine for cervical and lumbar pain, should be assessed, along with associated

TABLE 1 Upper and Lower Extremity Nerve Distributions and Myotome Function

Nerve	Myotome Function
C5	Elbow flexion, shoulder abduction, and external rotators
C6	Wrist extension, forearm pronation, elbow flexion, shoulder external rotation
C7	Wrist pronation, elbow extension
C8	Thumb abduction, index finger extension, finger abduction and flexion
T1	Finger abduction
L2	Hip flexion
L3	Hip flexion, hip adduction, knee extension
L4	Knee extension, ankle dorsiflexion
L5	Great toe extension, ankle dorsiflexion, hip abduction, and internal rotation
S1	Ankle plantar flexion and toe flexion

upper and lower extremity joints correlating with cervical and lumbar spine pain.
- Both active and passive range of motion should be performed for complete evaluation with adequate documentation of symptoms and functional limitations associated with various range-of-motion examinations.
- Palpation of the relevant areas, including the cervical, thoracic, and lumbar midline spine and paraspinal areas, should be performed to evaluate local myofascial pain, bursitis, bony tenderness, bony step-off, and soft-tissue swelling/edema.

TABLE 2 Muscle Strength Grading Scale

Strength Grading	Muscle Strength and Range
0	No muscular contraction
1	Muscle contracture with minimal detectable strength
2	Active muscle contraction and strength without gravity
3	Active muscle contraction and range of motion against gravity
4	Active muscle contraction against gravity with resistance on strength testing
5	Active muscle contraction against gravity with full/normal strength against resistance

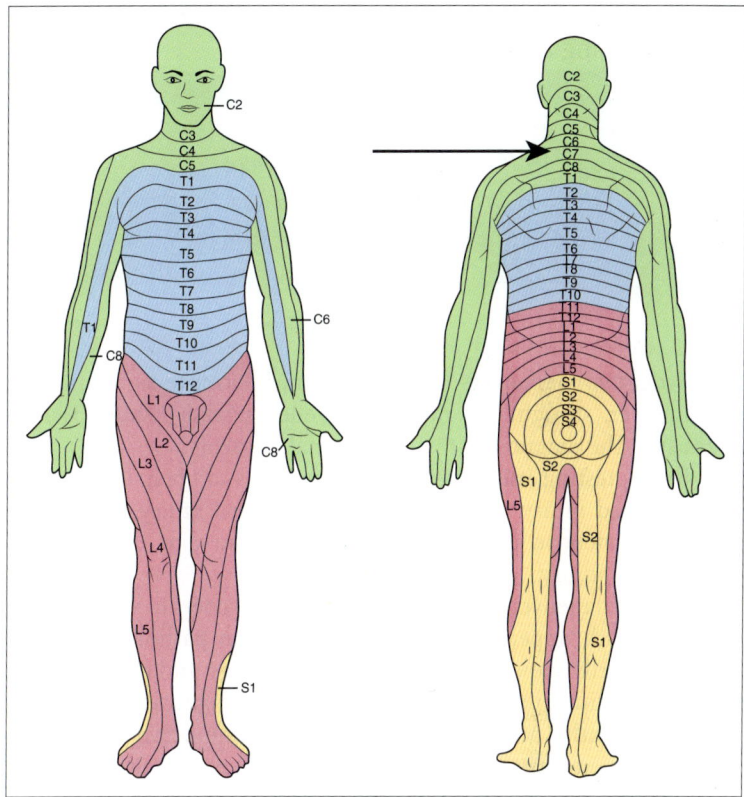

Figure 13 Illustrations show the anterior and posterior dermatomal distribution. (Reproduced with permission from Lippincott's Professional Development Programs, 2012. © Wolters Kluwer. All rights reserved.)

- Neuromuscular examination is critical to assess for spinal cord and nerve root function and myotome strength.
  - Palpation to light touch over various dermatomal distributions is performed with symmetric comparison to evaluate sensory changes and paresthesia associated with palpation over bilateral upper and lower extremities.
- Strength testing is performed over bilateral upper and or lower extremities and graded on a scale of 1 to 5 as indicated in **Table 2** with thorough understanding of the upper and lower extremity myotomes and nerve innervation.[6]

TABLE 3 Upper and Lower Extremity Nerve Roots and Corresponding Reflexes

Nerve Roots	Reflex
C5	Biceps reflex
C6	Brachioradialis reflex
C7	Triceps reflex
L4	Patellar tendon reflex
S1	Achilles tendon reflex

- Provocative maneuvers (Hoffman sign, Lhermitte sign, Spurling maneuver, straight leg raise) and reflex testing (**Table 3**) also assist in the diagnosis of various spinal ailments.
  - Reflex testing and provocative maneuvers can help localize spinal cord injury or the level of spinal cord injury with upper motor neuron pathology, nerve root injury, or lower motor neuron injury.
  - These maneuvers and reflexes may also generate signs associated with upper and lower motor neuron pathology but not necessarily indicate true injury or pathology and must be associated with spinal imaging for definitive diagnosis.
- Radiculopathy and myelopathy require cumulative association of the patient-reported symptoms, physical examination findings and signs, and correlation of the patient's symptoms with imaging findings as needed for definitive opinion and treatment.
  - Pain originating from the nervous system requires careful differentiation from osteoarthritis of the hip and knee or rotator cuff and nerve dysfunction in the upper extremity.
  - The differential diagnosis should also include neurogenic claudication, vascular claudication, diabetic neuropathy, and other systemic causes.
  - It is important that a diagnosis is made in a timely manner.
    - Most radiculopathy is self-limited and will resolve over weeks to months; the symptoms can be quite intense when they occur.
    - Symptoms of myelopathy, however, can be subtle and slowly progressive over time.
- The clinical syndromes of conus medullaris syndrome and cauda equina syndrome require a high index of suspicion in patients

presenting with severe bilateral lower extremity symptoms, including pain, paresthesias, bowel and bladder symptoms, and require careful evaluation and MRI for definitive diagnosis.[7]

Relevant Imaging

- Complete evaluation of back pain and various spinal pathologies sometimes requires spinal imaging for definitive diagnosis in addition to the patient's reported symptoms and physical examination findings.
  - The most commonly used imaging modalities include plain radiography, CT, and MRI.
- Standard plain radiographs are widely available and often the first line of imaging for evaluation of various spinal conditions.
  - Radiographs are limited to the evaluation of the bony anatomy, fractures, dislocation, and disk height and do not provide any direct visualization of neuromuscular structures including the muscle, spinal cord, and nerve roots. Initial imaging will often include a standard AP radiograph and lateral radiograph of the cervical, thoracic, and lumbar spine for cervical, thoracic, and lumbar spine pathology, respectively.
  - Dynamic imaging including flexion and extension radiographs are often used to evaluate for flexibility or instability of the spine in the preoperative setting and for evaluation of spondylolisthesis.
  - Oblique images can be used to evaluate for spondylolysis or pars defect in the lumbar spine.
- CT provides a more detailed evaluation of bony anatomy.
  - Most valuable in the trauma setting because of limitations associated with radiographs especially in the cervical and thoracic spine.
  - Valuable in evaluating the bony anatomy for patients with congenital bony abnormalities and/or patients with previous spinal surgery.
  - Limited to evaluation of the bony anatomy without clear visualization of the nerve roots and spinal cord or soft tissue within the epidural space or neuroforamen.
  - Most effective at evaluating spine trauma patients in addition to patients with spondylolysis.
  - CT with myelogram provides indirect interpretation of the patency of the spinal canal and limited evaluation of the nerve

roots within the neuroforamen for patients in whom MRI cannot be performed for evaluation of spinal cord and nerve root compression.
- MRI is the gold standard for evaluation of the neuromuscular spine and intervertebral disk.
  - Most effective at evaluation of the patency of the central canal, including the epidural space, spinal cord and the neuroforamen, and nerve roots.
  - Various causes of spinal cord and nerve root compression, including disk herniation, hematoma, fat, and spinal tumor, are easily visualized using MRI.
  - Contraindicated for some patients with noncompatible pacemakers, spinal stimulators, retained metal fragments, etc.
  - Interpretation of MRI is also limited for patients with extensive metal hardware from previous surgery.
    - CT myelogram is often used for these patients for indirect evaluation of the patency of the central canal and neuroforamen.

Nonsurgical Measures

- Treatment of various spinal pathologies requires understanding of the natural history of various spinal conditions—back pain, neck pain, radiculopathy, stenosis, etc.[8,9]
  - It is also critical to evaluate for nonspinal etiology of pain to formulate the differential diagnosis.
  - Comprehensive evaluation of the patient is most ideal for best patient care.
- Deformities such as Scheuermann disease, adult degenerative scoliosis, and early-onset or adolescent idiopathic scoliosis are evaluated in a clinical setting.
  - For these disorders, nonsurgical measures relate to the risk of progression and associated symptoms, and metrics such as Risser sign to assess growth or radiographic parameters delineate the switch to consider surgical options.
- There is no single clearly defined or specific nonsurgical measure for the management of spinal pain, but various nonsurgical modalities have been described with some success.
- Nonsurgical treatment often includes a combination of multiple modalities including observation, physical therapy, use of spinal

injections, bracing, neuromodulation medications, and various analgesics including NSAIDs or narcotics.[10,11]
- Should be tailored to the patient's symptoms and best available medical evidence for treatment.

Surgical Intervention

- Surgical intervention for most spinal pathologies is often indicated as a last resort after nonsurgical management has failed.
  - May be indicated in emergency situations such as spine trauma, acute neurologic compromise from various pathologies, including cauda equina syndrome, intractable nerve pain, metastatic lesions with spinal cord injury, or nerve root injury.
- The overall goal of spinal surgical intervention is to halt and/or reverse the progression of neurologic injury/deterioration and deficit, to restore spinal function and stability, and pain control.
  - Generally accomplished through surgical decompression of the neural elements including the spinal cord and nerve roots, spinal fusion, or combined decompression and fusion.
- Surgical decompression can be achieved through either direct spinal or indirect approach or a combination of both.
  - Can be achieved through an anterior approach, posterior approach, lateral approach to the spine, or a combination of the various approaches.
  - Direct decompression involves targeted removal or resection of the inciting factors, which can include disk herniation, tumor lesion, bony or cartilaginous lesions, hematoma, epidural fat, etc.
  - Indirect decompression involves expansion of the spinal canal or neuroforamen without necessarily resecting the incident factors leading to nerve root or spinal cord compression.
    - Indirect decompression can be achieved through bony resection, diskectomy, and use of mechanical devices to restore disk height and foraminal height through distraction.
  - Decompression through a direct or indirect approach can sometimes lead to spinal instability requiring spinal instrumentation with or without spinal fusion.
    - Can be achieved with use of various mechanical devices including disk arthroplasty, screws, rods, wiring, and various spinal implants and biologics.

- The decision for surgical approach or surgical plan is based on best evidence available based on the patient's pathology, minimizing morbidity associated with surgical intervention and thorough understanding of the treatment goals and expectations.

Top 10 Knowledge Drops for Your Rotation

1. It is critical to both clinical evaluation of the spine and treatment strategies/options to understand the bony and ligamentous anatomy of the spine including the anterior, middle, and posterior column and its relationship to the joint surfaces, ligaments, and nerve roots.
2. Cervical, thoracic, and lumbar nerve distributions/dermatomal distributions are key to evaluating spinal etiology of various spine-related pathologies.
3. Spinal pathologies are often manifested as radiculopathy, myelopathy, or pain or a combination of the three.
4. Degenerative disk disease, disk herniation, and nerve compression are not always symptomatic and must be correlated with the patient's reported history.
5. Patient history and physical examination must be correlated with imaging modalities including radiography, CT, and MRI as needed to determine the etiology of the symptoms for adequate treatment.
6. MRI is the gold standard for evaluating various spinal cord and nerve root–related spine pathologies, with CT myelogram for patients for whom MRI is contraindicated.
7. Most spine pathologies can be managed with a nonsurgical/conservative approach.
8. Surgical approach including decompression with or without fusion is determined by the extent of the pathology and stability of the spine.
9. Direct versus indirect surgical approach is determined based on pathology, number of levels involved, and morbidity associated with each approach.
10. The goal of surgical and nonsurgical management of spinal disease is to arrest deterioration in physical function and pain and or relieve pain and restore physical function.

References

1. Martin BI, Deyor RA, Mirza SK, et al: Expenditures and health status among adults with back and neck problems. *JAMA* 2008;299(6):656-664.
2. Denis F: The three-column spine and its significance in the classification of acute thoracolumbar spinal injuries. *Spine [Phila Pa 1976]* 1983;8(8):817-831.
3. Vleeming A, Schuenke MD, Masi AT, Carreiro JE, Danneels L, Willard FH: The sacroiliac joint: An overview of its anatomy, function and potential clinical implications. *J Anat* 2012;221(6):537-567.
4. Kirchmair L, Lirk P, Colvin J, Mitterschiffthaler G, Moriggl B: Lumbar plexus and psoas major muscle: Not always as expected. *Anesth Pain Med* 2008;33(2):109-114.
5. Tezuka F, Sakai T, Nishisho T, et al: Variations in arterial supply to the lower lumbar spine. *Eur Spine J* 2016;25(12):4181-4187.
6. Bates B: *A Guide to Physical Examination and History Taking*, ed 5. JB Lippincott, 1991.
7. Radcliff KE, Kepler CK, Delasotta LA, et al: Current management review of thoracolumbar cord syndromes. *Spine J* 2011;11(9):884-892.
8. Lees F, Turner JW: Natural history and prognosis of cervical spondylosis. *Br Med J* 1963;2(5373):1607-1610.
9. Johnsson KE, Rosén I, Udén A: The natural course of lumbar spinal stenosis. *Clin Orthop Relat Res* 1992;279:82-86.
10. Rhee JM, Yoon T, Riew KD: Cervical radiculopathy. *J Am Acad Orthop Surg* 2007;15(8):486-494.
11. Madigan L, Vaccaro AR, Spector LR, Milam AR: Management of symptomatic lumbar degenerative disk disease. *J Am Acad Orthop Surg* 2009;17(2):102-111.

13

Tumor ABCs

Tessa Balach, MD, FAAOS
Cara A. Cipriano, MD, MSc, FAAOS
Sheila Ann Conway, MD, FAAOS, FAOA
Ginger E. Holt, MD, FAAOS

Introduction

Malignant bone and soft-tissue masses are exceedingly rare. Because of the rarity of bone and soft-tissue tumors, their diagnosis is often delayed as a result of a lack of education on the practitioner's part.

Epidemiology

- Malignant primary bone tumors account for approximately 0.2% of all malignancies.[1]
- Soft-tissue sarcomas comprise less than 1% of all malignancies.[2]
  - These tumors arise from a mesenchymal cell origin and thus, behave differently than other tumors.
  - Primarily, this is manifested as a location in the bones, muscles, fat, nerves, and walls of vessels.
  - The metastatic pattern of hematogenous spread, with lung metastases being the primary site (as opposed to lymph nodes)

Dr. Balach or an immediate family member serves as a board member, owner, officer, or committee member of the Accreditation Council for Graduate Medical Education (ACGME), the American Orthopaedic Association, the Musculoskeletal Oncology Research Initiative, and the Musculoskeletal Tumor Society. Dr. Cipriano or an immediate family member serves as a paid consultant to or is an employee of DePuy, a Johnson & Johnson Company and Link Orthopaedics and serves as a board member, owner, officer, or committee member of the American Association of Hip and Knee Surgeons, the Musculoskeletal Tumor Society, and the Ruth Jackson Orthopaedic Society. Dr. Conway or an immediate family member serves as an unpaid consultant to DePuy, a Johnson & Johnson Company. Dr. Holt or an immediate family member serves as a board member, owner, officer, or committee member of the Musculoskeletal Tumor Society.

- Carcinoma (prostate, breast, etc) comprises 64% of all cancers, with 4.8% of these patients having skeletal metastases at 1 year.
- Benign bone tumors (osteochondromas) and benign soft-tissue tumors (lipomas) are far more common, with an incidence of approximately 1 per 1,000.

Pertinent Anatomy

- Orthopaedic tumors affect the entire musculoskeletal system.
- Rather than learning a few standard approaches, relevant anatomy is best studied on a case-by-case basis.
- When reviewing imaging or preparing for a surgery, the structures surrounding the tumor should be the focus.
- The physician should be familiar with the location and function of the muscles in the compartment, as well as any nerves or vessels that may be in the surgical field.
- Tumors often distort anatomy, so identifying known anatomic structures first as a framework is important.

Age at Presentation

- Younger than 5 years
  - Malignant
    - Langerhans cell histiocytoses (Letterer-Siwe disease; Hand-Schüller-Christian disease)
    - Metastatic rhabdomyosarcoma
    - Metastatic neuroblastoma
  - Benign
    - Osteomyelitis
    - Osteofibrous dysplasia
- Younger than 30 years
  - Malignant
    - Ewing sarcoma (**Figure 1**)
    - Osteosarcoma (**Figure 2**)
  - Benign
    - Osteoid osteoma (**Figure 3**)
    - Osteoblastoma
    - Chondroblastoma
    - Aneurysmal bone cyst (**Figure 4**)
    - Langerhans cell histiocytosis

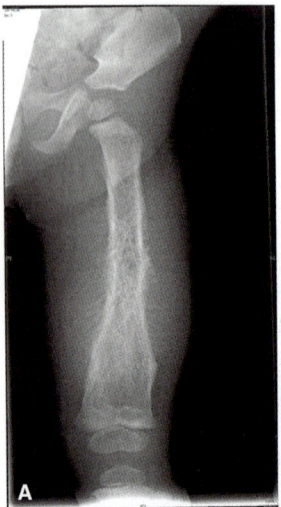
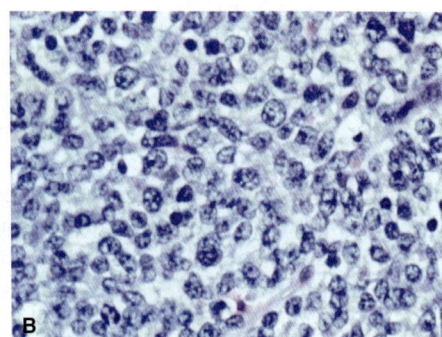

Figure 1 Ewing sarcoma. **A**, AP radiograph shows left femur with diaphyseal lesion with aggressive pattern periosteal reaction (hair on end). **B**, Histologic image showing small round blue cells of Ewing sarcoma.

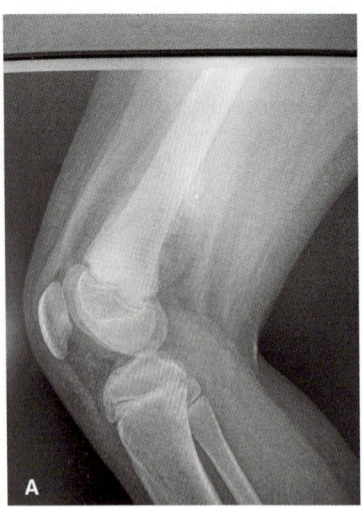
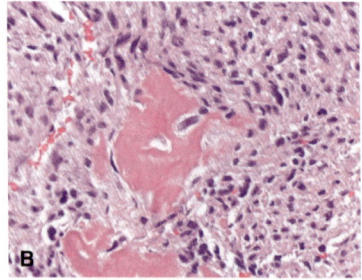

Figure 2 Osteosarcoma. **A**, Lateral radiograph with distal femur lesion characterized by osseous mineralization pattern and large soft-tissue mass. **B**, Histologic image showing pathology characterized by osteoid formation and malignant spindle cells.

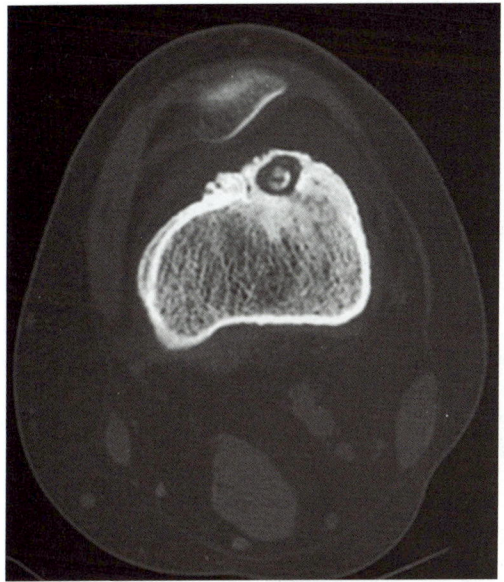

Figure 3 Osteoid osteoma. Axial CT image of the distal femur demonstrating the classic nidus in the anterior cortex.

- Osteofibrous dysplasia
- Nonossifying fibroma (**Figure 5**)
- Older than 30 years
  - Malignant
    - Chondrosarcoma (**Figure 6**)
    - Metastases (**Figure 7**)
    - Lymphoma
    - Myeloma (**Figure 8**)
    - Chordoma
    - Adamantinoma (**Figure 9**)
  - Benign
    - Giant cell tumor (**Figure 10**)
    - Paget disease

Pertinent History/Physical Examination Findings

- The patient history should be considered along with epidemiology, physical examination, and available imaging to determine the next appropriate steps of workup.

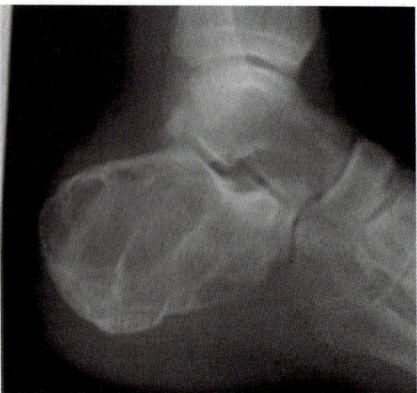

Figure 4 Aneurysmal bone cyst. Lateral radiograph with lytic lesion with a multilocular cystic appearance.

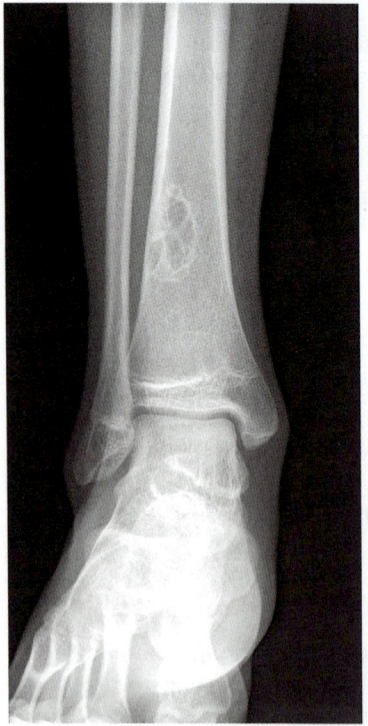

Figure 5 Nonossifying fibroma. AP radiograph of distal tibia characterized by eccentric location, lobular appearance, and sclerotic margin.

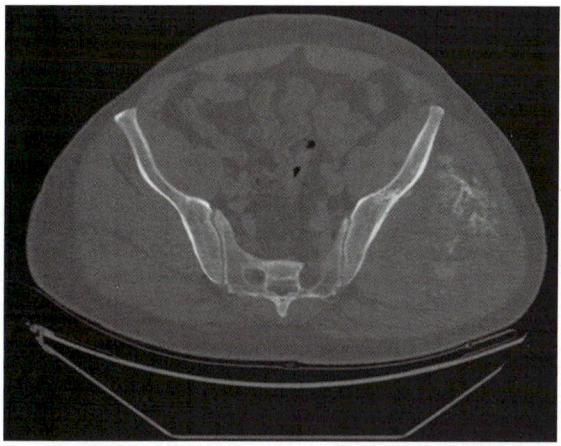

Figure 6 Chondrosarcoma. Axial CT image of the pelvis with left ilium lesion and associated large soft-tissue mass with cartilage mineralization pattern.

- When evaluating a patient with a soft-tissue mass or bone tumor, it is important to ask:
  - How long it has been present?
  - Has it changed in size?
  - Is it painful?

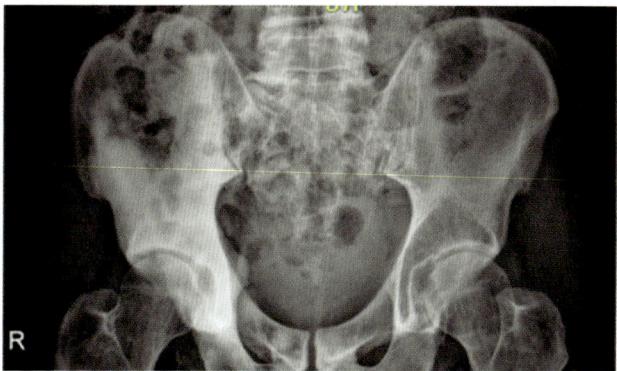

Figure 7 Pelvic radiograph demonstrating multiple osseous blastic metastases in the pelvis.

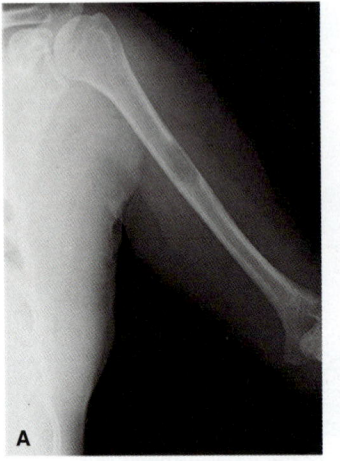
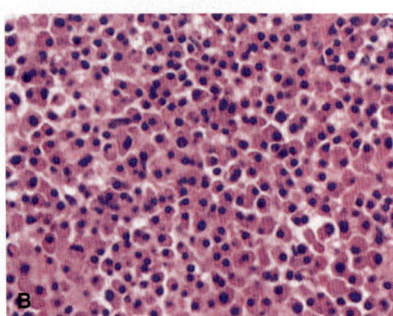

Figure 8 Multiple myeloma. **A**, AP radiograph with lytic lesion of the diaphysis of the humerus with cortical thinning. **B**, Histologic image demonstrates sheets of malignant plasma cells.

- Confounding factors may confuse the presentation.
  - It is not uncommon for patients to report an injury at the time they first noticed a mass or pain.
  - Although the incident draws patients' attention to the problem, it is not necessarily the underlying cause.
  - History of a traumatic onset does not necessarily rule out an oncologic issue.
  - Taking a complete medical, surgical, and social history is important.
  - Symptoms such as fevers, chills, or unintentional weight loss are important as these may help to narrow the differential diagnosis.
- Common syndromes associated with bone and soft-tissue tumors:[1]
  - Li-Fraumeni syndrome
    - Disease: sarcoma, breast, leukemia, and adrenal gland syndrome
    - Musculoskeletal neoplasm: osteosarcoma
    - Genetic association: P53

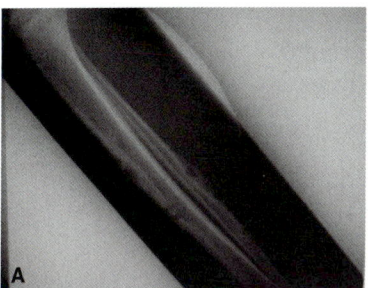 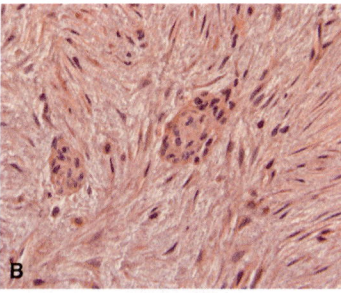

Figure 9 Adamantinoma. **A**, Lateral radiograph with multiple lytic cortically based lesions of the tibia and fibula. **B**, Histologic image showing biphasic pathology with spindle cell background and clusters of epitheloid cells.

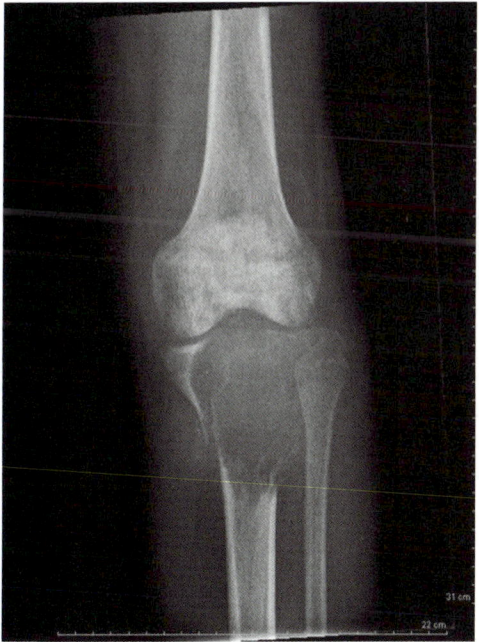

Figure 10 Giant cell tumor of bone. AP radiograph with lytic lesion of the metaphysis and epiphysis of proximal tibia.

- Retinoblastoma
  - Disease: bilateral malignant tumor of the eye in children
  - Musculoskeletal neoplasm: osteosarcoma
  - Genetic association: RB1
- Multiple hereditary exostoses
  - Disease: multiple osteochondromas
  - Musculoskeletal neoplasm: chondroblastoma
  - Genetic associations: EXT 1, EXT 2
- Stewart-Treves syndrome
  - Disease: chronic lymphedema
  - Musculoskeletal neoplasm: angiosarcoma
  - Genetic association: none
- Neurofibromatosis (type 1)
  - Disease: multiple neurofibromas
  - Musculoskeletal neoplasm: malignant peripheral nerve sheath tumor
  - Genetic association: NF1

Bone Tumors

- Benign bone tumors (including neoplasms, cysts, and metabolic processes)
  - Present either with pain or as incidental image findings
  - Lesions that are benign can be painful if they weaken the bone.
  - Some benign latent or active lesions (eg, large unicameral bone cysts, fibrous dysplasia, or even occasionally nonossifying fibromas) can compromise mechanical stability enough to cause discomfort, particularly related to weight-bearing activities.
  - Weakness of the bone from a lesion can also lead to pathologic fracture, sometimes with relatively minor trauma.
  - Benign aggressive lesions (eg, aneurysmal bone cysts and giant cell tumors) are often inherently painful even before they mechanically compromise the bone.
  - Other causes for pain associated with a benign bone tumor include:
    - Prominence (as with osteochondromas) or
    - Prostaglandin release (as with osteoid osteomas)

- Many benign bone tumors are found incidentally.
  - The lesion is noticed on imaging performed during workup of another issue.
  - Example: nonossifying fibroma in the distal tibia of a child with a sprained ankle while playing soccer.
  - Most tumors discovered in this fashion are latent and can be expected to remain stable or resolve without any intervention, and do not require further workup or monitoring.
  - Less commonly, additional follow-up imaging, or even biopsy, may be required.
- Most benign bone tumors are contained within the bone itself, so size is not measureable on physical examination.
  - Osteochondromas are an exception.
    - Often subcutaneous and can be palpated.
    - Grow until skeletal maturity, so a size change can be expected.
- **Table 1** summarizes the key features of common benign bone tumors (osteochondroma, enchondroma, giant cell tumor).
- Malignant primary bone tumors (ie, bone sarcomas)
  - Most commonly present as a painful mass.
  - Patients may describe a gradual onset of pain or start noticing it after a specific event.

TABLE 1 Comparison of Benign Bone Tumors

	Osteochondroma	Enchondroma	Giant Cell Tumor
Age	Younger than 30 yr	Any age	Older than 30 yr
Presentation	Pain or incidental	Incidental	Pain
Imaging	• Looks like cauliflower with stalk from bone and flower cap • Intramedullary canal is confluent with the lesion • Common location metaphyseal/pelvis and scapula	• Stippled calcifications • Arcs and rings • No endosteal scalloping or erosion	• Lytic bone lesion • Metaphyseal location • May be collision with aneurysmal bone cyst
Histology	• Mature bone blends into a mature cartilage stalk	• Bland minimally cellular binucleate cells in a light blue background	• Multinucleated giant cells with nuclei that appear the same as the stromal cells
Biology	Benign	Benign	Benign-aggressive
Treatment	Observe or surgical resection if painful	Observe	Intralesional resection/curettage

- The pain becomes severe and unrelenting.
- Pain that occurs at night and pain unrelated to activity is concerning for malignancy (a notable exception to this is osteoid osteoma).
- Growth of a mass (other than a known osteochondroma in a child) is also a concerning finding.
- In contrast with carcinomas or hematologic malignancies, bone sarcomas are not associated with systemic symptoms.
  - It is less relevant to ask or report about general symptoms such as weight loss or fatigue.
  - Exception: Ewing sarcoma
    - Can present with inflammatory signs/symptoms
    - Example: elevated erythrocyte sedimentation rate/C-reactive protein and malaise
  - **Table 2** summarizes the key features of the primary bone sarcomas (osteosarcoma, chondrosarcoma, and Ewing sarcoma)
- Metastatic bone disease
  - Causes musculoskeletal symptoms based on the location and extent of osseous involvement
  - It is important to assess the location and degree of pain to guide clinical decisions.
  - Pain with weight-bearing suggests mechanical weakness in the affected extremity, which may warrant intervention.
  - A cancer history is important to obtain.
    - Not sufficient to distinguish between primary and metastatic bone tumors
    - Patients with bone metastases may not have a history of cancer at the time of presentation, as orthopaedic complaints frequently lead to the initial diagnosis.
  - A solitary bone lesion in a patient with a history of cancer may not necessarily be a metastasis, so appropriate workup is needed to rule out a primary bone tumor.[3]
  - For a patient with a history of cancer, ask:
    - When was the cancer diagnosed?
    - Is the cancer active or in remission?
    - What prior or current treatments have been given?
    - Relevant risk factors (history of smoking)?

TABLE 2 Comparison of Primary Bone Sarcomas

	Osteosarcoma	Chondrosarcoma	Ewing Sarcoma
Age	Younger than 30 yr and older than 60 yr	Older than 30 yr	Younger than 30 yr
Presentation	Pain	Pain	Pain May be accompanied by fever, elevated white blood cell count
Imaging	• Mixed lytic/destructive aggressive intramedullary bone producing lesion • Common location metaphyseal	• Metadiaphyseal long bone or flat bone • Popcorn calcifications with arcs and rings, endosteal scalloping and erosion, mixed appearance lytic and arc/rings • May arise in the setting of multiple hereditary exostosis, Ollier disease	• Sunburst saucerized surface lesion • Diaphyseal • Characteristic location femur or tibia or flat bones—pelvis and scapula
Histology	• Poorly arranged osseous trabeculae with malignant rimming osteoblasts • Atypical spindle cells	• Osseous trabeculae • Chondroblastic elements	• Small round blue cells • Pseudorosettes • CD99 positive • EWS-FLI1 positive
Biology	65% 5-yr survival	90% 5-yr survival	80% 5-yr survival
Treatment	Chemotherapy Limb salvage surgery (when possible)	Limb salvage surgery (when possible)	Chemotherapy Limb salvage surgery (when possible)

- Patients may also experience systemic symptoms that are:
  - Generalized: weight loss, fatigue
  - Specific: to their primary disease
    - Cough, hemoptysis—lung cancer
    - Urinary symptoms, retention—prostate cancer
    - Bloody stools—colon cancer

Soft-Tissue Tumors

- Patients of all ages will present with lumps, bumps, and masses that are concerning to them.
- The clinician is charged with finding those that are truly worrisome (ie, malignant, versus those that are not).

- Mass characteristics that should give rise for concern:[4]
  - Larger than 5 cm in the extremity (1.5 cm in the hand or foot)
  - Deep to fascia
  - Immobile/fixed and firm and
  - Growing
- Evaluation of a concerning mass[4]
  - Ultrasonography may be beneficial in defining the size and characterizing of a small, superficial mass (useful to confirm a diagnosis of suspected cyst or lipoma).
  - MRI is most helpful in determining the tissue composition, location, and extent of a mass relative to surrounding structures.
  - MRI performed to assess a mass should include the entire mass and be done with and without intravenous contrast.
  - If a patient cannot undergo MRI (pacemaker or brain clips), then CT may be performed.
- Benign soft-tissue tumors
  - Pain
    - Commonly painless
    - Exception: benign nerve tumors (neurofibromas and schwannomas) are and can be very sensitive to pressure.
    - Lipomas and other benign masses are classically painless, but in some situations may cause symptoms because of mass effect (ie, pressure or tension exerted on surrounding structures).[5]
    - When examining a patient with a lipoma and complaints of pain, it is important to carefully consider and rule out any other sources before concluding that the tumor is responsible.
  - Growth
    - Stable or long-standing masses are more likely to be benign, but this is not always the case.
    - Rapidly growing soft-tissue tumors are suspicious for malignancy.
    - Waxing and waning: vascular malformations often fill with blood and become symptomatic with activity, then recede with rest.
    - Shrinking: masses that are consistently shrinking are more likely to be inflammatory or traumatic than neoplastic.
- Malignant primary soft-tissue tumors (ie, soft-tissue sarcomas)
  - Most commonly present as an enlarging mass
  - Typically, painless (in contrast to bone sarcomas)

- No systemic symptoms (similar to bone sarcomas)
- Rapid growth is concerning.
- Physical examination
  - Visual: inspect the quality and condition of the skin, any defects, wounds or deformity, and the neurovascular condition.
  - Note the size and location of the mass.
  - Assess the consistency of the mass.
    - Soft: vascular
    - Doughy: lipoma
    - Firm: fibromatosis or sarcoma
  - Mobile or fixed
    - With the overlying muscles relaxed and off tension, feel whether the mass moves freely beneath the skin and over the bone.
    - If a tumor feels mobile with the muscle relaxed and remains mobile with the muscle flexed, it is superficial.
    - If a tumor feels fixed when the muscle is flexed, it is likely deep to fascia.
    - Determine whether the mass is tender.
- Unlike in most other orthopaedic subspecialties, the physical examination is much more dependent on inspection than palpation, rather than strength and range of motion. As such, be sensitive to patients and do not overly manipulate a limb that is obviously painful.

Relevant Imaging

- Radiographs
  - Plain radiographs in two planes should be completed on an extremity where a bone lesion is suspected.
  - For bone tumors, radiographs are the most important imaging test to help determine the diagnosis.
  - There are four questions to be asked when reviewing the radiographs as taught by Enneking:
    - What is the location?
      - Location refers to location within the bone (eg, epiphyseal, metaphyseal, diaphyseal; **Table 2**).
    - What is the tumor-bone interaction?
      - Lodwick described the tumor and bone interaction as how aggressive is the tumor, is it moving so fast as to destroy

the bone (metastases), forming a soft-tissue mass outside of the bone (lymphoma) or slow growing?
- What is the bone-tumor interaction?
  - The bone reaction refers to processes such as onion skinning (Ewing sarcoma), or endosteal scalloping and erosion (chondrosarcoma).
- What is the matrix?
  - The matrix refers to what type of extracellular matrix the tumor is making such as osteoid or bone in osteosarcoma, cartilage in chondrosarcoma, or fibrous matrix in fibrous dysplasia.
- The answers to these four questions will help create a radiographic differential diagnosis for a bone tumor.
- MRI[6]
  - MRI is the imaging modality of choice for soft-tissue tumors.
  - Helps to provide detailed information about the precise size of the location and characteristics of both bone and soft-tissue tumors.
  - It can determine whether a soft-tissue mass originates from a primary bone location or if a soft-tissue mass is externally compressing a bone.
  - MRI also helps to show the relationship between the tumor and surrounding neurovascular structures.
  - Common MRI findings are:
    - T1 lesion isointense with muscle
    - T2 enhancement
    - T2 fat saturation—does not suppress
- CT[6]
  - CT is used to assess the chest, abdomen, and pelvis when looking for the source of a carcinoma that has metastasized to bone.
  - It is also used to look for pulmonary metastases in the setting of a sarcoma of bone or soft tissue.
  - CT of the extremities is used to assess an osseous matrix, specifically when looking for the diagnostic nidus of an osteoid osteoma.
- Whole-body bone scan; technetium-99 scan[6]
  - A whole-body bone scan is used to assess the skeleton completely for the presence of metastases, in adults with metastatic carcinoma and in younger patients to look for skip metastases in Ewing sarcoma and osteosarcoma.

- Positron emission tomography[6]
  - Positron emission tomography is used to evaluate for metastases or in the staging of melanoma or lymphoma. It should be ordered if the aforementioned tests do not reveal the necessary information.
- Findings on imaging
  - Bone tumors have a predilection for certain locations in the bone.
  - Tumors by radiographic location[1]
    - Epiphyseal
      - Chondroblastoma
      - Giant cell tumor (**Figure 10**)
      - Clear cell chondrosarcoma (femoral head)
    - Metaphyseal
      - Osteosarcoma (**Figure 2**)
      - Chondrosarcoma (**Figure 6**)
      - Metastatic disease (**Figure 7**)
    - Diaphyseal
      - A = adamantinoma (**Figure 9**)
      - E = eosinophilic granuloma
      - I = infection
      - O = osteoid osteoma/osteoblastoma (**Figure 3**)
      - U = Ewing sarcoma (**Figure 1**)
      - Y = mYeloma, lYmphoma, fibrous dYsplasia
    - Flat bones
      - Chondrosarcoma
      - Fibrous dysplasia
      - Hemangioma
      - Paget disease
      - Ewing sarcoma
    - Spine
      - Anterior
        - Giant cell tumor
        - Metastatic disease
      - Posterior
        - Osteoid osteoma/osteoblastoma
        - Aneurysmal bone cyst
    - Sacrum
      - Midline: chordoma
      - Eccentric: aneurysmal bone cyst/giant cell tumor/metastatic disease

Biopsy

- Principles of biopsy[1]
  - Understanding when and how to biopsy are complex cognitive skills.
  - The timing, location, orientation, and interpretation of a biopsy are critical to patient longevity and outcome.
  - Ideally, the surgeon who will eventually perform the definitive surgical procedure should perform the biopsy.
- Principles of musculoskeletal biopsy
  - Longitudinal incision in line with future resection—longitudinal incision is extensile and the tract can be excised with final resection.
  - Critical structures, for example, neurovascular bundles, should be avoided—contamination of critical structures precludes limb salvage.
  - The soft-tissue component should be biopsied when present—bone is weakened when its cortex is disrupted.
  - Strict hemostasis should be maintained: increased contamination outside of the biopsy tract by iatrogenic tumor spread should be avoided.

Surgical Treatment

- Benign soft-tissue tumors
  - The indication for resection of a benign soft-tissue tumor is management of a symptomatic and/or enlarging mass.
  - Marginal excision is sufficient.
  - If a mass is stable and nonsurgical treatment is favored, formal monitoring is usually not indicated; however, patients should be instructed to follow up if they notice the size of the mass increasing.
  - Vascular lesions, such as hemangiomas or vascular malformations, may be managed nonsurgically with gentle compression during activity to minimize swelling and associated pain. Sclerotherapy or embolization is also effective in some cases.
- Benign bone tumors
  - Latent or active can be managed nonsurgically if asymptomatic and not at risk of fracture. Observation with serial radiographs may be indicated if there is concern for progression.

- Pathologic fracture of the upper extremity (ie, through a unicameral bone cyst or fibrous dysplasia), immobilization in an appropriate cast, splint, or sling. The bone will heal reliably, and cysts will often resolve in the process. If the underlying lesion persists and appears to be at risk for refracture after the bone has healed, surgery can be considered. Pathologic fractures of the lower extremity are more frequently managed surgically, except in very young children.
- For active and aggressive benign bone tumors (eg, aneurysmal bone cyst or giant cell tumors of bone), surgical treatment is indicated to prevent further bone destruction and provide mechanical stabilization of the bone.
- Metastatic bone disease
- The indication for surgical treatment of benign soft-tissue tumors is management of a symptomatic mass or a mass that is increasing in size.
- For active and aggressive benign bone tumors (eg, aneurysmal bone cyst or giant cell tumors of bone), surgical treatment is indicated to prevent further bone destruction and provide mechanical stabilization of the bone.
  - Patients with metastatic bone tumors are treated with surgery to manage pathologic fractures, or more preferably, to prophylactically stabilize impending pathologic fractures with plate-and-screw constructs, intramedullary nails, or arthroplasty-type procedures.
  - In the setting of metastatic spine lesions, surgery is indicated to treat patients with structural instability or neurocompressive symptoms related to the tumor.
- Primary bone and soft-tissue sarcoma
- The goal of the treatment of malignant bone and soft-tissue tumors is to remove the lesion with minimal risk of local recurrence.
  - Limb salvage surgery is wide-margin surgical resection excising a cuff of normal tissue.
  - Is performed when two essential criteria are met:
    - Adequate local control can be achieved.
    - The function of the remaining limb must be at least as good as the amputation.
- Surgical margins are defined as follows:
  - Intralesional margin
    - The plane of dissection goes directly through the tumor.

- Appropriate only for benign tumors such as giant cell tumor of bone or aneurysmal bone cyst.
- Marginal margin
  - The line of resection goes through the reactive zone of the tumor; the reactive zone contains inflammatory cells, edema, fibrous tissue, and possibly satellites of tumor cells.
  - This may be used in areas of malignant tumors where critical structures are preserved (ie, large nerve or artery).
  - This is used commonly for atypical lipomas and well differentiated liposarcomas.
  - Unplanned marginal resection can result in a local recurrence rate of 25% to 50%.
- Wide margin
  - Also known as wide excision, this margin uses a wide line of surgical resection is accomplished when the entire tumor is removed with a cuff of normal tissue surrounding it and is the most common margin for a soft-tissue sarcoma.
  - The local recurrence rate drops below 10% when a wide margin is achieved.
- Radical margin
  - A radical margin is achieved when the entire tumor and its compartment (all surrounding muscles, ligaments, and connective tissues) are removed.
  - Examples include some amputations and resection of the entire anterior thigh compartment (rectus fem vastus intermedius, lateralis, and medialis).

Adjuvant Treatment

- Bone sarcomas[4]
  - Managed with a combination of surgery and chemotherapy.
  - Systemic treatments can be used for micrometastatic disease (present but not detectable), more than 90% of cases are limb salvage, and rate of survival is approximately 70%.
  - Classic chemotherapy agents for bone sarcomas include methotrexate, doxorubicin, ifosfamide, and cisplatin, administered both before and after surgical resection of the primary tumor.
  - The application of neoadjuvant chemotherapy allows for the biologic response to treatment to be assessed on histologic inspection of the resected tumor, which has an implication on prognosis.

- With few exceptions (eg, nonresectable Ewing sarcoma), radiation is not used in the management of bone sarcomas.
- Metastatic bone disease (**Table 3**)
  - Managed nonsurgically with systemic therapies, radiation, diphosphonates, and pain medications.[7]
  - If the risk of fracture is very high, or if a pathologic fracture has occurred, surgery is often indicated.
  - In lower risk situations, a low dose of radiation (20 to 30 Gy), usually given over the course of 2 weeks (10 fractions) can be used to manage the tumor.
    - Radiation leads to pain relief and allows for eventual recovery of the bone. Even if the patient does undergo surgery, adjuvant radiation is indicated postoperatively to manage residual tumor and decreases the risk of local recurrence.
    - Some malignancies (eg, multiple myeloma) respond more reliably to radiation than others (eg, renal cell carcinoma), and this should be accounted for when considering and planning surgery.
    - Weight-bearing restrictions should be implemented to reduce the risk of fracture until the bone has recovered or been surgically stabilized.

TABLE 3 Evaluation of Patients Older Than 40 Years With a Lytic Bone Lesion

Test	Purpose	Pearls
CT of the chest, abdomen, pelvis	Locate primary site in metastatic bone disease	Breast, kidney, lung, prostate, and thyroid common solid organ tumors that metastasize to bone
Whole-body bone scan	Sites of metastatic or primary skeletal disease show increased radiotracer uptake	Metastatic bone disease is characterized by multifocal osseous disease of the axial and appendicular skeleton
Serum protein electrophoresis/urine protein electrophoresis	Evaluate for abnormal electrophoresis spike (M spike) seen in multiple myeloma	Immunoglobulin G and immunoglobulin A are the most common types of multiple myeloma
Prostate-specific antigen	Serum antigen elevated in prostate cancer	—
Bone biopsy	Tissue sampling to determine diagnostic pathology	Required in metastatic bone sites of unknown primary origin

- Patients with metastatic disease should undergo systemic treatment (eg, chemotherapy, hormone therapy, and immune therapy) based on their primary disease, as well as diphosphonate treatment to minimize further osteoclast-mediated bone loss and lower the risk of pathologic fracture.
- Pain medication is often part of the treatment of bone metastases.
- Soft-tissue sarcomas
  - Managed with surgical excision and radiation.
    - Radiation is most commonly used as external beam radiation either before or after surgery.
    - Radiation is typically administered over the course of 5 weeks.
  - Preoperative radiation is 50 Gy administered to the tumor and immediately adjacent tissues.
    - Preoperative radiation is associated with more frequent wound healing complications and infection (up to 40%) because of local tissue damage that impairs the healing process.
  - Postoperative radiation is 60 Gy given to the entire surgical field.
    - Higher volume and dose of postoperative radiation leads to more severe long-term complications, such as soft-tissue fibrosis and nerve toxicity. Radiation-induced sarcoma is a rare but devastating long-term sequela.
  - Chemotherapy treatments for soft-tissue sarcomas are not as effective as for bone sarcomas, and therefore not universally used.

Top 10 Knowledge Drops for Your Rotation

1. Primary bone tumors most commonly present with pain.
2. Soft-tissue sarcomas are commonly painless.
3. Common genetic mutations associated with sarcomas are P53, RB1, EXT1/2, and NF1.
4. Characteristics of a lump, bump, or mass that are concerning for a sarcoma include:
   - Size greater than 5 cm or greater than 1.5 cm in the hand/foot (although sarcomas can be smaller)
   - Enlarging over time

- Deep to fascia (although sarcomas can be superficial)
- Recurs after resection

5. Metastatic bone disease is the most common entity that creates skeletal destruction and lytic bone lesions in patients older than 40 years.
   - The evaluation of a patient with a lytic bone lesion should include:
     - Detailed history to include a personal or family history of cancer
     - CT of the chest, abdomen, and pelvis
     - Whole-body bone scan
     - Laboratory studies (serum protein electrophoresis and urine protein electrophoresis, prostate-specific antigen)
     - Biopsy
6. The five carcinomas that are most likely to metastasize to bone are those of the breast, lung, thyroid, kidney, and prostate (mnemonic: BLT and a kosher pickle).
7. The most common primary malignant bone tumors are osteosarcoma, chondrosarcoma, and Ewing sarcoma (in descending order).
8. The most common benign bone tumors are osteochondroma, enchondroma, and giant cell tumor of bone (in descending order).
9. Primary bone tumors (osteosarcoma and Ewing sarcoma) are managed with chemotherapy and surgical resection.
10. Soft-tissue sarcomas are managed with radiation and surgery.

References

1. Biermann JS, Seigel GW: *Orthopaedic Knowledge Update: Musculoskeletal Tumors*, ed 4. American Academy of Orthopaedic Surgeons, 2021.
2. Lans J, Yue K, Castelein RM, et al: Soft-tissue sarcoma of the hand. patient characteristics, treatment, and oncologic outcomes. *J Am Acad Orthop Surg* 2020;29(6):e297-e307.
3. Peabody TD, Attar S: *Orthopaedic Oncology: Primary and Metastatic Tumors of the Skeletal System*. Cancer Treatment and Research. Springer International Publishing, 2014.
4. Pollock RE, Randall RL, O'Sullivan B: *Sarcoma Oncology: A Multidisciplinary Approach*. People's Medical Publishing House, 2019.

5. Johnson CN, Ha AS, Chen E: Lipomatous soft-tissue tumors. *J Am Acad Orthop Surg* 2018;26(22):779-788.
6. Miller BJ: Use of imaging prior to referral to a musculoskeletal oncologist. *J Am Acad Orthop Surg* 2019;27(22):e1001-e1008.
7. Voskuil RT, Mayerson JL, Scharschmidt TJ: Management of metastatic disease of the upper extremity. *J Am Acad Orthop Surg* 2021;29(3):e116-e125.

14 Pediatrics

Monica Kogan, MD, FAAOS, FAOA
Brian Scannell, MD, FAAOS
Mara S. Karamitopoulos, MD, FAAOS

Introduction

Slipped capital femoral epiphysis (SCFE) is the most common hip disorder affecting adolescents between the ages of 9 and 16 years. The etiology is multifactorial and may vary with ethnicity, sex, and region. The practitioner should have a high index of suspicion for any patient who presents at ages 9 to 16 years with hip pain, knee pain, or a limp (either painless or painful). The diagnosis is made with plain radiographs or rarely MRI is performed when SCFE is suspected but the plain radiographs are inconclusive. Prompt identification is of utmost importance because SCFE may lead to devastating long-term consequences. Once identified, the treatment is surgical intervention. Developmental dysplasia of the hip includes acetabular dysplasia, hip subluxation dislocation. It previously was referred to as congenital dislocation of the hip; however, it was found to be a dynamic disorder. Routine screening is not indicated unless infants have known risk factors such as oligohydramnios, breech presentation, family history of developmental dysplasia of the hip, or an abnormal examination. Initial treatment is traditionally performed with a Pavlik harness, with excellent results. Infants in whom nonsurgical management failed are treated with surgical intervention and this may include a closed reduction and spica casting versus open hip reduction (medial or anteriorly) versus open hip reduction/femoral

---

Neither of the following authors nor any immediate family member has received anything of value from or has stock or stock options held in a commercial company or institution related directly or indirectly to the subject of this chapter: Dr. Kogan, Dr. Scannell, and Dr. Karamitopoulos.

osteotomy/acetabular osteotomy depending on the stability, severity, and patient's age. These patients need to be followed for years to ensure that the dysplasia resolved and did not return. Clubfoot (talipes equinovarus) is a congenital disorder of the foot. The four aspects of the clubfoot include forefoot cavus, adductus, hindfoot varus, and equinus of the foot. Treatment with the Ponseti casting technique is the most common form of treatment with excellent results. Rarely do children require further intervention because of recurrence. Compliance with the Ponseti treatment protocol by the caregivers has been associated with improved, outcomes. Supracondylar humerus fractures in children are one of the most common elbow fractures in pediatric patients. Treatment depends on the severity of the injury. Nonsurgical management is reserved for nondisplaced fractures and surgical management reserved for fractures with displacement. An accurate physical examination is imperative, including the documentation of neurovascular status. Timing of surgical intervention is dependent on neurologic status (urgent) versus vascular status (emergent). Surgical treatment most commonly includes closed reduction and percutaneous pinning and rarely requires an open reduction and fixation. Intoeing is a common reason for pediatric orthopaedic evaluation. It refers to walking with the toes pointing inward (pigeon toed). For most children, the intoeing will resolve on its own by age 10 years. In a small number of children, intoeing will persist; however, it will not cause issues with function/activities/future problems. Reassurance is the most common recommendation for parents.

SLIPPED CAPITAL FEMORAL EPIPHYSIS

- Slipped capital femoral epiphysis (SCFE) is the most common hip disorder affecting adolescents between the ages of 9 and 16 years.[1]
- It is defined as the displacement of the femoral head relative to the femoral neck and shaft in the physis.
- The proximal femoral neck and shaft move anteriorly and rotate outwardly relative to the femoral head, leaving the femoral head within the acetabulum.[2]

- Etiology is multifactorial:
  - Structural issues
  - Obesity
  - Hormonal causes
  - Seasonal and geographic variations[1]
- Presenting symptoms may include a history of a limp, and hip or knee pain with or without a history of trauma.
- Clinical examination findings may be subtle and a heightened sense of awareness is required in order for the diagnosis to be made in a timely manner; treatment delays can lead to worse outcomes.
- Radiographs are obtained to confirm the diagnosis and if a SCFE is identified, prompt surgical stabilization is required.
- Development of underlying health issues as patients age has been identified in patients treated for SCFE.
- Educating adolescent patients on healthy lifestyle choices may help to prevent these issues from developing in the future.

Epidemiology

- The incidence of SCFE is approximately 10 cases per 100,000 children.[1]
- Incidence varies with ethnicity, sex, and region, ranging from 4.4 to 10.8 cases per 100,000 children.
- Highest incidence of SCFE is in those with a Polynesian background (4.5 times higher than white children,) followed by black children (2 times higher).
- Children of Indonesian-Malay and Indo-Mediterranean backgrounds have lower incidences of SCFE than white children (0.5 and 0.1, respectively).[3]
- Hormonal or systemic diseases, such as hypothyroidism, growth hormone supplementation, and hypogonadal abnormalities have been associated with weakening of the physis and may result in SCFE.[4]
- Boys are affected more often than girls, with a ratio 1.43:1.[3]
- The average age for boys is 12.0 years and for girls is 11.2 years,[5] attesting to the influence that hormones have on the physis.
- A correlation has been identified between obesity and SCFE.
- Cadaver studies have suggested that increased forces may lead to SCFE in obese children.[6]

- Patients with severe obesity at age 11 to 12 years have been found to have a 17.0 times higher risk of SCFE than those who did not have obesity.[7]
- Shearing forces exerted on the hips, especially in boys younger than 12 years and girls younger than 11 years, resulting in slippage of the epiphysis, especially when the perichondral ring is damaged.
- Obesity is present in more than 50% of the children affected at any age.
- Obesity was reported to be more prevalent in children with SCFE who were younger than 10 years and above the 97th percentile body mass index for age.[8]
- Patients more commonly present with a unilateral SCFE.
- Bilateral may occur in 20% to 40% of which those with bilateral involvement tend to occur at younger age.[3] More than 80% of those presenting with a unilateral SCFE in whom a contralateral SCFE subsequently develops will do so within 18 months.[9]
- Seasonal variations both north and south have been found to be associated with SCFE.
- Geographic locations north of 40° latitude had 57.4% of SCFEs occur during the summer months.
- 57.3% of SCFEs presented during the winter months south of 40° latitude. This seasonal variation is thought to be linked to vitamin D production at different times of the year.[5]

Public Health Consideration

- Long-term issues for patients with SCFE have been well documented and should be understood.
- Regardless of the severity of slip, patients who have had a SCFE have been found to have a higher likelihood of underlying systemic disease and long-term health issues 20 years after presentation.[10]
- Obesity has been found to continue into adulthood, with the patient's mean body mass index over the study period increasing from 27 kg/m^2 to 37 kg/m^2.
- When patients with SCFE were in their 30s, 8% to 16% of the patients were found to have diabetes, elevated blood glucose level, chest pain, and hypertension.[10]

- These findings highlight the need for an increased surveillance of adult patients with a history of SCFE.[11]
- It is important for the treating physician to begin stressing the importance of a healthy lifestyle to the patients and parents when they first present with SCFE to prevent medical comorbidities as the patients enter adulthood.
- Other long-term issues have been seen in adult patients who sustained SCFE during their youth.
- A deformity of the proximal femur may develop in patients with SCFE as a result of the epiphysis slipping and has been associated with premature hip osteoarthritis, hip pain, decreased range of motion, impingement, and long-term disability.[12,13]

Pertinent Anatomy/Pathoanatomy

- SCFE occurs through the proximal femoral physis, in the hypertrophic zone.
- Weakening in the physis results in anterior displacement of the femoral neck in relation to the proximal femoral epiphysis, which remains in the acetabulum.[2]
- It is important to remember that it is the metaphysis that displaces relative to the femoral head and that the femoral head remains in the acetabulum.
- Anatomic associations have been identified in patients with SCFE:
  - Abnormalities of the epiphyseal tubercle and physis result in weakening, femoral acetabular retroversion,[12] and obliquity of the physis.[13]
- Histologically, SCFE is characterized by physeal widening of the hypertrophic zone, enlargement of chondrocytes, cellular column disorganization, higher proteoglycan and extracellular matrix concentrations in the physis, and widespread disruption in chondrocyte differentiation and endochondral ossification.[14]
- The retinacular vessels are the main blood supply to the epiphysis.
- These vessels may be predisposed to disruption with displacement of the femoral metaphysis causing kinking or compression on the vessels.
- The cause of osteonecrosis in unstable SCFE is unknown; however, multiple possible mechanisms have been proposed:[15]
  - Frank vascular laceration of the lateral ascending branch of the medial femoral circumflex artery

- Vascular kinking
- Spasm
- Thrombosis due to infolding of the posterior soft-tissue envelope following epiphyseal displacement
- Vascular tamponade due to increased intracapsular pressure beyond the perfusion pressure of the femoral head vascular supply
- The epiphyseal tubercle has gained increasing attention over the years.
  - Located in the posterosuperior quadrant of the epiphysis
  - Believed to give mechanical strength to the physis and is believed to be crucial for physeal stability[6]
  - Epiphyseal tubercle decreases in size and surface area during childhood and adolescence[14]
- Mechanical studies have revealed that childhood obesity may generate forces sufficient to overcome the yield point of the physis.
- Peak age of SCFE is around puberty, and rapid growth of the bone is believed to lower the mechanical yield point for physeal injury.
- Obesity around puberty, rather than earlier in childhood, is the most important time point in the development of the disease.[7]

Pertinent History/Physical Examination Findings

- Presentation of SCFE may be obvious or subtle.
- The clinician should always have a high index of suspicion for a SCFE in any patient who presents with a history of hip/thigh/knee pain, limp, or inability to bear weight,[16] especially in a child age 10 to 15 years.
- A delay in diagnosis may result in a worse outcome for the patient.
- SCFE should always be high on differential diagnosis when a patient presents with the stated symptom.[5]
- Other physical examination findings:
  - Outtoeing gait on the affected side
  - Obligate outward rotation of the hip when flexing the hip (Drehmann sign)
  - Limited inward rotation of hip when the hip is flexed 90°
    - Limited inward rotation of the hip is due to the anterolateral and superior displacement of the metaphysis relative to the epiphysis[11]

- Unilateral SCFE is more common; however, involvement of both hips may occur in 40% of children. The patients who present with both hips involved tend to present at a younger age.
- Bilateral SCFE can be present at the initial visit and more than 80% of those presenting with a unilateral SCFE in whom a contralateral SCFE subsequently develops will do so within 18 months.[9]
  - Parents should be advised to have a heightened awareness of any subtle symptoms in the opposite hip of the child.
- Significant risk factors for contralateral SCFE:[17]
  - Patients younger than 10 years
  - Body mass index 95th percentile or higher
  - Presence of an endocrine abnormality
  - Higher posterior sloping angle of the unaffected hip
  - Lower modified Oxford score

Relevant Imaging

- AP pelvis and frog-lateral radiographs of the hip should be obtained if there is a concern for SCFE.
- Including the unaffected hip for comparison may also serve to identify if any findings of asymptomatic SCFE on the opposite side.
- Radiographic findings suggestive of SCFE include:[18]
  - Subtle widening of the physis
  - Relative decreased height of the epiphysis
  - Loss of intersection of the epiphysis by a lateral cortical line along the femoral neck (Klein line) (**Figure 1**)
  - Double density detected at the metaphysis (Steel sign, which is caused by posterior slip of the epiphysis)
  - Southwick classification is a radiographic method that can be used to assess the magnitude of the slip.[19]
    - Angle measured on an AP or the frog-lateral view of the bilateral hips
    - Line drawn perpendicular to a line connecting two points at the posterior and anterior tips of the epiphysis at the physis, on the lateral radiograph, or inferior and superior edge of the epiphysis on the AP radiograph
    - Third line is drawn down the axis of femur

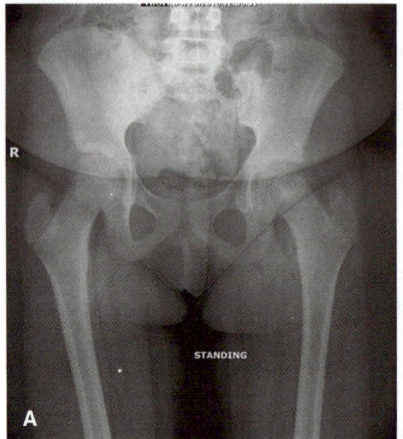
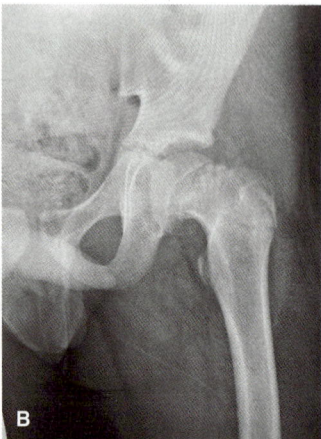

Figure 1 **A** and **B**, Radiographs showing Klein line. On the right side normal alignment is revealed; on the left side the line does not intersect the femoral head.

- Angle between the perpendicular line and the femoral shaft line is Southwick angle; measured bilaterally
- Slipped side then subtracted from the normal side, which is measured in the same manner
- In the case of bilateral involvement, 12° is the normal reference value for the lateral view and 145° on the AP view as a reference for the unaffected hip.
- The number calculated determines the severity.
  - Mild, less than 30°
  - Moderate, 30° to 50°
  - Severe slip, greater than 50°
- Others use a grading system based on percentage of slippage of the epiphysis on the metaphysis, with mild zero to 33%, moderate 34% to 50%, and severe slips being >50% slippage.
- The peritubercle lucency sign on radiographs is considered to be accurate and reliable for the early diagnosis of SCFE.[20]
  - On AP radiographs, the epiphyseal tubercle is usually found in the central one-third of the epiphyseal plate.
  - On lateral radiographs, the tubercle is usually located at the posterior third quadrant of the epiphyseal plate.

- The peritubercle luceny sign includes focal changes around the tubercle including widening or enlargement of the corresponding metaphyseal fossa, with or without adjacent osteolysis or sclerosis.[20]
- Most recently, it was reported that the peritubercle lucency sign on radiographs is accurate and reliable for the early diagnosis of SCFE compared with MRI as the gold standard.[20]
- If there is a clinical suspicion of a SCFE and radiographs are negative, MRI can be performed and has been considered the gold standard.
  - MRI findings consistent with a SCFE can include:
    - Physeal widening
    - Greater signal intensity of the proximal femoral physis compared with the physis of the greater trochanter
    - Bone marrow edema can also be seen[21] (**Figure 2**).
- SCFE can be classified in three ways:
  - Radiographically
  - By the length of symptoms

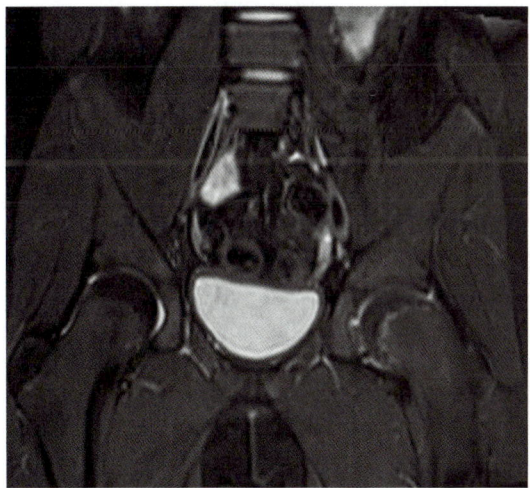

Figure 2 MRI was performed because of vague symptoms on the right side with radiographic findings of slipped capital femoral epiphysis on the left. Edema in the physis on the left along with physeal widening seen compared with the normal right side.

- By the ability or inability to bear weight even with the use of crutches (Loder classification)
- Depending on the length of symptoms, SCFE can be classified as acute, acute-on-chronic, and chronic.
  - An acute SCFE is characterized by the presence of symptoms for less than 3 weeks.
    - Pain that occurs suddenly
  - A chronic SCFE has symptoms for more than 3 weeks.
    - Represents most patients who present with SCFE
  - Acute-on-chronic SCFE is diagnosed when symptoms are present for more than 3 weeks but with an abrupt exacerbation of pain and/or inability to walk.
- Loder classification is often used and is based on the ability/inability to walk either with or without crutches (stable versus unstable). This classification system is important because those with unstable SCFEs have been found to have worse outcomes than those with stable SCFEs.
  - Patients who are unable to walk either with or without crutches are classified as having an unstable SCFE.
  - Patients who are able to walk with or without crutches are classified as having a stable SCFE.

Nonsurgical Measures

- For historical purposes only, SCFEs had been managed by removal of load and traction of the limb followed by immobilization in a plaster cast or observation[22] because it was thought that this would be enough to halt the progression of the SCFE.
- Nonsurgical management of SCFE, however, was found to lead to increased rates of chondrolysis, which was as high as 28% in patients with moderate slips.
- 17% of SCFE cases progressed with additional slippage when they were treated nonsurgically.
- Continued presence of an open epiphyseal plate constituted a risk of progression to slippage after diagnosis.
- Currently, nonsurgical management is not the standard of care and these patients are treated with surgical stabilization.

Chapter 14: Pediatrics

Surgical Intervention

- Surgical intervention is indicated for any SCFE identified in a patient, regardless of the length of symptoms, severity of slip, ability/inability to bear weight, or radiographic findings. The goal of treatment is to prevent further slippage, achieve stable closure of the proximal femoral physis, improve the alignment of the epiphysis on the femoral neck, and to prevent chondrolysis and osteonecrosis.[1]
- Surgical intervention is the standard of care when a patient presents with a SCFE.
- There are different approaches depending on the stability of the slip as well as the surgeon's comfort level and experience with the procedures.
- The most common treatment for SCFE (stable and unstable) remains percutaneous in situ fixation using single-screw or double-screw fixation.
- The goal of all treatment is to prevent further slippage.
- Traditionally, fixation is performed without attempting a formal reduction of the slip, which can leave the epiphysis in a displaced position.
  - Positional or an incidental reduction may occur while the patient is positioned; however, a formal reduction maneuver is never performed.
- Both single-screw and double-screw fixation has been described.
- Excellent results have been reported when using a single screw in cases of mild and moderate slippage, with success rates of 91% to 95%.[11,13]
- Double-screw fixation is another option in the management of both stable and unstable SCFEs; however, it has not shown any biomechanical or clinical advantage to placement of a single screw.[23]
  - For this reason, as well as technical challenges of placing double screws, single-screw placement is more commonly performed.
- An increase in the intracapsular pressure in hips with unstable SCFE has been found to be twice that of the nonaffected hip.
  - Drastic pressure increases have been seen with manipulation and then normalization after capsulotomy.[24]

- A capsulotomy can be performed either through aspiration or through open capsulotomy to decompress the joint before in situ pinning.
- In situ pinning is the more common surgery performed; it does not always reach the goal of prevention of hip arthritis because it does not improve the alignment of the epiphysis.[25]
- Osteonecrosis rates vary between 10% and 40% with this technique[26] depending on the stability of the SCFE.
- The surgical hip dislocation or modified Dunn procedure allows for an anatomic reorientation of the epiphysis.
- Acute, unstable, and chronic, as well as stable, SCFE can be successfully managed with the modified Dunn procedure.
- Complication rate is statistically higher in patients with stable SCFE, specifically both osteonecrosis rate and postoperative instability.
- The modified Dunn procedure allows for an anatomic reorientation of the epiphysis.
  - It is a procedure with a steep learning curve.
  - It should be performed only in a referral center as a statistically significant association between surgeon experience and osteonecrosis has been identified.[27]
- The technique permits the surgeon to manage associated lesions, such as early acetabular labrum and cartilage damage or the metaphyseal bump that limits internal rotation, leading to femoroacetabular impingement, which can occur even in mild slips.
- Early reports were encouraging, with restoration of alignment of the proximal femoral epiphysis and low rates of complications such as osteonecrosis.
- Recent publications have documented higher complication rates resulting in decreased enthusiasm for this procedure.[28]

Technique: In Situ Pinning

- SCFE is pinned in situ, which means pinning without a formal reduction.
- A positional or serendipitous reduction can occur when an unstable slip reduces to some degree by placing the patient on the fracture table with the patella facing anteriorly and the surgical limb in neutral or slight abduction.

- Positional reduction and pinning remain the gold standard, especially in mild to moderate stable and unstable slips because it yields reliable functional and radiographic outcomes at long-term follow-up (**Figure 3**).
- Preferred entry point for the screw should be lateral to the intertrochanteric line on the AP view to ensure the screw heads will be extracapsular to avoid impingement.
- Ideally the screw(s) are placed perpendicular to the physis.
- For the severe slips, to keep the screw within the femoral head a more oblique trajectory may be necessary.
- The goal is for 40% to 60% of the threads to cross the physis into the epiphysis as this provides the greatest load to failure.

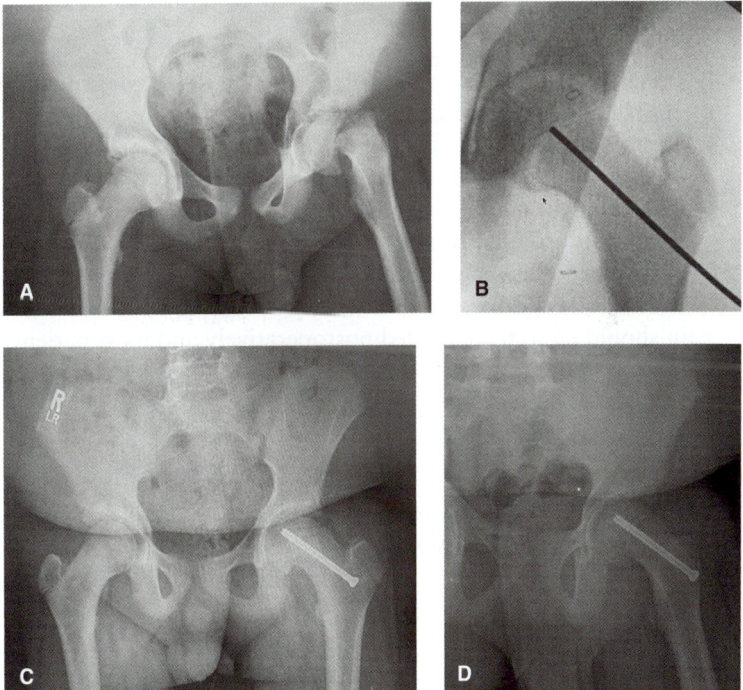

Figure 3 **A**, Radiograph showing left unstable slipped capital femoral epiphysis presenting with acute pain and inability to bear weight. **B**, Intraoperative fluoroscopic view after incidental reduction. **C** and **D**, Postoperative AP and lateral views are shown.

- This can be done with a fully threaded or 32-mm partially threaded cannulated screw.
- Once the screw is secured, the approach withdrawal technique is then used to ensure a safe screw tip–subchondral bone distance, 2.5 to 5 mm from the subchondral bone.
  - The hip is brought from maximum internal rotation to maximum external rotation.
  - As the limb is moved through this arc of motion, the screw appears to move closer to the subchondral bone (approach) and then appears to move further from it (withdrawal).
  - The point at which the screw appears to transition from approach to withdrawal represents the closest position to the joint and can reveal unrecognized screw penetration.[29]

Postoperative Orders

- Postoperatively the patient's weight-bearing status depends on the procedure performed and the stability of the slip.
  - In stable SCFE managed with in situ pinning, the patient should practice partial weight bearing for 4 to 6 weeks and then progress to full weight bearing. Sports and running can resume at 3 to 6 months.
  - In instable SCFE, the patient does not bear weight for 4 to 6 weeks, followed by progressive weight bearing with crutches.
- Pain should be well controlled postoperatively and most patients require acetaminophen and ibuprofen. Stronger narcotics are usually not required.

Pearls and Pitfalls

- The incidence of osteonecrosis is most strongly associated with the stability of the slip at presentation.[30]
- A prompt diagnosis is an important measure to prevent these sequelae.
- It is imperative to have a heightened suspicion for a SCFE in children age 10 to 15 years with a limp, hip pain, or knee pain as increased duration of symptoms before diagnosis is associated with greater slip angles.
- Slip angle may be associated with an impaired Harris hip score and higher radiographic grades of osteoarthritis later in life.[31]

- Placing the screw in the center of the epiphysis is important.
  - Screws placed in the posterior superior quadrant of the femoral neck are associated with a high incidence of osteonecrosis as it can affect the perfusion coming from the lateral epiphyseal vessels.
- The screw should not penetrate the joint because persistent pin penetration into the hip joint has been associated with chondrolysis.[32]
- Care should also be taken to ensure that the entry point is not below the level of the lesser trochanter as this can predispose the patient to a fracture.
- The screw ideally should be placed lateral to the intertrochanteric line to avoid impingement of the screw head with the acetabulum.

Outcomes

- In situ fixation is the most common treatment performed for stable/unstable hips with mild to moderate slips.
- Greater slips can be managed with in situ pinning; however, the risk of impingement from the residual deformity may be higher and may warrant an anatomic realignment to restore hip anatomy (**Figure 4**).
- A formal closed manipulation to achieve anatomic realignment is no longer performed because it does not allow direct control of the retinacular vessels and can result in a higher incidence of osteonecrosis.
- The modified Dunn procedure is safe, efficient, and reproducible, but should be performed by surgeons experienced with the procedure.
- Timing of surgery is thought to be crucial to the development of osteonecrosis. It is also thought that surgery should be performed within 24 hours from the onset of symptoms.[33]
- Bilateral involvement in SCFE ranges from 14% to 63%.
- Risk can increase to up to 80% when diagnosed at a very young age and up to 100% when endocrinopathies are associated.
- Prophylactic surgical treatment remains controversial as reports of osteonecrosis in the contralateral asymptomatic hip have been reported, resulting in devastating outcomes (**Figure 5, A** and **B**).
- Prophylactic treatment of an asymptomatic hip without radiographic findings should be reserved for a selected cohort of

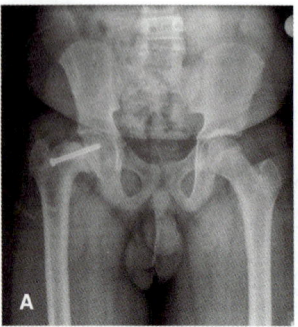 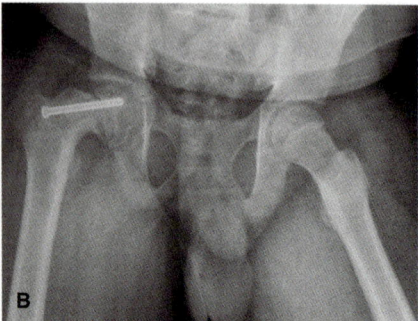

Figure 4 **A**, Radiograph of stable slipped capital femoral epiphysis pinned in situ with residual deformity. **B**, Radiograph showing prominence of lateral metaphysis.

patients, such as very young children, presence of endocrinopathy, patients with obesity, and those whose follow-up is thought to be difficult.
- Osteonecrosis in unstable SCFE was found to be as high as 21%.
- More recent studies show promising results with a lower osteonecrosis rate after urgent reduction, decompression and fixation, or open reduction and fixation.
- Presence of an increased intracapsular hip pressure and the effect of joint decompression have been studied in unstable hips with SCFE with divergent conclusions.[24]
  - The role of increased intracapsular pressure in the development of osteonecrosis in unstable SCFE remains unclear, although a recent prospective series with precapsulotomy and postcapsulotomy vascular flow measurements suggests that capsulotomy with confirmed return of blood flow to the femoral head entirely removes the risk of osteonecrosis.[34]
  - In patients with unstable SCFE, the increase in intracapsular pressure can simulate a compartment syndrome–like phenomenon in the joint capsule, with postcapsulotomy pressures lower than predecompression reading.[24]
  - Other studies have not been able to confirm that capsular decompression lowered the rate of osteonecrosis following unstable SCFE, but recommended the surgeon weigh the minor

Chapter 14: Pediatrics

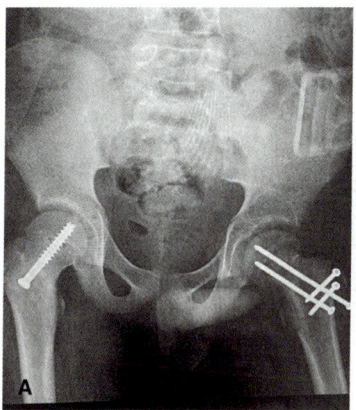
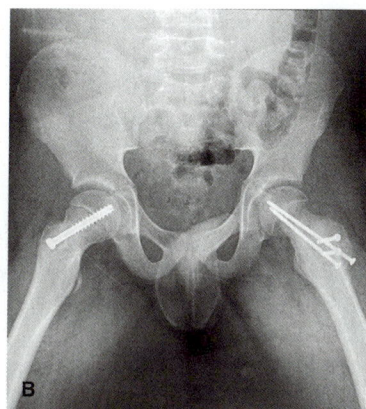
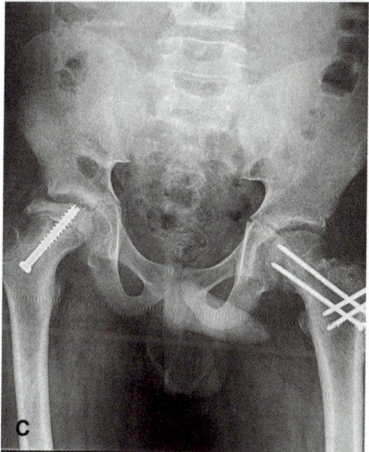

Figure 5 AP and lateral radiographs from a 9-year-old boy who presented with an unstable left slipped capital femoral epiphysis. **A**, Modified Dunn procedure on the left hip and because of the patient's young age a prophylactic pinning was performed on the right hip. **B**, Lateral radiographs of bilateral hips 2 weeks postoperatively. **C**, Six months postoperatively the patient presented with pain in the right hip with osteonecrosis present and screw penetration into the hip joint.

  risks of this added procedure against the lack of conclusive evidence showing a lower osteonecrosis rate.[35]
- Mild SCFE deformity has been shown to contribute to abnormal joint kinematics and the development of degenerative arthritis of the hip.[36]

- In one recent study at 20-year follow-up, 5% of patients with SCFE were found to have undergone total hip arthroplasty, revealing an increased risk of degenerative joint disease compared with the average population.[37]

Top 10 Knowledge Drops for Your Rotation

1. It is important to remember that it is the metaphysis that displaces relative to the femoral head and that the femoral head remains in the acetabulum.
2. Osteonecrosis is more common with unstable SCFE.
3. The most common treatment for stable and unstable SCFE is in situ pinning. Surgical hip dislocation/modified Dunn procedure should be performed in patients with unstable SCFE by surgeons with experience in the procedure.
4. The surgical hip dislocation/modified Dunn procedure has a higher risk of osteonecrosis and postoperative hip instability when performed on stable SCFE.
5. For in situ pinning of a SCFE, one screw is just as effective as two screws.
6. For in situ pinning, full threaded or 32-mm threaded screws are preferred and shoudl cross the physis.
7. SCFE can present with knee pain and it is important to have a heightened sense of awareness when examining the hip in any patient age 10 to 15 years who presents with a limp/knee pain/hip pain.
8. For in situ pinning procedures, a formal reduction is not recommended; however, an incidental reduction is often seen while positioning the patient on the table.
9. More than 80% of those presenting with a unilateral SCFE in whom a contralateral SCFE subsequently develops will do so within 18 months; patients should be counseled that any sort of discomfort in the contralateral hip should be worked up.
10. At patient presentation, an AP and frog-lateral pelvis radiograph should be obtained of both hips to ensure that there is not a SCFE on the contralateral side, because 20% to 40% of children will present with bilateral involvement.

DEVELOPMENTAL DYSPLASIA OF THE HIP

- Developmental dysplasia of the hip (DDH) spans a wide range of disorders including acetabular dysplasia, hip subluxation, and dislocation of the hip.
- Previously DDH was referred to as congenital dislocation of the hip; it is now understood that it is a dynamic disorder and a developmental issue versus a congenital one.
- Early diagnosis is important to help improve results and decrease future issues.
- Nonsurgical management with a Pavlik harness is the most common treatment with very good outcomes.
- Surgical intervention is reserved for hips in which nonsurgical management fails.
- Long-term issues can be seen and include persistent dysplasia, osteonecrosis, and early osteoarthritis.

Epidemiology

- Incidence of DDH is variable and is multifactorial.
- Approximately 1 in 1,000 children is born with a dislocated hip, and 10 in 1,000 may have hip subluxation.[38]
- Prenatal and postnatal factors are found to be associated with DDH.
- Prenatal factors include breech presentation, female sex, positive family history, firstborn status, and oligohydramnios.
- The most important risk factors are intrauterine position, sex, race, and positive family history.
- The left hip is more commonly involved (60% of children) because of the common intrauterine positioning of left occiput anterior, which results in the left hip adducted against the mother's sacrum.
- The right hip is affected in 20% of children, and 20% of children have both hips affected.[39]
- Females are affected more than males because of the increased ligamentous laxity secondary to the circulating maternal hormones and the additional effect of estrogens that are produced by the female infant's uterus.
- A family history positive for DDH may be found in 12% to 33% of affected patients.

- Risk for DDH to develop in a child is 6% if one of their siblings has DDH, 12% if one of their parents has DDH, and 36% if both a parent and a sibling have DDH.[40]
- DDH is common in children who present in the breech position.[39]
  - In utero knee extension of the infant in the breech position results in sustained hamstring forces around the hip and contributes to subsequent hip instability.
- Firstborn children are affected twice as often as subsequent siblings, presumably because of an unstretched uterus and tight abdominal structures in the mother.
- Postnatal positioning also can play a role in DDH.
  - In cultures in which swaddling with the legs extended is practiced (Native American and Asian), there is a higher incidence of DDH.
  - In these positions the legs are extended, which forces the hips into adduction and extension resulting in abnormal forces within the joint.
  - Cultures where the infants/children are carried astride the hips (African/Eskimo) have a very low incidence of DDH.[41]
- One in 60 newborns has hip instability, and more than 60% of them stabilize in the first week without any treatment, and a total of 88% stabilize within the first 2 months. The remaining 12% have DDH that will persist.[42]
- Timely and successful reduction of the hip(s) yields acceptable outcomes into adulthood.
- A delay in treatment can result in persistence of hip dysplasia into adolescence and adulthood, which may result in abnormal gait, decreased strength, limb-length discrepancy with a flexion/adduction deformity of the hip, increased rate of degenerative hip joint disease, postural scoliosis, back pain, and ipsilateral genu valgum with consequent arthritis of the knee.[43]

Pertinent Anatomy/Pathoanatomy

- Bony and soft-tissue anatomy may block the reduction of the hip.
  - Blocks to a concentric reduction include inverted labrum, presence of a limbus, hypertrophied ligamentum teres, pulvinar, contracted capsule, contracted transverse acetabular ligament (TAL), and contracted iliopsoas.

- The femoral head stimulates the acetabulum to develop and vice versa.
  - The longer the femoral head is not anatomically positioned, the more severe is the dysplasia.
- Anatomic findings on the femoral side include femoral anteversion and a smaller femoral ossific nucleus (**Figure 6**).
- Soft-tissue adaptations develop at the labrum, limbus, ligamentum teres, pulvinar, TAL, iliopsoas tendon, and hip-joint capsule.
- The acetabular labrum, a fibrocartilaginous structure located at the acetabular rim, enhances the depth of the acetabulum by 20% to 50% and contributes to the growth of the acetabular rim.
- As the femoral head migrates proximally, the labrum gradually everts and hypertrophies because of the abnormal pressure.
- The limbus (fibrous tissue) develops secondary to mechanical stimulation of the dislocated hip and merges with the hyaline cartilage of the acetabulum at its rim.
- The limbus may then prevent concentric reduction of the hip.
- With dislocation of the hip(s), the ligamentum teres lengthens, hypertrophies, and may block concentric reduction of the femoral head in the acetabulum.
- Pulvinar, a fibrofatty tissue, within the acetabulum, may prevent acceptable reduction of the femoral head within the acetabulum.
- The ligamentum teres inserts on the TAL, located at the base of the acetabulum.

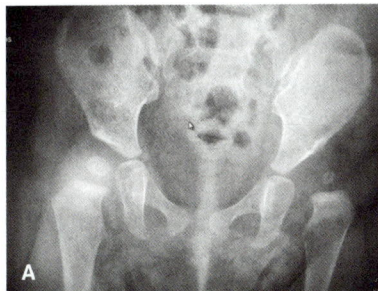 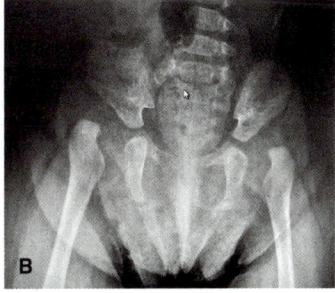

Figure 6 **A**, Radiograph shows small femoral head with a dysplastic acetabulum. **B**, Radiograph shows bilateral dislocation and lack of development of the femoral head.

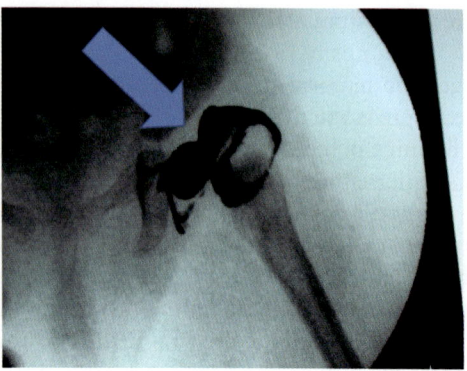

Figure 7 Arthrogram shows hourglass constriction caused by the iliopsoas tendon overlying the hip capsule (arrow).

- As the hip displaces, the femoral head migrates proximally, the ligamentum teres pulls on the TAL, causing it to contract, and results in a narrowing of the acetabulum. Incising the TAL is essential for complete reduction of the hip because it is a major block to concentric reduction.
- As the hip displaces, the iliopsoas contracts and can prevent the reduction of the hip.
- The hourglass constriction often seen on an arthrogram is caused by the tight iliopsoas overlying and compressing the capsule (**Figure 7**).
- Understanding the anatomy in a patient with DDH is crucial to ensure that the obstacles to a concentric reduction have been addressed, allowing the femoral head to seat well within the acetabulum.

Pertinent History/Physical Examination Findings

- DDH is a dynamic process and encompasses a range of findings.
- It is important to understand the terminology used when describing these patients.
- A dislocated hip is one where there is no articular contact between the femoral head and the acetabulum, which may be irreducible or reducible.

Chapter 14: Pediatrics

- A subluxated hip is present when the femoral head is partially displaced from its normal position, but some degree of contact with the acetabulum still remains.
- The hip is called dislocatable when application of a posteriorly directed force on the hip positioned in adduction leads to complete displacement of the femoral head from the margins of the acetabulum. Similarly, the hip is called subluxatable, if the femoral head is able to glide but not completely lose contact with the acetabulum.
- Acetabular dysplasia describes the abnormality in the development of the acetabulum, including an alteration in size, shape, and organization.[44]
- The physical examination begins with a complete assessment of the child from head to toes.
- DDH may be considered a packaging disorder, and associated conditions such as torticollis, metatarsus adductus, and clubfoot should be ruled out.
- Hip examination begins with the inspection for asymmetrical gluteal or thigh skin folds.
- Unequal skin folds do not confirm a dislocated hip; patients with a dislocated hip will often have asymmetrical skin folds but not all children with asymmetric thigh folds will have a dislocated hip (**Figure 8**).
- Assessment of a limb-length inequality is performed by placing the child in a supine position with the hips and knees flexed. Unequal knee heights might be noticed (Galeazzi sign), revealing

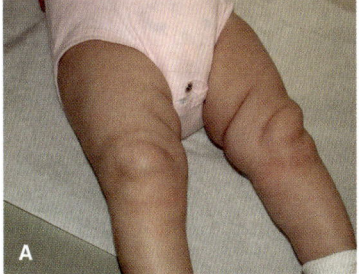
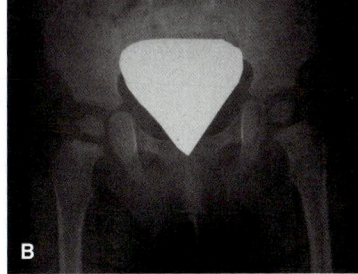

Figure 8 **A**, Photograph shows asymmetrical femoral skin folds. **B**, Radiograph showing normal presentation of the hips of a patient with asymmetrical skin folds.

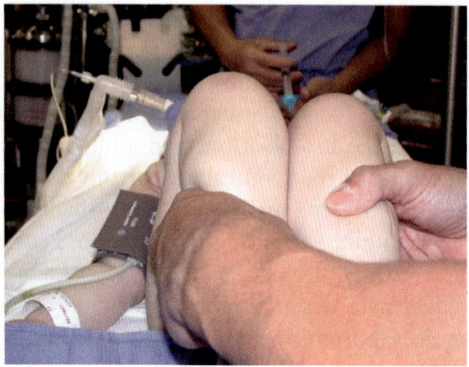

Figure 9 Photograph shows Galeazzi sign revealing an apparent limb-length inequality in the patient's left leg, which has a dislocated hip.

an apparent limb-length inequality with a subluxated or dislocated hip (**Figure 9**).
- Understanding the normal range of hip abduction is important; as with bilateral hip dislocations the hip examination may not show asymmetry but abnormality may still be present.
- Hip range of motion should be assessed for any asymmetry or restricted hip abduction.
- In an infant, maximal abduction of the hips should be greater than 60°; if it is less, a dislocated hip should be suspected.
- The next steps in the physical examination are provocative dynamic tests that assess stability, such as the Ortolani and Barlow maneuvers.[45]
- Each hip must be examined separately.
- The Ortolani maneuver reduces a dislocated hip into the acetabulum.
- The child should be supine with the hips flexed to 90°. The examiner should place their index and long fingers laterally over the child's greater trochanter with the thumb medially along the inner thigh near the groin crease.
- The pelvis is stabilized by holding the contralateral hip still while performing the examination.
- The examiner gently abducts the hip being tested while simultaneously exerting an upward force through the greater trochanter laterally.

Chapter 14: Pediatrics

- The sensation of a palpable clunk is a positive Ortolani test and represents the reduction of a dislocated hip into the bony acetabulum.
- The Barlow test subluxates or dislocates the hip posteriorly from a reduced position.
- To perform the Barlow test, the pelvis is held stable and the patient is positioned in a manner similar to the Ortolani test.
- The examiner adducts the hip and exerts a gentle downward force (toward the examining table) in an attempt to subluxate or dislocate an unstable hip posteriorly.
- These tests generally are only useful in infants 3 months or younger because after this time period soft-tissue contractures may limit the motion of the hip.
- In children older than 3 months, asymmetry or limitation of abduction becomes the most reliable sign associated with DDH and if noted a further workup is warranted.
- It should be noted that in an ambulating child, a limp may also be seen on the physical examination as the limb is apparently short.
- Children with bilateral hip dislocations may be difficult to identify and the clinician should have a heightened sense of awareness of the clinical findings in this scenario.
- These children may have a Trendelenburg sign, waddling gait, hyperlumbar lordosis, and symmetrical but decreased hip abduction[46] (**Figure 10**).
- DDH is not a cause for walking delay in children; a recent controlled study suggested that even though the median time to the age of independent walking was 1 month less in healthy control patients compared with that of children with late presentation of DDH, it was clinically insignificant because they all walked within the expected time.[47]
- DDH is an evolving process; a normal physical examination finding as an infant does not preclude a subsequent diagnosis of DDH.[46] Any changes in a physical examination (eg, range of motion of hip/gait abnormalities/limp) should warrant a further workup.

Relevant Imaging

- Ultrasonography is the study of choice to evaluate children younger than 6 months becuse it can identify dysplasia of the cartilaginous portion of the acetabulum, confirm subluxation of

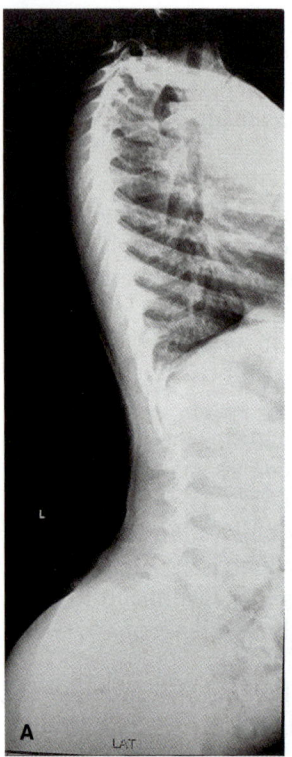
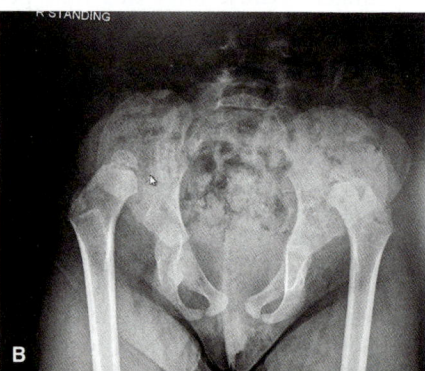

Figure 10 **A**, Lateral radiographs from a patient with bilateral hip dislocations who presented with hyperlordosis. **B**, AP pelvis radiograph demonstrates bilateral hip dislocations found in a patient who presented for evaluation of hyperlordosis.

the hip, and document reducibility and stability of the hip in the infant being treated for DDH (**Figure 11**).
- A normally positioned femoral head is covered by the acetabulum by at least 50%.
- The angle that is formed between the bony line and the base line is known as the alpha angle.
- The angle that is formed between the cartilage roof line and the base line is called the beta angle.
- An alpha angle of 60° or greater in infants older than 3 months or between 50° and 59° in infants younger than 3 months is considered normal.

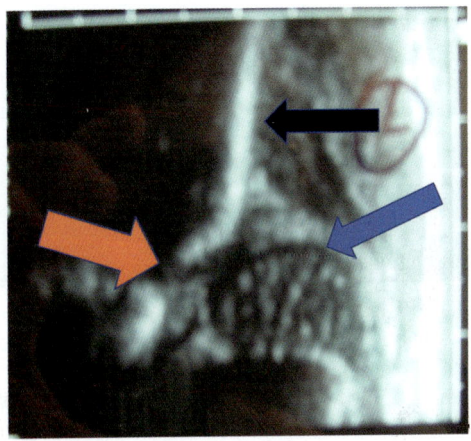

Figure 11 Ultrasonographic image of a displaced femoral head. Black arrow shows the lateral edge of the ilium. Blue arrow shows the femoral head. Orange arrow points to the acetabulum.

- The beta angle quantifies the depth of cartilaginous acetabular roof and is formed between the cartilaginous acetabulum and the cortical margin of the ilium.
- A beta angle of 55° or less is considered normal. Although the beta angle better represents femoral head coverage, the high variability in the interreader measurements makes the beta angle less reliable and thus less clinically practical.[48]
- Ultrasonography is overly sensitive as a universal screening tool in the first 6 weeks of life, and in general should not be ordered unless there are risk factors or a clinical examination that is concerning for DDH.[49]
- Infants with risk factors for DDH should have an ultrasonography performed.
- 60% to 80% of the hips of newborns identified as abnormal or as suspicious for DDH by physical examination and more than 90% of those identified by ultrasonography in the newborn period resolve spontaneously, requiring no intervention.
- Femoral heads ossify at 4 to 6 months of age and plain radiographs are not ordered until that time.
- Once the AP radiograph is ordered, several reference lines and angles are used to evaluate the radiograph.

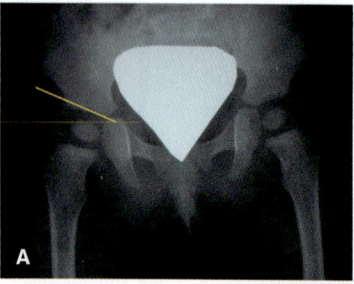 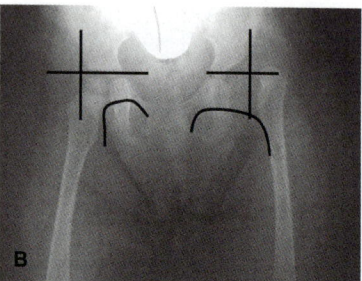

Figure 12 **A**, Radiograph depicts lines representing the acetabular index. **B**, Radiograph showing horizontal line through the triradiate cartilage representing Hilgenreiner line. Perpendicular line to the lateral edge of the acetabulum represents Perkins line. The femoral head should be in the inferior medial quadrant. Shenton line from the obturator foramen should hit the femoral neck. On the left side, the line hits the femoral shaft indicating a dislocated femoral head.

- If subluxation or dislocation is present, then a frog-lateral view is used to determine reducibility of the femoral head.
- The acetabular index is formed by the junction of Hilgenreiner line and a line drawn along the acetabulum.
- Newborns with no hip abnormality can have an acetabular index average of 27.5°.
- By age 2 years, it normalizes at around 20°, with 30° being the upper limit of normal[50] (**Figure 12**).
- Hilgenreiner line is drawn horizontally through the triradiate cartilages of the pelvis.
- Perkins line is drawn perpendicular to the lateral edge of each acetabulum.
- The femoral head should lie within the inferomedial quadrant formed by Hilgrenreiner and Perkins lines. Shenton line is curvilinear and runs from the superior border of the obturator foramen to the femoral neck.
- If there is displacement of the femoral head from the bony acetabulum, the Shenton line will align with the femoral shaft and not the femoral neck.
- MRI can be used for preoperative planning or to check reduction after surgery; however, other imaging typically is not needed for the initial diagnosis and management of DDH.

- Four radiographic findings can be followed as the child grows to ensure that a reduction was successful: improvement in the acetabular index, a sharp (not rounded) lateral border of the acetabulum, a narrow teardrop, and an intact Shenton line.
- The development of the teardrop after reduction of the dislocated hip may be the earliest radiographic sign that a stable, concentric reduction of the hip had been accomplished.
- For the teardrop to develop, the femoral head needs to be positioned within the acetabulum.
- An abnormal teardrop appearance on radiographs can include the absence of the acetabular line, persistent widening, or a V-shaped teardrop.
- The presence of the teardrop at 6 months after reduction predicted a satisfactory outcome in 93% of hips.[51]

Nonsurgical Measures

- Appropriate Use Criteria were developed to help guide the practitioner in their decision-making process for treating patients referred to them for DDH[52] because of the variability in treatment protocols for DDH.
- The goal of treatment of DDH is to achieve and maintain reduction of the femoral head in the true acetabulum by nonsurgical or surgical methods.
- The earlier the treatment is initiated, the greater the success and the lower the incidence of residual dysplasia and long-term complications.
- Subluxation of the hip at birth often corrects spontaneously and may be observed for 2 weeks without treatment.
- Wearing double or triple diapers did not demonstrate improved results when compared with no intervention at all.
- In newborns and infants up to 6 months of age, the first step in treatment is the Pavlik harness.
- The Pavlik harness is a dynamic brace that hold the hips in a flexed and abducted position while allowing motion at the knees and ankles (**Figure 13**).
- Reduction of the hip should be confirmed by ultrasonography within 3 weeks of harness placement.
- Treatment usually is continued for at least 6 weeks full-time and 6 weeks part-time in young infants and possibly longer in older children.

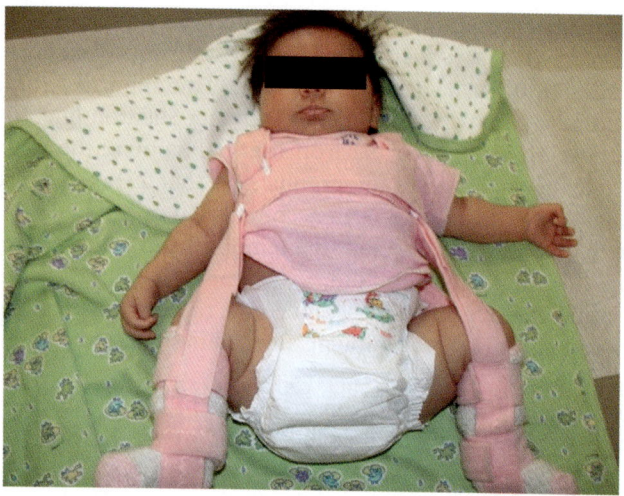

Figure 13 Clinical photograph showing the Pavlik harness.

- The endpoint of brace treatment is a stable hip with normal imaging studies.
- It is imperative for caregivers to be educated on how to appropriately place the harness as extreme positions such as hyperabduction and hyperflexion have been associated with osteonecrosis and femoral nerve palsy, respectively.[53,54]
- If a dislocated hip is not reduced within 3 weeks, the harness should be discontinued, and an alternative treatment selected.
- If persistent instability or dysplasia is present after Pavlik harness treatment or the ultrasonography at 4 weeks still shows the hip to be dislocated, a hip abduction brace can be trialed; however, if not reduced in a month, then the brace should be discontinued.[55]
- Despite the widespread acceptance of the use of the Pavlik harness as the initial management for DDH, variation exists in the literature as to the specific treatment protocols, frequency of clinic visits, and the daily wear duration in the first month of treatment.
- Risks and complications of osteonecrosis are seen only in hips that have been managed with either nonsurgical (bracing) or surgical methods and avoiding this complication is imperative to a good outcome for the child.

Surgical Intervention

- Surgical treatment is indicated if nonsurgical treatment fails.
- The two main goals of surgical treatment are (1) obtaining a stable concentric reduction and (2) limiting the risk of osteonecrosis or the need for secondary procedures.
- Surgical treatment is divided into closed and open procedures.
- In children younger than 12 months, an attempt at closed reduction and spica casting is typically performed first, with or without an intraoperative adductor tenotomy.
- If this fails, then an open reduction of the hip with or without bony procedures is needed.
- As children grow older, the ability of the hip to remodel in response to soft-tissue procedures diminishes, and more aggressive treatments are indicated.
- In children age 12 months to 3 years, residual bony deformity can be corrected with either a femoral or pelvic osteotomy in addition to open reduction.
- Increasing surgical complexity is typically required with increasing age at presentation of patients with DDH.

Closed Reduction

- If nonsurgical management fails, the next steps are usually (1) closed reduction (with or without adductor tenotomy), (2) arthrogram, and (3) spica casting, which is performed in the operating room under general anesthesia.
- The closed reduction maneuver consists of flexion, abduction, and gentle traction.
- Slight anterior pressure may be directed to the greater trochanter to assist in reduction.
- Reduction is confirmed with an arthrogram.
- If the femoral head is well seated in the acetabulum, there will be less than 5 to 6 mm of dye pool noted[56] (**Figure 14**).
- An hourglass constriction can often be seen because of the iliopsoas overlying the capsule (**Figure 15**).
- After reduction is confirmed, the surgeon must select the most stable position of immobilization for spica casting.
- The position most commonly used consists of approximately 90° to 100° of flexion, and approximately 55° of abduction (**Figure 16**).

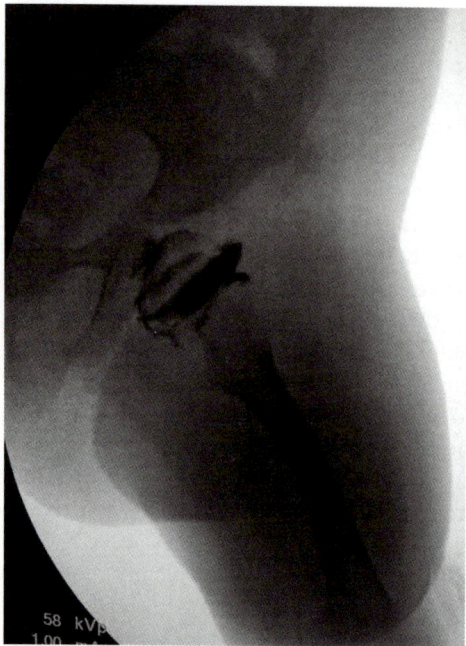

Figure 14 Arthrogram with less than 5 to 6 mm of dye pool confirming a well-seated femoral head within the acetabulum.

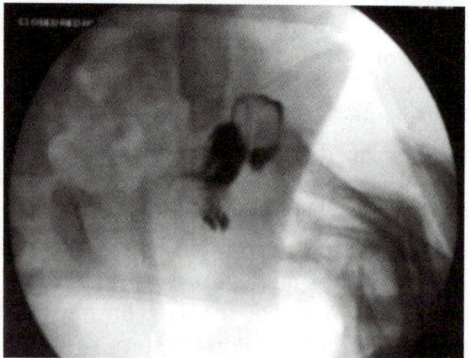

Figure 15 Intraoperative fluoroscopic arthrogram of the left hip demonstrating the hourglass constriction.

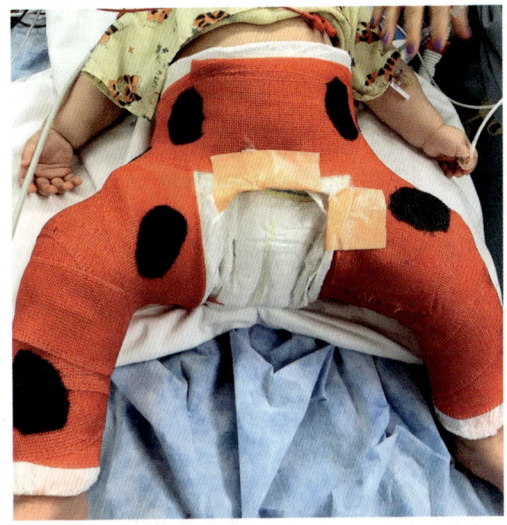

Figure 16 Clinical photograph shows spica cast in the human position, avoiding excessive hip abduction and flexion.

- The safe zone is a descriptor used to evaluate the stability of the hip when it is reduced.
- It is evaluated by ranging the hip from a reduced position in abduction and adducting the leg until the hip dislocates.
- From the reduced abducted position, if the hip dislocates by adducting the leg slightly, it is considered a narrow safe zone, which indicates that the hip reduction is unstable.
- A wide safe zone is desired.
- The degree of abduction that is required to hold the hip stable should also be noted. Excessive abduction should be avoided to decrease the risk of osteonecrosis as mobilization of the hips in greater than 55° of abduction has been associated with an increased risk of osteonecrosis, especially in patients younger than 6 months.[57,58]
- An adductor tenotomy helps release soft-tissue contracture and increases the safe zone of abduction and is often performed as well.
- After a stable position of reduction has been obtained, the child's hips are immobilized in a spica cast.

- Plain radiographs can be obtained in the operating room to confirm reduction after the cast is applied.
- Postoperatively, advanced imaging studies are often performed to further confirm the reduction.
- MRI is the preferred modality to assess the reduction as the hip can be visualized with the least amount of radiation when compared with a CT scan.
- Immobilization in a spica cast continues for 3 months, with a cast change at 6 weeks to assess hip reduction and stability (and for hygienic purposes).

Open Reduction

- When closed reduction has failed, the obstacles to obtaining and maintaining a reduction are addressed with an open reduction.
- The blocks to reduction include (1) hypertrophied ligamentum teres, (2) pulvinar, (3) inverted labrum, (4) TAL, and (5) contracted hip capsule, psoas tendon, or adductor tendons.
- The open approach can be performed through an anterior or medial approach and may depend on the age of the patient and the surgeon's preference and comfort level.
- All of the obstacles can be addressed with both medial and anterior approaches; however, a capsulorrhaphy, which is often required in patients older than 12 months, cannot be performed with a medial approach.
- The anterior open hip reduction is performed through a bikini-type incision using the Smith-Petersen approach.
- The oblique muscles are elevated; the iliac apophysis is split or elevated off the iliac crest.
- Once the rectus femoris tendon is detached from the anterior inferior iliac spine, the hip capsule is visualized, a T-capsulotomy is performed, and the obstacles to reduction are addressed.
- The capsulorrhaphy is performed to stabilize the hip.
- Immobilization in a spica cast is for a total of 3 months, with a cast change at 6 weeks to assess stability and for hygienic purposes, similar to immobilization after closed reduction.
- Benefits of anterior open reduction include anatomy that is familiar to the surgeon and the ability to perform acetabular bony procedures, if indicated.

- The downside of the anterior approach is weakness that can occur in the abductors, which although resolves over time, is important to warn the caregivers that a temporary limp may be noticed.
- The medial approach is performed through a longitudinal incision in the groin.
- The adductor longus tendon is released and the capsule is visualized.
- The medial femoral circumflex vessels are identified overlying the capsule and should be preserved.
- The capsule is incised, and impediments to reduction are assessed. A capsulorrhaphy cannot be performed with a medial approach and for this reason is reserved for patients younger than walking age.
- Benefits of the medial open reduction include a cosmetic scar, abductors of the hip are unaffected, obstacles to reduction can be easily accessed, and bilateral procedures can be undertaken in one setting.

Osteotomies
- Pelvic and femoral osteotomies are used in patients with DDH who demonstrate dysplasia or dislocation and are typically performed in children older than 12 months.

Femoral Osteotomies
- Femoral osteotomies are usually performed in patients older than 12 months, because associated soft-tissue contractures are often present and result in excessive traction or force required to seat the femoral head within the acetabulum.
- The femoral osteotomy shortens the femur, which decreases excessive contact pressure after reduction, reducing the risk of osteonecrosis.
- Varus correction of valgus is not commonly performed in the treatment of patients with idiopathic pediatric DDH and is reserved for patients with neuromuscular disorders.
- The proximal femur is approached laterally.
- The osteotomy is performed, and the femoral head is placed in the acetabulum.

- The amount of shortening is determined by the amount of overlap between the femoral shaft and resected to avoid excessive contact pressure on the reduced femoral head in the acetabulum.
- The bone ends are held in place with a plate and screws.

Pelvic Osteotomies
- Pelvic osteotomies are used in the surgical management of pediatric hip dysplasia to directly improve femoral head coverage by the acetabulum.
- The choice of pelvic osteotomy largely depends on the surgeon's preference.
- Three types of pelvic osteotomies are used in the management of pediatric DDH: redirectional orientation osteotomies (eg, Salter, triple), volume-reducing osteotomies (eg, Dega, Pemberton), and salvage osteotomies (eg, shelf, Chiari).
- For the redirectional and volume-reducing pelvic osteotomies, the hip must be well reduced before the pelvic osteotomy is performed.
- The Salter innominate osteotomy starts in the sciatic notch, ends at the anterior inferior iliac spine, and is traditionally performed with a Gigli saw.
- The distal fragment is orientated to allow for improvement of anterior and lateral coverage of the femoral head, and hinges through the symphysis pubis.
- The Salter osteotomy typically performed in younger patients as the symphysis pubis begins to become less mobile as a child ages.
- The Salter osteotomy requires internal fixation for stabilization.
- The Pemberton pericapsular osteotomy (or acetabuloplasty) uses the triradiate cartilage as a hinge and is used to improve anterior coverage.
- The Pemberton osteotomy consists of an incomplete cut through the acetabulum, and no internal fixation is required.
- Children whose triradiate cartilage is closed require other acetabular osteotomies.
- The Dega osteotomy is a pericapsular osteotomy; however, it primarily improves anterior and lateral coverage by hinging on the medial cortex of the ilium.
- It is described as a semicircular cut through the lateral wall of the ilium directed toward but not through the medial cortex of the ilium.

- Treatment can be especially difficult in patients who have bilateral DDH at walking age and require bilateral open reduction.
- With bilateral DDH, patients older than 9 to 10 years should be treated nonsurgically because a good result may be able to be achieved on one side with redislocation on the other resulting in a limb-length inequality.
- A unilateral dislocation in an older child, however, should be managed surgically, usually requiring an anterior open hip reduction, femoral shortening, and pelvic osteotomy.
- After an open or closed hip reduction, a dreaded complication is the redislocation of the hip(s).
- Reasons for the hip redislocating can include an insufficient release of the anteromedial capsule, an insufficiently released TAL, or a residual limb of the ligamentum teres.
- Osteonecrosis is not part of the natural history of DDH as osteonecrosis can develop only in hips that have undergone treatment (by any modality).
- Osteonecrosis is one of the most feared complications in children with DDH and can have lifelong repercussions.
- Some think that reducing a hip before the ossific nucleus ossifying is a risk factor; however, studies have not show any conclusive evidence to support this.[59]

Outcomes

- Comparing the anterior open reduction with the medial open reduction, no association has been found between the surgical approach and rates of osteonecrosis or the need for secondary surgery.
- Regardless of the surgical approach used, failure of closed reduction was associated with a sixfold increase in the risk of requiring secondary surgery.[60]
- Including a pelvic osteotomy as part of the surgical procedure has been found to more effectively improve the acetabular index than in patients who underwent an open hip reduction and femoral osteotomy.[61]
- It may be difficult to identify if osteonecrosis has developed as well as to predict if it will improve or worsen.
- Radiographic findings consistent with osteonecrosis include failure of the femoral head to ossify (or failure of an ossific nucleus

to grow) within 1 year after reduction, broadening of the femoral neck, an increase in density of the femoral head followed by fragmentation, and residual deformity after ossification is complete.
- Confirming the diagnosis may take 1 to 2 years posttreatment.[62]
- Treatment can be especially difficult in patients who have bilateral DDH at walking age and require bilateral open reduction.
- Patient age and severity of dislocation were found to be risk factors for osteonecrosis.
- In patients with bilateral DDH, the poor outcomes are not the result of the bilaterality itself but of the severity of the disease and the age at which surgical intervention is undertaken.[63]

Top 10 Knowledge Drops for Your Rotation

1. A Pavlik harness is the initial treatment of choice for DDH.
2. DDH is a spectrum of disorders ranging from dysplasia to subluxation to dislocation and can be present at birth or develop as a child grows.
3. Universal ultrasonography screening is not recommended unless the patient has risk factors for DDH.
4. Only patients who have undergone treatment for DDH (nonsurgical and/or surgical) are at risk for osteonecrosis.
5. Bilateral hip dislocations in children younger than 9 years should be treated with surgical intervention; those older than 9 years should be treated nonsurgically.
6. The presence of the teardrop at 6 months after reduction predicts a satisfactory outcome.
7. The medial open hip reduction approach allows for all of the obstacles to reduction to be addressed; however, a capsulorrhaphy cannot be performed.
8. Children older than 12 months typically require an anterior open hip reduction with/without femoral osteotomy, with/without acetabular osteotomy.
9. Anterior open hip reduction weakens the abductors for a period of time.
10. 1 to 2 years after treatment may be required before an appropriate diagnosis of osteonecrosis can be confirmed.

CLUBFOOT (CONGENITAL TALIPES EQUINOVARUS)

- Clubfoot is a common congenital condition of the foot.
- Clubfoot refers to a combination of pathologies: cavus, adductus, varus, and equinus foot position. The mnemonic CAVE is typically used to remember the four aspects of the deformity.
- It is most commonly corrected by a series of casts popularized by Dr. Ignacio Ponseti and is referred to as Ponseti casting.

Epidemiology

- Occurs in 1 to 2 per 1,000 live births[64]
- Family history has a strong association (680% increased odds).[65]
- Mothers who take selective serotonin reuptake inhibitors, have maternal obesity, and are smoking have also been shown to confer increased risk.[65]
- Bilateral in 50% of patients[66]
- Males affected more than females (2:1 ratio)[67]
- Many genes have shown involvement in the development of clubfoot, including *HOX*, *PITX1*, and *TBX4* (genes involved in limb development).[67]

Pertinent Anatomy/Pathoanatomy

- Clubfoot can often be seen on prenatal ultrasonography and is visible at birth.
- Characterized by four components: cavus, forefoot adductus, hindfoot varus, equinus (CAVE)
- The deformity can vary from very mild and flexible to severe and rigid (**Figure 17**).
- Both bony and soft-tissue structures are affected.[68]
- The calcaneus is medially rotated and in varus.[68]
- The navicular is medially displaced.
- The talar head is prominent.
- The posterior and medial ligaments are thick and shortened.[5]
- Clubfoot can involve the whole lower extremity. Commonly, decreased calf musculature will be seen (although this is sometimes difficult to assess until baby is a bit older).

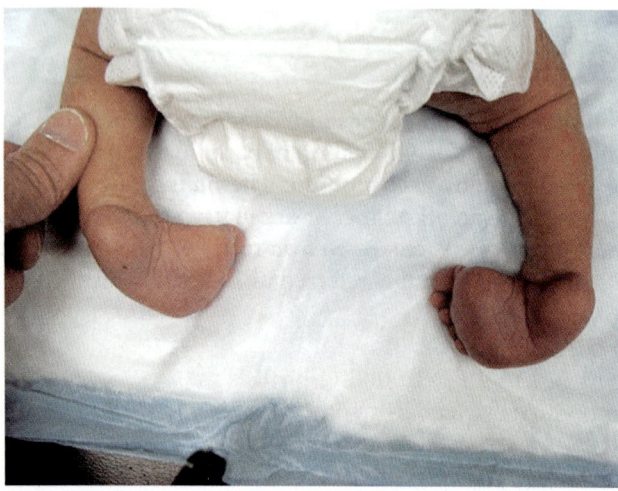

Figure 17 Clinical photograph showing idiopathic clubfoot in an infant demonstrates the characteristic deformities of cavus, metatarsus adductus, hindfoot varus, and equinus. (Reproduced from Nemeth BA, Noonan KJ: Treatment of clubfoot using the Ponseti method, in Colvin AC, Flatow E, eds: *Atlas of Essential Orthopaedic Procedures,* ed 2. American Academy of Orthopaedic Surgeons, 2019, p 950.)

Pertinent History/Physical Examination Findings

- Clubfoot can be unilateral or bilateral.
- Clubfoot can be isolated (most commonly) or associated with other syndromes.
- A thorough history and physical examination are essential to ensure that the clubfoot deformity is isolated and not associated with other clinical syndromes.
- Common syndromes associated with clubfeet include myelomeningocele (spina bifida) and arthrogryposis. Spine examination should be performed to look for sacral dimpling or hairy patches. Neurologic examination as well as an assessment of the entire lower extremity is needed.
- Range of motion of upper and lower extremity should be noted (stiffness can be associated with arthrogryposis).
- As mentioned previously, CAVE deformities are seen. Feet will often have a prominent medial crease and posterior crease. The

heel pad can often be empty (because of position of calcaneus), and the talar head is typically prominent.
- Leg length discrepancy can be seen in children who have a unilateral clubfoot,[69] and leg lengths should be assessed at each visit in older children.
- Some studies have linked clubfoot with an increased incidence of hip dysplasia. Careful physical examination of the hips is critical. Some orthopaedic surgeons will perform a screening ultrasonography of the hips in all babies with clubfoot (although this is controversial).[70,71]

Relevant Imaging

- Radiographs are often not obtained in infants with clubfoot because they can be difficult to interpret.
- However, radiographs are useful in preoperative planning or in examining infants and children who are not progressing well with casting.
- Reduced dorsiflexion seen on forced dorsiflexion lateral foot radiograph is associated with increased recurrence risk.[72]
- Some pediatric orthopaedic surgeons will perform hip ultrasonography on babies with clubfoot.
- Weight-bearing foot radiographs are essential for preoperative planning.

Nonsurgical Measures

- Ponseti casting technique is most commonly used for treatment.
- Ponseti casting consists of a series of long leg manipulative casts that align the foot. Casts are typically changed every week.
- Deformities are corrected in a specific order. The cavus is first corrected with forefoot supination and upward pressure under the first metatarsal. The remaining deformities are corrected over the remaining casts by applying pressure over the head of the talus while abducting the supinated foot. All manipulation should be gentle and guided by the flexibility of the foot.
- The goal for abduction after the fourth cast is 50°.[73]
- The final cast is used to correct the residual equinus. Percutaneous Achilles tenotomy is often performed at the time the last cast is fitted. Tenotomy is required in more than 90% of cases,[73] and many practitioners perform this procedure in the office. The

posttenotomy cast is kept in place for 3 weeks with the foot in 5° to 10° of dorsiflexion and 70° of abduction.[73]
- Ponseti casting is 90% effective.[68]
- The goal of treatment is to provide a plantigrade, pain-free foot.[74]
- Once casting has been completed, long-term abduction bracing over several years is recommended for optimal results.[75]
- Braces are worn full-time for 3 months and then at night until age 4 years.[75]
- Ponseti casting method has been used with success even in older children.[76,77]
- Feet should be scored at every visit to document initial severity and progress with casting.
- Two common scoring systems include the Diméglio et al[78] and Pirani et al scoring systems.[79] Both scoring systems account for the major clinical features of the deformity, including posterior and medial creases, amount of adductus, and amount of equinus. The Pirani scoring system may be most pragmatic at the medical student and resident level because of its ease of use (**Table 1**).
- Nonidiopathic (syndromic) clubfeet can also be managed with Ponseti casting, but parents should be cautioned that more casts may be required and the need for future surgical procedures is higher.[80]

TABLE 1 Pirani Scoring System

Pirani Score	
1	Posterior crease
2	Empty heel pad
3	Rigid equinus
4	Medial crease
5	Curvature of lateral border
6	Position of talar head

Minimum total score is 0 and the maximum total score is 6. A high Pirani score indicates a severe deformity.
Reproduced with permission from Pirani S, Outerbridge H, Sawatzky B, Stothers K, eds: *A Reliable Method of Clinically Evaluating a Virgin Clubfoot Evaluation.* 21st SICOT Congress, 1999.

Surgical Intervention

- Before the popularity of Ponseti casting, surgical intervention via a large posteromedial release used to be the mainstay of treatment. Long-term outcomes of these surgical patients have shown stiffness, subtalar arthritis, and decreases in strength.[81,82]
- More recently, surgical procedures have been reserved for relapses that cannot be corrected with repeat casting or for feet that cannot be fully corrected with meticulous casting technique (more commonly syndromic feet).
- Surgeons now prefer a more individualized approach, as opposed to the traditional large posteromedial release, addressing only the components of the deformity that are uncorrected.
- A Z-plasty of the Achilles tendon or a gastrocnemius recession can address the equinus.
- Plantar fascia release can help address the cavus.
- Transfer of the tibialis anterior to the lateral cuneiform is one of the most commonly performed procedures in children who relapse. It is typically performed in children who have dynamic supination in the swing phase of gait.[83-85]

Outcomes

- Results of Ponseti casting are excellent, with 90% rate of initial correction.[86]
- However, relapses can occur in up to 40% of patients.[83]
- The most common cause of relapse after Ponseti casting is decreased compliance with abduction bracing.[87] Parental education and reeducation is critical to success!
- The initial severity of the foot can be predictive of relapse.[83]
- Many relapses can be managed with a course of recasting using Ponseti technique.[83,88]
- Deformities can return in the reverse order of the **CAVE** mnemonic. Equinus is typically the first deformity to return.

Top 10 Knowledge Drops for Your Rotation

1. Clubfoot is one of the most common congenital deformities of the lower extremity.
2. Family history is the most important risk factor.
3. **CAVE** mnemonic is for deformities (**C**avus, **A**dductus, **V**arus, **E**quinus).
4. A thorough physical examination is required to rule out other underlying syndromes.
5. Spina bifida and arthrogryposis are the most common syndromes associated with clubfoot.
6. Ponseti casting is the first-line treatment and has a 90% success rate.
7. Abduction bracing is initiated after casting and should continue until age 4 years.
8. The biggest predictor of relapse is nonadherence to long-term bracing. Parental education is key!
9. Repeat course of casting is undertaken for relapses before surgical intervention.
10. Surgical intervention is individualized and should address residual components of deformity.

SUPRACONDYLAR HUMERUS FRACTURES

- Supracondylar humerus fractures (SCHFs) in children are one of the most common elbow fractures in pediatric patients.

Epidemiology

- SCHFs are one of the most common pediatric elbow fractures accounting for 55% to 80% of such fractures.[89]
- Most of these injuries occur from a fall onto an outstretched hand and typically a fall from a height.[90,91]
- The most common age is 5 to 7 years.
- Fracture types fall into two broad categories:
  - Extension type:
    - Typically occurs from a fall on an outstretched hand with the elbow extended and results in posterior displacement of the fracture

- Accounts for 98% of SCHF[92]
- Flexion type:
  - Typically occurs from a fall onto a flexed elbow and results in anterolateral displacement of the distal portion of the fracture
  - Accounts for 2% of SCHF[92]
- Neurologic injury occurs in more than 10% of these injuries.[93]

Pertinent Anatomy/Pathoanatomy

- A basic understanding of proximity of soft-tissue, neurologic, and vascular structures is necessary in the management of SCHF.
- Periosteum:
  - Periosteum in and around the distal humerus typically fails on the tension side. For example, in an extension-type SCHF, the periosteum typically fails anteriorly. For minimally displaced SCHF, the periosteum typically remains intact posteriorly on extension-type fractures.
- Muscle: The brachialis muscle sits just anterior to the supracondylar humerus. With an extension-type SCHF, the metaphyseal (or proximal) portion can buttonhole through the brachialis causing dimpling or puckering of the antecubital fossa (**Figure 18**).
- Neurologic
  - The adjacent neurologic structures are at risk with displaced SCHF. The direction of the fracture displacement will stretch the nerves on the concavity of the deformity.
  - The most commonly injured nerve in extension type SCHF is the anterior interosseous nerve followed by a complete median nerve palsy.[94]
  - The most commonly injured nerve in flexion type SCHF is the ulnar nerve.[94]
- Vascular
  - The brachial artery sits anterior at the elbow and is at risk.
  - The prevalence of a vascular injury in patients with displaced SCHF is 15%.[93]

Pertinent History/Physical Examination Findings

- The important aspects of the history include mechanism of injury, age, prior injuries to the elbow, handedness, and activities (important for discussion of returning to activities after recovery).

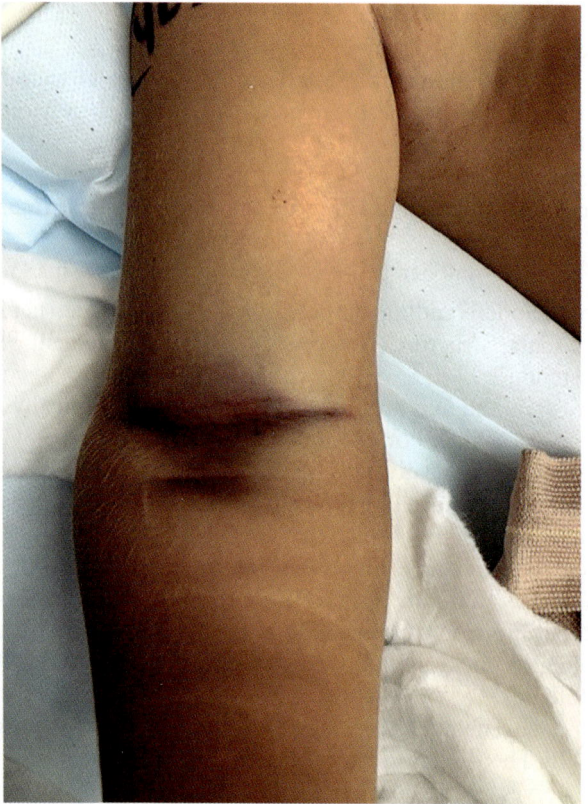

Figure 18 Clinical photograph showing brachialis sign that occurred when the proximal fracture fragment has pierced through the brachialis muscle into the deep dermis, resulting in puckering of the skin.

- Examination:
  - Soft-tissue signs of trauma
    - Ecchymosis in and around the elbow, in particular in the antecubital fossa
    - Swelling
    - Brachialis sign (**Figure 18**)
    - Observe for swelling or tenderness elsewhere in the extremity as concomitant forearm or wrist injuries occur[95]
  - Neurologic and motor

- A thorough examination is paramount; however, it can be difficult to obtain an examination in children
- Sensory examination[93]
  - Sensation can be obtained with light touch or pin prick
  - Radial: obtained best at the dorsal aspect of the first web space
  - Median: obtained best at the volar aspect of the index finger
  - Ulnar: obtained best at the volar aspect of the small fingertip
- Motor examination
  - Radial: Observe for digital extension and thumb interphalangeal joint extension (posterior interosseous nerve)
  - Median:
    - Observe for finger flexion and grip
    - Observe for thumb interphalangeal joint and index distal interphalangeal joint flexion (anterior interosseous nerve); isolation of the thumb on examination can aid in detecting thumb interphalangeal joint flexion (**Figure 19**)
  - Ulnar: Observe for finger abduction and adduction
- Vascular:
  - Assessment includes:
    - Palpation of radial artery

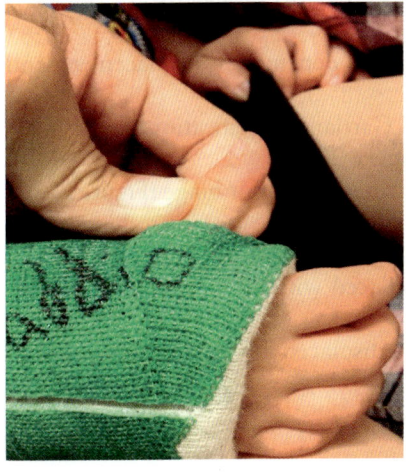

Figure 19 Photograph shows isolation of the thumb interphalangeal joint can help in detecting a nerve palsy. Inability of thumb interphalangeal joint extension suggests a posterior interosseous or radial nerve injury. Inability of thumb interphalangeal joint flexion suggests an anterior interosseous or median nerve injury.

- Assessment of capillary review
    - Doppler ultrasonography of radial artery
- Categories of vascular injury in SCHF[93]
    - Normal perfusion: The hand is well perfused and has a palpable radial pulse.
    - Perfused, pulseless: Radial pulse is not palpable, but capillary refill is normal, less than 2 seconds; this type may or may not have normal findings on Doppler ultrasonography of the radial artery.
    - Ischemic: Radial pulse is not palpable and capillary refill is not normal. This type may present with a poorly perfused hand that appears lighter than baseline.

Relevant Imaging

- Radiographic assessment should include:
    - AP and lateral elbow radiographs
        - In a normal lateral view of the elbow, the anterior humeral line should bisect the capitellum (**Figure 20, A**).
        - AP assessment should evaluate Baumann angle to ensure no varus or valgus deformity. Baumann angle should not be more than 10°.
        - Contralateral elbow radiographs can be used for assessment if needed.
    - Forearm radiographs (AP and lateral) should also be obtained to rule out any ipsilateral injury.
- Classification of the radiographs depends on displacement and direction of displacement.
    - Extension type—Modified Gartland classification
        - Type I: nondisplaced (**Figure 20, B**)
        - Type IIA: displaced with intact posterior hinge (**Figure 20, C**)
        - Type IIB: displaced with intact posterior hinge and malrotation/impaction
        - Type III: completely displaced with no intact posterior cortex (**Figure 20, D**)
        - Type IV: completely displaced with multidirectional instability
    - Flexion type (**Figure 20, E**)

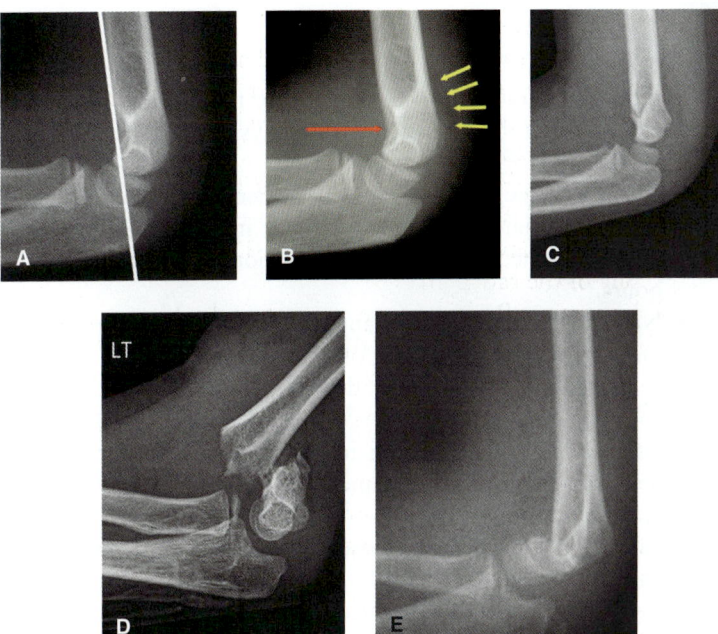

Figure 20 **A**, Lateral radiograph without a fracture demonstrates that the anterior humeral line bisects the capitellum. **B**, Lateral radiograph of a type I extension supracondylar humerus fracture (SCHF)—fracture line is seen (red arrow) and a posterior fat pad sign is seen (yellow arrows). **C**, Lateral radiograph of a type IIa extension SCHF—anterior humeral line does not bisect through the capitellum but the posterior cortex is intact. **D**, Lateral radiograph of a type III extension SCHF—complete displacement of the posterior cortex is seen. **E**, Lateral radiograph of a flexion-type SCHF.

Nonsurgical Measures

- Indications for nonsurgical management include nondisplaced SCHF, that is, type I SCHF.[95]
- SCHF can be managed with 3 to 4 weeks of immobilization.
- Typical immobilization would include a long arm cast for the duration of treatment.
- Immobilization of the elbow should be no more than 90°.

Surgical Intervention

- Timing
  - Type II: There is no surgical urgency for type II fractures; these can be successfully managed within days of the injury.
  - Type III:
    - No neurologic injury: There is no emergency to perform surgery immediately and no difference in outcome when performed immediately after presentation or greater than 12 hours.[96,97]
    - Neurologic injury: Most authors recommend more urgent management in the setting of a neurologic injury.[98]
      - Progressive neurologic deficits should result in more urgent timing for surgery.[97]
    - Vascular injury: Any suspicion for a vascular injury should result in emergent management.
- Surgical management
  - Most SCHF can undergo closed reduction and percutaneous pinning.
    - Very few require open reduction and pinning.
    - Type III SCHF and most type II SCHF require surgical management.
  - Positioning:
    - Patients are positioned in a supine position on the operating room table.
    - The elbow is placed on a radiolucent arm board and the patient's arm must be positioned as far onto the arm board to ensure full radiographic evaluation intraoperatively.
  - Reduction
    - With the patient positioned supine, longitudinal traction is pulled on the arm and the fracture is aligned in regard to varus, valgus, and translation.
    - The elbow is then flexed while applying an anteriorly directed pressure on the olecranon.
      - The forearm is rotated into pronation for posteromedial displaced fractures.
      - The forearm is rotated into supination for posterolateral displaced fractures.
    - The reduction is then assessed radiographically on both the AP and lateral views.

- Pin location, number, and configuration
  - Location:
    - Most elbows can undergo successful fixation with a lateral-entry pin technique (**Figure 21**).
    - Cross-pinning with medial and lateral pins can also be performed.
      - In this setting, pinning is typically performed first laterally and then the elbow is extended and a small incision is made to avoid injury to the ulnar nerve. When the elbow is extended the ulnar nerve relaxes, placing it in a better position for medial pin placement. The open incision makes this a safer procedure.[99]
  - Number of pins:
    - Typically, two pins are adequate for type II fractures and three pins are recommended for type III fractures.[95]
  - Pin configuration:
    - Biomechanical data demonstrate no significant torsional stability when comparing all-lateral entry pins to cross pin configuration.[100]

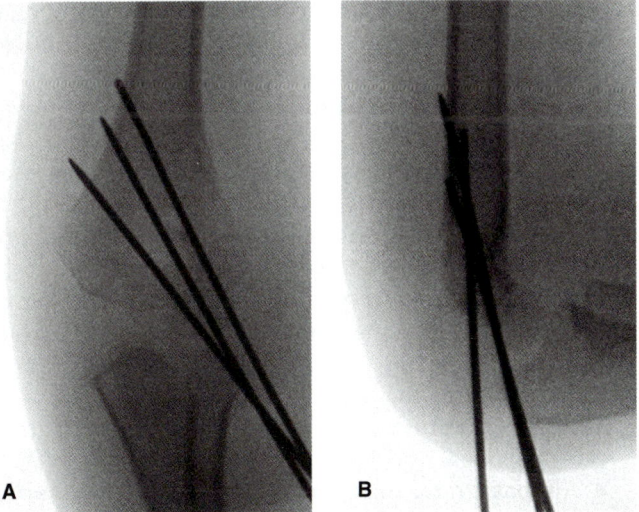

Figure 21 Pins typically are placed from an all-lateral entry start point with a goal of divergent pins in the AP view (**A**) and lateral view (**B**).

- The goal of pin placement should be to achieve spread of the pins in regard to where they cross the fracture site and to ensure achieving bicortical fixation with at least two pins[101] (**Figure 21**).
- Pins are then bent outside of the side and sterile dressing is placed around them.
- Intraoperative assessment of vascular status
  - Following closed reduction and percutaneous pinning, vascular status should be reevaluated.
    - Palpation of radial pulse
    - Evaluation of capillary refill
    - If there is a change in vascular status, exploration of the antecubital fossa may be necessary.
- Open reduction
  - Indications for open reduction:
    - Unable to obtain adequate reduction
    - Anterior fracture gap after reduction (suggesting entrapped neurologic and vascular structures)
    - Change/decline in perfusion after reduction and pinning or continued poor perfusion after reduction and pining
  - Approach: Transverse incision in the antecubital fossa, which can be extended medially and proximally or distal and laterally as needed[102]
- Special circumstances: The pink pulseless SCHF
  - These fractures require prompt treatment with initial reduction and pinning.[103-105]
    - Treatment algorithms for the well-perfused, pulseless SCHF have been developed to help treating surgeons.[95,103,104]
  - Nearly half of the pulseless SCHF that undergo initial reduction and pinning have a return of a palpable pulse.[105]
  - If patients have a well-perfused extremity/hand after closed reduction and pinning, most authors recommend watchful waiting or close observation for 24 to 48 hours.[106-110]
  - In cases where the upper extremity is still not well perfused, exploration of the antecubital fossa is strongly recommended.
    - Although rare, some patients will require intraoperative vascular consultation.

- Postoperative follow-up
  - Cast and pin removal typically occurs 3 to 4 weeks after surgery in the office setting.
  - Follow-up radiographs including AP and lateral of the elbow are obtained to assess healing.
  - Children can progress back to range of motion after the pins are removed.
- Complications:
  - Infection: Pin tract infections can occur but are rare;[111] pin removal is recommended by 4 weeks postoperatively to help avoid this complication.
  - Stiffness: Most patients regain full elbow range of motion after a SCHF.
  - Malunion:
    - Cubitus varus
    - Extension or flexion deformities may affect elbow range of motion.
  - Osteonecrosis: There are reports of osteonecrosis occurring postoperatively and resultant fishtail deformities.[110]
  - Compartment syndrome

Top 10 Knowledge Drops for Your Rotation

1. SCHFs are classified as extension or flexion types.
2. Neurologic injury occurs in approximately 10% of SCHFs.
3. The most injured nerve in extension type SCHFs is the anterior interosseous nerve.
4. The most injured nerve in flexion type SCHFs is the ulnar nerve.
5. The prevalence of a vascular injury in patients with a displaced SCHF is 15%.
6. Thorough neurologic, motor, and vascular examination can be difficult to perform in a child but it is important to identify any potential injuries.
7. Patients with type I SCHFs can undergo treatment in a long arm cast.
8. Surgical management commonly entails closed reduction and percutaneous pinning with a goal of restoring varus/valgus,

translation (coronal and sagittal plane), and flexion/extension (sagittal alignment) through the evaluation of the anterior humeral line.
9. Type III SCHFs with a neurologic injury or progressive neurologic deficit should undergo urgent closed reduction and percutaneous pinning.
10. Type III well-perfused, pulseless SCHFs should undergo emergent closed reduction and percutaneous pinning with reevaluation of the pulse. Patients with return of a pulse or stable vascular examination can be observed in the hospital for 24 to 48 hours. Patients with a poorly perfused hand or a decrease in perfusion will require open exploration.

INTOEING

- Intoeing is a common reason for pediatric orthopaedic evaluation.
- Intoeing refers to a walking pattern where children walk with their feet turned in (internal foot progression).
- Intoeing can arise from three different locations (**Table 2**):
  - Hips (femoral anteversion)
  - Lower leg (internal tibial torsion [ITT])
  - Feet (metatarsus adductus)
- In most cases, intoeing will resolve on its own without treatment.
- Bracing or surgical intervention is seldom needed.

TABLE 2 Different Pathologies That Can Cause Intoeing

Location	Medical Name	Common Age at Presentation	Associations	Treatment
Hip	Femoral anteversion	3-6 yr	Ligamentous laxity	None
Leg	Tibial torsion	1-4 yr	None	None
Foot	Metatarsus adductus	At birth (often mistaken for a clubfoot)	Torticollis Hip dysplasia	None Casting only if rigid

Epidemiology

- Metatarsus adductus is the most common foot deformity in newborns, occurring in 1 to 2 per 1,000 births.[112]
- ITT is the most common cause of intoeing identified between the ages of 1 to 4 years (although the condition can present during infancy). It is typically seen from birth but not always noted by families until the child begins to walk. There is no identified cause or sex predilection.[113]
- Femoral anteversion is the third most common cause of intoeing, and children typically present between the ages of 3 and 6 years. Anteversion is more common in females.[114]
- 95% of children presenting for intoeing were found to have a benign cause (neurotypical children expected to improve with time).[115]

Pertinent Anatomy/Pathoanatomy

- Intoeing can be linked to intrauterine positioning.
- In metatarsus adductus, soft tissues at the level of the tarsometatarsal joints are contracted, which makes the forefoot adduct (face inward) in relation to the hindfoot.[112] Deformity is typically present at birth.
- ITT involves medial rotation of the tibial shaft and is the most common cause of intoeing.
- Femoral version describes the difference angular difference between the femoral neck and the transcondylar axis of the knee.[116] Anteversion is higher in children than it is in adults. Babies are born with 30° to 40° of anteversion that decreases to 10° to 15° by adolescence.

Pertinent History/Physical Examination Findings

- Birth history is important! Be sure to ask if the child was born in the breech position or at full term, or if there were any pregnancy complications.
- Make sure a child's height and weight are taken. Height below the fifth percentile may be associated with genetics.
- Ask about developmental milestones! Depending on the child's age, ask if they are meeting their motor milestones. Delays may be a red flag for other conditions that should not be missed (genetic or neurologic conditions not related to their intoeing).

- Children often present to the physician because of caregiver concerns regarding tripping, falling, being bowlegged, or cosmesis.[117]
- Many children can have a family history of intoeing (ie, parent or sibling). Historically, many rotational deformities were treated with bracing and/or casting. Relatives may remember having this treatment themselves.
- These deformities should be symmetric. Asymmetry may also raise concerns about developmental or neurologic conditions.
- Some children can have a combination of pathologies that contribute to their gait.
- Remember to examine the entire lower extremity!

Metatarsus Adductus

- Metatarsus adductus is often present at birth. Often, the foot will appear bean shaped. Only the forefoot is involved.
- The condition is often mistaken for clubfoot by physicians who are not orthopaedic surgeons.
- Metatarsus adductus can be classified as mild, moderate, or severe. This classification is in relation to the heel bisector line and to whether the foot is flexible, partially flexible, or rigid.
- The heel bisector line can be measured with the baby/child supine or in the caregiver's lap if needed. It is a clinical measurement looking at the foot from the plantar aspect. Normally, the center of the heel should bisect the second and third toes.[118]
- In mild adductus, the line bisects the third toe.
- In moderate adductus, the line bisects between the third and fourth toes.
- In severe adductus, the line bisects lateral to the fourth toe.
- The flexibility of the foot should also be assessed. With gentle pressure on the first ray, the adductus can be completely flexible, partially flexible, or rigid.
- Because adductus can be associated with other packaging disorders, a thorough neck (for sternocleidomastoid tightness) and hip examination are required to identify other associated conditions.

Internal Tibial Torsion

- The child will walk with the patellae pointing straight ahead but the feet pointing inward.

- The thigh-foot angle is often measured for assessment of ITT. With the child prone, the axis of the thigh is compared with the axis of the foot with the leg bent and hindfoot held in neutral.[118]
- The cover-up test[8] can be used to differentiate ITT (bowing of the tibial shaft) from early infantile Blount disease (bowing of the proximal tibia called tibia vara). It is performed with the child sitting or supine. The knee is physically covered by the examiner's hand. If covering the knee takes away the appearance of bowing, the source of the bowing is the proximal tibia. If the tibia still appears bowed with the knee covered, the deformity is coming from the tibia shaft (ITT).[119]
- This distinction is important because bracing is effective in tibia vara, whereas bracing is not used for children with ITT and the condition resolves spontaneously.

Femoral Anteversion

- The child typically has more than 30° of mismatch between internal and external hip rotation (more internal than external).[120] This is best measured in the prone position (**Figures 22** and **23**).
- On standing examination, patellae face inward (kissing patellae).[121]
- On sitting examination, children will be able to sit in a "W" position (**Figure 24**).
- Children can have a circumduction gait when walking but more often with running.
- Internal foot progression angle (how many degrees from neutral feet point in while walking) is also measured. It should be symmetric bilaterally.
- Evaluate for ligamentous laxity, which can be common in children with anteversion.

Relevant Imaging

- Imaging is not obtained in many cases on initial evaluation[122] with some notable exceptions:
  - For babies with metatarsus adductus, hip ultrasonography is performed to evaluate for DDH, as both are packaging disorders.
  - For children with femoral anteversion, an AP radiograph of the pelvis should be obtained if there is any asymmetry on

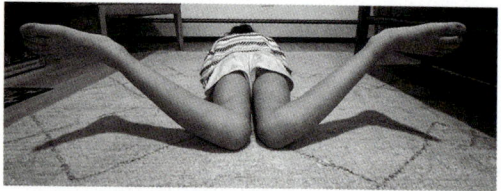

Figure 22 Photograph shows prone hip rotation examination showing internal rotation.

examination or if there are other history/examination findings concerning for hip dysplasia (ie, family history, breech presentation).
- In rare cases of older children needing surgery, standing radiographs of the lower extremity can be helpful for surgical planning.
- CT version studies or MRI can also be used for evaluation of femoral anteversion in older children in whom surgery is planned.[123]

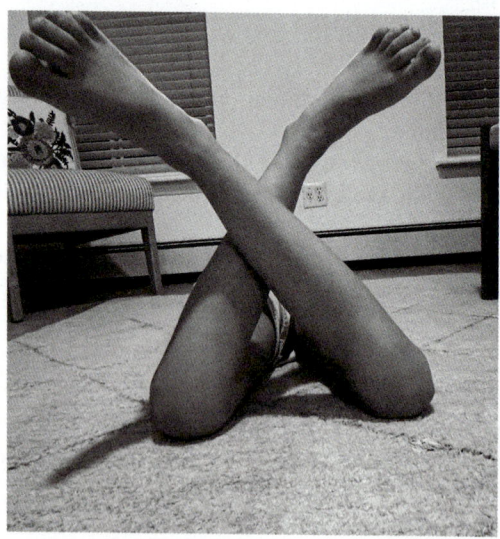

Figure 23 Photograph shows prone hip rotation examination showing external rotation.

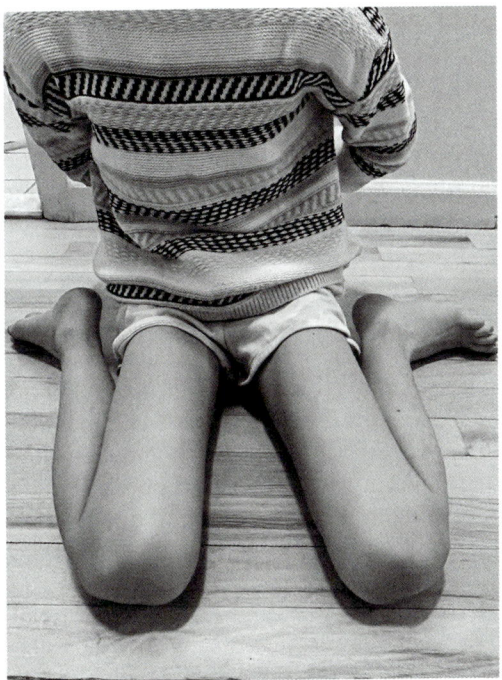

Figure 24 Photograph shows the demonstration of "W" sitting.

Nonsurgical Treatment

Metatarsus Adductus

- Flexible metatarsus adductus will often resolve on its own without treatment.[124]
- There is some evidence that caregiver stretching may help.[124] Stretching may also allow caregivers to feel ownership over treatment and outcome.
- Casting can be initiated for less flexible deformities in cases that do not improve over the first 6 months of life. Typically, long leg casting is used to control tibial rotation and because of the small size of the baby.[121]

Internal Tibial Torsion

- There is no effective brace treatment that is agreed on for ITT.[125]

Femoral Anteversion

- Historically, femoral anteversion was treated with braces. These are no longer widely used and have shown limited effectiveness.[125-127]
- Physical therapy has not been shown to correct intoeing but can be helpful when the child is not meeting developmental milestones or has issues relating to balance and/or coordination.[117]

Surgical Intervention/Outcomes

- Often not required as many children improve with time.
- Surgical intervention for metatarsus adductus is very rare, as even most rigid cases can be treated with casting.
- Derotational osteotomies may be warranted in children with significant torsional deformities (ITT or femoral anteversion) that impair their ability to walk without tripping.[128]
- Most authors recommend waiting until age 8 years to consider surgical intervention to allow for maximal natural correction of deformity.[129]
- Femoral derotational osteotomies can be performed proximally or distally in the femur.[116]
- In most children the deformity resolves with time and growth.
- Outcomes of tibial osteotomy are very good at improving deformity but not all gait parameters.[128]
- Outcomes of femoral derotation osteotomy show a decrease in patellofemoral knee pain in improvement in overall alignment.[116]

Top 10 Knowledge Drops For Your Rotation

1. Birth and developmental history matter! Inquire about all patients presenting with intoeing.
2. Intoeing can come from three different locations (hip, lower leg, foot). Examine the whole lower extremity.
3. Recognize associated conditions with metatarsus adductus (torticollis and DDH).
4. The heel bisector line should be measured to assess severity of metatarsus adductus.
5. Prone examination (best assessment of hip rotation) can be difficult in small children. Supine examination or examination on

the caregiver's lap can substitute if a small child is resistant or fearful.
6. Asymmetric hip motion should warrant an AP radiograph of the pelvis.
7. Babies with metatarsus adductus should undergo hip ultrasonography.
8. Bracing is not effective for intoeing.
9. Casting can be effective in babies with rigid or partially flexible metatarsus adductus.
10. There are surgical options for adolescents, but these interventions are rarely needed.

References

1. Lehmann CL, Arons RR, Loder RT, Vitale MG: The epidemiology of slipped capital femoral epiphysis: An update. *J Pediatr Orthop* 2006;26(3):286-290.
2. Burrows HJ: Slipped upper femoral epiphysis; characteristic of a hundred cases. *J Bone Joint Surg Br* 1957;39-B(4):641-658.
3. Loder RT: The demographics of slipped capital femoral epiphysis. An international multicenter study. *Clin Orthop Relat Res* 1996;322:8-27.
4. Witbreuk M, Van Kemenade FJ, Van Der Sluijs JA, Jansma EP, Rotteveel J, Van Royen BJ: Slipped capital femoral epiphysis and its association with endocrine, metabolic and chronic diseases: A systematic review of the literature. *J Child Orthop* 2013;7(3):213-223.
5. Aprato A, Conti A, Bertolo F, Massè A: Slipped capital femoral epiphysis: Current management strategies. *Orthop Res Rev* 2019;11:47-54.
6. Aversano MW, Moazzaz P, Scaduto AA, Otsuka NY: Association between body mass index-for-age and slipped capital femoral epiphysis: The long-term risk for subsequent slip in patients followed until physeal closure. *J Child Orthop* 2016;10(3):209-213.
7. Perry DC, Metcalfe D, Lane S, Turner S: Childhood obesity and slipped capital femoral epiphysis. *Pediatrics* 2018;142(5):e20181067.
8. Davids JR, Blackhurst DW, Allen BL Jr: Clinical evaluation of bowed legs in children. *J Pediatr Orthop B* 2000;9(4):278-284.
9. Stasikelis PJ, Sullivan CM, Phillips WA, Polard JA: Slipped capital femoral epiphysis. Prediction of contralateral involvement. *J Bone Joint Surg Am* 1996;78(8):1149-1155.

10. Escott BG, De La Rocha A, Jo CH, Sucato DJ, Karol LA: Patient-reported health outcomes after in situ percutaneous fixation for slipped capital femoral epiphysis: An average twenty-year follow-up study. *J Bone Joint Surg Am* 2015;97(23):1929-1934.
11. Hailer YD: Fate of patients with slipped capital femoral epiphysis (SCFE) in later life: Risk of obesity, hypothyroidism, and death in 2,564 patients with SCFE compared with 25,638 controls. *Acta Orthop* 2020;91(4):457-463.
12. Bland DC, Valdovino AG, Jeffords ME, Bomar JD, Newton PO, Upasani VV: Evaluation of the three-dimensional translational and angular deformity in slipped capital femoral epiphysis. *J Orthop Res* 2020;38(5):1081-1088.
13. Abraham E, Gonzalez MH, Pratap S, Amirouche F, Atluri P, Simon P: Clinical implications of anatomical wear characteristics in slipped capital femoral epiphysis and primary osteoarthritis. *J Pediatr Orthop* 2007;27(7):788-795.
14. Georgiadis AG, Zaltz I: Slipped capital femoral epiphysis: How to evaluate with a review and update of treatment. *Pediatr Clin North Am* 2014;61(6):1119-1135.
15. Upasani VV, Badrinath R, Farnsworth CL, et al: Increased hip intracapsular pressure decreases perfusion of the capital femoral epiphysis in a skeletally immature porcine model. *J Pediatr Orthop* 2020;40(4):176-182.
16. Uvodich M, Schwend R, Stevanovic O, Wurster W, Leamon J, Hermanson A: Patterns of pain in adolescents with slipped capital femoral epiphysis. *J Pediatr* 2019;206:184-189.e1.
17. Swarup I, Goodbody C, Goto R, Sankar WN, Fabricant PD: Risk factors for contralateral slipped capital femoral epiphysis: A meta-analysis of cohort and case-control studies. *J Pediatr Orthop* 2020;40(6):e446-e453.
18. Herman MJ, Martinek M: The limping child. *Pediatr Rev* 2015;36(5):184-195.
19. Loder RT: Slipped capital femoral epiphysis. *Am Fam Physician* 1998;57(9):2135-2142, 2148-2150.
20. Maranho DA, Bixby SD, Miller PE, et al: What is the accuracy and reliability of the peritubercle lucency sign on radiographs for early diagnosis of slipped capital femoral epiphysis compared with MRI as the gold standard? *Clin Orthop Relat Res* 2020;478(5):1049-1059.
21. Balch Samora J, Adler B, Druhan S, et al: MRI in idiopathic, stable, slipped capital femoral epiphysis: Evaluation of contralateral pre-slip. *J Child Orthop* 2018;12(5):454-460.
22. Betz RR, Steel HH, Emper WD, Huss GK, Clancy M: Treatment of slipped capital femoral epiphysis. Spica-cast immobilization. *J Bone Joint Surg Am* 1990;72(4):587-600.

23. Kibiloski LJ, Doane RM, Karol LA, Haut RC, Loder RT: Biomechanical analysis of single- versus double-screw fixation in slipped capital femoral epiphysis at physiological load levels. *J Pediatr Orthop* 1994;14(5):627-630.

24. Herrera-Soto JA, Duffy MF, Birnbaum MA, Vander Have KL: Increased intracapsular pressures after unstable slipped capital femoral epiphysis. *J Pediatr Orthop* 2008;28(7):723-728.

25. Castañeda P, Macías C, Rocha A, Harfush A, Cassis N: Functional outcome of stable grade III slipped capital femoral epiphysis treated with in situ pinning. *J Pediatr Orthop* 2009;29(5):454-458.

26. Loder RT, Aronsson DD, Weinstein SL, Breur GJ, Ganz R, Leunig M: Slipped capital femoral epiphysis. *Instr Course Lect* 2008;57:473-498.

27. Upasani VV, Matheney TH, Spencer SA, Kim YJ, Millis MB, Kasser JR: Complications after modified Dunn osteotomy for the treatment of adolescent slipped capital femoral epiphysis. *J Pediatr Orthop* 2014;34(7):661-667.

28. Sankar WN, Vanderhave KL, Matheney T, Herrera-Soto JA, Karlen JW: The modified Dunn procedure for unstable slipped capital femoral epiphysis: A multicenter perspective. *J Bone Joint Surg Am* 2013;95(7):585-591.

29. Upasani V, Kishan S, Oka R, et al: Biomechanical analysis of single screw fixation for slipped capital femoral epiphysis: Are more threads across the physis necessary for stability? *J Pediatr Orthop* 2006;26(4):474-478.

30. Loder RT, Richards BS, Shapiro PS, Reznick LR, Aronson DD: Acute slipped capital femoral epiphysis: The importance of physeal stability. *J Bone Joint Surg Am* 1993;75(8):1134-1140.

31. Castañeda P, Ponce C, Villareal G, Vidal C: The natural history of osteoarthritis after a slipped capital femoral epiphysis/the pistol grip deformity. *J Pediatr Orthop* 2013;33(suppl 1):S76-S82.

32. Lubicky JP: Chondrolysis and avascular necrosis: Complications of slipped capital femoral epiphysis. *J Pediatr Orthop B* 1996;5(3):162-167.

33. Kohno Y, Nakashima Y, Kitano T, et al: Is the timing of surgery associated with avascular necrosis after unstable slipped capital femoral epiphysis? A multicenter study. *J Orthop Sci* 2017;22(1):112-115.

34. Schrader T, Jones CR, Kaufman AM, Herzog MM: Intraoperative monitoring of epiphyseal perfusion in slipped capital femoral epiphysis. *J Bone Joint Surg Am* 2016;98(12):1030-1040.

35. Kaushal N, Chen C, Agarwal KN, Schrader T, Kelly D, Dodwell ER: Capsulotomy in unstable slipped capital femoral epiphysis and the odds of AVN: A meta-analysis of retrospective studies. *J Pediatr Orthop* 2019;39(6):e406-e411.

36. Mathew SE, Larson AN: Natural history of slipped capital femoral epiphysis. *J Pediatr Orthop* 2019;39(6 suppl 1):S23-S27.
37. Larson AN, Sierra RJ, Yu EM, Trousdale RT, Stans AA: Outcomes of slipped capital femoral epiphysis treated with in situ pinning. *J Pediatr Orthop* 2012;32(2):125-130.
38. Tredwell SJ: Neonatal screening for hip joint instability. Its clinical and economic relevance. *Clin Orthop Relat Res* 1992;281:63-68.
39. Dunn PM: Perinatal observations on the etiology of congenital dislocation of the hip. *Clin Orthop Relat Res* 1976;119:11-22.
40. Wynne-Davies R: Acetabular dysplasia and familial joint laxity: Two etiological factors in congenital dislocation of the hip. A review of 589 patients and their families. *J Bone Joint Surg Br* 1970;52(4):704-716.
41. Salter RB: Etiology, pathogenesis and possible prevention of congenital dislocation of the hip. *Can Med Assoc J* 1968;98(20):933-945.
42. Barlow TG: Early diagnosis and treatment of congenital dislocation of the hip. *Proc R Soc Med* 1963;56:804-806.
43. Thomas SR: A review of long-term outcomes for late presenting developmental hip dysplasia. *Bone Joint J* 2015;97-B(6):729-733.
44. Guille JT, Pizzutillo PD, MacEwen GD: Development dysplasia of the hip from birth to six months. *J Am Acad Orthop Surg* 2000;8(4):232-242.
45. Ortolani M: Congenital hip dysplasia in the light of early and very early diagnosis. *Clin Orthop Relat Res* 1976;119:6-10.
46. Vitale MG, Skaggs DL: Developmental dysplasia of the hip from six months to four years of age. *J Am Acad Orthop Surg* 2001;9(6):401-411.
47. Kamath SU, Bennet GC: Does developmental dysplasia of the hip cause a delay in walking? *J Pediatr Orthop* 2004;24(3):265.
48. Carbonell PG, de Puga DB, Vicente-Franqueira JR, Ortuño AL: Radiographic study of the acetabulum and proximal femur between 1 and 3 years of age. *Surg Radiol Anat* 2009;31(7):483-487.
49. U.S. Preventive Service Task Force: Screening for developmental dysplasia of the hip: Recommendation statement. *Am Fam Physician* 2006;73(11):1992-1996.
50. Copuroglu C, Ozcan M, Aykac B, Tuncer B, Saridogan K: Reliability of ultrasonographic measurements in suspected patients of developmental dysplasia of the hip and correlation with the acetabular index. *Indian J Orthop* 2011;45(6):553-557.
51. Smith JT, Matan A, Coleman SS, Stevens PM, Scott SM: The predictive value of the development of the acetabular teardrop figure in developmental dysplasia of the hip. *J Pediatr Orthop* 1997;17(2):165-169.
52. Schaeffer E, Lubicky J, Mulpuri K: AAOS appropriate use criteria: The management of developmental dysplasia of the hip in infants up to six months of age – Intended for use by orthopaedic specialists. *J Am Acad Orthop Surg* 2019;27(8):e369-e372.

53. Tiruveedhula M, Reading IC, Clarke NM: Failed Pavlik harness treatment for DDH as a risk factor for avascular necrosis. *J Pediatr Orthop* 2015;35(2):140-143.
54. Murnaghan ML, Browne RH, Sucato DJ, Birch J: Femoral nerve palsy in Pavlik harness treatment for developmental dysplasia of the hip. *J Bone Joint Surg Am* 2011;93(5):493-499.
55. Hedequist D, Kasser J, Emans J: Use of an abduction brace for developmental dysplasia of the hip after failure of Pavlik harness use. *J Pediatr Orthop* 2003;23(2):175-177.
56. Race C, Herring JA: Congenital dislocation of the hip: An evaluation of closed reduction. *J Pediatr Orthop* 1983;3(2):166-172.
57. Schur MD, Lee C, Arkader A, Catalano A, Choi PD: Risk factors for avascular necrosis after closed reduction for developmental dysplasia of the hip. *J Child Orthop* 2016;10(3):185-192.
58. Smith BG, Millis MB, Hey LA, Jaramillo D, Kasser JR: Postreduction computed tomography in developmental dislocation of the hip: Part II – Predictive value for outcome. *J Pediatr Orthop* 1997;17(5):631-636.
59. Roposch A, Ridout D, Protopapa E, Nicolaou N, Gelfer Y: Osteonecrosis complicating developmental dysplasia of the hip compromises subsequent acetabular remodeling. *Clin Orthop Relat Res* 2013;471(7):2318-2326.
60. Hoellwarth JS, Kim YJ, Millis MB, Kasser JR, Zurakowski D, Matheney TH: Medial versus anterior open reduction for developmental hip dislocation in age-matched patients. *J Pediatr Orthop* 2015;35(1):50-56.
61. Spence G, Hocking R, Wedge JH, Roposch A: Effect of innominate and femoral varus derotation osteotomy on acetabular development in developmental dysplasia of the hip. *J Bone Joint Surg Am* 2009;91(11):2622-2636.
62. Murphy RF, Kim YJ: Surgical management of pediatric developmental dysplasia of the hip. *J Am Acad Orthop Surg* 2016;24(9):615-624.
63. Wang TM, Wu KW, Shih SF, Huang SC, Kuo KN: Outcomes of open reduction for developmental dysplasia of the hip: does bilateral dysplasia have a poorer outcome? *J Bone Joint Surg Am* 2013;95(12):1081-1086.
64. Dobbs MB, Gurnett CA: Genetics of clubfoot. *J Pediatr Orthop B* 2012;21:7-9.
65. Chen C, Kaushal N, Scher DM, Doyle SM, Blanco JS, Dodwell ER: Clubfoot etiology: A meta-analysis and systematic review of observational and randomized trials. *J Pediatr Orthop* 2018;38(8):e462-e469.
66. Zionts LE, Jew MH, Ebramzadeh E, Sangiorgio SN: The influence of sex and laterality on clubfoot severity. *J Pediatr Orthop* 2017;37:e129-e133.

67. Yau A, Doyle SM: Clubfoot for the primary care physician: Frequently asked questions. *Curr Opin Pediatr* 2020;32(1):100-106.
68. Ponseti IV, Smoley EN: Congenital club foot: The results of treatment. *J Bone Joint Surg Am* 1963;45:261-344.
69. Shimode K, Miyagi N, Majima T, Yasuda K, Minami A: Limb length and girth discrepancy of unilateral congenital clubfeet. *J Pediatr Orthop B* 2005;14(4):280-284.
70. Zhao D, Rao W, Zhao L, et al: Is it worthwhile to screen the hip in infants born with clubfeet? *Int Orthop* 2013;37(12):2415-2420.
71. Perry DC, Tawfiq SM, Roche A, et al: The association between clubfoot and developmental dysplasia of the hip. *J Bone Joint Surg Br* 2010;92(11):1586-1588.
72. O'Halloran C, Halanski M, Nemeth B, Zimmermann C, Noonan K: Can radiographs predict outcome in patients with idiopathic clubfeet treated with the ponseti method? *J Pediatr Orthop* 2015;35(7):734-738.
73. Dobbs MB, Gurnett CA: Update on clubfoot: Etiology and treatment. *Clin Orthop Relat Res* 2009;467(5):1146-1153.
74. Ponseti IV: Treatment of congenital club foot. *J Bone Joint Surg Am* 1992;74(3):448-454.
75. Chu A, Lehman WB: Treatment of idiopathic clubfoot in the Ponseti era and beyond. *Foot Ankle Clin* 2015;20:555-562.
76. Digge V, Desai J, Das S: Expanded age indication for Ponseti method for correction of congenital idiopathic talipes equinovarus: A systematic review. *J Foot Ankle Surg* 2018;57:155-158.
77. Spiegel DA, Shrestha OP, Sitoula P, et al: Ponseti method for untreated idiopathic clubfeet in Nepalese patients from 1 to 6 years of age. *Clin Orthop Relat Res* 2009;467:1164-1170.
78. Diméglio A, Bensahel H, Souchet P, Mazeau P, Bonnet F: Classification of clubfoot. *J Pediatr Orthop* 1995;4:129-136.
79. Dyer PJ, Davis N: The role of the Pirani scoring system in the management of club foot by the Ponseti method. *J Bone Joint Surg Br* 2006;88(8):1082-1084.
80. Janicki JA, Narayanan UG, Harvey B, Roy A, Ramseier LE, Wright JG: Treatment of neuromuscular and syndrome-associated (nonidiopathic) clubfeet using the Ponseti method. *J Pediatr Orthop* 2009;29(4):393-397.
81. Aronson J, Puskarich CL: Deformity and disability from treated clubfoot. *J Pediatr Orthop* 1990;10(1):109-119.
82. Graf A, Hassani S, Krzak J, et al: Long-term outcome evaluation in young adults following clubfoot surgical release. *J Pediatr Orthop* 2010;30(4):379-385.

83. Masrouha K, Chu A, Lehman W: Narrative review of the management of a relapsed clubfoot. *Ann Transl Med* 2021;9(13):1102.
84. McKay SD, Dolan LA, Morcuende JA: Treatment results of late-relapsing idiopathic clubfoot previously treated with the Ponseti method. *J Pediatr Orthop* 2012;32:406-411.
85. Zionts LE, Ebramzadeh E, Morgan RD, et al: Sixty years on: Ponseti method for clubfoot treatment produces high satisfaction despite inherent tendency to relapse. *J Bone Joint Surg Am* 2018;100:721-728.
86. Laaveg SJ, Ponseti IV: Long-term results of treatment of congenital club foot. *J Bone Joint Surg Am* 1980;62(1):23-31.
87. Dobbs MB, Rudzki JR, Purcell DB, Walton T, Porter KR, Gurnett CA: Factors predictive of outcome after use of the Ponseti method for the treatment of idiopathic clubfeet. *J Bone Joint Surg Am* 2004;86(1):22-27.
88. van Praag VM, Lysenko M, Harvey B, et al: Casting is effective for recurrence following ponseti treatment of clubfoot. *J Bone Joint Surg Am* 2018;100:1001-1008.
89. Choi PD, Melikian R, Skaggs DL: Risk factors for vascular repair and compartment syndrome in the pulseless supracondylar humerus fracture in children. *J Pediatr Orthop* 2010;30(1):50-56.
90. Carson S, Woolridge DP, Colletti J, Kilgore K: Pediatric upper extremity injuries. *Pediatr Clin North Am* 2006;53(1):41-67.
91. Farnsworth CL, Silva PD, Mubarak SJ: Etiology of supracondylar humerus fractures. *J Pediatr Orthop* 1998;18(1):38-42.
92. Cheng JC, Lam TP, Maffulli N: Epidemiological features of supracondylar fractures of the humerus in Chinese children. *J Pediatr Orthop B* 2001;10(1):63-67.
93. Scannell BP, Brighton BK, Vanderhave KL: Neurological and vascular complications associated with supracondylar humeral fractures in children. *JBJS Rev* 2015;3(12):e2.
94. Babal JC, Mehlman CT, Klein G: Nerve injuries associated with pediatric supracondylar humeral fractures: A meta-analysis. *J Pediatr Orthop* 2010;30(3):253-263.
95. Abzug JM, Herman MJ: Management of supracondylar humerus fractures in children: Current concepts. *J Am Acad Orthop Surg* 2012;20:69-77.
96. Gupta N, Kay RM, Leitch K, Femino JD, Tolo VT, Skaggs DL: Effect of surgical delay on perioperative complications and need for open reduction in supracondylar humerus fractures in children. *J Pediatr Orthop* 2004;24(3):245-248.

97. Mehlman CT, Strub WM, Roy DR, Wall EJ, Crawford AH: The effect of surgical timing on the perioperative complications of treatment of supracondylar humeral fractures in children. *J Bone Joint Surg Am* 2001;83(3):323-327.
98. Ramachandran M, Skaggs DL, Crawford HA, et al: Delaying treatment of supracondylar fractures in children: Has the pendulum swung too far? *J Bone Joint Surg Br* 2008;90(9):1228-1233.
99. Rees AB, Schultz JD, Wollenman LC, et al: A mini-open approach to medial pinning in pediatric supracondylar humeral fractures may be safer than previously thought. *J Bone Joint Surg Am* 2022;104(1):33-40.
100. Larson L, Firoozbakhsh K, Passarelli R, Bosch P: Biomechanical analysis of pinning techniques for pediatric supracondylar humerus fractures. *J Pediatr Orthop* 2006;26(5):573-578.
101. Sankar WN, Hebela NM, Skaggs DL, Flynn JM: Loss of pin fixation in displaced supracondylar humeral fractures in children: Causes and prevention. *J Bone Joint Surg Am* 2007;89(4):713-717.
102. Ay S, Akinci M, Kamiloglu S, Ercetin O: Open reduction of displaced pediatric supracondylar humeral fractures through the anterior cubital approach. *J Pediatr Orthop* 2005;25:149-153.
103. Franklin CC, Skaggs DL: Approach to the pediatric supracondylar humeral fracture with neurovascular compromise. *Instr Course Lect* 2013;62:429-433.
104. Shah AS, Waters PM, Bae DS: Treatment of the "pink pulseless hand" in pediatric supracondylar humerus fractures. *J Hand Surg Am* 2013;38(7):1399-1403.
105. White L, Mehlman CT, Crawford AH: Perfused, pulseless, and puzzling: A systematic review of vascular injuries in pediatric supracondylar humerus fractures and results of a POSNA questionnaire. *J Pediatr Orthop* 2010;30(4):328-335.
106. Garbuz DS, Leitch K, Wright JG: The treatment of supracondylar fractures in children with an absent radial pulse. *J Pediatr Orthop* 1996;16(5):594-596.
107. Pirone AM, Graham HK, Krajbich JI: Management of displaced extension-type supracondylar fractures of the humerus in children. *J Bone Joint Surg Am* 1988;70(5):641-650.
108. Ramesh P, Avadhani A, Shetty AP, Dheenadhayalan J, Rajasekaran S: Management of acute 'pink pulseless' hand in pediatric supracondylar fractures of the humerus. *J Pediatr Orthop B* 2011;20(3):124-128.
109. Sabharwal S, Tredwell SJ, Beauchamp RD, et al: Management of pulseless pink hand in pediatric supracondylar fractures of humerus. *J Pediatr Orthop* 1997;17(3):303-310.

110. Scannell BP, Jackson JB III, Bray C, Roush TS, Brighton BK, Frick SL: The perfused, pulseless supracondylar humeral fracture: Intermediate-term follow-up of vascular status and function. *J Bone Joint Surg Am* 2013;95(21):1913-1919.
111. Bloomer AK, Coe KM, Brandt AM, Roomian T, Brighton B, Scannell BP: Hold the antibiotics: Are preoperative antibiotics unnecessary in the treatment of pediatric supracondylar humerus fractures? *J Pediatr Orthop* 2022;42(5):e474-e479.
112. Williams CL, James A, Tran T: Metatarsus adductus: Development of a non-surgical treatment pathway. *J Paediatr Child Health* 2013;49(9):E428-E433.
113. Gonzales AS, Saber AY, Ampat G, et al: Intoeing, in *StatPearls*. StatPearls Publishing, 2022.
114. Dobbe AM, Gibbons PJ: Common paediatric conditions of the lower limb. *J Paediatr Child Health* 2017;53(11):1077-1085.
115. Faulks S, Browne K, Birch JG: Spectrum of diagnosis and disposition of patients referred to a pediatric orthopaedic center for a diagnosis of intoeing. *J Pediatr Orthop* 2017;37(7):e432-e435.
116. Nelitz M: Femoral derotational osteotomies. *Curr Rev Musculoskelet Med* 2018;11(2):272-279.
117. Berry KM: Evidence-based management of in-toeing in children. *Clin Pediatr (Phila)* 2018;57(11):1261-1265.
118. Jones S, Khandekar S, Tolessa E: Normal variants of the lower limbs in pediatric orthopedics. *Int J Clin Med* 2013;4:12-17.
119. Davids JR, Blackhurst DW, Allen BL Jr: Clinical evaluation of bowed legs in children. *J Pediatr Orthop B* 2000;9(4):278-284.
120. Rerucha CM, Dickison C, Baird DC: Lower extremity abnormalities in children. *Am Fam Physician* 2017;96(4):226-233.
121. Staheli LT: Rotational problems in children. *Instr Course Lect* 1994;43:199-209.
122. Staheli LT: Torsion–treatment indications. *Clin Orthop Relat Res* 1989;247(1):61-66.
123. Georgiadis AG, Siegal DS, Scher CE, Zaltz I: Can femoral rotation be localized and quantified using standard CT measures?. *Clin Orthop Relat Res* 2015;473(4):1309-1314.
124. Rushforth GF: The natural history of hooked forefoot. *J Bone Joint Surg Br* 1978;60-B:530-532.
125. Harris E: The intoeing child: Etiology, prognosis, and current treatment options. *Clin Podiatr Med Surg* 2013;30(4):531-565.
126. Sass P, Hassan G: Lower extremity abnormalities in children. *Am Fam Physician* 2003;68(3):461-468.

127. Uden H, Kumar S: Non-surgical management of a pediatric "intoed" gait pattern – A systematic review of the current best evidence. *J Multidiscip Healthc* 2012;5:27-35.
128. Davids JR, Davis RB, Jameson LC, Westberry DE, Hardin JW: Surgical management of persistent intoeing gait due to increased internal tibial torsion in children. *J Pediatr Orthop* 2014;34(4):467-473.
129. Staheli LT, Corbett M, Wyss C, King H: Lower-extremity rotational problems in children. Normal values to guide management. *J Bone Joint Surg Am* 1985;67(1):39-47.

Index

Note: Page numbers followed by "*f*" indicate figures and "*t*" indicate tables.

A

Achilles tendinopathy and tendon rupture
  anatomy/pathoanatomy, 533–534
  clinical outcomes, 543
  epidemiology, 533
  fixation strategies, 543
  imaging, 535–537, 536*f*
  insertional tendinopathy, 534–535, 539–540
  nonsurgical measures, 537–539, 538*f*
  patient history, 534–535
  pearls and pitfalls, 544
  physical examination, 534–535
  postoperative orders, 543–544
  rupture, 540–543, 540*f*–542*f*
  surgical intervention, 539
  venous thromboembolism prophylaxis, 544
Acromioclavicular joint separation
  anatomy/pathophysiology, 182
  epidemiology, 181–182
  imaging, 182, 183*f*
  nonsurgical measures, 183
  patient history, 182
  physical examination, 182
  surgical intervention, 183–185
Active assisted range of motion, 2–3
Active range of motion, 2
Adhesive capsulitis
  anatomy/pathoanatomy, 250
  epidemiology, 250
  imaging, 251–252
  nonsurgical management, 252
  patient history, 250–251
  physical examination, 250–251
  surgical intervention, 252–256
Adult forearm fractures
  anatomy/pathoanatomy, 207
  epidemiology, 207
  imaging, 208
  nonsurgical measures, 208
  patient history, 207–208
  physical examination, 207–208
  surgical intervention, 208–209
Ankle fractures
  anatomy/pathoanatomy, 114–116
  classification of, 117–119, 118*f*
  epidemiology, 114
  imaging, 116–117
  initial management, 119–120
  nonsurgical measures, 120
  patient history, 116
  pearls and pitfalls, 125–126
  physical examination, 116
  surgical intervention, 120–125, 121*f*–123*f*
Aortic bifurcation, 575
Articular cartilage, 26*t*, 38–39, 40*f*
Artifacts, MRI in, 39–41, 42*f*
Atlantoaxial complex, 565

B

Benign bone tumors, 587, 594–595, 595*t*, 602–603
Benign soft-tissue tumors, 598
Bennett fracture, 220
Biopsy, 34, 250, 595, 602
Bone marrow edema, 28–30, 36, 37*f*
Bone tumors, 594–597, 595*t*, 597*t*
Both-bone forearm fracture, 207
Boxer's fracture, 220

C

Calcaneus fractures
  anatomy/pathoanatomy, 141–144, 142*f*, 144*f*

Index

Calcaneus fractures *(continued)*
   classification, 144–146, 145*f*–146*f*
   imaging, 149–151, 149*f*–150*f*
   initial management, 151–152, 153*f*
   patient history, 146–148, 148*f*
   patient outcomes, 158–159
   treatment, 153–158, 157*f*
Calcium deposition, 36
Carpal tunnel syndrome
   anatomy/pathoanatomy, 314–315
   epidemiology, 313–314
   imaging, 318
   nonsurgical measures, 318–319
   patient history, 315–318
   physical examination, 315–318
   surgical intervention, 319–323
Cheilectomy
   approaches, 519, 519*f*
   clinical outcomes, 520–521
   indications, 520
   pearls and pitfalls, 520
   postoperative orders, 520
Chevron bunionectomy, 504–505, 505*f*
   indications for, 506
   fixation strategies, 506
   outcomes, 506–507
   pearls and pitfalls, 506
   postoperative orders, 506
Clavicle fractures
   anatomy/pathoanatomy, 169
   epidemiology, 168–169
   nonsurgical measures, 169
   patient history, 169
   physical examination, 169
   surgical intervention, 169–171, 170*f*
Clubfoot
   anatomy/pathoanatomy, 647, 648*f*
   clinical outcomes, 651
   epidemiology, 647
   imaging, 649
   nonsurgical measures, 649–650, 650*t*
   patient history, 648–649
   physical examination, 648–649
   surgical intervention, 651

Computed tomography (CT)
   ankle fractures, 117
   arthrography, 22, 22*f*
   calcaneus fractures, 149–151
   distal radius fractures, 210
   fracture characterization and complications, 21–22
   hip fractures, 63
   intoeing, 666
   lateral ankle instability, 548
   Lisfranc injury, 110
   malignant bone tumors, 600
   meniscus tears, 411
   multiplanar reformations, 18–19
   myelography, 23, 23*f*
   patellofemoral pain, 393
   pelvic fractures, 51–52
   perilunate injuries, 213
   pilon fractures, 97
   posterior tibial tendon dysfunction, 529
   proximal humerus fractures, 172
   proximal radius fractures, 194
   scout image, 16–18
   soft-tissue evaluation, 19, 20*f*
   spine-related pain, 581–582
   talar fractures, 133
   terrible triad injuries, 203
   three-dimensional representations, 16, 18*f*, 77*f*, 81*f*, 151, 180*f*, 203, 243, 529
   tibial plateau fractures, 76
   tibial shaft fractures, 86
   two-dimensional representations, 16, 18*f*
Coronoid fractures, 197
Cruciate and collateral ligament injuries
   anatomy/pathoanatomy, 423–426, 424*f*–426*f*
   epidemiology, 422
   imaging, 430, 431*f*
   nonsurgical measures, 431
   patient history, 427
   physical examination, 427–429
   surgical intervention, 432–437
CT. *See* Computed tomography (CT)

Index

D
Deep vein thrombosis, 36, 58
Developmental dysplasia of the hip (DDH)
- anatomy/pathoanatomy, 628–630, 629f–630f
- clinical outcomes, 645–646
- closed reduction, 639–642, 640f–641f
- epidemiology, 627–628
- imaging, 633–637, 635f–636f
- nonsurgical measures, 637–638, 638f
- open reduction, 642–643
- osteotomies
  - femoral osteotomies, 643–644
  - pelvic osteotomies, 644–645
- patient history, 630–633, 632f
- physical examination, 630–633, 632f
- surgical intervention, 639

Diffusion tensor imaging, 42
Distal biceps tendon rupture
- anatomy/pathoanatomy, 293–294
- epidemiology, 293
- history/physical examination, 294–295
- imaging, 295, 296f
- nonsurgical measures, 296
- surgical intervention, 296–301, 301f

Distal humerus fractures
- anatomy/pathoanatomy, 189–190
- epidemiology, 189
- imaging, 190, 191f
- nonsurgical measures, 190–192
- patient history, 190
- physical examination, 190
- surgical intervention, 192–193

Distal radius fractures
- anatomy/pathoanatomy, 209
- epidemiology, 209
- imaging, 210
- nonsurgical measures, 210
- patient history, 207–208
- physical examination, 207–208
- surgical intervention, 211

E
Elbow injuries
- distal humerus fractures, 189–193
- proximal radius fractures, 193–196
- proximal ulna fracture, 196–198
- simple elbow dislocation, 198–201
- terrible triad injuries, 202–205

Elbow pain
- carpal tunnel syndrome, 313–323
- distal biceps tendon rupture, 292–301
- flexor tendon injuries, 330–334
- lateral epicondylitis, 270–282
- medial epicondylitis, 283–291
- thumb carpometacarpal arthritis, 336–341
- trigger finger, 324–329
- ulnar nerve compression, 302–309

F
Femoral anteversion, 668
Femoral osteotomies, 643–644
Femoroacetabular impingement (FAI)
- anatomy/pathoanatomy, 347, 348f
- epidemiology, 346–347
- imaging, 350–351
- nonsurgical measures, 351–352
- patient history, 348–349, 349f–350f
- physical examination, 348–349, 349f–350f
- surgical intervention, 352–356, 353f–354f

Fifth metacarpal fractures, 220
First metatarsophalangeal joint fusion
- approaches, 522–523
- clinical outcomes, 525
- fixation strategies, 524
- indications, 523–524
- pearls and pitfalls, 524–525
- postoperative orders, 524

Flexor tendon injuries
- anatomy/pathoanatomy, 330–331
- epidemiology, 330
- surgical intervention, 331–334, 334f

Index

G
Galeazzi fractures, 207
Glenohumeral dislocations
  anatomy/pathoanatomy, 178–179
  epidemiology, 178
  imaging, 179, 180f
  nonsurgical measures, 180–181
  patient history, 179
  physical examination, 179
  surgical intervention, 181
Glenohumeral osteoarthritis
  anatomy/pathoanatomy, 257
  epidemiology, 257
  imaging, 258–260, 258f–261f
  patient history, 257–258
  physical examination, 257–258
  surgical intervention, 261–266, 263f, 265f–266f
Gluteal injuries
  anatomy/pathoanatomy, 376–377
  epidemiology, 376
  imaging, 378–379, 379f–380f
  nonsurgical measures, 379
  patient history, 377–378
  physical examination, 377–378
  surgical intervention, 379–382, 380f–381f

H
Hallux rigidus
  anatomy/pathoanatomy, 513–514
  cheilectomy
    approaches, 519, 519f
    clinical outcomes, 520–521
    indications, 520
    pearls and pitfalls, 520
    postoperative orders, 520
  classification, 515–516, 515t
  clinical outcomes, 518
  demographics, 513
  epidemiology, 513
  first metatarsophalangeal joint fusion
    approaches, 522–523
    clinical outcomes, 525
    fixation strategies, 524
    indications, 523–524
    pearls and pitfalls, 524–525
    postoperative orders, 524
  imaging, 517
  incidence, 513
  interposition arthroplasty
    approaches, 521
    clinical outcomes, 522
    indications, 521
    pearls and pitfalls, 521–522
    postoperative orders, 521
  nonsurgical measures, 517–518
  patient history, 514
  physical examination, 514–515
  surgical interventions, 518
Hallux valgus
  anatomy/pathoanatomy, 498–500, 499f
  bony structures, 500–501, 500f
  chevron bunionectomy, 504–505, 505f
    fixation strategies, 506
    indications, 506
    outcomes, 506–507
    pearls and pitfalls, 506
    postoperative orders, 506
  clinical outcomes, 503–504
  deformity, classification of, 503
  demographics, 497–498
  epidemiology, 497
  imaging, 501–503
  incidence, 497
  Lapidus bunionectomy
    approaches, 510–511
    clinical outcomes, 511–512
    fixation strategies, 511
    indications, 511
    pearls and pitfalls, 511
    postoperative orders, 511
  nonsurgical measures, 503
  patient history, 501
  physical examination, 501
  public health considerations, 498
  scarf bunionectomy
    approaches, 507–508
    clinical outcomes, 509–510
    fixation strategies, 509
    indications, 509
    pearls and pitfalls, 509

postoperative orders, 509
surgical intervention, 504
Hamstrings injuries
  anatomy/pathoanatomy, 366–367
  epidemiology, 365
  imaging, 368–369, 369f
  nonsurgical measures, 370–371
  patient history, 367–368
  physical examination, 367–368
  surgical intervention, 371–375, 373f
Hand fractures
  metacarpal fractures, 216–220, 219t
  phalangeal fractures, 216–220
Hill-Sachs lesion, 30–32
Hip fractures
  anatomy/pathoanatomy, 61, 62f
  epidemiology, 60–61
  imaging, 63, 64f
  nonsurgical measures, 64–65
  patient history, 61–63
  physical examination, 61–63
  surgical intervention, 65–73, 66f–67f, 69f–72f
Hip pain
  femoroacetabular impingement, 346–356
  gluteal injuries, 376–382
  hamstrings injuries, 365–375
  iliopsoas disorders, 357–364
Humeral shaft fractures
  anatomy/pathoanatomy, 174–175
  epidemiology, 174
  imaging, 175
  nonsurgical measures, 175–176
  patient history, 175
  physical examination, 175
  surgical intervention, 177–178, 177f

I

Iliopsoas disorders
  anatomy/pathoanatomy, 358–359
  epidemiology, 357
  imaging, 361
  nonsurgical measures, 361–362
  patient history, 359–360
  physical examination, 359–360
  surgical intervention, 362–364, 363f

Instability
  anatomy/pathoanatomy, 237–239, 237t, 238f
  epidemiology, 237
  imaging, 241–243, 242f
  nonsurgical management, 243
  patient history, 239–241
  physical examination, 239–241
  surgical intervention, 244–249
Internal tibial torsion, 667
Interposition arthroplasty
  approaches, 521
  clinical outcomes, 522
  indications, 521
  pearls and pitfalls, 521–522
  postoperative orders, 521
Intoeing, 662t
  anatomy/pathoanatomy, 663
  epidemiology, 663
  femoral anteversion, 665, 666f–667f, 668
  imaging, 666
  internal tibial torsion, 664–665, 667
  metatarsus adductus, 664, 667
  patient history, 663–664
  physical examination, 663–664
  surgical intervention, 668

J

Joint-depression type fracture, 145, 145f
Joint replacement
  anatomy/pathoanatomy, 441–446
  epidemiology, 441
  imaging, 447, 448f
  patient history, 446–447
  periprosthetic fractures, 482–492
  periprosthetic joint infection, 470–480
  physical examination, 446–447
  risk factors, 441–446
  total hip arthroplasty, 462–469
  total knee arthroplasty, 449–460

K

Kienböck disease, 37
Knee pain
  cruciate and collateral ligament injuries, 421–437
  meniscus tears, 405–420
  patellofemoral pain, 387–403

L

Lapidus bunionectomy
  approaches, 510–511
  clinical outcomes, 511–512
  fixation strategies, 511
  indications, 511
  pearls and pitfalls, 511
  postoperative orders, 511
Lateral ankle instability
  anatomy/pathoanatomy, 546
  epidemiology, 545–546
  imaging, 548, 548f
  nonsurgical intervention, 549
  patient history, 546–548, 547f
  physical examination, 546–548, 547f
  surgical intervention, 549–550, 550f
Lateral epicondylitis
  anatomy/pathoanatomy, 271–273, 272f
  epidemiology, 271
  imaging, 274
  nonsurgical measures, 274–278
  patient history, 273
  physical examination, 273
  surgical intervention, 278–282, 280f
Li-Fraumeni syndrome, 592
Lisfranc injuries
  anatomy/pathoanatomy, 106, 107f–108f
  epidemiology, 106
  imaging, 108–110, 110f–111f
  nonsurgical measures, 110
  patient history, 108
  physical examination, 108
  surgical intervention, 111–113, 112f
Lower extremity trauma
  ankle fractures, 114–126
  calcaneus fractures, 140–159
  hip fractures, 60–73
  Lisfranc injuries, 105–113
  pelvic fractures, 45–59
  pilon fractures, 95–104
  talar fractures, 127–138
  tibial plateau fractures, 74–82
  tibial shaft fractures, 83–93
Lumbosacral junction, 570

M

Magnetic resonance imaging (MRI)
  articular cartilage, 26t, 27, 38–39, 39f
  artifacts, 39–41, 41f
  black bone, 37–38, 38f
  bone marrow edema, 28–30, 29f–30f, 34, 315, 617
  calcium deposition, 36
  chronic spondylolysis, 36
  cruciate and collateral ligament injuries, 430
  deep vein thrombosis, 36
  diffusion tensor imaging, 42
  distal biceps tendon rupture, 295
  fat-suppressed sequence, 27–28
  glenohumeral dislocations, 179
  gluteal injuries, 378
  hamstring injuries, 368–369
  hip fractures, 63
  iliopsoas disorders, 361
  intoeing, 666
  Kienböck disease, 37
  lateral ankle instability, 548
  lateral epicondylitis, 274
  Lisfranc injury, 110
  malignant bone tumors, 600
  medial epicondylitis, 287
  meniscus tears, 411
  musculoskeletal infection, 32, 474
  neuropathic arthropathy, 34
  occult fractures, 215
  osteoid osteoma, 29, 30f, 36, 589, 596
  patellofemoral pain, 392–393
  pelvic fractures, 52
  posterior tibial tendon dysfunction, 529

pulse sequences, 25–27, 26t, 37–38, 38f, 41
rotator cuff injuries, 186
spine-related pain, 581–582
talar fractures, 134
tibial plateau fractures, 76
total joint arthroplasty, 447
ultrashort echo time pulse sequences, 42
zero echo time, 42
Malignant bone tumors, 595–596
adjuvant treatment, 604–606, 605t
biopsy, 602
surgical treatment, 602–604
Malignant soft-tissue tumors, 598–599
Medial epicondylitis
anatomy/pathoanatomy, 284–285
epidemiology, 283–284
imaging, 286–287
nonsurgical measures, 287–289
patient history, 285–286
physical examination, 285–286
surgical intervention, 289–291, 290f
Meniscus tears
anatomy/pathoanatomy, 405–409, 407f
arthroscopic partial meniscectomy, 413–416, 415f
epidemiology, 405
imaging, 410–411
meniscus repair, 416–419
meniscus root repair, 419–420
nonsurgical measures, 411–412
patient history, 409
physical examination, 409–410
surgical intervention, 412
Metastatic bone disease, 596–597
Metatarsus adductus, 667
Monteggia fractures, 207
Motor and neurovascular evaluation, 3
MRI. *See* Magnetic resonance imaging (MRI)
Multiple hereditary exostoses, 594
Musculoskeletal infection, magnetic resonance imaging in, 32
Myelopathy, 557

N
Neck and back pain. *See* Spine-related pain
Neural elements, 570–576, 571f–575f
Neurofibromatosis, 594
Neuropathic arthropathy, magnetic resonance imaging in, 34

O
Olecranon fractures, 197
Osteoarthritis, 29, 251, 258, 410, 440–442, 444–446, 613, 627
Osteoid osteoma, magnetic resonance imaging in, 29, 30f, 36
Osteotomies
femoral osteotomies, 643–644
pelvic osteotomies, 644–645

P
Pars articularis, 562
Passive range of motion, 2, 192, 197, 288, 332, 399, 428, 578
Patellofemoral pain
anatomy/pathoanatomy, 388–389, 390f
cartilage restoration, 399–403, 403f
epidemiology, 388
imaging, 392–393, 393f–394f
medial patellofemoral ligament reconstruction, 395–397
nonsurgical measures, 394–395
patient history, 389–392
physical examination, 389–392
surgical intervention, 395
tibial tubercle osteotomy, 398–399, 400f
Pelvic fractures
anatomy/pathoanatomy, 46, 47f–48f
epidemiology, 46
imaging, 50–52, 51f–54f, 54t
inspection, 47–48
neurologic examination, 49
nonsurgical measures, 53–55, 54t
patient history, 47–48, 49f
physical examination, 47–48, 49f
surgical intervention, 55–59, 56f

Pelvic osteotomy, 644–645
Periprosthetic fractures
　anatomy/pathoanatomy, 483–485, 486*f*
　epidemiology, 480–483, 483*t*
　patient history, 486
　physical examination, 486
　treatment, 487–492, 491*f*
Periprosthetic joint infections, 474–478, 475*f*, 476*t*, 477*f*
　epidemiology, 470–472, 472*t*
　microbiology, 472–473
　nonsurgical measures, 478
　patient history, 473–474
　surgical intervention, 478–480
Physical examination
　inspection and observation, 1–2
　neurovascular evaluation, 3–4
　palpation, 2
　range of motion, 2–3
Pilon fractures
　anatomy/pathoanatomy, 96–97, 96*f*
　epidemiology, 95–96
　imaging, 97–98, 98*f*–99*f*
　nonsurgical measures, 98
　patient history, 97
　physical examination, 97
　surgical intervention, 99–104, 103*f*
Posterior tibial tendon dysfunction
　anatomy/pathoanatomy, 527
　classification, 529–530
　epidemiology, 526–527
　imaging, 529, 530*f*
　nonsurgical measures, 530–531
　patient history, 528
　physical examination, 528
　surgical intervention, 531–532
Proximal humerus fractures
　anatomy/pathoanatomy, 171–172
　epidemiology, 171
　imaging, 172, 173*f*
　nonsurgical measures, 172
　patient history, 172
　physical examination, 172
　surgical intervention, 172–174

Proximal radius fractures
　anatomy/pathoanatomy, 193
　epidemiology, 193
　imaging, 194
　nonsurgical measures, 194–195
　patient history, 193–194
　physical examination, 193–194
　surgical intervention, 195–196
Proximal ulna fracture
　anatomy/pathoanatomy, 196
　epidemiology, 196
　imaging, 197, 197*f*
　nonsurgical measures, 197
　patient history, 196–197
　physical examination, 196–197
　surgical intervention, 198

Q
Quantitative magnetic resonance techniques, 42

R
Radial head arthroplasty, 195, 205
Radial head fractures, 204
Radiculopathy, 557
Radiography
　after arthroplasty, 7
　ankle fractures, 116–117
　cervical spine, 11
　cruciate and collateral ligament injuries, 430
　distal biceps tendon rupture, 295
　gluteal injuries, 378
　hip fractures, 63
　image manipulation, 9–11
　lateral epicondylitis, 274
　malignant bone tumors, 599–600
　medial epicondylitis, 286
　meniscus tears, 410
　oblique views, 14*f*
　pelvic fractures, 50–51
　pilon fractures, 97
　posterior tibial tendon dysfunction, 529
　proximal humeral physis, 15
　radiation safety, 6

Index

slipped capital femoral epiphysis, 615–616
subtle stress/insufficiency fractures, 13
talar fractures, 131–133
tibial plateau fractures, 76
total joint arthroplasty, 447
trauma setting, 16
ulnar nerve compression, 304
views of, 13
Retinoblastoma, 594
Rotator cuff
  anatomy/pathoanatomy, 224–227
  epidemiology, 223
  imaging, 228–229
  injuries
    anatomy/pathoanatomy, 185
    epidemiology, 185
    imaging, 186
    nonsurgical management, 186, 230
    patient history, 185–186
    physical examination, 185–186
    surgical intervention, 187–188
  patient history, 227–228
  physical examination, 227–228
  surgical intervention, 230–235, 231f–232f

S

Scarf bunionectomy
  approaches, 507–508
  clinical outcomes, 509–510
  fixation strategies, 509
  indications, 509
  pearls and pitfalls, 509
  postoperative orders, 509
SCFE. *See* Slipped capital femoral epiphysis (SCFE)
Sensory neurovascular evaluation, 3, 210, 289, 293, 302
Shoulder injuries
  acromioclavicular joint separations, 181–185, 184f
  clavicle fractures, 168–171, 170f
  glenohumeral dislocations, 178–181, 180f
  humeral shaft fractures, 174–178, 176f, 177f
  proximal humerus fractures, 171–174, 173f
  rotator cuff injuries, 185–188, 187f
Simple elbow dislocation
  anatomy/pathoanatomy, 199–200
  epidemiology, 198
  imaging, 200
  nonsurgical measures, 200–201
  patient history, 200
  physical examination, 200
  surgical intervention, 201
Slipped capital femoral epiphysis (SCFE), 610–611
  anatomy/pathoanatomy, 613–614
  clinical outcomes, 623–626, 624f–625f
  epidemiology, 611–612
  imaging, 615–618, 616f–617f
  nonsurgical measures, 618
  patient history, 614–615
  pearls and pitfalls, 622–623
  postoperative orders, 622
  public health consideration, 612–613
  in situ pinning technique, 620–622, 621f
  surgical intervention, 619–620
Soft-tissue tumors, 597–599
Spine-related pain
  anatomy/pathoanatomy, 558–576, 559f–560f
    anterior and middle structures, 561–562
    neural elements, 570–576, 571f–575f
    posterior structures, 562–569, 564f–568f, 570f
    vertebral structure, 558–561
  epidemiology, 557
  imaging, 581–582
  nonsurgical measures, 582–583
  patient history, 576–581, 578t, 579f, 580t
  surgical intervention, 583–584
Spondylolysis, chronic, 36, 37f

Stuart-Treves syndrome, 594
Supracondylar humerus fractures
  anatomy/pathoanatomy, 653, 654f
  epidemiology, 652–653
  imaging, 656, 657f
  nonsurgical measures, 657
  patient history, 653–656, 655f
  physical examination, 653–656, 655f
  surgical intervention, 658–661, 659f

T

Talar fractures
  anatomy/pathoanatomy, 128–130, 129f–130f
  classification, 134
  epidemiology, 127–128
  imaging, 131–134, 132f–133f
  nonsurgical measures, 134–136
  patient history, 130–131
  surgical intervention, 136–138, 139f
Terrible triad injuries
  anatomy/pathoanatomy, 202–203
  epidemiology, 202
  imaging, 203
  nonsurgical measures, 203–204
  patient history, 203
  physical examination, 203
  surgical intervention, 204–205
THA. *See* Total hip arthroplasty (THA)
Thoracolumbar junction, 568
Thumb carpometacarpal arthritis
  anatomy/pathoanatomy, 336
  epidemiology, 336
  imaging, 338
  nonsurgical measures, 338
  patient history, 336–337, 337f
  physical examination, 336–337, 337f
  surgical intervention, 338–341, 339f–341f
Tibial plateau fractures
  anatomy/pathoanatomy, 74, 75f
  epidemiology, 74
  imaging, 76–78, 76f–78f
  neurologic examination, 76
  nonsurgical measures, 79
  patient history, 74–75
  physical examination, 74–75
  surgical intervention, 79–82, 80f–81f
Tibial shaft fractures
  anatomy/pathoanatomy, 84, 85f
  epidemiology, 83
  imaging, 86, 88f
  nonsurgical measures, 87–89
  patient history, 84, 86f
  physical examination, 84, 86f
  surgical intervention, 89–93, 94f, 94t
Total hip arthroplasty (THA)
  cementing in, 467–469
  indications, 462
  postoperative management, 469
  technique, 466–467
  templating, 462–464
Total joint arthroplasty (TJA)
  anatomy/pathoanatomy, 441–446, 444f
  epidemiology, 441
  imaging, 447, 447f–448f
  pathophysiology, 441–446
  patient history, 446–447
  physical examination, 446–447
  risk factors, 441–446
Total knee arthroplasty (TKA)
  nonsurgical measures, 450
  patient history, 449–450
  physical examination, 449–450
  surgical intervention, 450–460, 452f, 454f–455f, 457t, 458f
Trigger finger
  anatomy/pathoanatomy, 324
  clinical outcomes, 328–329
  epidemiology, 324
  nonsurgical measures, 326, 326f
  patient history, 325
  physical examination, 325
  surgical intervention, 327–328, 327f
Tumors
  age at presentation, 587–589, 588f–593f
  bone tumors, 594–597, 595t, 597t
  epidemiology, 586–587
  imaging, 599–601
  patient history, 589–594

physical examination, 589–594
soft-tissue tumors, 597–599

U

Ulnar nerve compression
  anatomy/pathoanatomy, 303
  epidemiology, 302
  imaging, 304–305
  nonsurgical measures, 305
  patient history, 303–304
  physical examination, 303–304
  surgical intervention, 305–309, 306f–307f
Ultrashort echo time pulse sequences, 42
Ultrasonography
  carpal tunnel syndrome, 318
  developmental dysplasia of the hip, 633–634
  distal biceps tendon rupture, 295
  lateral epicondylitis, 274
  medial epicondylitis, 286

Upper extremity trauma
  adult forearm fractures 207–209
  distal radius fractures, 209–211
  elbow injuries, 189–205
  hand fractures, 216–220
  shoulder injuries, 168–188
  wrist injuries, 212–215

V

Vascular, neurovascular evaluation, 3, 116
Venous thromboembolism prophylaxis, 544

W

Wrist injuries
  perilunate injuries, 212–214, 213f
  scaphoid fractures, 214–215

Z

Zero echo time imaging, 42, 42f